HESI

Comprehensive Review for the NCLEX-RN® Examination

Edition 7

HESI

Comprehensive Review for the NCLEX-RN® Examination

EDITOR

Denise M. Korniewicz, PhD, RN, FAAN
School of Nursing
Interim Dean and Professor
Bouvé College of Health Sciences,
Northeastern University
Boston, Massachusetts

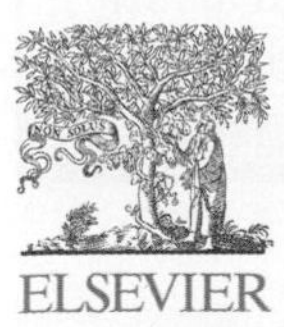

Elsevier
3251 Riverport Lane
St. Louis, Missouri 63043

HESI COMPREHENSIVE REVIEW FOR THE NCLEX-RN®
EXAMINATION, SEVENTH EDITION
ISBN: 978-0-323-83193-2

Previous editions copyrighted 2020, 2017, 2014, 2011, and 2008.

Content Strategist: Heather Bays-Petrovic
Content Development Specialist: Casey Potter
Publishing Services Manager: Deepthi Unni
Senior Project Manager: Kamatchi Madhavan
Design Direction: Bridget Hoette

Printed in India

Last digit is the print number: 9 8 7 6 5 4 3 2 1

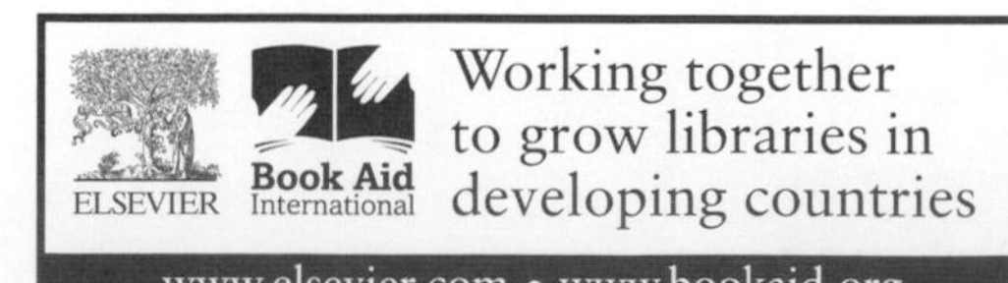

CONTRIBUTORS

Denise M. Korniewicz, PhD, RN, FAAN
School of Nursing
Interim Dean and Professor
Bouvé College of Health Sciences
Northeastern University
Boston, Massachusetts

Mary Wyckoff, PhD, RN, NNP-BC, ACNP-BC, FNP-BC, CCNS, CCRN, FAANP
Neonatal Nurse Practitioner, Family Nurse Practitioner, Acute Care Nurse Practitioner & Neonatology Nurse Practitioner
University of California, Davis;
Professor Nursing
Samuel Merritt University
Sacramento, California

Charlene Romer, PhD, RN, CNE, CNEcl
BSN Faculty Nursing
Herzing University
Menomonee Falls, Wisconsin

Carol Patton, DrPH, FNP-BC, CRNP, CNE
Director of Nursing Research
St. Peter's Hospital
New Brunswick, New Jersey;
Professor of Nursing
Director of the Doctor of Nursing Practice Program
Waynesburg University
Waynesburg, Pennsylvania

Maridee Shogren, DNP, CNM, CLC
Clinical Professor
College of Nursing and Professional Disciplines;
Interim Dean, College of Health and Nursing
University of North Dakota;
Don't Quit the Quit-PI
Grand Forks, North Dakota

James J. Weidel, PhD, FNP-BC, PMHNP-BC
Adjunct Professor
Nicole Wertheim College of Nursing and Health Sciences
Florida International University
Miami, Florida

PREFACE

Welcome to *HESI Comprehensive Review for the Next Generation NCLEX-RN (NGN)* exam with online study exams by HESI. The NCLEX-RN Next Generation (NGN) exam asks critically thinking questions that helps nurses make the right decisions.

This outstanding review manual with online study exams is designed to prepare nursing students for what is very likely the most important examination they will ever take—the *Next Generation NCLEX-RN (NGN)* Licensing Examination. *HESI Comprehensive Review for the NCLEX-RN® Examination* allows the nursing student to prepare for the NCLEX-RN (NGN) Next Generation licensure examination in a structured way.

NEXT GENERATION NCLEX (NGN) AND CLINICAL JUDGMENT

In July of 2017, the National Council of State Boards of Nursing (NCSBN) began including a special research section to select candidates after they completed the exam. The data collected from this section has been used to help determine new item types that may be included in a future version of the NCLEX. This initiative is known as the Next Generation NCLEX-RN (NGN). (More information can be found at http://www.ncsbn.org/next-generation-nclex.htm.) An important piece of the NGN is the clinical judgment model. Clinical judgment is important for all nurses, and this book helps nursing students by reviewing information and skills that nurses must master to practice clinical judgment. Additionally, NCLEX practice questions on the Evolve website written at higher levels of Bloom's taxonomy help students practice applying their clinical judgment knowledge. Finally, a Clinical Judgment Scenario with practice NGN questions is included in Chapters 2 to 8 to familiarize students with these types of questions.

In preparation to take any major test, you will need to systematically think about how to organize the content you review. Consistent study habits help you to be able to critically analyze each content area for a clear systematic review. Keep in mind the following when studying for the *NCLEX-RN® Examination*:

- Organize previously learned basic nursing knowledge.
- Review content learned during basic nursing curriculum.
- Identify deficits in content knowledge so that study effort can be focused appropriately.
- Develop test-taking skills to demonstrate application of safe nursing practice.
- Reduce anxiety level by increasing predictability of ability to correctly answer Next Generation (NGN)—Style item types.
- Boost test-taking confidence by being well prepared and knowing what to expect.

ORGANIZA[illegible]KE TESTS

Chapter 1, Introduction to Test-Taking Strategies and the *Next Generation NCLEX-RN* (NGN), gives an overview of the *Next Generation NCLEX-RN (NGN)* Licensing Examination history and test plan for the examination. The focus of this chapter is to understand the purpose and development of the new *Next Generation NCLEX-RN (NGN)* the type of content that will be included on the items. One of the most important areas that will be discussed includes the clinical judgement model. Discussion includes the six cognitive processes related to the clinical judgement model. These include: recognize cues, analyze cues, prioritize hypothesis, generate solutions, take action, and evaluate outcomes.

Chapter 2, Leadership and Management, reviews the legal aspects of nursing, leadership and management, and disaster nursing. Additionally, this chapter introduces the use of the Next-Generation (NGN)—Style Examination item type "bow-tie". The importance of this type of item is that it helps you to learn how to think and solve complicated nursing problems.

Chapter 3, Advanced Clinical Concepts, presents a cadre of nursing concepts that are essential in the understanding of the nursing process. The major areas of assessment, analysis, planning and intervention, using the clinical judgment model to critically understand the higher levels of practice are presented. Topics reviewed include respiratory failure, shock, disseminated intravascular coagulation, resuscitation, fluid and electrolyte balance, intravenous therapy, acid–base balance, electrocardiogram, perioperative care, HIV, pain, and death and grief. The review questions assist you in conceptually understanding the clinical concepts and are located at the end of content section. Again, the example of a "bowtie" NGN test item helps you reflect on one of the content areas and think about how to answer similar items when you sit for the examination.

Chapters 4 through 8, **Medical-Surgical Nursing, Pediatric Nursing, Maternity Nursing, Psychiatric Nursing, and Gerontologic Nursing**, are presented in traditional clinical areas. Each clinical area is divided into physiologic components, with essential knowledge about basic anatomy, growth and development, pharmacology and medication calculation, nutrition, communication, client and family education, acute and chronic care, leadership and management, complementary and alternative interventions, cultural and spiritual diversity, and clinical decision making threaded throughout the different components. For each of the content areas are review questions to prepare you for the essential content that may be on the NCLEX-RN Examination. At the end of each chapter is a "bowtie" item that will test your conceptual knowledge of the essential content.

For each chapter, there are a group of questions that are used to expand your knowledge about the content area. These items are important because the offer you a comprehensive approach to the content area. Several learning opportunities are used to assist you to prepare for the exam. These strategies include:

- Reading the manual
- Discussing content with others
- Answering the review items
- Practicing the "bowtie" items to get used to the type of new items.

These learning experiences are all different ways that students should use to prepare for the *NCLEX-RN® Examination.* The purpose of the questions appearing at the end of the chapter is not a focused practice session on managing *NCLEX-RN (NGN)*—style questions, but rather a learning approach that allows for critical thinking about specific topics in the chapter. The use of the "bowtie" style questions allows you to begin to make decisions based on the evidence presented in the cases at the end of each chapter. Multiple-choice questions alone cannot provide the essential analysis needed to know how to process nursing content that may be complicated by the questions at the end of the chapter. In addition, the questions presented at the end of the chapter provide a summary experience that helps students focus on the main topics that were covered in the chapter. Teachers use open-ended questions to stimulate the critical-thinking process, and *HESI Comprehensive Review for the NCLEX-RN® Examination* facilitates the critical-thinking process by posing the same type of questions the teacher might ask.

EVOLVE

When students need to practice multiple-choice questions, the online study exams on Evolve offer extensive opportunities for practice and skill building to improve their test-taking abilities. The online study exams include six content-specific exams (Medical-Surgical Nursing, Pharmacology, Pediatrics, Fundamentals, Maternity, and Psychiatric-Mental Health Nursing) and two comprehensive exams for additional study. Next Generation (NGN)—Style Questions, including single-episode and unfolding questions, are also provided for students to practice the new item formats. The online study exams on Evolve can be accessed as many times as necessary until students feel comfortable. The purpose of the study exams is to provide practice and exposure to the critical thinking—style questions that students will encounter on the NCLEX-RN exam. However, the study exams should not be used to predict performance on the actual NCLEX-RN exam. Only the HESI Exit Exam, a secure, computerized exam that simulates the NCLEX-RN exam has evidence-based results from numerous research studies indicating a high level of accuracy in predicting NCLEX-RN exam success, is offered as a true predictor exam. Students are allowed unlimited practice on each online study exam so that they can be sure to have the opportunity to review all of the rationales for the questions.

Here is a plan for a student to use with the online study exam:

1. Organize your knowledge.
2. Identify weaknesses in content knowledge to help focus your study time.
3. Review need-to-know content learned in nursing school.
4. Develop strong test-taking skills to demonstrate your knowledge.
5. Reduce your level of anxiety by dissecting test questions and using your foundational knowledge to arrive at the correct answer.
6. Know what to expect. Remember that knowledge is power. You are powerful when you are well prepared and know what to expect.
7. Take the RN study exam without studying for it to see your strengths and weaknesses.
8. After going over the content that relates to the study questions in a particular clinical area (e.g., Pediatrics, Medical-Surgical, or Maternity), review that section of the manual and take the test again to determine whether you have been able to improve your scores.
9. Purposely miss every question on the exam so that you can view the rationales for every question.
10. Take the exam again under timed conditions at the pace that you would have to progress.
11. Put the exam away for a while and continue review and remediation with other textbooks, resources, and results of any HESI secure exams that you have taken at your school. Then, take the study exams again to see if your performance improves after in-depth study and following a few weeks' break from these questions.

HESI RN PRODUCTS

Additional assistance for you to study includes using a variety of online products in the Elsevier family. Many nursing schools have also adopted the following:

- *HESI Examinations*—A comprehensive set of examinations designed to prepare nursing students for the *Next Generation NCLEX-RN (NGN) examination.* They include customized electronic remediation from current Elsevier textbooks and multimedia, as well as additional practice questions. Each student is given an individualized report detailing exam results and is allowed to view questions and rationales for items that were answered incorrectly. The electronic remediation, a complementary feature of the specialty and exit exams, can be filed by the student for later study.
- *HESI Practice Test*—This is the ideal way to practice for the *Next Generation NCLEX-RN (NGN) examination.* With more than 1200 practice questions included in this online test bank, nursing students can access practice exams 24 hours a day, 7 days a week. *HESI Practice Test* questions are written at the critical-thinking level so that students are tested not for memorization but for their skills in clinical application. Students select a test option (either a clinical specialty or a comprehensive exam), and *HESI Practice Test* automatically supplies a series of critical-thinking practice questions. NCLEX exam-style questions include

multiple-choice and alternate-item formats and are accompanied by correct answers and rationales.

- *HESI RN Case Studies*—These prepare students to manage complex patient conditions and make sound clinical judgments. These online case studies cover a broad range of physiologic and psychosocial alterations, plus related management, pharmacology, and therapeutic concepts.
- *HESI Patient Reviews*—These are designed to teach and assess students' retention of core nursing content. These online interactive reviews provide a firsthand look at safe and effective nursing care.
- *HESI Live Review*—A live review course is presented by an expert faculty member who has additional instruction in working with students who are preparing to take the NCLEX exam. Students are presented with a workbook and practice NCLEX-style questions that are used during the course.
- *Evolve eBooks*—Online versions of all of the Mosby, Saunders, and Elsevier textbooks used in the student's nursing curriculum are presented. Search across titles, highlight, make notes, and more—all on your computer.
- *Elsevier Simulations*—Virtual versions simulate the clinical environment. These multilayered, complex, supplemental simulations enable students to experience clinical assignments without the need for actual clinical space.
- *Elsevier Courses*—These are created by experts using instructional design principles. This interactive content engages students with reading, animation, video, audio, interactive exercises, and assessments.

CONTENTS

1

Introduction to Test-Taking Strategies and the NGN-NCLEX-RN

Congratulations! You have made the wise decision to prepare, in a structured way, for the Next Generation NCLEX®-RN EXAM (National Council of State Boards of Nursing, NCSBN, 2019).

A. Since you have successfully completed a basic nursing program and are well acquainted with your test-taking skills and ability to apply your clinical knowledge, you already have the basic knowledge required to pass the licensing examination. Throughout your nursing education, you have learned that there is a systematic way of thinking to solve clinical problems and make clinical decisions. The problem-solving process has used a "scientific, clinical reasoning approach to patient care that has included assessment, analysis, implementation and evaluation (National Council of State Boards of Nursing [NCSBN], 2018, p. 5)". As a result, you have learned to organize your thoughts and systematically approach a client's problem. These skills will help to ensure your success in passing the Next Generation Nursing [NGN] NCLEX-RN EXAM.

B. Following these general test taking guidelines will help ensure your success.
   1. Organize your knowledge.
   2. Identify weaknesses in content knowledge to help focus your study time.
   3. Review need-to-know content learned in nursing school.
   4. Develop strong test-taking skills to demonstrate your knowledge.
   5. Reduce your level of anxiety by dissecting test questions and using your foundational knowledge to arrive at the correct answer.
   6. Know what to expect. Remember that knowledge is power. You are powerful when you are well prepared and know what to expect.

TEST-TAKING STRATEGIES

These test-taking strategies help you focus your study so that you can concentrate on what the exam questions are asking instead of being distracted by extraneous information that is not needed to answer the questions.

A. The Next Generation NCLEX-RN EXAM aims to assess your overall readiness for practice. The National Council of State Boards of Nursing (NCSBN, 2018b) encompasses ways to measure your clinical judgment. This will assist you in being able to meet the nursing practice demands and clinical decisions that have an impact on client outcomes. The NCSBN (2018a) Clinical Judgement Model (CJMM; Betts, Muntean, Kim, Jorion, & Dickison, 2019) provides a framework to assess your clinical judgment when providing safe client care. The CJMM model helps you to develop your critical thinking, decision making, and clinical judgment skills. Based on the CJMM framework, several core concepts will be included such as recognizing cues, analyzing cues, prioritizing hypotheses, generating solutions, taking action, and evaluating client outcomes. For example, a question may appear to be a medical-surgical or pediatric question, but the question can also cover such topics as communication, nutrition, growth and development, medication, client and family education, and safety.

> **HESI HINT** The most questions element of nursing care is client safety.

B. Understand the question.
   1. Determine whether the question is written in a positive or negative style.
      a. A *positive* style question may ask what the nurse should do or ask for the best or first nursing intervention to implement.
      b. A *negative* style question may ask what the nurse should avoid, which prescription the nurse should question, or which behavior indicates the need for reteaching the client.

> **HESI HINT** Most questions are written in a positive style under.

> **HESI HINT** Negative style questions contain keywords that denote the negative style.
>
> **Examples**
> 1. "Which response indicates to the nurse a need to *reteach* the client about heart disease?" (Which information or understanding by the client is incorrect?)
> 2. "Which medication order should the nurse *question*?" (Which prescription is unsafe, not beneficial, inappropriate to this client's situation?)

C. Identify keywords.
   1. Ask yourself which words or phrases provide the critical information.

2. This information may include the age of the client, the setting, the timing, a set of symptoms or behaviors, or any number of other factors.
   a. For example, the nursing actions for a 10-year-old postop client are different from those for a 70-year-old postop client.

D. Rephrase the question.
1. Rephrasing the question helps eliminate nonessential information in the question to help you determine the correct answer.
   a. Ask yourself, "What is this question *really* asking?"
   b. While keeping the options covered, rephrase the question in your own words.
2. Rule out options.
   a. Based on your knowledge, you can most likely identify one or two options that are clearly incorrect.
   b. Physically mark through those options on the test booklet if allowed. Mentally mark through those options in your head if using a computer.
   c. Differentiate between the remaining options, considering your knowledge of the subject and related nursing principles, such as roles of the nurse, nursing process, ABCs (airway, breathing, circulation), CAB (circulation, airway, breathing for cardiopulmonary resuscitation [CPR]), and Maslow's hierarchy of needs.

E. Implement these guidelines.
1. Consider the content of the question and what specifically the question is asking.
2. Generally, an assessment of the client occurs before an action is taken, except in the case of an emergency, for example, if a client is bleeding profusely, stop the bleeding. Or, if a client is having difficulty breathing, open the airway, then assess the client.
3. Identify the least invasive intervention before taking action.
4. Gather all the necessary information and complete the necessary assessments before calling the healthcare provider.
5. Determine which client to assess first (e.g., most at risk, most physiologically unstable).
6. Identify opposites in the answers.
   a. Example: prone versus supine; elevated versus decreased.
   b. Read *VERY* carefully; one opposite is likely to be the answer, but not always.
   c. If you do not know the answer, choose the most likely of the "opposites" and move on.
7. Consider a client's lifestyle, culture, and spiritual beliefs when answering a question.

F. Use your critical thinking skills.
1. Respond to questions based on
   a. Client safety
   b. ABCs
   c. CAB for CPR
   d. Caring
   e. Incorporation of culture and spiritual practices
   f. Scientific, behavioral, and sociologic principles
   g. Communication (spoken and written [documentation]) with client, family, colleagues, and other members of the healthcare team
   h. Principles of teaching and learning
   i. Maslow's hierarchy of needs
   j. Nursing Clinical Judgement
   k. Focus on what information is in the stem. Do not focus on information not included in the question. Do not read more into the question than is already there.
2. Do not respond to questions based on
   a. YOUR past client care experiences or your employer's policies
   b. A familiar phrase or term
   c. "Of course, I would have already"
   d. What you think is realistic; perceptions of realism are subjective
   e. Your children, pregnancies, parents, personal response to a drug, etc.
   f. The "what-ifs"
   g. Keep memorization to a minimum.
3. Don't try to memorize all the material found in your textbooks because it isn't possible. Only memorize core concepts.
   a. Growth and developmental milestones
   b. Death and dying stages
   c. Crisis intervention
   d. Immunization schedules
   e. Principles of teaching and learning
   f. Stages of pregnancy and fetal growth
   g. Nurse Practice Act: Standards of Practice and Delegation
   h. Ethical practices and standards
   i. Commonly used laboratory test values:
      1. Review Appendix A.
      2. Hemoglobin and hematocrit (H&H)
      3. White blood cells (WBCs), red blood cells (RBCs), platelets
      4. Electrolytes: K^+, Na^+, Ca^{++}, Mg^{++}, Cl^-, PO_4^-
      5. Blood urea nitrogen (BUN) and creatinine
      6. Relationship of Ca^{++} and PO_4^-
      7. Arterial blood gases (ABGs)
      8. The SED rate is defined as the amount of transparent fluid present at the top portion of the vertical tube after one hour. An increased SED rate detects diseases that cause inflammation in the body. Some conditions or medications affect the speed at which red blood cells fall. An example of a disease with an increase in SED rate may be rheumatoid arthritis.

HESI HINT Remember not to confuse prothrombin time (PT), partial thromboplastin time (PTT), and activated partial thromboplastin time (aPTT).

   j. Nutrition
      1. High or low Na^+
      2. High or low K^+
      3. High PO_4^-

4. Iron
5. Vitamin K
6. Proteins
7. Carbohydrates
8. Fats

k. Foods and diets related to
1. Body system disturbances (cardiac, endocrine, gastrointestinal)
2. Chemotherapy, radiation, surgery
3. Pregnancy and fetal growth needs
4. Dialysis
5. Burns

l. Nutrition concepts
1. Introduce one food at a time for infants and clients with allergies.
2. Progression to "as tolerated" foods and diets

G. Understand medication administration.
1. Safe medication administration requires more than knowing the name, classification, and action of the medication.
a. The Six Rights, including techniques of skill execution
b. Drug interactions
c. Vulnerable organs to medication effects
1. Know what to assess (kidney function, vital signs)
2. Know which laboratory values relate to specific organs and their functions
d. Client allergies
e. Presence of infections and superinfections
f. Concepts of peak and trough levels
g. How you would know if
1. The drug is working
2. There is a problem
h. Nursing actions
i. Client education
1. Safety
2. Empowerment
3. Compliance

THE NEXT GENERATION NCLEX-RN EXAMINATION

A. The main purpose that the Next Generation NCLEX-RN examination is given is to protect the public.
B. Next Generation NCLEX-RN
1. Was developed by the National Council of State Boards of Nursing (NCSBN, 2019) (referred to as "The Council" throughout this book)
2. Is administered by the State Board of Nurse Examiners
3. Is designed to test candidates'
a. Capabilities for safe and effective nursing practice
b. Essential entry-level nursing knowledge
c. Ability to problem solve by applying critical thinking skills
d. Proficiency in measuring your clinical judgment skills

JOB ANALYSIS STUDIES

In 2002, Smith and Crawford reported that 50% of entry-level nurses were involved in practice errors following graduation. Brennan and Safran (2005) found that 65% of entry-level nurse errors were related to poor clinical decision making. It is interesting to note that although graduates were taught to clinically problem solve by using the nursing process (assessment, analysis, implementation, and evaluation) they still performed poorly during their first year especially in making clinical decisions that were unsafe for patients.

A further study by Saintsing (2011) reported that only 20% of employers were not satisfied with the decision-making abilities of entry-level nurses. In 2017, newly licensed RNs, RN educators, and RN supervisors completed the *RN Nursing Knowledge Survey* distributed by the NCSBN (2019) and found that there was overall consistency with previous research showing that clinical judgment was essential to the safe practice of nursing at the entry level. As a result of these studies, the NCSBN decided to revise the NCLEX RN test to clearly measure the clinical judgment skills of graduate nurses.

HESI HINT The Council wants to ensure that the licensing examination measures current entry-level nursing behaviors. For this reason, job analysis studies are conducted every 3 years. These studies determine how frequently various types of nursing activities are performed, how often they are delegated, and how critical they are to client safety, with criticality given more value than frequency.

NGN-NCLEX-RN CLINICAL JUDGMENT MODEL

In 2017, Kavanaugh and Szweda completed a study of novice nurses (n = 5000) and found that new graduates were not competent in basic clinical reasoning and judgment skills. As a result, the National Council State Board of Nursing (NCSBN) identified six cognitive processes that were essential for clinical judgment. These included recognizing cues, analyzing cues, prioritizing hypotheses, generating solutions, taking action, and evaluating outcomes (Fig. 1.1, Level 3). The important changes that have occurred in the NGN-NCLEX-RN test include not only the nursing process but concepts related to clinical judgment (Table 1.1).

The Next Generation NCLEX (NGN) requires you to critically think and apply best practices by using safe, clinical judgments (see Fig. 1.1, Level 3). The clinical judgment nursing model provides a clear, systematic approach to making correct clinical judgments. The clinical judgment model has four layers: zero: Title, NCSBN model; one: clinical judgment (satisfied or not satisfied); two: form, refine, and evaluate hypotheses; three: recognize, analyze, prioritize, generate solutions, take actions, and evaluate outcomes; and four: environmental and individual factors that influence clinical judgments (see Fig. 1.1). Layer four indirectly impacts the

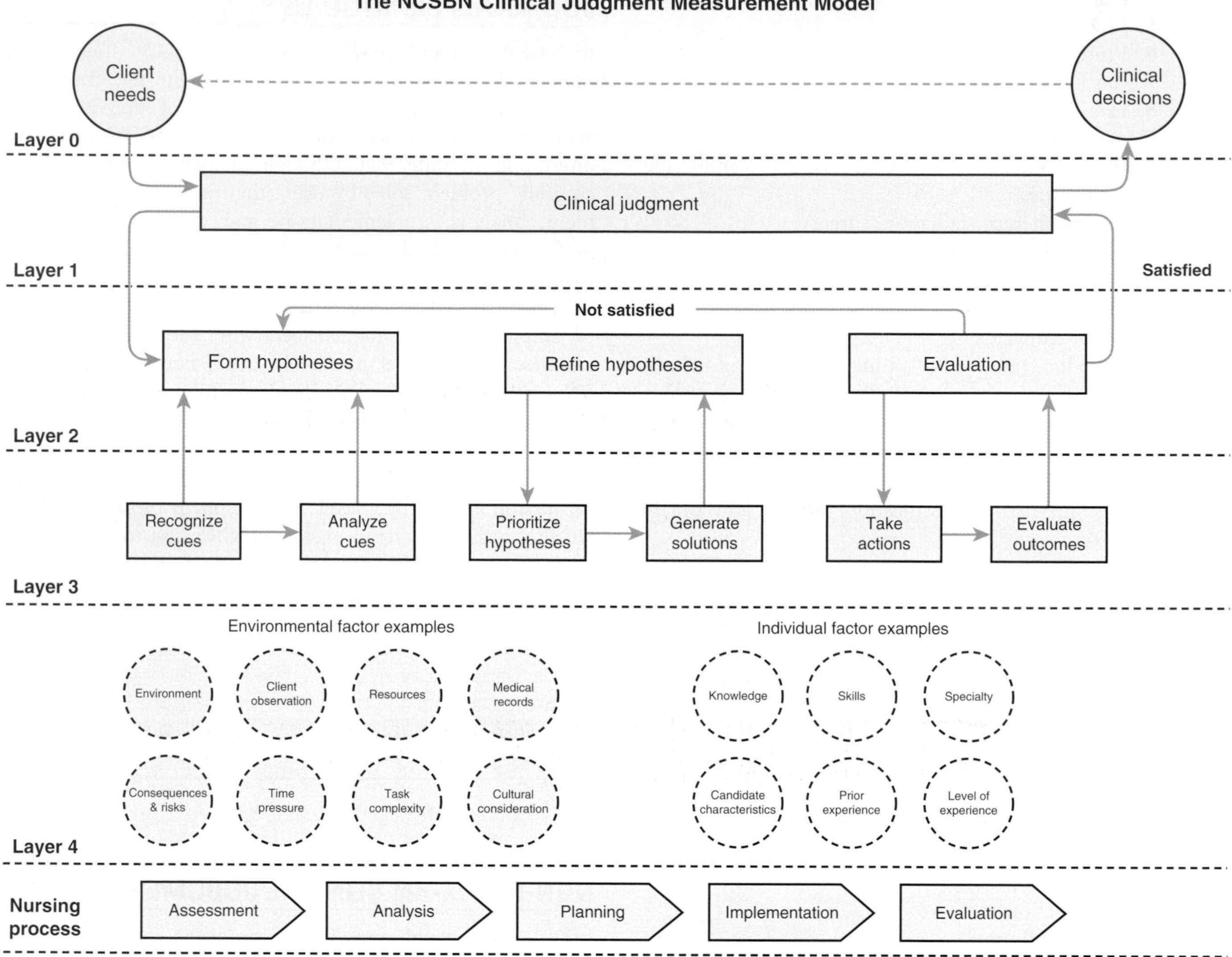

Fig. 1.1 Clinical Judgment Measurement Model. (Courtesy of NCSBN.)

patient, but may be just as important as layer three depending on the patients' needs. Environmental may include client observation, resources, medical records, and cultural preferences whereas an individual may include knowledge, skills, or prior experience.

The clinical judgment model was developed by researchers at the NCSBN who wanted to be able to measure the cognitive processes required for clinical judgment. For many years, clinical judgment and decision making have been important content in most prelicensure education programs; however, the ability to measure and isolate these traits with psychometric rigor was not readily demonstrated. Therefore, the NCSBN research teams were able to develop effective test items that measured sound clinical judgment and demonstrated that candidates could provide safe patient care.

As a result of these conceptual changes, the members of the NCSBN have developed several different ways of writing test items. For you to study and pass the new licensure examination, it is important to be knowledgeable about the way the test items are written. In the past, the NCLEX-RN test items were predominantly multiple-choice type questions; however; the Next Generation NCLEX-RN examination will have a variety of test items that have been written and pre-tested to ensure that the critical thinking skills and overall nursing judgment actions are reflected.

The result of this work was an evidence-based framework for developing, classifying, and scoring test items that were not only technologically attainable but feasible within the current computerized adaptive testing (CAT) model of the NCLEX. The psychometric rigor associated with the NCSBN Clinical Judgment Measurement Model (NCJMM) was developed by practicing nurses and psychometricians who were able to develop a high-stakes exam that measured and validated clinical judgment and decision making. The test items reflect the ability of the nurse to focus on the clinical judgment and decision-making processes that may be encountered in clinical practice. The test is not only composed of multiple-choice items but includes several types of new

TABLE 1.1 Comparison and Definitions of the Nursing Process Steps With Clinical Judgment Cognitive Skills and Definitions

Nursing Process Steps	Definition Nursing Process	Clinical Judgment Skills	Definition of Clinical Judgment
Assessment	Assessment includes the physiological, psychological, sociocultural, spiritual, economic, and lifestyle factors of the patient.	*Recognize cues*	Cues are elements of assessment data that provide important information for the nurse as a basis for making client decisions. In a clinical situation, the nurse determines which data are relevant (directly related to the client's outcomes or the priority of care) and of immediate concern to the nurse, or irrelevant (unrelated to client outcomes or priority of).
Assessment	The underlying part of the process is to identify what is abnormal compared to what is normal for the patient. Attention to detail and critical thinking skills are essential.	*Analyze cues*	When using this skill, the nurse considers the context of the client's history and situation and interprets how the identified relevant cues relate to the client's condition. Data that support or contradict a particular cue in the client's situation are determined, and potential complications are identified.
Analysis	The nurse's ability to make a clinical judgment about the client's response to actual or potential health conditions or needs.	*Prioritize hypotheses*	The urgency and risk for the client are considered for each possible health condition. The nurse determines which client conditions are the most likely and most serious, and why. For this skill, the nurse needs to examine all possibilities about what is occurring in the client's situation
Nursing Process Steps	**Definition Nursing Process**	**Clinical Judgment Skills**	**Definition of Clinical Judgment**
Planning	The nurse sets measurable and achievable short- and long-range goals for this patient.	*Generate solutions*	To generate solutions, the nurse first identifies expected client outcomes. Using the prioritized hypotheses, the nurse then plans specific actions that may achieve the desired outcomes. Actual or potential evidence-based actions that should be avoided or are contraindicated are also considered because some actions could be harmful to the client in the given situation.
Implementation	Nursing care is implemented according to the care plan, so continuity of care for the patient during hospitalization and in preparation for discharge needs to be ensured. Care is documented in the patient's record.	*Take action*	Using this skill, the nurse decides which nursing actions will address the highest priorities of care and determines in what priority these actions will be implemented. Actions can include, but are not limited to, additional assessment, health teaching, documentation, requested primary healthcare provider orders, the performance of nursing skills, and consultation with healthcare team members.
Evaluation	The patient's status is evaluated based on the effectiveness of the nursing care. Must be continuously evaluated, and the care plan modified as needed.	*Evaluate outcomes*	After implementing the best evidence-based nursing action, the nurse evaluates the actual client outcomes in the situation and compares them to expected outcomes. The nurse then decides if the selected nursing actions were effective, ineffective, or made no difference in how the client is progressing.

Adapted from Ignatavicius, D., & Silvestri L. (2019). *Developing clinical judgment in nursing: A primer, developed for Elsevier, 2019.* Data from NCSBN.

questions that require you to critically think and prioritize your nursing care (see Table 1.1). Notice that the nursing process undergirds the overall model, provides an evidence-based approach, and offers a consistent method for scoring the test items (see Fig. 1.1).

NEXT GENERATION NCLEX-RN COMPUTER ADAPTIVE TESTING

A. Computer adaptive testing (CAT) is used for implementation of the Next Generation NCLEX-RN.

TABLE 1.2 Maslow's Hierarchy of Needs

Need	Definition	Nursing Implications
Physiologic	Biological needs for food, shelter, water, sleep, oxygen, sexual expression	The primary biologic need is breathing (i.e., an open airway). If asked to identify the *most important* action, identification needs to be associated with physiologic integrity (e.g., providing an open airway) as the most important nursing action.
Safety	Avoiding harm; attaining security, order, and physical safety	Ensuring that the client's environment is safe is a priority (e.g., teaching an older client to remove throw rugs that pose a safety hazard when ambulating has a greater priority than teaching the client how to use a walker). The first priority is safety, followed by coping skills.
Love and Belonging Esteem and Recognition	Giving and receiving affection; companionship; identification with a group Self-esteem and respect of others; success in work; prestige	Although these needs are important, they are less important than physiological or safety needs. For example, it is more important for a client to have an open airway and a safe environment for ambulating than it is to assist him or her to become part of a support group. However, assisting the client in becoming a part of a support group has a higher priority than assisting in the development of self-esteem. The sense of belonging comes first, and such a sense may help in developing self-esteem.
Self-Actualization Aesthetic	Fulfillment of unique potential. Search for beauty and spiritual goals	It is important to understand the last two needs in Maslow's hierarchy. They could deal with client needs associated with health promotion and maintenance, such as continued growth and development and self-care, as well as those associated with psychosocial integrity. However, you will probably not be asked to prioritize needs at this level. Remember, it is the goal of the Council to ensure *safe* nursing practices, and such practice does not usually deal with the client's self-actualization or aesthetic needs.

B. The CAT is administered at a testing center selected by the Council.
C. Pearson VUE is responsible for adapting the NCLEX-RN to the CAT format, processing candidate applications, and transmitting test results to its data center for scoring.
D. The testing centers are located throughout the United States.
E. The Council generates the Next Generation NCLEX-RN questions.

> **HESI HINT** Answering NCLEX-RN questions often depends on setting priorities, making judgments about priorities, analyzing the data, and formulating a decision about care based on priorities. Using Maslow's hierarchy of needs can help you set nursing priorities (Table 1.2).

How Computerized Adaptive Testing Works

A. The candidate is presented with a variety of test items and possible answers.
B. Clinical Judgment will be measured two ways on the Next Generation NCLEX (NGN), *Case Studies:* real-world nursing scenario accompanied by multiple test items.
Standalone Items: Individual items are not part of the case.
All items will be presented on a computer screen.
C. The Next Generation NCLEX-RN Test Design includes the length of the exam, type of items, and total score needed to pass the exam.
D. The Next Generation NCLEX-RN Exam Test Design compared to the NCLEX-RN exam will take 5 hours; however, the items may be different. See Table 1.3 to review the difference in examinations.
E. Scoring for the Next Generation NCLEX-RN Exam may include partially correct answers and receive partial credit, for example, points possible: 0, 1, 2, 3, 4, etc. This is a new approach to scoring; therefore, you will need to be able to differentiate between clinical symptoms and clinical judgment.
F. Partial credit scoring allows for more complex item types and allows for more precise measurement. Additionally,

TABLE 1.3 Next Generation NCLEX Test Design

Design Specification	NCLEX Today	NGN Minimum Length Exam	NGN Maximum Length Exam
Time Allowed	5 h	5 h	5 h
Case Studies	N/A	3 (i.e., 18 items)	3 (i.e., 18 items)
Clinical Judgment Standalones	N/A	0	Approx. 7[a]
Knowledge Items	60–130	52	Approx. 110
Total Scored Items	60–130	70	135
Unscored (Pretest) Items	15	15	15
Delivery method	CAT	CAT[b]	CAT[b]

NGN, Next Generation NCLEX.
[a]Approximately 10% of the final 65 items on the exam
[b]Items within a Case Study are static, not adaptive
Courtesy of NCSBN.

having multiple ways to assign partial credit reduces the impact of random guessing.

G. The first optional break is offered after 2 hours of testing. The second optional break is offered after 3.5 hours of testing. The computer will automatically tell candidates when these scheduled breaks begin.
   1. All breaks count against testing time.
   2. When candidates take breaks, they must leave the testing room, and they will be required to provide a palm vein scan before and after the breaks.

H. A specific passing score is recommended by the Council. All states require the same score to pass so that if you pass in one state, you are eligible to practice nursing in any other state. However, states do differ in their requirements regarding the number of times a candidate can take the Next Generation NCLEX-RN EXAM.

I. Although the Council can determine a candidate's score at the time of completion of the examination, it has been decided that it would be best for candidates to receive their scores from their individual Board of Nurse Examiners. The Council does not want the testing center to be in a position of having to deal with candidates' reactions to scores, nor does the Council want those waiting to take their examinations to be influenced by such reactions.

J. The candidate must answer each question to proceed. You cannot omit a question or return to an item presented earlier. There is no going back; this works in your favor!

K. The examination is written at a tenth-grade reading level.

L. The NCSBN Candidate Bulletin is available at https://www.ncsbn.org/1213.htm. Select **NCLEX & Other Exams > Before the Exam > Candidate Bulletin & Information > NCLEX Candidate Bulletin**

General Examination Formats

A. Several different types of examination items are presented on the Next Generation NCLEX-RN EXAM. Many of the questions are multiple-choice items with four answer choices from which the candidate is asked to choose one correct answer. There are seven alternate format item types of questions.
   1. Multiple-response items require the candidate to select one or more responses. The item will instruct the candidate to select all that apply.
   2. Fill-in-the-blank questions require the candidate to calculate the answer and type in numbers. A drop-down calculator is provided.
   3. Hot-spot items require the candidate to identify an area on a picture or graph and click on the area.
   4. Chart or exhibit formats present a chart or exhibit that the candidate must read to be able to solve the problem.
   5. Drag-and-drop items require a candidate to rank order or move options to provide the correct order of actions or events.
   6. Audio format items require the candidate to listen to an audio clip using headphones and then select the correct option that applies to the audio clip.
   7. Graphic format items require the candidate to choose the correct graphic option in response to the question.

Next Generation NCLEX-RN Exam Items

The importance of clinical judgment was rated between "important" and "critically important" by newly licensed RNs, RN educators, and RN supervisors. As a result, the NCSBN developed a variety of new test items that are more consistent with clinical decisions and clinical judgment. Table 1.4 provides an overview of the type of test items, a simple description, and the cognitive skills that would be measured if using the item. Notice that under the NGN items, over 10 new types of items will be used. It is important that you practice how to answer these items since the scoring may depend on the number of correct responses as well as a deduction of points for the number of wrong answers for the item. One example of a new type of NGN item would be using a case study and asking the student to highlight the "Enhanced Hot Spots" listed within the case (Figs. 1.2 and 1.3). For this example, the "hot spots" have been highlighted as changes in the client's vital signs and her history of hemorrhaging from a previous vaginal delivery. The second example of a Next Generation NCLEX (NGN) item would be the Cloze (Drop-Down) format, which is much like a fill-in-the-blank, except the responses are available in a drop-down list. The blank spaces may be in a sentence, table, or chart and the choices may be single words or phrases (Figs. 1.4 and 1.5). Review Table 1.4 so that you will become familiar with other types of items that will be available.

GENERAL PRINICIPLES TO REMEMBER

A. Be sure to take care of yourself. If you don't, you may be susceptible to illness that can cause you to miss the exam.

B. Eat well. Consume lots of fresh fruits, vegetables, and lean protein, and avoid high-fat foods and sugars. Processed sugar can cause blood sugar levels to spike and then plummet, which can cause brain fogginess.

C. Get enough sleep. This includes getting enough sleep the week of, not just the night before, the exam. The week of the exam is not the time to cram or to party.

D. Eliminate alcohol and other mind-altering drugs. These substances can inhibit your performance on the examination.

E. Schedule study times. During the weeks leading up to the examination, review nursing content, focusing on areas that you have identified as your weakest areas. Use a study schedule to block out the time needed for studying.

F. Be prepared. Assemble all necessary materials the night before the examination (admission ticket, directions to the testing center, identification, money for lunch, glasses, or contacts).

G. Bring the necessary items to the exam. Candidates are only allowed to bring a form of identification into the testing room. Watches, candy, chewing gum, food, drinks, purses, wallets, pens, pencils, beepers, cellular phones, Post-it notes, study materials or aids, and calculators are not permitted. A test administrator will provide each candidate with an

TABLE 1.4 Examples of NCLEX-RN Exam Questions Versus the Next Generation NCLEX-RN Items

NCLEX-RN Exam Items	NCLEX Description	Next Generation NCLEX-RN (NGN) Items	NextGen NCLEX Description
Multiple Choice	Standard "NCLEX-style" question with four options	Standalone	Items include components of recognizing, analyzing, prioritizing hypotheses, generating solutions, taking action, and evaluating outcomes.
Multiple Response	Your choices include any of the options that are correct. Additionally, this is known as "select all that apply" (SATA). The correct response includes all the options, one of the options, or anything in between.	Enhanced Multiple Response	These items may give you a patient scenario and ask you to provide a list of options that should be taken for the nursing actions that need to be completed.
Image or "Hot Spot" Questions	These questions usually have an image (illustration, table, or chart). You will need to click on the "hot spot" that answers the question.	Enhanced Hot Spots	These items may be illustrations, case studies, or chart data and you will need to click on the information provided to demonstrate that you know what is important to make your decision.
NCLEX-RN Exam Items	**NCLEX Description**	**Next Generation NCLEX-RN (NGN) Items**	**NextGen NCLEX Description**
Fill-in-the-Blank	These items include dosage calculations, I/O calculation, or some other kind of medical math. You will type your answer into the answer box.		
Drag and Drop	These items will ask you to place the steps to an intervention in the proper order.	Extended Drag and Drop	These items will assess your ability to make sound clinical judgments based on your drag-and-drop choices. There can be 3 to 5 options in each drop-down.
Graphic Questions	Your answer will be images, not words.		
Chart-Based Questions	These items use a patient chart, and you will need to click around on various tabs to find the information you need.		
Video and Audio	Items that may provide sounds and ask you to interpret what you hear.		
NCLEX-RN Exam Items	**NCLEX Description**	**Next Generation NCLEX-RN (NGN) Items**	**NextGen NCLEX Description**
		CLOZE (drop-down)	These items are short-answer and there are drop-down menus that contain a few options for your clinical choice.
		Drop-Down Rationale	Items include 1 sentence with 1 case and 1 effect OR 1 sentence with 1 cause and 2 effects; there will be a minimum of 1 sentence with 1 drop-down per sentence; a maximum of 5 sentences with 1 drop-down per sentence.
		Drop-Down Table	Items include a table of information with drop-down options.
		Dynamic Exhibit and Constructed Response	These items will provide patient data in a "dynamic exhibit" and ask a question in a short format.
		Matrix/Grid	These questions give you a list of options and ask you to classify them as essential, non-essential, or contraindicated for the patient.

NCLEX-RN Exam Items	NCLEX Description	Next Generation NCLEX-RN (NGN) Items	NextGen NCLEX Description
		Case Studies	These are unfolding key data cases that ask you to make careful planning to foster a decision. These questions require you to recognize which of the assessment findings and assess your ability to interpret lab/diagnostic results relevant that require action. You'll need to be able to focus on the most important data to make a clinical decision and be able to identify potential risks to the patient. You will need to demonstrate your ability to prioritize patient care and determine what needs to be addressed for the patient. Other test priorities will ask you to predict what types of treatments and interventions are needed as part of the patient's plan of care and show that you are able to act on that plan of care. Finally, you will need to be able to evaluate the patients' outcomes and determine if the patient is meeting their goals.
		Bowtie Items	These items provide a brief medical history and physician orders. You will need to prioritize the nursing actions, potential complications, and the health parameters that would be monitored based on your actions.

Case study example

Case study

The nurse is caring for a 28-year-old client who is gravida 4, para 2, is at 40 weeks gestation and is in active labor.

Nurses' notes

The client is receiving titrated intravenous oxytocin for augmentation of labor via the secondary line on an intravenous pump. The client is also receiving maintenance intravenous fluid of lactated Ringer's solution at 125 mL/hr via an intravenous pump. The client has a cervical dilatation of 5 cm and a cervical effacement of 100% with a fetal station of 0 in vertex presentation. Intact amniotic membranes are noted. Category I tracing of fetal heart rate (FHR) of 150 bpm, with moderate variability, and 3 accelerations of 15 bpm over the baseline lasting 15 seconds via external ultrasound. The client is experiencing contractions every 5 minutes, which are lasting 70 seconds with moderate intensity via tocotransducer. Vital signs: HR of 88, BP of 115/78, RR of 15, T of 100.4°F (38.0°C). Has a continuous epidural infusion of 0.25% bupivacaine with fentanyl running at 10 mL/hr. Pain 0/10 at this time. Client states, "I had postpartum hemorrhage with my last vaginal delivery and I required a blood transfusion." Medical history of hypothyroidism and asthma.

Fig. 1.2 Case Study Example. (Courtesy of NCSBN.)

Enhanced hot spot example

Case study

➤ Click to highlight the findings that would require follow-up.

Nurses' notes

The client is receiving titrated intravenous oxytocin for augmentation of labor via the secondary line on an intravenous pump. The client is also receiving maintenance intravenous fluid of lactated Ringer's solution at 125 mL/hr via an intravenous pump. The client has a cervical dilatation of 5 cm and a cervical effacement of 100% with a fetal station of 0 in vertex presentation. Intact amniotic membranes are noted. Category I tracing of fetal heart rate (FHR) of 150 bpm, with moderate variability, and 3 accelerations of 15 bpm over the baseline lasting 15 seconds via external ultrasound. The client is experiencing contractions every 5 minutes, which are lasting 70 seconds with moderate intensity via tocotransducer. Vital signs: HR of 88, BP of 115/78, RR of 15, T of 100.4°F (38.0°C). Has a continuous epidural infusion of 0.25% bupivacaine with fentanyl running at 10 mL/hr. Pain 0/10 at this time. Client states, "I had postpartum hemorrhage with my last vaginal delivery and I required a blood transfusion." Medical history of hypothyroidism and asthma.

Fig. 1.3 Enhanced Hot Spot Example (Courtesy of NCSBN.)

The nurse is caring for a 78-year-old female in the emergency department (ED).

Nurses' notes

1000: Client was brought to the ED by her daughter due to increased shortness of breath this morning. The daughter reports that the client has been running a fever for the past few days and has started to cough up greenish colored mucus and to complain of "soreness" throughout her body. The client was recently hospitalized for issues with atrial fibrillation 6 days ago. The client has a history of hypertension.
Vital signs: 101.1° F (38.4° C), P 92, RR 22, BP 152/86, pulse oximetry reading 94% on oxygen at 2 L/min via nasal cannula. Upon assessment, the client's breathing appear slightly labored, and course crackles are noted in bilateral lung bases.
Skin slightly cool to touch and pale pink in tone, pulse +3 and irregular. Capillary refill is 3 seconds. Client is alert and oriented to person, place, and time.
The client's daughter states, "Sometimes it seems like my mother is confused."

Fig. 1.4 Example of Cloze (Drop-Down) Item (Courtesy of NCSBN.)

➢ Complete the following sentence by choosing from the lists of options.

The client is at highest risk for developing [Select... ▾] as evidenced by the client's [Select... ▾]

Select...
Vital signs
Neurologic assessment
Respiratory assessment
Cardiovascular assessment

Select...
Hypoxia
Stroke
Dysrhythmias
A pulmonary embolism

Fig. 1.5 Available Options for Cloze Drop-Down Item (Courtesy of NCSBN.)

erasable note board that may be replaced as needed while testing. Candidates may not take their own note boards, scratch paper, or writing instruments into the examination. A calculator on the computer screen will be available for use.

H. Arrive early. Allow plenty of time to eat breakfast and travel to the testing center. It is better to be early than late. Allow for traffic jams and so forth. The candidate may consider spending the night in a hotel or motel near the testing center the night before the examination.

I. Dress comfortably. Dress in layers so that you can put on or take off a sweater or jacket as needed.

J. Avoid negative people. During the weeks leading up to the examination, stay away from those who share their anxieties with you or project their insecurities onto you. Sometimes this is a fellow classmate or even your best friend. The person will still be there when the examination is over. Stay focused and positive.

K. Do not discuss the exam. Avoid talking about the examination during breaks and while waiting to take the test.

L. Avoid distractions. Take earplugs with you and use them if you find that those around you are distracting you. The rattling of paper or a candidate getting up to leave the exam room can be distracting.

Think positively. Use the affirmation, "I am successful." Obtain a relaxation and affirmation recording and use it during rest periods or any time you feel the need to boost your confidence. Think, "I have the knowledge to successfully complete the Next Generation NCLEX-RN EX."

> **HESI HINT** The night before the NCLEX-RN, allow only 30 min of study time. This 30-min period should be designated for review of test-taking strategies only. Practice these strategies with various practice test items if you wish (for 30 min only; do not take an entire test). Spend the night before the examination doing something that you enjoy.

REFERENCES AND BIBLIOGRAPHY

Betts, J., Muntean, W., Kim, D., Jorion, N., & Dickison, P. (2019). Building a method for writing clinical judgment items for entry-level nursing exams. *Journal of Applied Testing Technology, 20*(S2), 21–36.

Brennan, P. F., & Safran, C. (2005). Empowered consumers. In *Consumer health informatics* (pp. 8–21). New York, NY: Springer.

Ignatavicius, D., & Silvestri, A. (2021). What we know about the Next Generation (NGN) NClex: getting read for the evolving journey. https://share.vidyard.com/watch/sogbMTJfbbWD5gwzKaV74T?chapter=1.

Kavanaugh, J. M., & Szweda, C. (2017). A crisis in competency: The strategic and ethical imperative to assessing new graduate nurses' clinical reasoning. *Nursing Education Perspectives, 38*(2), 57–62. https://doi.org/10.1097/01. NEP.0000000000000112. PMid: 29194297.

Maslow, A. H. (1943). A theory of human motivation. *Psychological Review, 50*(4), 370–396. http://psycnet.apa.org/record/1943-03751-001.

National Council of State Boards of Nursing (NCSBN). (2018). *Strategic Practice Analysis.* NCSBN Research Brief, 71. Chicago, IL: NCSBN. https://www.ncsbn.org/11995.htm.

National Council of State Boards of Nursing. (2018a). Measuring the right things: NCSBN's next generation NCLEX® endeavors to go beyond the leading edge. Winter. In *Focus*. Chicago, IL.

National Council of State Boards of Nursing (NCSBN). (2018b). *NCLEX RN® Examination Test Plan or the National lCouncil Licensure Examination for Registered Nurses*. Chicago, IL.

National Council of State Boards of Nursing (NCSBN). (2019). The clinical judgment model. *Next generation NCLEX News* (Winter), 1–6.

Saintsing, D., Gibson, L. M., & Pennington, A. W. (2011). The novice nurse and clinical decision-making: How to avoid errors. *Journal of Nursing Management, 19*(3), 354–359. https://doi.org/10.1111/j.1365-2834.2011.01248.x. PMid: 21507106.

2

Leadership and Management

Often, novice nurses think that if they do not desire to be nurse leaders or managers, they will be exempt from having to assume nurse leadership and management roles. The reality is that every nurse, regardless of whether they are a novice or an expert, must be ready to always apply leadership and management concepts. For example, there may be an emergency in the healthcare setting, in the community, or at the patient bedside requiring a novice, inexperienced nurse to act during a crisis.

Novice nurses need to apply leadership and management skills that are essential to healthcare organizations at multiple levels ranging from the bedside to the boardroom. For example, it is the nurse at the bedside who informs healthcare administrators about gaps in healthcare and the need to ensure patient safety and quality outcomes within a rapidly evolving healthcare delivery setting. Critical thinking is a vital component of every decision a nurse leader/nurse manager makes in every situation regardless of the level of simplicity or complexity of the required decision.

All nurses, regardless of whether they want to be a nurse leader or not, have to have leadership and management skills. It is requisite for every nurse to apply leadership and management skills in a logical and systematic manner within the changing healthcare system. For example, due to the rapidly changing technology, political processes, reimbursement, and regulatory changes within the healthcare delivery system, it is important that the nursing profession be at the decision-making processes that impact on safe patient outcomes. There are four major content areas that every nurse should become familiar with as a leader or manager within the nursing profession. These areas include:

1. Leadership and Management
2. Maintaining a Safe, Effective Work Environment
3. Legal and Ethical Issues Influencing Nursing
4. Disaster Nursing and Crisis Intervention

> **HESI HINT** There are several assumptions underpinning nursing leadership and management of the 21st century:
>
> Novice and expert nurses need to apply leadership and management knowledge, skills, and competencies to foster and promote safe, effective care and ensure quality outcomes.
>
> Healthcare delivery continues to migrate from acute care healthcare settings to outpatient and community-based settings.
>
> The healthcare workforce members and patients we care for are becoming increasingly diverse, adding complexity to patient care, particularly related to communication and safe outcomes.
>
> Every nurse is a leader, a manager, and a follower regardless of their designated title or role.
>
> Healthcare consumers and major stakeholders influence and shape nursing care and how healthcare is delivered.
>
> Safe, effective, and efficient nursing care is grounded in fundamental concepts of communication, collaboration, and teamwork.
>
> Change in nursing and healthcare is ever constant and inevitable.
>
> Nursing care is essential to a highly effective healthcare delivery system.

> **HESI HINT** Every nurse must know about and apply leadership and management concepts to clinical practice whether caring for individual patients, populations, or systems.

LEADERSHIP AND MANAGEMENT

Leadership and management are not synonymous terms. Leadership is comprised of aligning other nurses or staff and setting a direction with expected follow-up and outcomes. Leaders motivate, inspire, and provide resources that motivate and enable others to meet organizational goals for organizational success.

> **HESI HINT**
>
> Nurse leaders inspire and engage nurses, colleagues, and other workers.
>
> Seventy percent of American workers have negative feelings about their job.
>
> Nurse leaders positively influence and change the way nurses, colleagues, and workers feel about their work.

Leaders Versus Managers

Nurses desire and prefer to be led and not managed (Roussel, Thomas, & Harris, 2020, p. 25). Leaders inspire constituents through respecting one's dignity, autonomy, and self-esteem (Morriss, Ely, & Frei, 2014). Good leaders inspire and motivate others in healthcare settings to foster and promote worker satisfaction and take pride in meeting organizational goals and strategic plans. Not every nurse wants or aspires to be a formal nurse leader in a healthcare setting; however, there will be opportunities where one may have the required leadership knowledge, skills, and competencies to lead. For example, there will be times when we are asked to be the leader of a committee or task force on our unit. We can always improve our leadership and management skills by accepting these opportunities.

To become a stronger nurse leader, we must assess and identify our areas of weakness to strengthen ourselves to grow as a leader. Nurse leaders are made up of the sum of our personal and professional lives. For example, being a leader means the integration of who we are professionally and personally and how we perform as a leader. One way of knowing and understanding one's authentic self is reflection. Reflection is an active strategy that helps us examine and reflect on our experiences, actions, and reactions to strengthen our professional growth (Yoder-Wise, 2019, p. 81). For example, if there was an unfortunate patient event on your work unit and you had to act quickly, you would be exerting your nursing leadership skill. Thinking-on-action provides a recount of the scenario and allows us to evaluate and reflect on our actions related to the situation that occurred and our nursing leadership relevant to the event. Thinking-on-action is like debriefing and reflecting on our thoughts, actions, and behaviors in the given situation.

HESI HINT

Thinking-in-action allows us opportunity to guide our nursing behaviors prior to a situation or event.

Thinking-on-action allows us opportunity to reflect and debrief after an event to determine what else might have been done and the impact of our leadership actions on others by the way we intervened.

Thinking-in-action allows us opportunity when we use our existing knowledge to guide our nursing behaviors as a situation develops (Yoder-Wise, 2019, p. 81). For example, if you have been asked to chair a policy task force related to a policy change about patient safety in your facility, you may use thinking-in-action to prepare for how you will lead the policy task force and meet the goals by the due date.

There are several well-known and accepted leadership styles that nurse leaders apply (Table 2.1) such as authentic, autocratic, assertive, transformational, or shared governance. Authentic leadership is comprised of honest relationships (George, 2003). Authentic leadership is described as a direct model where truth and trust are essential to being an authentic leader. Being authentic means if we try to adopt characteristics or behave in a way that is not comfortable for us, chances are, we will not feel or behave in authentic ways. Being truly authentic means you have a true passion for helping others and the important work they do (Yoder-Wise, 2019, p. 86). No matter what leadership style we choose for formal or informal nursing leadership roles, we can always self-assess and develop strategies to assist us to self-reflect and identify strategies for improvement.

HESI HINT

Becoming an authentic and effective nurse leader means having self-awareness and insight to strengths and weaknesses

Reflection and journaling are strategies to know and understand one's authentic self

Effective strategies for gaining personal insight are to practice reflection daily.

Apply what you learn from daily reflection to guide and direct you.

Use evidence-based self-assessment tools, and use the outcomes to strengthen yourself.

Reflection helps to assess and review the impact of our choices, decision, and actions on self and others.

Essential Characteristics and Focus of Nurse Leaders

1. Encouraging, fostering, and promoting positive working relationships between and among members of the interprofessional healthcare team
2. Create a work environment facilitating and role modeling open communication and collaboration
3. Align leadership focus with the mission, philosophy, and strategic plan of the healthcare organization
4. Develop strategies to align worker talents with organizational needs with culturally diverse workers and patient populations
5. Serve as a role model to prevent and resolve conflict
6. Coach and mentor other members of the interprofessional healthcare teams involving creative, evidence-based problem solving and negotiation
7. Implement evidence-based strategies to prevent or minimize stress, burnout, and staff turnover
8. Prevent behaviors leading to hostile work environments and have a zero tolerance for incivility in the workplace

APPLICATION - Leadership case: Jamie was a new graduate nurse (GN) who just received her license. She was employed as a medical surgical nurse on a very busy 40-bed telemetry unit. She was delighted to be on the unit, but it seemed understaffed. However, because she was new to the facility, she did not want to question the charge nurse or supervisor.

After 3 months working on the unit, one afternoon when she reported to work, she was told that she would have to have an extra patient load because they could not get an extra nurse to cover; thus she would have five instead of four patients. Because the telemetry unit was always staffed with a 4:1 ratio, this load was a little more than normal. During the 12-hour shift, two of Jamie's patients experienced chest pain, one had a full code and subsequently died, and the other two patients were stable.

Jamie discussed the short staffing problem with the charge nurse on duty; however, he did not think that it was an issue (Table 2.2).

Managers

Managers are individuals who work to accomplish the goals of the organization. The nurse manager acts to achieve the goals of safe, effective client care within the overall goals of a healthcare facility (Table 2.3). Nurse managers provide skills such as delegation, supervision, critical thinking, and evaluation of the overall outcomes of patients as an aggregate.

TABLE 2.1 Common Nursing Leadership Styles, Leadership Style Characteristics, and Competencies

Leadership Styles	Leadership Style Characteristics	Competencies
Transformational	• Critical to successfully meeting organizational outcomes • Provides evidence-based innovative approaches critical to meeting organizational outcomes and the strategic plan and mission • Recognized by the Institute of Medicine (IOM) in reducing medical errors and improving patient quality and safety	• Management of attention • Management of meaning • Management of trust • Management of self as leader • Serving as a coach • Serving as a mentor
Strategic Leadership	• Provides opportunity for critical reflection • Is focused on root cause analysis and determining causes of challenge or failure • Based on skills of anticipation, challenge, interpretation, decision, alignment, and learning	• Being transparent • Seek information on changes and products from key stakeholders to new initiatives • Prepare for the unexpected • Examine trends of fast-growing rivals and competitors • Promote open-mindedness
Lateral Leadership	• Consists of broad networking with persons internal and external to the organization • Need to collaborate and consult with others whose key opinions are valued and needed • Focuses on coalition building and avoid functional silos that overlook other valued opinions and perspectives	• Being knowledgeable and skilled in constructive persuasion and negotiation • Consultation with persons whose "buy in" is needed • Be able to create and build coalitions • Network with others whose opinions are essential for success and from persons including other leaders and key stakeholders whose opinions are very valued
Quantum Leadership	• Design leadership • Change is dynamic and essential • Adaptation involves whole systems thinking and not linear thinking about separate components • Considers the whole, integration, synthesis, relatedness, and team action	• Includes knowledge, persuasion, decision, implementation, and confirmation • Individuals include innovators, adopters, early majority adopters, late majority adopters, and laggards • Concepts include design thinking, thinking inside the box, disruptive innovation, and scenario planning (Roussel, 2020, p. 83)
Innovative Leadership	• Leadership that prepares healthcare organizations and organizational systems for change (Roussel, 2020, p. 37). • Often referred to as "disruptive innovation" • Commonly characterized by vertical orientation, hierarchical structures, focus on control, and process driven actions	• Familiarity with systems and design thinking • Able to envision with innovation and technology • Knowledge and understanding and leading innovators, early and late majority adopters of change within the organization, and laggards to create change in healthcare organizational systems
Shared Governance Model	• Often a nursing leadership model used in healthcare organizations that either have or are seeking Magnet recognition (Yoders-Wise, 2019, p. 309) • Is an accountability-based leadership model • Consists of structural empowerment • Relies on evidence-based practice improvements and innovation(s)	• Emphasis is on team collaboration through creating and sustaining a supportive work environment • Success depends on how well and to what degree the organization provides human and financial resources to support the work • Nurse leaders are responsible and accountable for creating systems and monitoring the degree to which or how well the organization provides adequate resources to meet organizational needs
Situational Leadership Model	• Based on the work of Hersey (2006), nurse leaders and managers are required to behave or act differently depending on the specifics of situations or encounters (Yoders-Wise, 2019, p. 309).	• Ability to change behavior or actions for nursing leadership based on different situations or scenarios and circumstances • Ability to assess behavioral characteristics, competencies, and training of the employees to factor into decision making at different points in time • Ability of the nurse leader to critically think and determine the best leadership approach given the circumstances and situation needs now or point in time

Delegation

The registered nurse (RN) has authority, accountability, and responsibility for safe delegation. Delegation for an RN is based on the state nurse practice act, standards of professional nursing practice, policies of the healthcare organization, and ethical-legal models of behavior.

Delegation is not a simple matter of asking someone else on the healthcare team to help you out. Delegation involves legal components and is typically governed by state nurse practice

TABLE 2.2 Clinical Judgment Measures: Leadership

Clinical Judgment Measure	Assessment Characteristics
Recognize Cues	Number of nurses available less than standard of 4:1 ratio. Two patients had severe chest pain and needed immediate attention. One patient coded and died. Two patients remained stable.
Analyze Cues	Reported that 4:1 ratio was not being used; registered nurse (RN) overload Assessment of the two patients with severe chest pain, was it timely? Assessment of one patient who coded; did Jamie have time to complete all her patient assessments in a timely manner? Was the nurse staffing considered based on the sickness of patients?
Prioritize Cues	Determine if staffing was a problem in providing nursing care. Determine if patient assessment data was accurate. Did Jamie accurately determine which patient was the most serious? Did Jamie prioritize her plan of care for the assigned patients?
Actions	Did Jamie prioritize her nursing care based on the acuity of the patients? If her patient load was too difficult, did Jamie speak with the head nurse to change her duties for the shift?
Evaluate Outcomes	Outcomes for shift included: one patient died, two patients were relieved of pain and were stabilized, and two patients remained stable. Were the patient outcomes expected as compared with the assessment of telemetry patients?

TABLE 2.3 Skills, Characteristics of the Skill, and Characteristics of the Nurse Manager

Skills of the Nurse Manager	Characteristics of the Skills	Characteristics of the Nurse Manager
Organization	Plan evidence-based strategies to address the individual, group, or organizational issue or problem	Accountability
Supervision	Oversee, supervise care, and assess outcomes of care provided by other members of the healthcare team	Leadership
Evaluation	Provide timely qualitative and quantitative feedback to other members of the healthcare team who are direct reports	Leadership
Delegation	Identify members of the healthcare team to whom one can legally and ethically delegate components of care according to roles and responsibilities	Responsibility
Communication	Serve as a liaison between individuals and/or groups internal and external to the organization when issues or gaps in communication or processes occur Apply concepts and processes for written and verbal conflict management and resolution	Authority
Critical Thinking	Serve as a role model and resource for other members of the healthcare delivery team. Seek credible evidence-based sources to guide decisions.	Leadership

acts. For example, state nurse practice acts typically identify to whom nurses may delegate tasks to perform. The nurse leader must be certain delegation of tasks meets the state nurse practice acts and that there is accountability and documentation that the task or work delegated is performed in a timely, safe, and effective manner.

Delegation is a complex critical decision that requires critical thinking by the nurse. Delegation is an important responsibility and must be based on a firm scientific basis (Caputti, 2020, p. 79). Delegating consists of transferring responsibility for performing a task that you would do yourself to another member of the healthcare team. The nurse may delegate to other nurses as well as ancillary and unlicensed assistive personnel (UAP) under certain conditions. The person delegated to perform the task must be competent in performing the task, legally able to perform the task within the healthcare system, and accountable and competent for performing and completing the task safely, efficiently, and effectively. The nurse maintains ultimate responsibility, accountability, and supervision when assignments or tasks are delegated. Table 2.4 depicts key terms associated with delegation by the nurse to another member of the healthcare team.

When the nurse delegates a task or assignment to another person on the healthcare team, the nurse must make certain the five rights of delegation as defined by the National Council of State Boards of Nursing (NCSBN) are met. The act of delegation requires a great deal of critical thinking based on foundational knowledge known as the five rights of delegation NCSBN.

Table 2.5 indicates the rights and associated questions for each of the five rights of delegation by an RN. It is relevant and essential for nurses to be familiar with their state nurse

TABLE 2.4 Terms and Definition of Delegation

Term	Definition Delegation
Delegation	Delegating consists of transferring responsibility for performing a task yourself to another member of the healthcare team.
Responsibility	The obligation to complete the task or assignment delegated
Authority	The right to act or command actions of others
Accountability	Ability and willingness to assume responsibility for actions and related consequences according to the five rights of delegation as defined by the National Council of State Boards of Nursing (NCSBN)

TABLE 2.5 The Five Rights and Associated Questions for Delegation by the Registered Nurse

Right	Associated Questions
1. Right Task	Is this a task that can be delegated by the registered nurse?
2. Right Circumstance	Considering the setting and available resources, should this delegation take place?
3. Right Person	Is the task being delegated by the right person?
4. Right Direction/ Communication	Is the nurse providing a clear, concise description of the task, including limits and expectations?
5. Right Supervision	Once the task has been delegated, is appropriate supervision maintained?

practice act regarding to whom and when they can delegate to others.

Individual accountability is a major component of delegation for nurse leaders. Individual accountability refers to the individual nurse's ability to explain their actions and the results of those actions as measured against standards (Yoders-Wise, 2019, p. 309).

HESI HINT

The *Code of Ethics for Nurses with Interpretive Statements* is composed of nine provisions.

The *Code of Ethics for Nurses with Interpretive Statements* describes the ethical obligations of all nurses (Yoders-Wise, 2019, p. 309).

Nurses cannot delegate nursing activities or tasks related to nursing assessment and evaluation according to the fourth interpretive statement of the *Code of Ethics for Nurses with Interpretive Statements.*

Supervision is a major component of the RN role. The RN plays a major and essential role in supervising other members of the healthcare team. For example, the RN must monitor the performance of the task or assignment and monitor the level of adherence and degree to which the standards of professional practice, policies, and evidence-based procedures are met (Yoders-Wise, 2019, p. 306). The level of supervision must be well-linked to the task or assignment. To determine the level of supervision required, the RN must consider certain questions and observe certain behaviors for cues indicating the delegate's level of comfort performing the delegated task or activity. A trusting relationship with strong communication with the person to whom the task of activity is delegated is essential. The RN must be able to assess and determine if the UAP being asked to complete a delegated task feels comfortable or if the UAP needs support, guidance, or direct supervision when completing the task. Box 2.1 indicates examples of types of questions the RN should ask when delegating a task or assignment.

HESI HINT

Organizational accountability is an essential component of delegation (Yoders-Wise, 2019, p. 309).

The shared governance model is a relationship-based model of nursing leadership that fosters inter- and interprofessional communication, collaboration, and accountability.

The shared governance model fosters and promotes a positive culture in the work environment and is person-centric, promoting worker satisfaction and joy in the work environment.

The shared governance model creates requisite work environment characteristics essential for successful and effective delegation.

Supervision Skills

There are three basic aspects of supervision when the RN is delegating tasks or assignments to another healthcare team member. For example, the RN may be delegating according to the state Nurse Practice Act to a licensed practical nurse (LPN), a GN, novice, inexperienced nurse, student nurse, or UAP. Regardless of who is completing the delegated task or assignment, the RN is ultimately responsible for supervision and outcome. Supervisory skills of the RN must include clear direction and guidance, evaluation/monitoring, and follow-up with the person to whom the delegation has been made. Table 2.6 highlights specific parameters and characteristics to be considered with the three basic aspects of supervision.

HESI HINT The registered nurse (RN) must give clear explicit directions and guidance when communicating or delegating a task or activity to other healthcare personnel.

For example, the RN must adhere to the three components of supervision including licensed practical nurses (LPNs), graduate nurses (GNs), student nurses (SNs), and unlicensed assistive personnel (UAP)

BOX 2.1 Types of Supervisory Questions the Registered Nurse Should Ask When Delegating a Task

1. Has the task/activity been completed?
2. What patient changes or outcomes did you observe after completing the task/activity?
3. How did the patient respond before, during, and after you completed the task/activity?

TABLE 2.6 Specific Parameters to Be Considered With the Three Basic Aspects of Supervision

Specific Parameters	Characteristics to Be Considered With the Three Basic Aspects of Supervision
A. Direction/ Guidance	1. Clear, concise, specific direction and communication
	2. Clearly articulated specific outcomes
	3. Time frame
	4. Limitations
	5. Verification/validation of the task or assignment
B. Evaluation/ Monitoring	1. Frequent check-in
	2. Open, clear, and mutually agreed upon communication lines and processes
	3. Achievement
C. Follow-up	1. Was the task completed in a timely manner?
	2. Is the patient stable as a result?

Delegation is a high-level skill that requires a high degree of critical thinking and decision making. Delegation is based on several key components and considerations that include assessment, planning, assignment, supervision, and follow-up evaluation (Caputi, 2020, p. 77). Critical thinking in delegation requires the nurse to think about what may/can happen when you delegate a task to another person. Think also about what might go wrong or happen in the context when you delegate a task to another person or persons. Table 2.7 provides an overview of key components and considerations to consider relative to delegation in nursing.

HESI HINT Delegating to the right person requires the nurse is aware of the qualifications and job description of the person delegated to perform the task. For example, the nurse must be certain the person to whom they are delegating the task has the requisite documented education, training, knowledge, skills, experience, and competencies to complete the delegated task. Unlicensed assistive personnel (UAP) generally are not allowed or permitted by the state nurse practice act to perform sterile procedures or invasive procedures.

HESI HINT Some tasks may not be delegated to unlicensed assistive personnel (UAP). For example, delegated activities fall within the implementation phase of the nursing process and may not be delegated to UAP. The implementation phase of the nursing process consists of assessment, analysis, diagnosis, planning, and evaluation. Any activity or task requiring nursing judgment cannot be delegated to a UAP.

HESI HINT The nurse has the legal authority to delegate certain tasks or activities to a designated (delegate), competent individual, but the nurse is responsible for making certain the person to whom a task of activity is delegated is competent and duly supervised.

The nurse is ultimately responsible for the outcome of the activities delegated to others.

The nurse who delegates to the delegated must assess and evaluate the outcome(s) of the task(s) that have been delegated.

Collaboration: Interprofessional Healthcare Teams

Healthcare delivered in 21st century healthcare organizations involves a team of healthcare providers from diverse professions. This diverse team of healthcare professionals is

TABLE 2.7 Key Components of Delegation in Nursing

Key Components of Delegation	Rationale
• Delegation is a skill performed by registered nurses to other members of the healthcare team.	• Nurses are unable to perform each and every task involved in patient care by themselves.
• Delegation must be done according to the purview of the state nurse practice act.	• Delegation to others is a legal issue determined by the state nurse practice act. For example, the state nurse practice act determines who can delegate and to whom the person can delegate.
• Job descriptions are another important component of safe and legal delegation when delegating nursing tasks to other members of the healthcare team.	• Job descriptions indicate what each person's role and position responsibilities are and what specific tasks these persons are legally allowed to perform.
• The person delegated to perform the task must have documented knowledge, skills, and competencies and be legally able to perform the task they are being delegated.	• The nurse is legally responsible and accountable to make certain the task delegated is carried out in a timely, efficient, safe, and effective manner.
• Effective and clear communication is essential for safe delegation.	• The nurse delegating a task must provide clear, concise, timely, and reliable communication to be certain the delegated task is timely, efficient, safe, and in an effective manner.
• The ultimate responsibility in delegation lies with the nurse.	• There is a considerable amount of trust involved in delegation, but the nurse must have a body of knowledge and be a critical thinker to safely delegate to other members of the healthcare team.
• A nurse has the legal authority to delegate responsibility to complete certain designated tasks or activities to a designated, competent individual.	• The nurse who delegates responsibility to a designated, competent individual is accountable for ensuring that the person to whom the task or activity is delegated is competent, has the right skills and knowledge, and is properly and duly supervised.

referred to as *interprofessional healthcare teams*. The focus of interprofessional healthcare teams is to bring together a team that produces optimal patient outcomes. The key to having successful interprofessional healthcare teams is to understand the various roles of the interprofessional healthcare professionals.

Interprofessional healthcare teams must develop trust with one another and demonstrate mutual respect to achieve optimal patient outcomes and team satisfaction. Patients and families are also aware when interprofessional teams are or are not working well together in a cohesive, collaborative manner. The need for knowledge and understanding of interprofessional practice and relationships of interprofessional teams was so important that there were core competencies developed in 2016 by the Interprofessional Educational Collaborative (Yoders-Wise, 2020, p. 350). It is essential for every member of the interprofessional healthcare team to respect the unique roles of each team member and communicate effectively and efficiently to provide safe, quality patient care that enhances patient outcomes.

HESI HINT Interprofessional teams are composed of multiple healthcare professionals working together collaboratively to achieve high-quality, safe, patient outcomes based on the collective synergy and talents of each healthcare professional on the team.

Communication

Nursing leadership and management skills require nurse leaders to be assertive.

Assertive communication means there are clearly defined and articulated goals and expectations shared with the other person(s) with whom the nurse leader is communicating. Assertive communication includes congruence between verbal and nonverbal communication and messages or information the nurse leader shares. Assertive communication is foundational and essential for managing and leading as a nurse leader or manager.

HESI HINT

Communicating assertively means nurses care about the person and the person's feelings with whom they are communicating.

Communicating aggressively means nurses do not think or care about the person and the person's feelings with whom they are communicating.

Communication is the beginning of understanding. Therefore the nurse needs to be sure that all team members understand the outcomes necessary for quality healthcare. To provide a platform for effective communication, the nurse should understand that there are leadership skills necessary to be an effective change agent. Change theory is a commonly use theory used by nurses to lead change. Lewin's change theory includes three stages of change: unfreezing, moving, and refreezing. Examples of the application of these three stages can be found in Table 2.8.

Critical thinking strategies that promote decision making by nurse leaders and managers must focus on:

A. Application of the Clinical Judgment Model to problem solve and establish priorities
B. Apply the Clinical Judgment Model to:
   1. Determine assessment of the need or problem.
   2. Analyze the data and establish the highest priority.
   3. Plan to determine the established goals and outcomes that must be met.
   4. Determine resources needed to meet goals and outcomes.
   5. Implement the evidence-based best practice to meet the goals and outcomes.
   6. Evaluate the goals and outcomes to determine if effective or not.
   7. Modify the process or goals and outcomes if goals and outcomes are not met.

MAINTAINING A SAFE, EFFECTIVE WORK ENVIRONMENT

A. Nurse managers are responsible for addressing
   1. Workplace violence

TABLE 2.8 Three Stages of Lewin's Change Theory

Stages of Lewin's Change Theory	Characteristics of the Stage	Example of Application of the Stage
Unfreezing	Initiation of a change	• A new policy must be initiated in the healthcare setting due to changes in reimbursement by the Centers for Medicare and Medicaid (CMS). • Example: CMS will no longer reimburse healthcare facilities if a patient develops a catheter-associated urinary tract infection (CAUTI) from having an indwelling foley catheter.
Moving	Motivations toward the change	• The unit manager must coordinate the education of staff and share the needed change and new policy and why the change is necessary and required. • Example: The unit manager works with staff development nurse educators to schedule in-services and staff development sessions to educate nurses on the new evidence-based practice policy.
Refreezing	Implementation of the change	• The new policy is implemented and is spread throughout the healthcare facility and is monitored for sustainability and adherence. • Example: Retrospective chart audits are conducted for the next 6 months to assess incidence and prevalence of CAUTIs on the unit.

2. Nursing staff substance abuse.
3. Incivility and bullying
   a. Incivility and bullying include actions taken and not taken.
   b. Example: Refusing to share pertinent information with another nurse regarding a client's stats, thus jeopardizing the client's safety.
   c. Example: Deliberately withholding information pertinent to the client's well-being and safety, such as not telling a nurse that the healthcare personnel (HCP) requested that a client's medication should be held.
4. Inappropriate use of social media
5. Inappropriate nurse-client relationships

B. Nurse leaders and staff members must provide systems to educate staff for heightened awareness of common behaviors associated with the aforementioned items, as well as providing mechanisms for reporting.
   1. In dire cases, nurse managers must implement remediation and training to protect clients from these egregious behaviors that infringe on patients' safety.
   2. The Joint Commission, the American Nurses Association, and other entities are addressing the dangerous impact of incivility and bullying on patients.

LEGAL AND ETHICAL ISSUES INFLUENCING NURSING

Intentional Torts

A. Assault and battery
   1. Assault: Mental or physical threat (e.g., forcing [without touching] a client to take a medication or treatment).
   2. Battery: Actual and intentional touching of one another, with or without the intent to do harm (e.g., hitting or striking a client). If a mentally competent adult is forced to have a treatment he or she has refused, battery occurs.

B. Invasion of privacy: Encroachment or trespassing on another's body or personality.
   1. False imprisonment: Confinement without authorization
   2. Exposure of a person:
      a. Body: After death, a client has the right to be unobserved, excluded from unwarranted operations, and protected from unauthorized touching of the body.
      b. Personality: Exposure or discussion of a client's case or revealing personal information or identity.
   3. Defamation: Divulgence of privileged information or communication (e.g., through charts, conversations, or observations).

C. Fraud: Illegal activity and willful and purposeful misrepresentation that could cause, or has caused, loss or harm to a person or property. Examples of fraud include.
   1. Presenting false credentials for the purpose of entering nursing school, obtaining a license, or obtaining employment (e.g., falsification of records).
   2. Describing a myth regarding a treatment (e.g., telling a client that a placebo has no side effects and will cure the disease, or telling a client that a treatment or diagnostic test will not hurt, when indeed pain is involved in the procedure).

Crime

A. An act contrary to a criminal statute. Crimes are wrongs punishable by the state and committed against the state, with intent usually present. The nurse remains bound by all criminal laws.

B. Commission of a crime involves the following behaviors:
   1. A person commits a deed contrary to criminal law.
   2. A person omits an act when there is a legal obligation to perform such an act (e.g., refusing to assist with the birth of a child if such a refusal results in injury to the child).
   3. Criminal conspiracy occurs when two or more persons agree to commit a crime.
   4. Assisting or giving aid to a person in the commission of a crime makes that person equally guilty of the offense (awareness must be present that the crime is being committed).
   5. Ignoring a law is not usually an adequate defense against the commission of a crime (e.g., a nurse who sees another nurse taking narcotics from the unit supply and ignores this observation is not adequately defended against committing a crime).
   6. Assault is justified for self-defense. However, to be justified, only enough force can be used to maintain self-protection.
   7. Search warrants are required before searching a person's property.
   8. It is a crime *not* to report suspected child abuse.

> **HESI HINT** The nurse has a legal responsibility to report suspected child abuse.

Nursing Practice and the Law

Psychiatric Nursing

A. Civil procedures: Methods used to protect the rights of psychiatric clients.

B. Voluntary admission: The client admits himself or herself to an institution for treatment and retains civil rights.

C. Involuntary admission: Someone other than the client applies for the client's admission to an institution.
   1. This requires certification by a healthcare provider that the person is a danger to self or others. (Depending on the state, one or two healthcare provider certifications are required).
   2. Individuals have the right to a legal hearing within a certain number of hours or days.
   3. Most states limit commitment to 90 days.
   4. Extended commitment is usually no longer than 1 year.

D. Emergency admission: Any adult may apply for emergency detention of another. However, medical or judicial approval is required to detain anyone beyond 24 hours.

1. A person held against his or her will can file a writ of habeas corpus to try to get the court to hear the case and release the person.
2. The court determines the sanity and alleged unlawful restraint of a person.

E. Legal and civil rights of hospitalized clients
1. The right to wear their own clothes and to keep personal items and a reasonable amount of cash for small purchases.
2. The right to have individual storage space for one's own use.
3. The right to see visitors daily.
4. The right to have reasonable access to a telephone and the opportunity to have private conversations by telephone.
5. The right to receive and send mail (unopened).
6. The right to refuse shock treatments and lobotomy.

F. Competency hearing: Legal hearing that is held to determine a person's ability to make responsible decisions about self, dependents, or property.
1. Persons declared incompetent have the legal status of a minor—they cannot
   a. Vote
   b. Make contracts or wills
   c. Drive a car
   d. Sue or be sued
      i. Hold a professional license
2. A guardian is appointed by the court for an incompetent person. Declaring a person incompetent can be initiated by the state or the family.

G. Insanity: Legal term meaning the accused is not criminally responsible for the unlawful act committed because he or she is mentally ill.

H. Inability to stand trial: Person accused of committing a crime is not mentally capable of standing trial. He or she
1. Cannot understand the charge against himself or herself
2. Must be sent to the psychiatric unit until legally determined to be competent for trial.
3. Once mentally fit, must stand trial and serve any sentence, if convicted.

Patient Identification

A. The Joint Commission has implemented new patient identification requirements to meet safety goals (http://www.jointcommission.org/standards_information/npsgs.aspx).

B. Use at least two patient identifiers. Ask the client to tell you his or her name and date of birth (DOB) whenever taking blood samples, administering medications, or administering blood products.

C. The patient room number may *not* be used as a form of identification.

Surgical Permit

A. Consent to operate (surgical permit) must be obtained before any surgical procedure, however minor it might be.

B. Legally, the surgical permit must be
1. Written
2. Obtained voluntarily
3. Explained to the client (i.e., informed consent must be obtained)

C. Informed consent means the procedure and treatment, or operation has been fully explained to the client, including
1. Possible complications, risks, and disfigurements
2. Removal of any organs or parts of the body
3. Benefits and expected results

D. Surgery permits must be obtained as follows:
1. They must be witnessed by an authorized person, such as the healthcare provider or a nurse.
2. They protect the client against unsanctioned surgery, and they protect the healthcare provider and surgeon, hospital, and hospital staff against possible claims of unauthorized operations.
3. Adults and emancipated minors may sign their own operative permits if they are mentally competent.
4. Permission to operate on a minor child or an incompetent or unconscious adult must be obtained from a legally responsible parent or guardian. The person granting permission to operate on an adult who lacks capacity to understand information about the proposed treatment (e.g., because of advanced Alzheimer disease or unconscious adult) must be identified in a durable power of attorney or an advance health directive.

> **HESI HINT** Often an National Council Licensure Examination for Registered Nurses (NCLEX-RN®) question asks who should explain and describe a surgical procedure to the client, including both complications and the expected results of the procedure. The answer is the healthcare provider. Remember that it is the nurse's responsibility to be sure that the operative permit is signed and is in the client's medical record. It is not the nurse's responsibility to explain the procedure to the client. The nurse must document that the client was given the information and agreed to it.

Consent

A. The law does not *require* written consent to perform medical treatment.
1. Treatment can be performed if the client has been fully informed about the procedure.
2. Treatment can be performed if the client voluntarily consents to the procedure.
3. If informed consent cannot be obtained (e.g., client is unconscious) and immediate treatment is required to save life or limb, the emergency laws can be applied. (See the subsequent section, Emergency Care.)

B. Verbal or written consent
1. When verbal consent is obtained, a notation should be made.
   a. It describes in detail how and why verbal consent was obtained.
   b. It is placed in the client's record or chart.
2. Verbal or written consent can be given by

a. Alert, coherent, or otherwise competent adults
b. A parent or legal guardian
c. A person in loco parentis (a person standing in for a parent with a parent's rights, duties, and responsibilities) in cases of minors or incompetent adults

C. Consent of minors
1. Minors 14 years of age and older must agree to treatment along with their parents or guardians.
2. Emancipated minors can consent to treatment themselves. Be aware that the definition of an emancipated minor may change from state to state.

Emergency Care

A. Good Samaritan Act: Protects healthcare providers against malpractice claims for care provided in emergency situations (e.g., the nurse gives aid at the scene to an automobile accident victim).
B. A nurse is required to perform in a "reasonable and prudent manner."

> **HESI HINT** Often NCLEX-RN questions address the Good Samaritan Act, which is the means of protecting a nurse when she or he is performing emergency care.

Prescriptions and HealthCare Providers

A. A nurse is required to obtain a prescription (order) to carry out medical procedures from a healthcare provider.
B. Although verbal telephone prescriptions should be avoided, the nurse should follow the agency's policy and procedures. Failure to follow such rules could be considered negligence. The Joint Commission requires that organizations implement a process for taking verbal or telephone orders that includes a read-back of critical values. The employee receiving the prescription should write the verbal order or critical value on the chart or record it in the computer and then read back the order or value to the healthcare provider.
C. If a nurse questions a healthcare provider's (e.g., physician, advanced practice RN, physician's assistant, dentist) prescription because he or she believes that it is wrong (e.g., the wrong dosage was prescribed for a medication), the nurse should do the following:
1. Inform the healthcare provider.
2. Record that the healthcare provider was informed, and record the healthcare provider's response to such information.
3. Inform the nursing supervisor.
4. Refuse to carry out the prescription.

D. If the nurse believes that a healthcare provider's prescription was made with poor judgment (e.g., the nurse believes the client does not need as many tranquilizers as the healthcare provider prescribed), the nurse should:
1. Record that the healthcare provider was notified and that the prescription was questioned.
2. Carry out the prescription because nursing judgment cannot be substituted for a healthcare provider's judgment.

E. If a nurse is asked to perform a task for which he or she has not been prepared educationally (e.g., obtain a urine specimen from a premature infant by needle aspiration of the bladder) or does not have the necessary experience (e.g., a nurse who has never worked in labor and delivery is asked to perform a vaginal examination and determine cervical dilation), the nurse should do the following:
1. Inform the healthcare provider that he or she does not have the education or experience necessary to carry out the prescription.
2. Refuse to carry out the prescription.

> **HESI HINT** If the nurse carries out a healthcare provider's prescription for which he or she is not prepared and does not inform the healthcare provider of his or her lack of preparation, the nurse is solely liable for any damages.

3. If the nurse informs the healthcare provider of his or her lack of preparation in carrying out a prescription and carries out the prescription anyway, the nurse *and* the healthcare provider are liable for any damages.
4. The nurse cannot, without a healthcare provider's prescription, alter the amount of drug given to a client. For example, if a healthcare provider has prescribed pain medication in a certain amount and the client's pain is not, in the nurse's judgment, severe enough to warrant the dosage prescribed, the nurse cannot reduce the amount without first checking with the healthcare provider. Remember, nursing judgment cannot be substituted for medical judgment.

Restraints

A. Clients may be restrained only under the following circumstances:
1. In an emergency
2. For a limited time
3. To protecting the client from injury or from harm

B. Nursing responsibilities about restraints
1. The nurse must notify the healthcare provider immediately that the client has been restrained.
2. It is required and imperative that the nurse accurately document the facts and the client's behavior leading to restraint.

C. When restraining a client, the nurse should do the following:
1. Use restraints (physical or chemical) after exhausting all reasonable alternatives.
2. Apply the restraints correctly and in accordance with facility policies and procedures.
3. Check frequently to see that the restraints do not impair circulation or cause pressure sores or other injuries.

4. Allow for nutrition, hydration, and stimulation at frequent intervals.
5. Remove restraints as soon as possible.
6. Document the need for and application, monitoring, and removal of restraints.
7. Never leave a restrained person alone.

HESI HINT Restraints of any kind may constitute false imprisonment. Freedom from unlawful restraint is a basic human right and is protected by law. Use of restraints must fall within guidelines specified by state law and hospital policy.

Health Insurance Portability and Accountability Act of 1996

A. Congress passed the Health Insurance Portability and Accountability Act of 1996 (HIPAA) to create a national patient-record privacy standard.
B. HIPAA privacy rules pertain to healthcare providers, health plans, and health clearinghouses and their business partners who engage in computer-to-computer transmission of healthcare claims, payment and remittance, benefit information, and health plan eligibility information, and who disclose personal health information that specifically identifies an individual and is transmitted electronically, in writing, or verbally.
C. Patient privacy rights are of key importance. Patients must provide written approval of the disclosure of any of their health information for almost any purpose. Healthcare providers must offer specific information to patients that explains how their personal health information will be used. Patients must have access to their medical records, and they can receive copies of them and request that changes be made if they identify inaccuracies.
D. Healthcare providers who do not comply with HIPAA regulations or make unauthorized disclosures risk civil and criminal liability.
E. For further information, use this link to the Department of Health and Human Services (DHHS) website, Office of Civil Rights, which contains frequently asked questions about HIPAA standards for privacy of individually identifiable health information: http://aspe.hhs.gov/admnsimp/final/pvcguide1.htm.

REVIEW OF LEGAL ASPECTS OF NURSING

1. What types of procedures should be assigned to professional nurses?
2. Negligence is measured by reasonableness. What question might the nurse ask when determining such reasonableness?
3. List the four elements that are necessary to prove malpractice (professional negligence).
4. Define an *intentional tort,* and give one example.
5. Differentiate between voluntary and involuntary admission.
6. List five activities a person who is declared incompetent cannot perform.
7. Name three legal requirements of a surgical permit.
8. Who may give consent for medical treatment?
9. What law protects the nurse who provides care or gives aid in an emergency?
10. What actions should the nurse take if the nurse questions a healthcare provider's prescription (i.e., believes the prescription is wrong)?
11. Describe the nurse's legal responsibility when asked to perform a task for which he or she is unprepared.
12. Describe nursing care of the restrained client.
13. Describe six patient rights guaranteed under HIPAA regulations that nurses must be aware of in practice.

See Answer Key at the end of this text for suggested responses.

DISASTER NURSING AND CRISIS INTERVENTION

Disaster Nursing

A. The role of the nurse takes place at all three levels of disaster management:
   1. Disaster preparedness.
   2. Disaster response.
   3. Disaster recovery.
B. To achieve effective disaster management,
   1. Organization is the key.
   2. All personnel must be trained.
   3. All personnel must know their roles.

Levels of Prevention in Disaster Management

A. Primary prevention
   1. Participate in the development of a disaster plan.
   2. Train rescue workers in triage and basic first aid.
   3. Educate personnel about shelter management.
   4. Educate the public about the disaster plan and personal preparation for disaster.
B. Secondary prevention
   1. Triage
   2. Treatment of injuries
   3. Treatment of other conditions, including mental health
   4. Shelter supervision
C. Tertiary prevention
   1. Follow-up care for injuries
   2. Follow-up care for psychological problems
   3. Recovery assistance
   4. Prevention of future disasters and their consequences

Triage

A. A French word meaning "to sort or categorize".

TABLE 2.9 Triage Color Code System

	Red	Yellow	Green	Black
Urgency	Most urgent, first priority	Urgent, second priority	Third priority	Dying or dead
Injury Type	Life-threatening injuries	Injuries with systemic effects and complications	Minimal injuries with no systemic complications	Catastrophic injuries
May Delay Treatment?	No	For 30–60 mins	Several hours	No hope for survival, no treatment

B. Goal: Maximize the number of survivors by sorting the injured according to treatable and untreatable victims (Table 2.9).
C. Primary criteria used:
  1. Potential for survival
  2. Availability of resources

Clinical Judgment and Roles in Triage

A. Triage duties using a systematic approach such as the simple triage and rapid treatment (START) method (Fig. 2.1).
B. Treatment of injuries
  1. Render first aid for injuries.
  2. Provide additional treatment as needed in definitive care areas.
C. Treatment of other conditions, including mental health
  1. Determine health needs other than injury.
  2. Refer for medical treatment as required.
  3. Provide treatment for other conditions based on medically approved protocols.

Shelter Supervision

A. Coordinate activities of shelter workers.
B. Oversee records of victims admitted and discharged from the shelter.
C. Promote effective interpersonal and group interactions among victims in the shelter.
D. Promote independence and involvement of victims housed in the shelter.

Bioterrorism

A. Learn the symptoms of illnesses that are associated with exposure to likely biologic and chemical agents.
B. Understand that the symptoms could appear days or weeks after exposure.
C. Nurses and other healthcare providers would be the first responders when victims seek medical evaluation after symptoms manifest. First responders are critical in identifying an outbreak, determining the cause of the outbreak, identifying risk factors, and implementing measures to control and minimize the outbreak.
D. Possible agents (Table 2.10)
  1. Biologic agents:
    a. Anthrax
    b. Pneumonic plague
    c. Botulism
    d. Smallpox
    e. Inhalation tularemia
    f. Viral hemorrhagic fever
  2. Chemical agents:
    a. Biotoxin agents: ricin
    b. Nerve agents: sarin
  3. Radiation

HESI HINT In a disaster the nurse must consider both the individual and the community.

Clinical Nursing Judgment

A. Community-disaster risk assessment
B. Measures to mitigate disaster effect
C. Exposure symptom identification

Clinical Nursing Judgment and Interventions

A. Participate in development of a disaster plan.
B. Educate the public on the disaster plan and personal preparation for disaster.
C. Train rescue workers in triage and basic first aid.
D. Educate personnel on shelter management.
E. Practice triage.
F. Treat injuries and illness.
G. Treat other conditions, including mental health.
H. Supervise shelters.
I. Arrange for follow-up care for injuries.
J. Arrange for follow-up care for psychological problems.
K. Assist in recovery.
L. Work to prevent future disasters and their consequences.

Ebola

A. The risk of contracting Ebola in the United States is very low, even when working with West African communities in the United States.
B. Ebola is spread by direct contact with blood or body fluids of a person who is ill with Ebola or has died from Ebola or has had contact with objects such as needles that have been contaminated with the virus.
  1. It is also possible that Ebola virus can be transmitted through the semen of men who have survived infection.

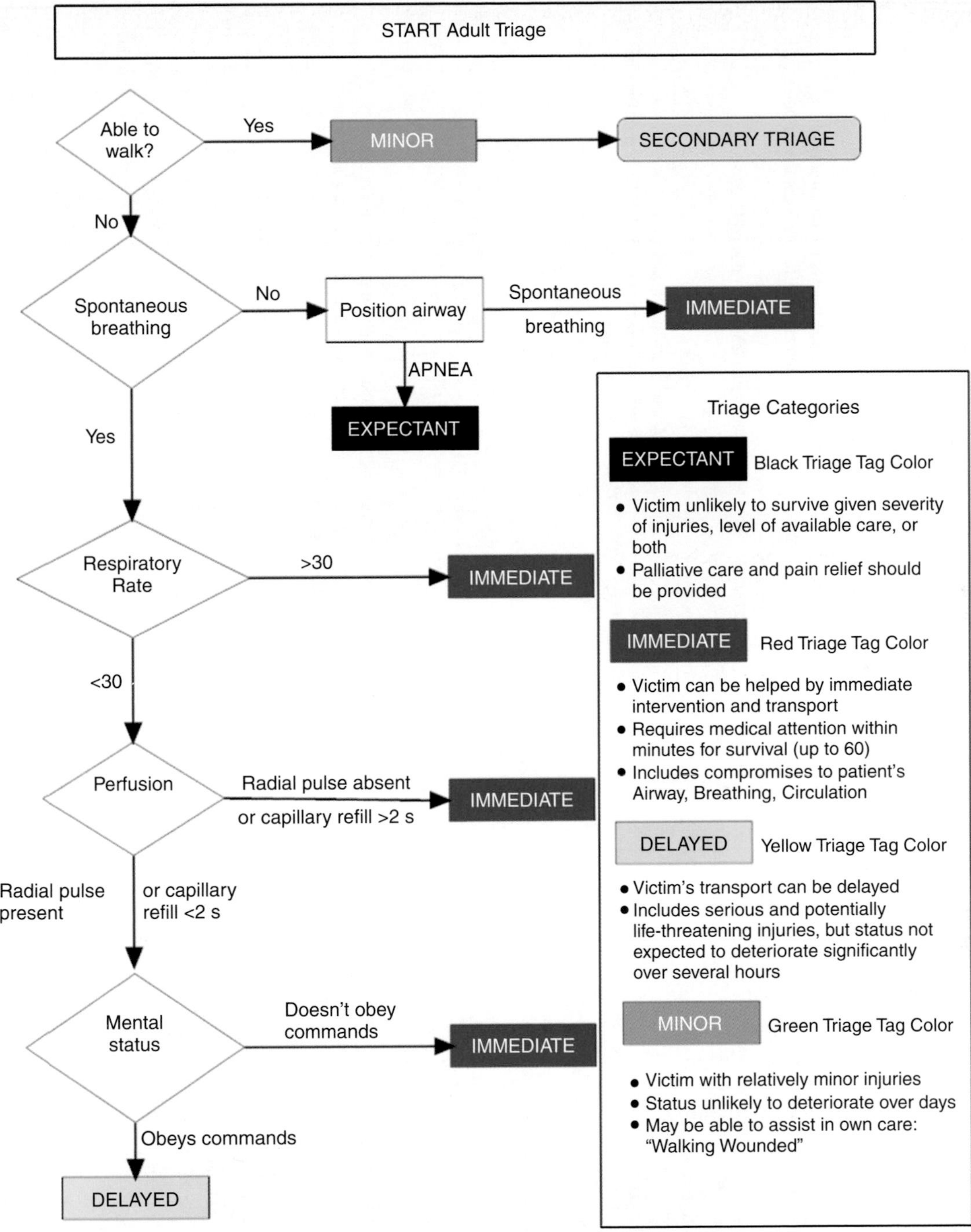

Fig. 2.1 Simple Triage and Rapid Treatment (START) Method of Triage.

C. The Centers for Disease Control and Prevention (CDC) implemented entry screening at five US airports for travelers arriving from Guinea, Liberia, and Sierra Leone, as well as other African countries. The CDC strongly recommends that travelers from these countries be actively monitored for symptoms by state or local health departments for 21 days after returning from any of these countries.

D. People of West African descent are not at more risk than other Americans if they have not recently traveled to the region. Neither ethnic nor racial backgrounds have anything to do with becoming infected with the Ebola virus.

E. Even if travelers were exposed, they are only contagious after they start to have symptoms (e.g., fever, severe headache, muscle pain, diarrhea, vomiting, and unexplained bleeding).

F. Symptoms:
   1. Fever of greater than 38.6°C or 101.5°F
   2. Severe headache
   3. Muscle pain

TABLE 2.10 Signs, Symptoms, and Treatments of Biologic and Chemical Agents and Radiation

	BIOLOGIC AGENTS		
	Anthrax	**Pneumonic Plague**	**Botulism**

Agent	• *Bacillus anthracis*
	• Bacterium that forms spores
	• Three types:
	  • Cutaneous
	  • Inhalation
	  • Digestive
		• *Yersinia pestis*
		• Bacterium found in rodents and their fleas
			• *Clostridium botulinum*
			• Toxin made by a bacterium

Transmission	• Inhalation of powder form • Inhalation of spores from infected animal products (e.g., wool) • Handling of infected animals • Eating undercooked meat from infected animals • Not spreadable from person to person	• Aerosol release into the environment • Respiratory droplets from an infected person (6-ft range) • Untreated bubonic plague sequelae	• Food: a person ingests preformed toxin • Wound: infection by *C. botulinum* that secretes the toxin • Not spreadable from person to person
Incubation Period	• Within 7 days (all types) • Inhalation incubation: period extends to 42 days	• 1–6 days	• A few hours to a few days • Foodborne: most commonly 12–36 h, but range is 6 h to 2 weeks
Signs and Symptoms	• Cutaneous: sores that develop into painless blisters, then ulcers with black centers • Gastrointestinal: nausea, anorexia, bloody diarrhea, fever, severe stomach pain • Inhalation: cold and flu symptoms, including sore throat, mild fever, muscle aches, cough, chest discomfort, shortness of breath, tiredness, muscle aches	• Fever • Weakness • Rapidly developing pneumonia • Bloody or watery sputum • Nausea, vomiting • Abdominal pain • Without early treatment, will see shock, respiratory failure, and rapid death	• Double and/or blurred vision • Drooping eyelids • Slurred speech • Difficulty swallowing • Descending muscle weakness
Treatment	• Prevention after exposure consists of the use of antibiotics, such as ciprofloxacin, doxycycline, or penicillin, and vaccination • Treatment after infection is usually a 60-day course of antibiotics • Success of treatment after infection depends on the type of anthrax and how soon the treatment begins	• If close contact with infected person and within 7 days of exposure, treatment is with antibiotics prophylactically • Recommended antibiotic treatment within 24 h of first symptom; treat for at least 7 days • Oral: tetracyclines, fluoroquinolones • IV: streptomycin or gentamycin	• Antitoxin to reduce severity of disease (most effective when administered early in course of disease) • Supportive care • May require mechanical ventilation
Miscellaneous	• Vaccine available, but not to the general public • Given to those who may be exposed, such as certain members of the US armed forces, laboratory workers, and workers who enter or reenter contaminated areas	• Easily destroyed by sunlight and drying • In air can survive up to 1 h • No vaccine available	• No vaccine available
	Smallpox	**Inhalation Tularemia**	**Viral Hemorrhagic Fever**
Agent	• Variola virus • Orthopoxvirus	• *Francisella tularensis* • Highly infectious bacterium	• Five families of viruses (e.g., Ebola, Lassa, dengue, yellow, Marburg) • RNA viruses enveloped in a lipid coating

Transmission	• Aerosol release into the environment • Contact with infected person (direct and prolonged, face to face) • Bodily fluids • Contaminated objects • Air in enclosed settings (rare)	• Insect (usually tick or deerfly) bites • Handling of sick or dead infected animals • Consuming of contaminated food or water • Inhalation of airborne bacterium • Cannot be spread from person to person	• From viral reservoirs such as rodents and arthropods or an animal host; some hosts remain unknown • May be transmitted person to person via close contact or bodily fluids • Objects contaminated by bodily fluids
Incubation Period	• 7–17 days	• Most commonly 3–5 days, but may range from 1 to 14 days	• 2–21 days (varies according to virus)
Signs and Symptoms	• High fever • Head and body aches • Vomiting • Rash that progresses to raised bumps and pus-filled blisters that crust and scab, then fall off in about 3 weeks, leaving a pitted scar	• Skin ulcers • Swollen and painful lymph glands • Sore throat • Mouth sores • Diarrhea • Pneumonia • If inhaled: abrupt onset of fever and chills, headache, muscle aches, joint pain, dry cough, and progressive weakness • If pneumonia develops: may exhibit chest pain, difficulty breathing, bloody sputum, and respiratory failure	• Varies by individual virus but common symptoms exist: • Marked fever • Exhaustion • Muscle aches • Loss of strength • As disease worsens, more severe symptoms emerge: • Bleeding under skin, in internal organs, or from body orifices (mouth, eyes, ears) • Shock • Central nervous system malfunction • Seizures • Coma • Renal failure
Treatment	• No proven treatment • Supportive therapy • Antibiotic treatment for secondary infections • Research being done with antivirals	• Antibiotics for 10–14 days • Oral: tetracyclines, fluoroquinolones • IM or IV: streptomycin, gentamicin	• Supportive therapy • Generally no established cure • May use ribavirin with Lassa fever
Miscellaneous	• A fragile virus; if aerosolized, dies within 24 h (quicker if in sunlight) • Vaccine available	• Can remain alive in water and soil for 2 weeks • No vaccine available	• Need a reservoir to survive; humans are not the natural reservoir, but once infected by the host, can transmit to one another • Once geographically restricted to where the host lived; increasing international travel brings outbreaks to places where the viruses have never been seen before • No vaccines available except for Argentine and yellow fever

CHEMICAL AGENTS AND RADIATION

	Ricin	Sarin	Radiation
Agent	• Poison made from waste left over from processing castor beans • Forms include powder, mist, pellet • Dissolved in water or weak acid	• Human-made chemical • Similar to, but far more potent than, organophosphate pesticides • Clear, odorless, and tasteless liquid that can evaporate into a gas and spread into the environment	• Form of energy both human-made and natural

Continued

TABLE 2.10 Signs, Symptoms, and Treatments of Biologic and Chemical Agents and Radiation—cont'd

CHEMICAL AGENTS AND RADIATION			
	Ricin	**Sarin**	**Radiation**
Transmission	• Deliberate act of poisoning by inhalation or injection (need minuscule amount [500 mcg] to kill) • Deliberate act of contamination of food and water supply (requires greater amount to kill) • Cannot be spread from person to person through casual contact	• Agent in air: exposed through skin, eyes, inhalation • Ingested in water or food • Clothing can release sarin for approximately 30 mins after contact	• External exposure comes from the sun or from human-made sources such as x-rays, nuclear bombs, and nuclear disasters (e.g., Chernobyl) • Small quantities in air, water, food, cause internal exposure
Incubation Period	• Inhalation: within 8 h • Ingestion: <6 h	• Vapor: a few seconds • Liquid: a few minutes to 18 h	• Exposure is cumulative; low-dose exposure effects may not be seen for several years. • High dose received in a matter of minutes results in ARS
Signs and Symptoms	• Inhalation: respiratory distress, fever, nausea, tightness in chest, heavy sweating, pulmonary edema, decreased blood pressure, respiratory failure, death • Ingestion: vomiting and diarrhea that becomes bloody, severe dehydration, decreased blood pressure, hallucinations, seizures, hematuria; within several days, liver, spleen, and kidney failure occur • Skin and eyes: redness and pain	• Runny nose • Watery eyes • Pinpoint pupils • Eye pain and blurred vision • Drooling • Excessive sweating • Respiratory symptoms • Diarrhea • Altered level of consciousness • Nausea and vomiting • Headache • Decreased or increased blood pressure • In large doses: loss of consciousness, convulsions, paralysis, respiratory failure, death	• ARS: nausea, vomiting, diarrhea; then bone marrow depletion, weight loss, loss of appetite, flulike symptoms, infection, and bleeding • Mild effects include skin reddening • May lead to cancers (with low dose and in those surviving ARS)
Treatment	• Supportive care	• Remove from body as soon as possible • Supportive care • Antidote available: most effective if given as soon as possible after exposure	• Dependent on dose and type of radiation • Supportive care
Miscellaneous	• Stable agent; not affected by very hot or very cold temperatures • Death usually occurs in about 36–72 h • If victim survives for 3–5 days, usually recovers • No vaccine available	• A heavy vapor, this agent sinks to low-lying areas • Mildly or moderately exposed people usually recover completely • Severely exposed people usually do not survive • May experience neurologic problems lasting 1–2 weeks after exposure	• Survival dependent on dose • Full recovery may take a few weeks to a few years

Note: For further information, go to https://emergency.cdc.gov/agent/agentlist-category.asp.
ARS, Acute radiation syndrome; *IM*, intramuscular; *IV*, intravenous.

4. Vomiting
5. Diarrhea
6. Abdominal pain
7. Unexplained hemorrhage

G. Diagnosis
1. Centers for Disease Control recommends testing for all persons with onset of fever within 21 days of having a high-risk exposure. A high-risk exposure includes any of the following:
   a. Percutaneous or mucous membrane exposure or direct skin contact with body fluids of a person with a confirmed or suspected case of Ebola without appropriate personal protective equipment (PPE).
   b. Laboratory processing of body fluids of suspected or confirmed Ebola cases without appropriate PPE or standard biosafety precautions.
   c. Participation in funeral rites or other direct exposure to human remains in the geographic area where the outbreak is occurring without appropriate PPE.

H. Clinical Judgement interventions
1. Obtain a thorough history, including recent travel from areas where the virus is present.
2. Monitor vital signs.
3. Place the client in strict isolation for 21 days, using special precautions identified by the CDC and state.
4. Notify the CDC.

I. Healthcare provider protection
1. Healthcare providers should wear gloves, gown (fluid resistant or impermeable), shoe covers, eye protection (goggles or face shield), and a facemask.
2. Additional PPE might be required in certain situations (e.g., copious amounts of blood, other body fluids, vomit, or feces present in the environment), including but not limited to double gloving, disposable shoe covers, and leg coverings.
3. Avoid aerosol-generating procedures. If performing these procedures, PPE should include respiratory protection (N95 filtering face piece respirator or higher), and the procedure should be performed in an airborne isolation room.
4. Diligent environmental cleaning, disinfection, and safe handling of potentially contaminated materials is paramount because blood, sweat, emesis, feces, and other body secretions represent potentially infectious materials.

Coronavirus disease (COVID-19)

A. COVID-19 information
1. CDC Guidelines: https://www.cdc.gov/coronavirus/2019-ncov/index.html

B. Agent
1. Coronavirus disease (**COVID-19**) is an infectious disease caused by the SARS-CoV-2 virus.

C. Transmission
1. Close personal contact
2. Droplet infection
3. Heating and ventilation ductwork spread

D. Signs and symptoms
1. Fever
2. Nasal and sinus congestion
3. Cough
   a. Stomach upset and nausea/vomiting
   b. Chills

E. Treatment
1. Primary and secondary prevention with vaccination
2. Tertiary prevention depends on symptoms and patient age
3. For most children and adults with symptomatic SARS-CoV-2, the virus that causes COVID-19, infection, isolation, and precautions can be discontinued 10 days after symptom onset and after resolution of fever for at least 24 hours and improvement of other symptoms.
4. For people who are severely ill (i.e., those requiring hospitalization, intensive care, or ventilation support) or severely immunocompromised, extending the duration of isolation and precautions up to 20 days after symptom onset and after resolution of fever and improvement of other symptoms may be warranted.
5. For people who are infected but asymptomatic (never develop symptoms), isolation and precautions can be discontinued 10 days after the first positive test.

F. Miscellaneous: Patients who have recovered from COVID-19 can continue to have detectable severe acute respiratory syndrome coronavirus 2 (SARS-CoV-2) RNA in upper respiratory specimens for up to 3 months after illness onset. However, replication-competent virus has not been reliably recovered and infectiousness is unlikely.

Review of Disaster Nursing

1. List the three levels of disaster management.
2. List examples of the three levels of prevention in disaster management.
3. Define *triage*.
4. Identify three bioterrorism agents.
5. Identify three infection control measures for Ebola.
6. Identify the agency to notify when providing care for a client with a suspected diagnosis of Ebola virus.

See Answer Key at the end of this text for suggested responses.

For more review, go to http://evolve.elsevier.com/HESI/RN for HESI's online study examinations.

NEXT-GENERATION NCLEX (NGN) EXAMINATION-STYLE QUESTION: BOWTIE QUESTION

Case Record

Sarah Lee, a 32-year-old emergency room nurse, was on her way home from the hospital when a major hurricane began to hit her hometown. Her car was pushed into the oncoming lane; however, she did not hit another victim; rather, she waited at the side of the road until most of the wind and rain receded. Because of her experience as a triage nurse, she immediately checked for her own injuries and began to assess her surroundings. She noted that several other people were walking around and were injured while others were laying in the middle of the road. Sara began to review her disaster training to initiate assistance to others in the area.

Disaster Principles

Invoke disaster training protocol.

Instructions

Complete the diagram by selecting from the choices below to specify which potential condition the client is most likely experiencing, 2 actions to take, and 2 parameters the nurse would monitor to assess the client's progress.

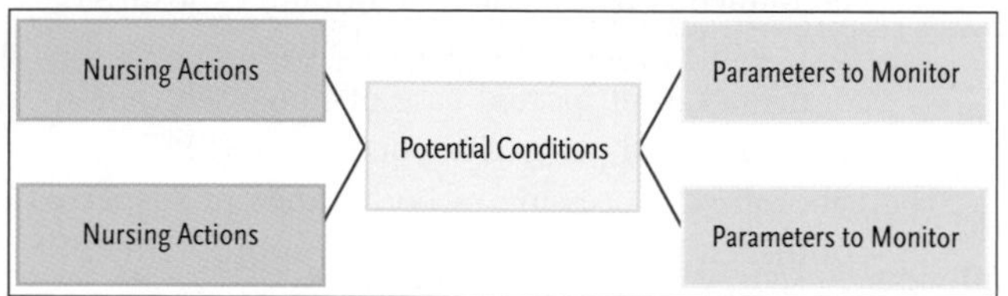

Actions to Take	Potential Conditions	Parameters to Monitor
Disaster preparedness, response, recovery	Blunt chest injuries	Infection control principles should be used
Monitor vital signs	Hypotension	Note any frank bleeding on any person
Initiate cardiopulmonary resuscitation (CPR)	Infection disease exposure	Monitor individuals who are treatable
Render first aid to injured	Constipation	Assess pain and monitor response
Provide water to the injured		Monitor bowel movements

Answers highlighted in Answer Key at the end of this text

REFERENCES AND BIBLIOGRAPHY*

Caputti, L. (2020). *Think like a nurse: A handbook.* Rolling Meadows, IL: Windy City Publishers (Revised Edition 2020).

George, B., Sims, P., McLean, A., & Mayer, D. (2007). *Discovering your authentic leadership.* Harvard Business Review, 3–4.

Hersey, P. (2006). *Situational leadership® model.* Escondido, CA: The Center for Leadership Studies, Inc. http://www.situational.com.

Morriss, A., Ely, R. J., & Frei, F. (2014, Fall). *Stop holding yourself back.* Harvard Business Review OnPoint. http://www.necf.org/whitepapers/HBR_Managing_Yourself.pdf.

Roussel, L. T., Thomas, P. L., & Harris, J. L. (2020). *Management and leaderhip for nurse administrators* (8th ed.). Burlington, MA: Jones & Bartlett, p. 4.

Yoder-Wise, P. (2019). *Leading and managing in nursing* (7th ed.). St. Louis, MO: Elsevier.

* asterics are used so reader knows it was first or to refer the reader to a specific note such as to refer to the first component of the topic or list.

3

Advanced Clinical Concepts

RESPIRATORY FAILURE

Acute respiratory distress syndrome (ARDS) is also known as acute lung injury (ALI), and noncardiac pulmonary edema.

Acute Respiratory Distress Syndrome

ARDS is a serious lung condition that causes hypoxemia in individuals who are usually ill due to another disease or a major injury. In ARDS, fluid builds up inside the alveoli causing inflammation and the breakdown of surfactant. These changes prevent the lungs from filling properly with air and moving enough oxygen into the bloodstream and throughout the body. The lung tissue may have decreased pulmonary compliance.

The first symptom of ARDS is usually dyspnea. Other signs and symptoms of ARDS are hypoxemia, tachypnea, and abnormal breath sounds.

The diagnosis of ARDS is made based on the following criteria: acute onset, bilateral lung infiltrates on chest radiograph of a non-cardiac origin, and a PaO/FiO ratio of less than 300 mm Hg. Further, ARDS is sub-classified into mild (PaO_2/FiO_2 200 to 300 mm Hg), moderate (PaO_2/FiO_2 100 to 200 mm Hg), and severe (PaO_2/FiO_2 less than 100 mm Hg) subtypes. Mortality and ventilator days increase with severity. A CT scan of the chest may be required in pneumothorax cases, pleural effusions, mediastinal lymphadenopathy, or barotrauma to properly identify infiltrates as pulmonic in location.

ARDS causes an exchange of oxygen (O_2) for carbon dioxide (CO_2) in the lungs that is inadequate for O_2 consumption and CO_2 production within the body's cells. The increased permeability of the alveolar membrane leads to fluid build-up in the alveoli and interferes with the exchange of CO_2 and O_2 at the capillary beds. Besides pulmonary infection or aspiration, extra-pulmonary sources include sepsis, trauma, massive transfusion, drowning, drug overdose, fat embolism, inhalation of toxic fumes, and pancreatitis. These extra-thoracic illnesses and/or injuries trigger an inflammatory cascade culminating in pulmonary injury (Fig. 3.1).

The causes of ARDS can be direct or indirect. Direct injuries include pneumonia, aspiration of stomach contents, near drowning, lung bruising from trauma (e.g., auto accident), and smoke inhalation. Indirect injuries may be associated with other underlying diseases such as inflammation of pancreas, medication reactions/overdose, sepsis, and blood transfusions. Regardless of the cause, the overall signs and symptoms of ARDS are the same and often can be life threatening.

Signs and symptoms for ARDS may include (American Lung Association):

1. Shortness of breath
2. Tachypnea
3. Tachycardia
4. Coughing that produces sputum
5. Cyanosis
6. Fatigue
7. Fever
8. Crackles and wheezes
9. Chest pain, especially when trying to breathe deeply
10. Hypotension
11. Confusion
12. Dense pulmonary infiltrates on radiography

A. Risk factors for ARDS
   1. History of smoking
   2. Alcohol abuse
   3. Recent chemotherapy
   4. O_2 use for previous lung conditions
   5. Recent high-risk surgery
   6. Obesity/ Lifestyle habits
   7. Environmental
   8. COVID-19

B. Complications of ARDS
   1. Acid-base imbalance in ARDS: respiratory and metabolic (Tables 3.1—3.3).
   2. Atelectasis: a complete or partial collapse of the lung. It may occur as a result of hospitalization.
   3. Complications of treatment in a hospital: may include a hypercoagulable state, muscle atrophy, infections, stress ulcers, and depression or other mood disorders. Confusion, memory, and judgment impairment also can result from the long-term use of sedative medicines.
   4. Multisystem organ failure: a condition in which two or more of major organs of the body begin to fail due to severe inflammation, infection, or injury.
   5. Pulmonary hypertension: a condition may occur when the blood vessel narrows as a result of damage from inflammation or mechanical ventilation. ARDS may also cause pulmonary embolism (PE).

HESI HINT Since ARDS is an unexpected, catastrophic pulmonary complication occurring in a person with no previous pulmonary problems, it is essential that the nurse perform a detailed clinical assessment. These critically ill patients are ventilated and are managed in an intensive care setting. The mortality rate in this population is 40%. Your assessment knowledge will be tested, and you will be asked questions about how to prioritize care for these clients on the examination (Singh, Gladdy, Chandy, & Sen, 2014).

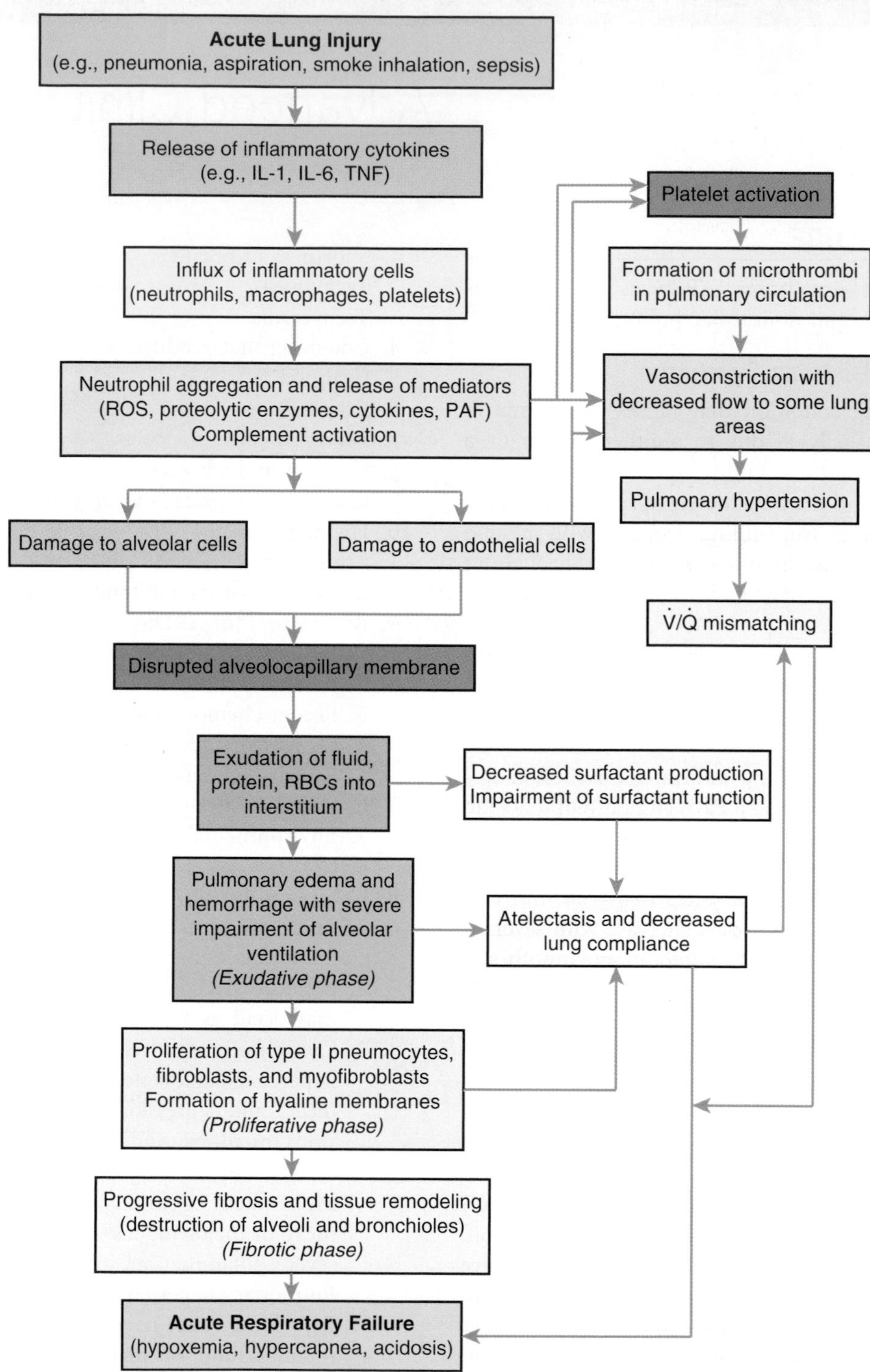

Fig. 3.1 Clinical Manifestations of Disrupted Acid-base Balance. (From Giddens, J. F. [2020]. *Concepts for nursing practice* [3rd ed.]. St. Louis: Mosby.)

HESI HINT The NGN-NCLEX-RN tests your ability to apply critical thinking skills when assessing and providing safe and appropriate nursing care for the client.

Example

Which action should the nurse take before drawing a sample for ABGs from the radial artery?

Perform the Allen test to assess collateral circulation. Make the client's hand blanch by obliterating both the radial and the ulnar pulses. Then release the pressure over the ulnar artery only. If flow through the ulnar artery is good, flushing will be seen immediately. The Allen test is then positive; therefore, the radial artery can be used for puncture. If the Allen test is negative, repeat on the other arm. If that test is also negative, seek another site for arterial puncture. The Allen test ensures collateral circulation to the hand if thrombosis of the radial artery should follow the puncture.

TABLE 3.1 **Clinical Judgment Measures: Acute Respiratory Distress Syndrome**

Clinical Judgment Measure	Assessment Characteristics
Recognize Cues	Monitor Lung sounds: Dyspnea, hyperpnea, crackles (or rales), wheezing or decreased breath sounds Assess for intercostal retractions or substernal retractions Note any cyanosis, pallor, mottled skin Determine if patient is hypoxic: partial pressure of $O_2(PO_2)$ <50 mm Hg with fraction of inspired O_2 (FiO_2) >60% 1. Increasing diminished breath sounds 2. Diffuse pulmonary infiltrates seen on chest radiograph as "white-out" appearance 3. Verbalization of anxiety, restlessness, confusion, and agitation
Analyze Cues	Determine if lung sounds are emergent. Notify intensivist/physician. Potential to improve oxygenation with mechanical ventilation Treat the underlying cause or injury.
Prioritize Cues	Determine if problem is emergent. Determine impact of problem on patient's overall health status.
Solutions	Prevent complications of clients on mechanical ventilation. Elevate head of bed (HOB) to at least 30 degrees. Assist with daily awakening ("sedation vacation"). Implement a comprehensive oral hygiene program. Monitor vital signs note any changes in cardiac function such as peaked T waves (early sign) as seen in hyperkalemia; as potassium levels become higher, there is increased Monitor PR intervals. Metabolic status through routine laboratory work. 1. Arterial blood gases (ABGs) routinely and interpret what ABGs indicate. 2. Monitor fluid and electrolyte balance. a. Monitor needs to determine whether the client is in a respiratory or metabolic state. b. The goal is to get the ABG pH level as close to normal as possible.
Actions	Suction oral cavity Give antibiotics as ordered Deep venous thrombosis (DVT) prophylaxis as ordered Stress ulcer prophylaxis Observe for barotrauma Monitor blood chemistry and fluid levels Nursing judgment measures for ARDS Intensivist for managing the patient on the ventilator and other ICU-related issues like pneumonia prevention, Deep vein thrombosis (DVT) prophylaxis, and gastric stress prevention. Position the client for maximal lung expansion, proning may be best option if ordered. Monitor the client for signs of hypoxemia and O_2 toxicity. Monitor vital organ status: central nervous system (CNS) level of consciousness, renal system (urinary output), and myocardium (apical pulse and blood pressure [BP]). Dietitian and nutritionist for nutritional support Respiratory therapist to manage the ventilator settings Pharmacist to manage the medications, which include antibiotics, anticoagulants, diuretics, among others Pulmonologist to manage the lung diseases Social worker to assess the patient financial situation transfer for rehab, and ensure there is an adequate follow-up Chaplain for spiritual care
Evaluate Outcomes	The chief treatment strategy is supportive care, along with adequate nutrition. Patients are mechanically ventilated, guarded against fluid overload with diuretics, and given nutritional support until evidence of improvement is observed. The mode in which a patient is ventilated affects lung recovery. Evidence suggests that some ventilatory strategies can exacerbate alveolar damage and perpetuate lung injury in the context of ARDS. Care is placed in preventing volutrauma (exposure to large tidal volumes), barotrauma (exposure to high plateau pressures), and atelectrauma (exposure to atelectasis).

ARDS, Acute respiratory distress syndrome.

RESPIRATORY FAILURE IN CHILDREN

Pediatric respiratory failure develops when the rate of gas exchange between the atmosphere and the blood is unable to match the body's metabolic demands. Acute respiratory failure remains an important cause of morbidity and mortality in children. Cardiac arrests in children frequently result from respiratory failure.

TABLE 3.2 Compensation With Blood Gas Values

pH →	$PaCO_2$ →	HCO_3 →	Compensation
Normal	*Abnormal*	*Abnormal*	FULLY
Abnormal	*Abnormal*	*Abnormal*	PARTIAL
Abnormal	Normal	*Abnormal*	UNCOMPENSATED
Abnormal	*Abnormal*	Normal	UNCOMPENSATED

TABLE 3.3 Clinical Manifestations of Disrupted Acid-Base Balance

	TOO MUCH ACID		TOO LITTLE ACID	
Types of Problem	**Too Much Carbonic Acid (Respiratory Acidosis)**	**Too Much Metabolic Acid (Metabolic Acidosis)**	**Too Little Carbonic Acid (Respiratory Alkalosis)**	**Too Little Metabolic Acid (Metabolic Alkalosis)**
Common clinical findings	Headache Decreased level of consciousness (LOC) Hypoventilation (cause of problem) Cardiac dysrhythmias If severe: hypotension	Decreased LOC Hyperventilation (compensatory mechanism) Abdominal pain Nausea and vomiting Cardiac dysrhythmias	Excitation and belligerence, lightheadedness, unusual behaviors; followed by decreased LOC if severe Perioral and digital paresthesias, carpopedal spasm, tetany Diaphoresis Hyperventilation (cause of problem) Cardiac dysrhythmias	Excitation followed by decreased LOC if severe Perioral and digital paresthesias, carpopedal spasm Hypoventilation (compensatory mechanism) Signs of volume depletion and hypokalemia if present
Blood gas findings	Blood gases; pH decreased (or low normal if fully compensated); $PaCO_2$ increased; HCO_3^- increased from compensation	Blood gases; pH decreased (or low normal if fully compensated); $PaCO_2$ decreased from compensation; HCO_3^- decreased	Blood gases; pH increased; $PaCO_2$ decreased; HCO_3^- decreased if compensation	Blood gases; pH increased; $PaCO_2$ increased from compensation; HCO_3— increased

From Giddens, J. F. (2017). *Concepts for nursing practice* (with Pageburst Digital Book Access on VST) (2nd ed., p. 81). VitalBook file. St. Louis: Mosby.

A. Causes of respiratory failure in children
   1. Congenital heart disease
   2. Respiratory distress syndrome
   3. Infection, sepsis
   4. Neuromuscular diseases
   5. Trauma and burns
   6. Aspiration
   7. Fluid overload and dehydration
   8. Anesthesia and narcotic overdose
   9. Structural anomalies resulting in obstruction of the airway
B. Risk factors for respiratory failure in children
   1. Choking
   2. Cardiac arrest
C. Complications of respiratory failure in children
   1. Death
D. Signs and symptoms of respiratory failure in children
   1. Signs and symptoms are not always evident and are difficult to recognize.
   2. Children may be lethargic, irritable, anxious, or unable to concentrate. Children with respiratory distress commonly sit up and lean forward to improve leverage for the accessory muscles and to allow for easy diaphragmatic movement. Children with epiglottitis sit upright with their neck extended and head forward while drooling and breathing through their mouth.

The respiratory rate and quality can provide diagnostic information, as exemplified by the following:

Bradypnea: most often observed in central control abnormalities

Tachypnea: fast and shallow breathing is most efficient in intrathoracic airway obstruction; it decreases dynamic compliance of the lung

Clinical Assessment:

- Stridor (an inspiratory sound)
- Wheezing (an expiratory sound)
- Crackles
- Decreased breath sounds (e.g., alveolar consolidation, pleural effusion)
- Paradoxical movement of the chest wall
- Accessory muscle use and nasal flaring (Hammer, 2013)

Refer to Table 3.2. See Pediatric chapter for further respiratory disease pathologies.

HESI HINT The NGN-NCLEX-RN tests your ability to assess the child's condition and then subsequently apply and implement actions to address acute life-threatening situations. For example, you need to know Acute **respiratory failure** describes any impairment in oxygenation or ventilation in which the arterial oxygen tension falls below 60 mm Hg (acute hypoxemia), the carbon dioxide tension rises above 50 mm Hg (acute hypercarbia, hypercapnia) and the pH drops below 7.35, or both (Hammer, 2013).

HESI HINT The NGN-NCLEX-RN asks many questions about clinical assessment and related pathophysiology.

Example

The nurse is assessing an infant who grunts during expiration. Which is the likely cause of this finding?

Infants and young children grunt during expiration as respiratory distress begins. Grunting is how the body attempts to create a form of "PEEP" (positive end-expiratory pressure) to help keep the alveoli open.

REVIEW OF RESPIRATORY FAILURE

The NGN-NCLEX-RN is NOT based on memorization. Nursing school graduates are expected to assess the elements of a given situation and subsequently develop a plan of action that meets the client's needs.

NGN-NCLEX-RN questions are designed for nursing school graduates to demonstrate their ability to apply critical thinking skills to meet the needs based on the contents of the questions.

1. What PO_2 value indicates respiratory failure in adults?
2. What blood value indicates hypercapnia?
3. Identify the condition that exists when the PO_2 is less than 60 mm Hg (acute hypoxemia), the carbon dioxide tension rises above 50 mm Hg (acute hypercarbia, hypercapnia) and the pH drops below 7.35, or both.
4. List three symptoms of respiratory failure in adults.
5. List four common causes of respiratory failure in children.
6. What percentage of O_2 should a child in severe respiratory distress receive?

See Answer Key at the end of this text for suggested responses.

SHOCK

Shock is defined as a state of cellular and tissue hypoxia due to either reduced oxygen delivery, increased oxygen consumption, inadequate oxygen utilization, or a combination of these processes. The state of shock will generally present as hypotensive but may also present as hypertensive or normotensive.

A. Types of shock:

B. Distributive—Distributive shock is characterized by severe peripheral vasodilatation (vasodilatory shock). Molecules that mediate vasodilatation vary, such as:
   1. Septic shock—Sepsis, defined as a dysregulated host response to infection resulting in life-threatening organ dysfunction, is the most common cause of distributive shock. Septic shock is a subset of sepsis associated with mortality in the 40% to 50% range that can be identified by the use of vasopressor therapy and the presence of elevated lactate levels (>2 mmol/L) despite adequate fluid resuscitation.
   2. Neurogenic shock—Hypotension and overt shock are common in patients with severe traumatic brain injury and spinal cord injury. Interruption of autonomic pathways, causing decreased vascular resistance and altered vagal tone, is responsible for distributive shock in patients.
   3. Anaphylactic shock—Shock from anaphylaxis is most commonly encountered in patients with severe, immunoglobulin-E (Ig-E) mediated, allergic reactions to insect stings, food, and drugs.

C. *Cardiogenic*—Cardiogenic shock is due to intracardiac causes of cardiac pump failure that result in reduced cardiac output (CO). Causes of cardiac pump failure are diverse, but can be divided into the following three categories: Cardiomyopathic, Arrhythmic, and Mechanical.

D. *Hypovolemic*—Hypovolemic shock is due to reduced intravascular volume (i.e., reduced preload), which reduces CO. Hypovolemic shock can be divided into two categories: hemorrhagic and nonhemorrhagic.

Hemorrhagic—Reduced intravascular volume from blood loss including blunt or penetrating trauma followed by hemorrhage.

Nonhemorrhagic—Reduced intravascular volume from fluid loss other than blood can cause shock. Volume depletion from loss of sodium and water can occur from a number of anatomic sites.

E. Obstructive—Obstructive shock is mostly due to extracardiac causes of cardiac pump failure and often associated with poor right ventricular output. The causes of obstructive shock can be divided into the following two categories:
   1. Pulmonary vascular—Most cases of obstructive shock are due to right ventricular failure from hemodynamically significant PE or severe pulmonary hypertension (PH). Patients with severe stenosis or with acute obstruction of the pulmonary or tricuspid valve may also fall into this category.
   2. Mechanical—Patients in this category present clinically as hypovolemic shock because their primary physiologic disturbance is decreased preload, rather than pump failure. Mechanical causes of obstructive shock include the following:
      a. Tension pneumothorax
      b. Pericardial tamponade
      c. Constrictive pericarditis
      d. Restrictive cardiomyopathy
      e. Abdominal compartment syndrome (ACS)
   3. Refer to Table 3.4 (Box 3.1).

F. Causes of shock
   1. Blood loss
   2. Trauma
   3. Allergic reaction
   4. Heatstroke
   5. Poisoning
   6. Severe burns

TABLE 3.4 Types of Shock

Types of Shock →		Cause →	End Result
Hypovolemic (most common)		Loss of **fluid** and/or blood → internal or externally	Refer to Table 3.3
Cardiogenic		Damaged **heart** → ischemia or impairment of tissue perfusion	Decreased cardiac output
Distributive	Anaphylactic	Reaction to an **allergen**	Excessive vasodilation and impaired distribution of blood flow
	Neurogenic	**Spinal cord** injury to descending sympathetic pathways	
	Septic	**Endotoxins** from bacteria	
Obstructive		Physical **obstruction** → tamponade, emboli, compartment syndrome	Impeded filling and outflow of blood resulting in decreased cardiac output

BOX 3.1 Clinical Manifestations of Respiratory Distress

Respiratory Acidosis	SEVERE Respiratory Acidosis	Respiratory Alkalosis	SEVERE Respiratory Alkalosis
Restlessness	Cyanosis	Lightheadedness	Confusion
Confusion	Dilated facial blood vessels	Anxiety	Syncope
Diaphoresis	Dilated conjunctival vessels	Circumoral numbness	Cardiac dysrhythmias
Tachypnea	Lethargy	Paresthesias	Seizures
Dyspnea	Ventricular dysrhythmias		Tetany
	Coma		

From Potter, P., Perry, A., Stockert, P., Hall, A., & Peterson, V. (2013). Clinical companion for fundamentals of nursing: Just the facts. In: VitalBook file (8th ed., p. 218). St. Louis: Mosby; Monahan, F. D. (2006). *Phipps' medical-surgical nursing: Health and illness perspectives* (8th ed., p. 364). St. Louis: Mosby.

7. Severe infection
8. Poisoning

B. Risk factors for shock
1. Very young and very old clients
2. Post–myocardial infarction (MI) or with severe dysrhythmia
3. Adrenocortical dysfunction
4. History of recent hemorrhage or blood loss
5. Burns
6. Massive or overwhelming infection (Ismail & Elbaih, 2017)

HESI HINT You will be tested on your ability to apply your knowledge of shock based on the information provided in the question or scenario. Remember that early signs of shock are agitation and restlessness resulting from cerebral hypoxia.

C. Complications of shock
1. Refer to Box 3.2

HESI HINT The examination may ask you a question about symptoms of a certain type of shock and then ask you to address the possible complications or impact described in the question or scenario. Remember that all types of shock can lead to systemic inflammatory response syndrome (SIRS) and result in multiple organ dysfunction syndrome (MODS).

D. Signs and symptoms of shock
1. Weak pulse
2. Rapid shallow breathing
3. Cold and clammy skin
4. Pale skin
5. Rapid heart rate
6. Oliguria/anuria
7. Confusion

E. Clinical assessment of shock
1. Refer to Table 3.4.

BOX 3.2 Complications of Shock

Early	Severe
Tachycardia	Organ dysfunction
Hypotension	Renal failure
Weakened peripheral pulses	Pleural effusion
Restlessness, agitation, confusion	Respiratory distress
Pale cool, clammy skin	Renal failure
Decreased urine output (M30 mL/hr)	Death

Data from Giddens, J. F. (2017). *Concepts for nursing practice* (with Pageburst Digital Book Access on VST). In: VitalBook file (2nd ed., p. 233). St. Louis: Mosby; Harkreader, H. (2007). *Fundamentals of nursing: caring and clinical judgment.* In: VitalBook file (3rd ed., p. 957). Philadelphia: Saunders.

F. Medical management of shock
1. Refer to Table 3.5.
2. Tissue perfusion
a. Oxygenation and ventilation
1) Optimize O_2 delivery and reduce demand on heart.
2) Increase arterial O_2 saturation with supplemental oxygenation and mechanical ventilation.
3) Space activities that decrease O_2 consumption.
2. Fluid resuscitation
a. Cause of shock dictates the type of treatment. Based on laboratory data, lactic acid infusion of volume-expanding fluids is the treatment for hypovolemic shock and anaphylactic shock.
b. Whole blood, plasma, plasma substitutes (colloid fluids) may be used.
c. Isotonic, (IV) solutions, such as Ringer's lactate solution and normal saline, may also be used.
d. If shock is cardiogenic in nature, infusion of volume-expanding fluids may be contraindicated and may result in pulmonary edema.
3. Drug therapy
a. Restoration of cardiac function should take priority. Drug selection is based on the effect of the shock on preload, afterload, or contractility.
1) Drugs that increase preload (e.g., blood products, crystalloids) or decrease preload (e.g., opioids such as morphine, nitrates, diuretics)
2) Drugs that increase afterload (e.g., vasopressors, stimulates alpha and beta 1 adrenergic and dominergic receptors such as dopamine) or decrease afterload (e.g., vasodilators/nitrates such as nitroprusside, angiotensin-converting enzyme inhibitor [ACE-I], angiotensin II receptor blocker [ARB])
3) Drugs that decrease contractility (e.g., beta blockers, calcium channel blockers) or increase contractility (e.g., antiarrhythmic inhibits sodium-potassium ATPase such as digoxin, beta 1 stimulator/mild chronotropic arrhythmogenic and vasodilative effects such as dobutamine, cAMP phosphodiesterase inhibitors such as milrinone). Milrinone is a phosphodiesterase 3 inhibitor that **increases cardiac inotropy, lusitropy, and peripheral vasodilatation.** In contrast, dobutamine is a synthetic catecholamine that acts as a β_1 and β_2-receptor agonist and improves blood pressure by increasing cardiac output.

G. Monitoring
a. Central monitoring system may be inserted for monitoring shock.
b. Continue to assess pulmonary function (using electrocardiogram [ECG], pulse oximetry, end-tidal CO_2 monitoring, ABGs, and hemodynamic monitoring urinary output, clinical assessment (i.e., mental status)) with close monitoring systems
c. Stabilizing and treating the underlying cause of the condition.

H. Clinical nursing judgment measures for shock
1. If cardiogenic shock exists in the presence of pulmonary edema (i.e., from pump failure), position client to reduce venous return (high Fowler position with legs down) to decrease further venous return to the left ventricle.
2. If an intra-aortic balloon pump (IABP) is used to decrease myocardial O_2 demand and improve myocardial perfusion, the nursing responsibilities are to monitor and assess the IABP (nurses must be educated on pump dynamics before being responsible for monitoring a patient with an IABP).
3. The nurse is also responsible for assessing for potential complications of this device such as limb ischemia, compartment syndrome, aorta dissection, plaque or emboli dislodgement, migration of the catheter, insertion site bleeding, rupture of the balloon, signs and symptoms of infection, and skin breakdown because the client has limited movement.
4. Monitor BP, pulse, respirations, and arrhythmias based on Intensive care unit (ICU) protocols.
5. Monitor arterial pressure by understanding the concepts related to arterial pressure (Table 3.6).
6. Assess urine output every hour to maintain at least 30 mL/h (roughly 0.5 mL/kg/h for 70-kg patient) and notify the healthcare provider if urine output drops below 30 mL/h (reflects decreased renal perfusion and may result in acute renal failure).
7. Administer fluids as prescribed by provider to improve preload: blood, colloids, or electrolyte solutions until designated central venous pressure (CVP) is reached.

(Table 3.7).

8. Remember client's bed position is dependent on cause of shock.
9. Administer medications IV (*not* intramuscular [IM] or subcutaneous) until perfusion improves in muscles and subcutaneous tissue.
10. Maintain warmth; increase heat in room and use warm blankets (not too hot).
11. Keep side rails up; due to mental confusion and high fall risk.
12. Obtain blood for laboratory work as prescribed. Anticipate: complete blood count (CBC), electrolytes, blood urea nitrogen (BUN), creatinine (renal damage), lactate (sepsis), and blood gases (oxygenation and ventilation).
a. When administering vasopressor, adrenergic stimulants, and or vasodilators.
b. Administer through volume-controlled pump.
c. Monitor hemodynamic status every 5 to 15 minutes or as ordered.
d. Watch IV site carefully for extravasation and tissue damage.
e. Ensure medications administered are for target MAP.
f. Glucose levels should be sustained based on orders and based on the shock.

TABLE 3.5 Clinical Assessment for Shock

NURSING ASSESSMENT	CARDIOGENIC	DISTRIBUTIVE			OBSTRUCTIVE		
		Analhpylatic	Neurogenic	Septic	Tamponade	Emboli	Compart-ment syndrome
Blood pressure	SBP < 90 mm Hg	SBP < 90 mm Hg	SBP < 90 mm Hg	SBP < 90 mm Hg	SBP < 90 mm Hg	Assessment varies dependent upon the locale	
Heart rate	> 100 BPM	> 100 BPM then <60 BPM	<60 BPM	>100 PM			
Pulse	Weak, thready			Full, bounding Widen pulse pressure	JVD Pulse paradoxus		
Heart	Diminished sounds Chest pain Dysrhythmias Decreased CO	Chest pain Decreased CO	Decreased CO	Increase CO initially, but then contractility fails → Decreased CO	Muffled heart sounds Decreased CO	Decreased CO	
Pulmonary	RR >24 Crackles	Throat tightening Cough Dyspnea Stridor Wheezing		>24 (early) <10 (late) Crackles			
Skin	Cool, pale	Warm Pruritus Redness Urticaria	Warm, dry	Pink, warm, flushed			
Mental status	Change in alertness	Appre-hensive Dizzy HA Confuse Syncope		Change in alertness			
GI/GU		N,V,D Abdominal cramping incontin		Decreased U.O.			

Table created by Katherine Ralph.

TABLE 3.6 Arterial Pressure

Concept	Definition
Mean arterial pressure (MAP)	• Level of pressure in the central arterial bed measured indirectly by blood pressure (BP) measurement • MAP = cardiac output × total peripheral resistance = systolic BP + 2 (diastolic BP)/3 • In adults, usually approaches 100 mm Hg • Can be measured directly through arterial catheter insertion
Cardiac output (CO)	• Volume of blood ejected by the left ventricle per unit of time • Stroke volume (amount of blood ejected per beat) × heart rate (normal: 4–6 L/min)
Peripheral resistance (PR)	• Resistance to blood flow offered by the vessels in the peripheral vascular bed
Central venous pressure (CVP)	• Pressure within the right atrium; normal CVP/RAP ranges from 2 to 6 mm Hg

TABLE 3.7 Administration of Blood Products

Component therapy has replaced the use of whole blood, which accounts for <10% of all transfusions.

BLOOD PRODUCTS

Description	Special Considerations	Indications for Use
Packed red blood cells (RBCs)	Less danger of fluid overload	Acute blood loss
Frozen RBCs: prepared from RBCs using glycerol for protection and then frozen	Must be used within 24 h of thawing	Auto transfusion: infrequently used because filters remove most of white blood cells
Platelets: pooled—300 mL One unit contains single donor—200 mL	Bag should be agitated periodically.	Bleeding caused by thrombocytopenia
Fresh-frozen plasma (FFP): liquid portion of whole blood separated from cells and frozen	The use of FFP is being replaced by albumin plasma expanders.	Bleeding caused by deficiency in clotting factors
Albumin: prepared from plasma and is available in 5% and 25% solutions	Albumin 25 g/100 mL is osmotically equal to 500 mL of plasma.	Hypovolemic shock, hypoalbuminemia
Cryoprecipitates and commercial concentrates: prepared from fresh-frozen plasma with 10–20 mL/bag	Used in treating hemophilia	Replacement of clotting factors, especially factor VIII and fibrinogen

TRANSFUSION REACTIONS

Reactions/Complications	Assessment	Nursing Judgment Measures
Acute hemolytic	Chills, fever, low back pain, flushing, tachycardia, hypotension progressing to acute renal failure, shock, and cardiac arrest	*Stop transfusion.* Change tubing, then continue saline intravenously (IV). Treat for shock if present. Draw blood samples for serologic testing. Monitor hourly urine output. Give diuretics as prescribed.
Febrile nonhemolytic (most common)	Sudden chills and fever, headaches, flushing, anxiety, and muscle pain	Give antipyretics as prescribed.
Mild allergic	Flushing, itching, urticaria (hives)	Give antihistamine as directed.
Anaphylactic and severe allergic	Anxiety, urticaria, wheezing, progressive cyanosis leading to shock and possible cardiac arrest	*Stop transfusion.* Initiate cardiopulmonary resuscitation (CPR).
Circulatory overload	Cough, dyspnea, pulmonary congestion, headache, hypertension	Place client in upright position with feet in dependent position and administer diuretics, O_2, morphine; slow IV rate.
Sepsis	Rapid onset of chills, high fever, vomiting, marked hypotension, or shock	Ensure a patent airway, obtain blood for culture, administer prescribed antibiotics, take vital signs every 5 min until stable.

Nursing Skills

- Obtain venous access; use central venous catheter or 19-gauge needle.
- Use only blood administration tubing to infuse blood products.
- Run blood products with saline solutions only. Dextrose solutions and Ringer's lactate solution will induce RBC hemolysis.
- Run infusion at prescribed rate and remain with client for the first 15–30 min of infusion.
- The blood should be administered as soon as it is brought to the client.
- Check vital signs frequently before, during, and immediately after the infusion; note any increase in temperature.
- Follow agency policy regarding specific timetable for blood infusion.
- Check and double-check the product before infusing to see that it is the:
  - Correct product, as prescribed; double-check with a second licensed person.
  - Correct blood type and Rh factor, matched with the client, and note expiration date.

13. Ensure the pulse oximetry probe is placed appropriately to ensure the probe is reading correctly and not cause necrosis due to decreased tissue perfusion.

I. Provide family support.
   a. Involve the family in care and facilitate a patient care support person, social worker, and spiritual support.
   b. Keep family updated.
   c. Collaborate with the healthcare provider before notifying family of medical interventions.

DISSEMINATED INTRAVASCULAR COAGAULATION

Description: Disseminated intravascular coagulation (DIC) is a life-threatening syndrome characterized by disseminated and often uncontrolled activation of coagulation. This syndrome is associated with a high risk of macro- and microvascular thrombosis and progressive consumption coagulopathy, which leads to an increased bleeding risk. Several pathological conditions may trigger DIC including but not limited to sepsis, cancer, trauma, and obstetric calamity ranking among the most frequent triggering factors (Papageorgiou et al., 2018).

DIC destroys the clotting factors, platelets, and red blood cells (RBCs).

A. DIC is a complication or an effect of the progression of other illnesses, is always secondary to an underlying disorder, and is associated with a number of clinical conditions, generally involving activation of systemic inflammation, such as sepsis and severe infection (including COVID-19), trauma (neurotrauma), organ destruction, malignancy, severe transfusion reactions.

B. DIC is most commonly observed in severe sepsis and septic shock. Indeed, the development and severity of DIC correlate with mortality in severe sepsis. Bacteremia, both gram-positive and gram-negative organisms, is most commonly associated with DIC. Other organisms (e.g., viruses, fungi, and parasites) may also cause DIC (Box 3.3).

C. The first phase involves abnormal clotting in the microcirculation, which uses up clotting factors and results in the inability to form clots, so hemorrhage occurs (Fig. 3.2).

D. The diagnosis is based on laboratory findings.
   1. Prothrombin time (PT): prolonged
   2. Partial thromboplastin time (PTT): prolonged
   3. Fibrinogen: decreased
   4. Platelet count: decreased
   5. Fibrin degradation (split) products (FSP or FDP): increased

Clinical Assessment

A. Petechiae, purpura, hematomas
B. Respiratory distress, tachypnea, dyspnea
C. Oozing from IV sites, drains, gums, and wounds
D. Gastrointestinal and genitourinary bleeding
E. Hemoptysis
F. Mental status change
G. Hypotension, tachycardia
H. Pain
I. ABGs and saturation

Clinical Nursing Judgment Measures

A. Treatment should primarily focus on addressing the underlying disorder
B. Monitor for bleeding.

BOX 3.3 Comparison of HELLP Syndrome and Disseminated Intravascular Coagulation

	HELPP SYNDROME	DIC
Signs and Symptoms	Nausea with or without vomiting Epigastric pain or pain in right upper abdominal quadrant Hypertension varying from mild to severe Malaise	Obvious signs of bleeding, such as hematuria or hematoma development at venipuncture sites, hemorrhage in the conjunctiva, and petechiae
Laboratory Blood Values	Increased aminotransferase, bilirubin, hemoglobin levels, and increased hematocrit Decreased platelet count	Elevated levels of fibrin degradation products, prothrombin time, and stimulated partial thromboplastin time
Treatment	Delivery of the fetus if the outcome of the mother or fetus is endangered Platelet administration if the cell count is $< 20,000/mm^3$ Monitoring of liver function Observation for organ systems dysfunction	Volume blood and clotting factor replacement Removal of the underlying precipitating factor to reverse the DIC Support for organ systems dysfunction

DIC, Disseminated intravascular coagulation.
From Bridges, E. J., Womble, S., Wallace, M., & McCartney, J. (2003). Hemodynamic monitoring in high-risk obstetrics patients, I. Expected hemodynamic changes during pregnancy. *Critical Care Nurse* 23, 53–62; Pourrat, O., Pierre, F., & Magnin, G. (2009). Le syndrome HELLP: les dix commandements. *La Revue de Médecine Interne 30*(1), 58–64; Beucher, G., Simonet, T., & Dreyfus, M. (2008). Point de vue d'expert Prise en charge du HELLP syndrome Management of HELLP syndrome. *Gynecologie Obstetrique Fertilite* 36, 1175–1190; Alspach, A. A. C. N. (2006). *Core curriculum for critical care nursing.* In: VitalBook file (6th ed.). St. Louis: Saunders.

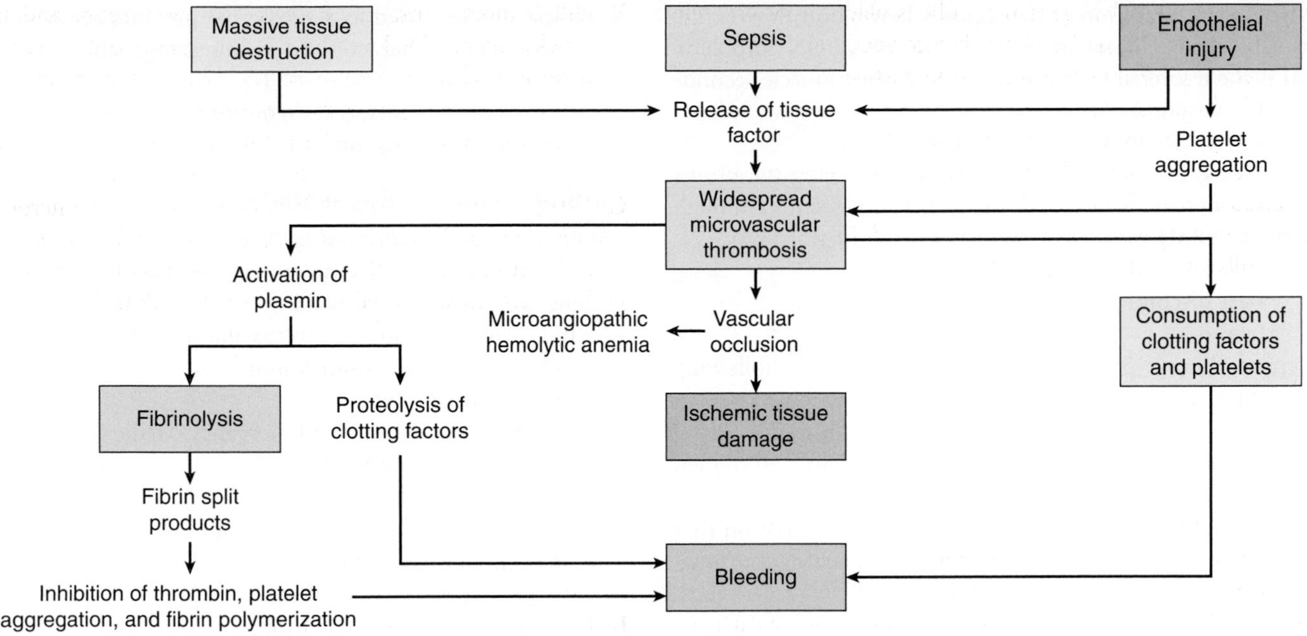

Fig. 3.2 Pathophysiology of Disseminated Intravascular Coagulation. (From Urden, L. D., Stacy, K. M., & Lough, M. E. [2020]. *Priorities in critical care nursing* [8th ed.]. St. Louis: Mosby.)

C. Monitor vital signs.
D. Monitor PT/international normalized ratio (INR).
E. Protect from injury and bleeding.
  1. Provide gentle oral care with mouth swabs.
  2. Minimize needle sticks; use smallest gauge needle possible.
  3. Turn frequently to eliminate pressure points.
  4. Minimize number of BP measurements taken by cuff.
  5. Use gentle suction to prevent trauma to mucosa.
  6. Apply pressure to any oozing site(s).
F. Provide emotional support to decrease anxiety.

HESI HINT The nurse is caring for a patient who sustained several fractures and internal injuries in a motor vehicle crash. The patient underwent exploratory laparotomy to control the bleeding. Several hours later, the nurse's assessment of the client reveals bleeding from the incision site; dyspnea; weak, thready pulse; cold, clammy skin; and hematuria.

The NGN-NCLEX-RN asks questions that begin with a detailed clinical scenario. To address this scenario, you must be able to address the typical signs and symptoms of DIC crisis. The nurse should immediately advise the surgeon for evaluation for further surgical intervention. Care would include administration of clotting factors, along with interventions to stop the hemorrhage (Papageorgiou et al., 2018).

REVIEW OF SHOCK AND DIC

1. Define *shock.*
2. What is the most common cause of shock?
3. What causes septic shock?
4. What is the goal of treatment for hypovolemic shock?
5. What intervention is used to restore cardiac output when hypovolemic shock exists? In this answer include the word warm: Rapid infusion of warm volume-expanding fluids.
6. It is important to differentiate between hypovolemic and cardiogenic shock. How might the nurse determine the existence of cardiogenic shock?
7. If a client is in cardiogenic shock, what might result from administration of volume-expanding fluids, and what intervention can the nurse expect to perform in the event of such an occurrence?
8. List five assessment findings that occur in most shock victims.
9. Once circulating volume is restored, vasopressors may be prescribed to increase venous return. List the main drugs that are used. Include milrinone in the answer to #9.
10. What is the established minimum renal output per hour?
11. List four measurable criteria that are the major expected outcomes of a shock crisis.
12. Define *DIC.*
13. What is the effect of DIC on PT, PTT, platelets, and FSPs.
14. What medication is used in the treatment of DIC?
15. Name four nursing judgment measures to prevent injury in clients with DIC.

See Answer Key at the end of this text for suggested responses.

RESUSCITATION

Cardiopulmonary Arrest

Occurs when the heart malfunctions and stops beating unexpectedly. Cardiac arrest is an "ELECTRICAL" problem.

Myocardial infarction (MI) occurs when blood flow to the heart is blocked. A heart attack is a "CIRCULATION" problem.

A. MI is the irreversible death/necrosis of heart muscle secondary to ischemia. Approximately 1.5 million cases of MI occur annually in the United States.
B. Patients with typical MI may have the following symptoms in the days or even weeks preceding the event (although typical STEMI may occur suddenly, without warning):
    1. Fatigue
    2. Chest discomfort
    3. Malaise
C. Typical chest pain in acute MI has the following characteristics:
    1. Intense and unremitting for 30 to 60 minutes
    2. Substernal, and often radiates up to the neck, shoulder, and jaw, and down the left arm
    3. Usually described as a substernal pressure sensation that also may be characterized as squeezing, aching, burning, or even sharp
    4. In some patients, the symptom is epigastric, with a feeling of indigestion or of fullness and gas
    5. Chest pain in a client with known coronary heart disease that is unrelieved by rest or nitroglycerin
D. Prehospital care
    1. For patients with chest pain, prehospital care includes the following:
    2. Intravenous (IV) access, supplemental oxygen if SaO_2 is less than 90%, pulse oximetry
    3. Immediate administration of nonenteric-coated chewable aspirin
    4. Nitroglycerin for active chest pain, given sublingually or by spray
E. Telemetry and prehospital ECG

The ECG is the most important tool in the initial evaluation and triage of patients in whom an acute coronary syndrome (ACS), such as MI, is suspected. It is confirmatory of the diagnosis in approximately 80% of cases. The information in this section is according to the 2020 ESC Guidelines for the Management of ACSs (Collet et al., 2020).

HESI HINT NGN-NCLEX-RN questions on cardiopulmonary resuscitation (CPR) often use critical thinking skills to determine prioritization of actions.
Question: What actions are required for each of the following situations?
- 24-year-old motorcycle accident victim with a ruptured artery of the leg who is pulseless and apneic
- 36-year-old first-time pregnant woman who arrests during labor
- 17-year-old with no pulse or respirations who is trapped in an overturned car that is starting to burn
- 40-year-old businessman who arrests 2 days after a cervical laminectomy

A. Chest pain in MI:
    1. Typical chest pain in acute MI has the following characteristics:
        a. Intense and unremitting for 30 to 60 minutes
        b. Substernal, and often radiates up to the neck, shoulder, and jaw, and down the left arm
    2. Usually described as a substernal pressure sensation that also may be characterized as squeezing, aching, burning, or even sharp
    3. In some patients, the symptom is epigastric, with a feeling of indigestion or of fullness and gas

Cardiopulmonary Resuscitation

The six links in the adult out-of-hospital Chain of Survival are:
- Recognition of cardiac arrest and activation of the emergency response system (calling 9-1-1 in the US)
- Early cardiopulmonary resuscitation (CPR) with an emphasis on chest compressions
- Rapid defibrillation
- Advanced resuscitation by Emergency Medical Services and other healthcare providers
- Post-cardiac arrest care
- Recovery (including additional treatment, observation, rehabilitation, and psychological support)

A strong Chain of Survival can improve chances of survival and recovery for victims of cardiac arrest.

Family presence during CPR benefits outweigh the risks. (Merchant et al., 2020)

HESI HINT The nurse must stay current with the AHA guidelines for basic life support (BLS) by being certified every 2 years, as required. See the AHA website for current CPR guidelines and locate a CPR class.

Major components of BLS consist of immediate recognition of cardiac arrest and activation of the emergency response system, CPR with emphasis on chest compression, and rapid defibrillation if indicated. There are several options for CPR known as Hands-Only CPR, High-Quality CPR, and In-Hospital CPR (Box 3.4).

HESI HINT Initiate CPR with basic life support (BLS) guidelines immediately; then move on to advanced cardiac life support.

PEDIATRIC RESUSCITATION

See "Maternity Nursing" (see Chapter 6) for Newborn Resuscitation.
- Rapid recognition of cardiac arrest, immediate initiation of high-quality chest compressions, and delivery of effective ventilations are critical to improve outcomes from cardiac arrest.
- Lay rescuers should not delay starting cardiopulmonary resuscitation (CPR) in a child with no "signs of life."
- Healthcare providers may consider assessing the presence of a pulse as long as the initiation of CPR is not delayed more than 10 s.
- Palpation for the presence or absence of a pulse is not reliable as the sole determinant of cardiac arrest and the need for chest compressions.
- In infants and children, asphyxia cardiac arrest is more common than cardiac arrest from a primary cardiac event; therefore, effective ventilation is important during resuscitation of children.
- When CPR is initiated, the sequence is compressions-airway-breathing.
- High-quality CPR generates blood flow to vital organs and increases the likelihood of return of spontaneous circulation (ROSC).
- The five main components of high-quality CPR:

1. adequate chest compression depth,
2. optimal chest compression rate,
3. minimizing interruptions in CPR (i.e., maximizing chest compression fraction or the proportion of time that chest compressions are provided for cardiac arrest)
4. allowing full chest recoil between compressions,
5. avoiding excessive ventilation.

- Compressions of inadequate depth and rate, incomplete chest recoil, and high ventilation rates are common during pediatric resuscitation.

From Topjian, A. A., Raymond, T. T., Atkins, D., Chan, M., Duff, J. P., Joyner, et al. (2021). Part 4: Pediatric Basic and Advanced Life Support 2020 American Heart Association Guidelines for Cardiopulmonary Resuscitation and Emergency Cardiovascular Care. *Pediatrics, 147* (Suppl 1), e2020038505D. https://doi.org/10.1542/peds.2020-038505D

For infants, single rescuers (whether lay rescuers or healthcare providers) should compress the sternum with two fingers or two thumbs placed just below the intermammary line.

For infants, the two-thumb—encircling hands technique is recommended when CPR is provided by two rescuers.

If the rescuer cannot physically encircle the victim's chest, compress the chest with two fingers.

For children, it may be reasonable to use either a one- or two-hand technique to perform chest compressions.

For infants, if the rescuer is unable to achieve guideline-recommended depths (at least one-third the anterior-posterior diameter of the chest), it may be reasonable to use the heel of one hand (Topjian et al., 2021).

The American Heart Association algorithms for CPR for adult and pediatric resuscitation can be downloaded from: https://cpr.heart.org/en/resuscitation-science/cpr-and-ecc-guidelines/algorithms

HESI HINT The pediatric cardiac arrest algorithm known as the reversible causes include the four "H's": **hypoxia**, **hypovolemia**, **hyperkalemia, hypokalemia, other electrolyte disturbances**, **and the four "Ts": T**ension pneumothorax, cardiac tamponade, drug toxicity and therapeutics, thromboembolism, and other outflow obstructions.

HESI HINT

- For infants and children provide chest compressions that depress the chest at least 1/3 of the anterior posterior diameter of the chest, use chest compression rate of ~100 to 120/min for infants and children.
- Single rescuers compression to ventilation rate 30:2; two rescuers 15:2

MANAGEMENT OF FOREIGN BODY AIRWAY OBSTRUCTION

Adults and Children

Foreign-body airway obstruction (FBAO), or choking, is an alarming and dramatic emergency.

To confirm a complete FBAO, ask the victim "Are you choking?" If the victim cannot speak or can only make weak, high-pitched sounds, perform abdominal thrust until the object is expelled or the victim becomes unresponsive.

A. Stand behind the victim
B. Make a fist with one hand
C. Place your fist on the victim's abdomen, slightly above the navel and well below the breastbone
D. Grasp your fist with your other hand
E. Deliver quick upward thrusts into the victim's abdomen (Heimlich maneuver)

BOX 3.4 Hands-Only CPR, High-Quality CPR, and In-Hospital CPR

Hands-Only CPR

Consists of two easy steps:

1. Call 9-1-1 (or send someone to do that)
2. Push hard and fast in the center of the chest

The focus is on early, high-quality chest compressions. The healthcare provider includes chest compressions before rescue breaths. "C-A-B" (Chest Compression, Airway, and Breathing) is now used for adults and children, whereas steps for the newborns remain "A-B-C" (Airway, Breathing, and Circulation).

Automated external defibrillators (AEDs) can greatly increase a cardiac arrest victim's chances of survival. To minimize the time to defibrillation for cardiac arrest victims, deployment of AEDs should not be limited to only trained people (although training is still recommended).

High-Quality CPR

High-quality CPR should be performed by anyone—including bystanders. There are five critical components:

1. Minimize interruptions in chest compressions
2. Provide compressions of adequate rate and depth
3. Avoid leaning on the victim between compressions
4. Ensure proper hand placement
5. Avoid excessive ventilation

In-Hospital Cardiac Arrest

1. For healthcare providers and those trained: conventional CPR using chest compressions and mouth-to-mouth breathing at a ratio of 30:2 compressions-to-breaths. In adult victims of cardiac arrest, it is reasonable for rescuers to perform chest compressions at a rate of 100 to 120/min and to a depth of at least 2 inches (5 cm) for an average adult, while avoiding excessive chest compression depths (greater than 2.4 inches [6 cm]).

CPR, Cardiopulmonary resuscitation.
Modified from What Is CPR. American Heart Association. Available at: https://cpr.heart.org/en/resources/what-is-cpr.

F. Deliver thrusts until the object is expelled or the victim becomes unresponsive. If a choking adult becomes unresponsive while you are doing abdominal thrust, you should ease the victim to the floor and send someone to activate the emergency response system.
G. When a choking victim becomes unresponsive, you begin the steps of CPR, starting with compressions.
H. The only difference is that each time you open the airway, look for the obstructing object before giving each breath.
I. Remove the object if you see it.
J. Chest thrust should be used in obese or pregnant patients.

Infants and Children

A. FBAO develops when an object becomes lodged in the airway and blocks the movement of air into and out of the lungs.
B. If the blockage is severe or complete, the victim will be unable to breathe and oxygenate blood supplying the brain, heart, and other vital organs with adequate oxygen to function normally.
C. If the blockage is not relieved, the victim will become unresponsive and can die.
D. Signs of severe or complete FBAO in infants and children include sudden onset of respiratory distress associated with weak or silent cough/cry, inability to speak, stridor or increasing respiratory difficulty.
E. These signs and symptoms of airway obstruction may also be caused by infections and croup.
F. Typically with FBAO these signs and symptoms will develop suddenly with no other signs of illness or infection.
G. If you suspect a severe (victim not passing air or ineffective cough/cry) or complete FBAO, follow these steps:
H. For a Responsive Infant
   1. Pick the infant up from a supine (lying face up) position by lifting the legs with one hand and sliding the other hand all the way to the infant's head. Once this is done, "sandwich" the infant by placing the opposite arm and hand on the infant's stomach and face, grasping the infant's facial cheeks.
   2. Supporting the infant—place them face down on your thigh—make sure the head is lower than the body.
   3. Deliver five back slaps with the heel of your free hand between the shoulder blades. "Sandwich" the infant between your arms once again and turn the infant over so that the infant is lying on their back along your arm which should be placed on your thigh for support.
   4. Deliver five chest thrusts in the same location used for CPR compressions. Alternate five back slaps and five chest thrusts until the object is expelled or the infant becomes unresponsive.
   5. If unresponsive, begin the steps of CPR—in this sequence—every time before you administer a breath—check the airway for foreign objects.
   6. For a Responsive Child—The steps for FBAO in a child are exactly the same, as you would use with an adult FBAO victim.
   7. Please review previous information.

REVIEW OF RESUSCITATION

1. What is the first priority when an adult with an unwitnessed cardiac arrest is found?
2. Define *myocardial infarction.*
3. What criteria should alert a client with known angina who takes nitroglycerin tablets sublingually to call EMS? Delete
4. After calling out for help and asking someone to dial for emergency services, what is the next action in CPR?
5. True or false? In feeling for presence of a carotid pulse, no more than 5 seconds should be used.
6. During one-rescuer CPR, what is the ratio of compressions to ventilations for an adult? During one-rescuer CPR, what is the ratio of compressions to ventilations for a child?
7. What is the first drug most likely to be used for an in-hospital cardiac arrest?
8. A client in cardiac arrest is noted on bedside monitor to be in pulseless ventricular tachycardia. What is the first action that should be taken?
9. How would the nurse assess the adequacy of compressions during CPR? How would the nurse assess the adequacy of ventilations during CPR?
10. If a person is choking, when should the rescuer intervene?
11. One should never make blind sweeps into the mouth of a choking child or infant. Why?

See Answer Key at the end of this text for suggested responses.

FLUID AND ELECTROLYTE BALANCE

Electrolytes play a vital role in maintaining homeostasis within the body.

- Electrolytes help to regulate myocardial and neurological functions, fluid balance, oxygen delivery, acid—base balance, and much more.
- The most serious electrolyte disturbances involve abnormalities in the levels of sodium, potassium, and/or calcium.
- Kidneys work to keep the electrolyte concentrations in the blood constant despite changes in the body.
- Homeostasis: The ability of a system or living organism to adjust its internal environment to maintain a stable equilibrium, such as the ability of warm-blooded animals to maintain a constant temperature.
- Electrolyte: Any of the various ions (such as sodium or chloride) that regulate the electric charge on cells and the flow of water across their membranes.
- Sodium: A chemical element with symbol Na (from Latin: natrium) and atomic number 11. It is a soft, silvery white, highly reactive metal and is a member of the alkali metals.

Importance of Electrolyte Balance

Electrolytes maintain voltages across their cell membranes, especially those of the nerves, heart, and muscle and to carry electrical impulses across nerve impulses, muscle contractions, and to other cells.

Electrolyte imbalances can develop from dehydration and over-hydration. The most common cause of electrolyte disturbances is renal failure. The most serious electrolyte disturbances involve abnormalities in the levels of sodium, potassium, and/or calcium.

Other electrolyte imbalances are less common, and often occur in conjunction with major electrolyte changes. Chronic laxative abuse or severe diarrhea or vomiting (gastroenteritis) can lead to electrolyte disturbances combined with dehydration. People suffering from bulimia or anorexia nervosa are especially at high risk for an electrolyte imbalance.

Kidneys work to keep the electrolyte concentrations in blood constant despite changes in your body. For example, during heavy exercise electrolytes are lost through sweating, particularly sodium and potassium, and sweating can increase the need for electrolyte (salt) replacement. It is necessary to replace these electrolytes to keep their concentrations in the body fluids constant.

Dehydration

There are three types of dehydration:

1. Hypotonic or hyponatremic (primarily a loss of electrolytes, sodium in particular).
2. Hypertonic or hypernatremic (primarily a loss of water).
3. Isotonic or isonatremic (an equal loss of water and electrolytes).
4. Most common type of dehydration is isotonic (isonatremic) dehydration, which effectively equates with hypovolemia; but the distinction of isotonic from hypotonic or hypertonic dehydration may be important when treating people with dehydration.
5. Physiologically, dehydration is both loss of water and solutes (mainly sodium) and lost in roughly equal quantities since they exist in blood plasma.
6. In hypotonic dehydration, intravascular water shifts to the extravascular space and exaggerates the intravascular volume depletion for a given amount of total body water loss.
7. Neurological complications can occur in hypotonic and hypertonic states and lead to seizures, and the latter can lead to osmotic cerebral edema upon rapid rehydration.
8. In more severe cases, the correction of a dehydrated state is accomplished by the replenishment of necessary water and electrolytes (through oral rehydration therapy or fluid replacement by IV therapy).
9. As oral rehydration is less painful, less invasive, less expensive, and easier to provide, it is the treatment of choice for mild dehydration.

Solutions used for IV rehydration must be isotonic or hypotonic. Fig. 3.3 illustrates the mechanism for the transportation of water and electrolytes across the epithelial cells in the secretory glands.

1. Review Table 3.8.

HESI HINT Most common type of dehydration is isotonic (isonatremic) dehydration, which effectively equates with hypovolemia; but the distinction of isotonic from hypotonic or hypertonic dehydration may be important when treating people with dehydration.

Physiologically, dehydration is both loss of water and solutes (mainly sodium) usually lost in roughly equal quantities as to how they exist in blood plasma.

HESI HINT

1. Hypotonic or hyponatremic (primarily a loss of electrolytes, sodium in particular).
2. Hypertonic or hypernatremic (primarily a loss of water).
3. Isotonic or isonatremic (an equal loss of water and electrolytes).

Fluid Volume Deficit: Dehydration

- *Fluid volume deficit* (FVD) or hypovolemia (may be acute or chronic): fluid output exceeds the fluid intake; the body loses both water and electrolytes from the ECF in similar proportions.
- Common sources of fluid loss are the gastrointestinal tract, polyuria, and increased perspiration.
- Risk factors for FVD: vomiting, diarrhea, GI suctioning, sweating, decreased intake, nausea, inability to gain access to fluids, adrenal insufficiency, osmotic diuresis, hemorrhage, coma, third-space fluid shifts, burns, ascites, and liver dysfunction
- Appropriate management is vital to prevent potentially life-threatening hypovolemic shock.
- Elderly patients are more likely to develop fluid imbalances.
- The goals of management are to treat the underlying disorder and return the extracellular fluid compartment to normal, to restore fluid volume, and to correct any electrolyte imbalances.

Causes of Fluid Volume Deficit

- Abnormal losses through the skin, GI tract, or kidneys.
- Decrease in intake of fluid (e.g., inability to intake fluid due to oral trauma)
- Bleeding
- Movement of fluid into third space
- Diarrhea
- Diuresis
- Abnormal drainage
- Inadequate fluid intake
- Increased metabolic rate (e.g., fever, infection)

Organ Function

A. Kidneys

1. Main function of the kidneys is to filter blood and adjust the amount and composition of fluids in the body. The total blood volume is determined by a client's gender, height, and weight. The average healthy adult has approximately 5.2 to 6 L of circulating blood in the body.
2. As a result of this filtration process, the kidney selectively maintains and excretes body fluids, producing approximately 1 to 2 L of urine (30 mL/h).

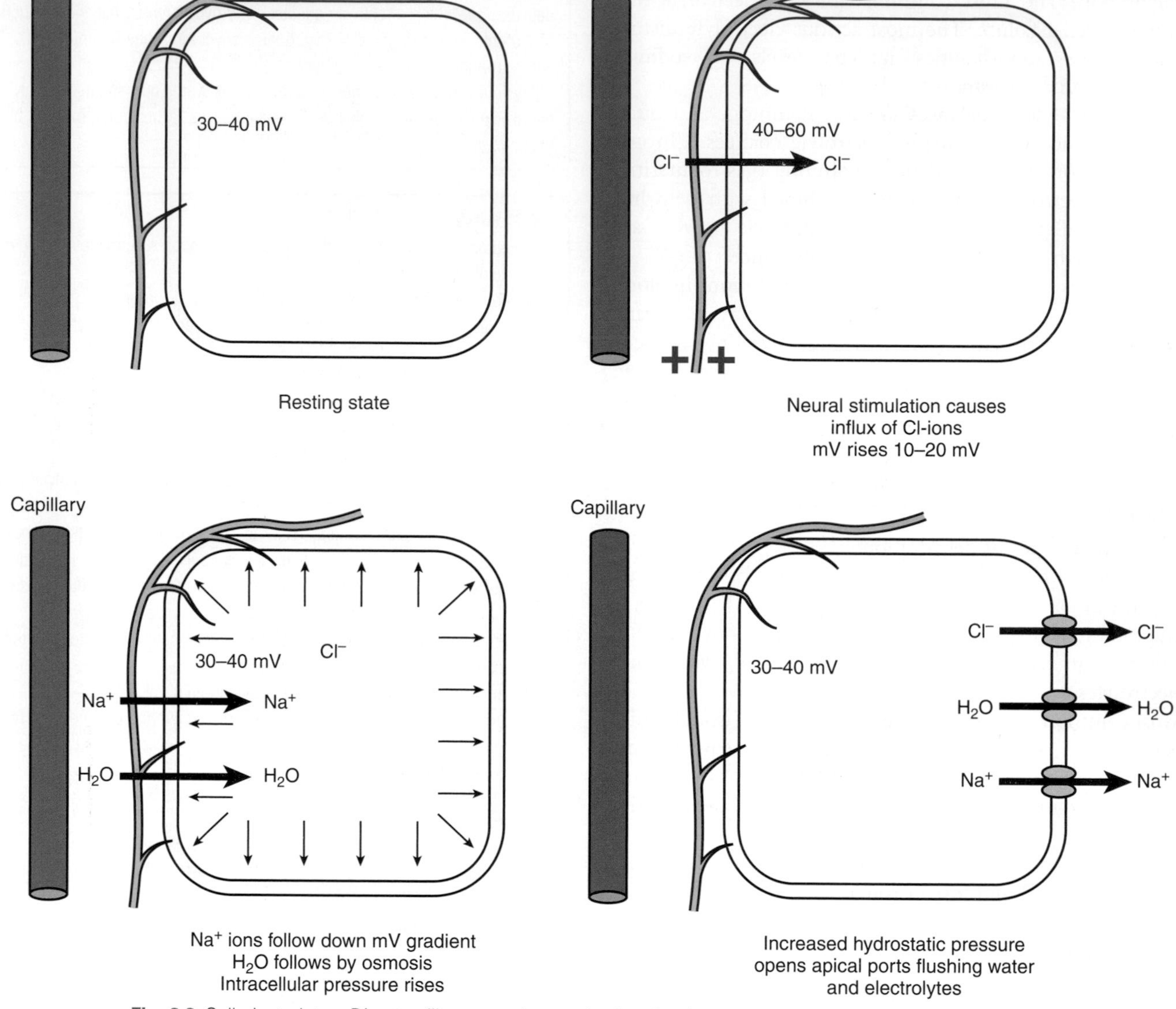

Fig. 3.3 Cell electrolytes: Diagram illustrates the mechanism for the transportation of water and electrolytes across the epithelial cells in the secretory glands. (From http://commons.wikimedia.org/wiki/File:Cell_electrolytes.png. License: CC BY: Attribution.)

3. Regulates sodium and potassium levels and maintains the pH level by excreting or maintaining hydrogen ions and bicarbonate.
4. Excretes metabolic wastes and toxic substances.
5. The kidneys are also responsible for manufacturing the hormone erythropoietin (EPO) (Fig. 3.4).

B. Lungs
1. Regulate CO_2 concentration as a result of O_2 and CO_2 gas exchange at the alveolar capillary beds, thus influencing the acid-base balance.
2. Water loss via lung is affected by the external temperature and humidity.

At 35°C and humidity at 75%, respectively, the loss of water via the lung during inspiration and expiration is ~7 mL/h. When the parameters change, for example, this can increase or decrease the lung excretion can change to minus 10°C and 25% lung excretion of H(2)O increases up to 20 mL/h. (Zieliński & Przybylski, 2012)

C. Heart
1. Pumps blood with sufficient force to perfuse the kidneys, allowing the kidneys to work effectively.
2. Potassium, sodium, and calcium electrolyte levels are crucial in maintaining adequate electrical conductivity to help with efficient myocardial pumping action.

D. Adrenal glands
1. Secretes aldosterone, when the body's BP becomes low, resulting in sodium retention (leading to water

TABLE 3.8 Fluid Volume

Variable	Deficit	Excess
Description	• Occurs when the body loses water and electrolytes isotonically—i.e., in the same proportion as exists in the normal body fluid • Serum electrolyte levels remain normal • Dehydration: state in which the body loses water and serum sodium levels increase	• Occurs when the body retains water and electrolytes isotonically • Water intoxication: state in which the body retains water and serum sodium levels decrease
Causes	• Vomiting • Diarrhea • Gastrointestinal suctioning • Sweating • Inadequate fluid intake • Massive edema, as in initial stage of major burns • Ascites • Older adults forgetting to drink	• Heart failure (HF) • Renal failure • Cirrhosis, liver failure • Excessive ingestion of table salt • Over-hydration with sodium-containing fluid • Poorly controlled intravenous (IV) therapy, especially in young and old clients
Symptoms	• Weight loss (1 L of fluid weight loss or gain is approximately equal to 2.2 pounds or 1 kg) • Decreased skin turgor • Oliguria (concentrated urine) • Dry and sticky mucous membranes • Postural hypotension or weak, rapid pulse	• Peripheral edema • Increased bounding pulse • Elevated BP • Distended neck and hand veins • Dyspnea; moist crackles heard when lungs auscultated • Attention loss, confusion, aphasia • Altered level of consciousness
Laboratory findings	• Elevated blood urea nitrogen (BUN) and creatinine • Increased serum osmolarity • Elevated hemoglobin and hematocrit	• Decreased BUN • Decreased hemoglobin and hematocrit • Decreased serum osmolality • Decreased urine osmolality and specific gravity
Treatment and nursing care	• Strict I&O • Replacement of fluids isotonically, preferably orally • Water is a hypotonic fluid. • If intravenous hydration is needed, isotonic fluids are used.	• Diuretics • Fluid restriction • Strict I&O • Sodium-restricted diet • Weighed daily • Serum K+ monitored

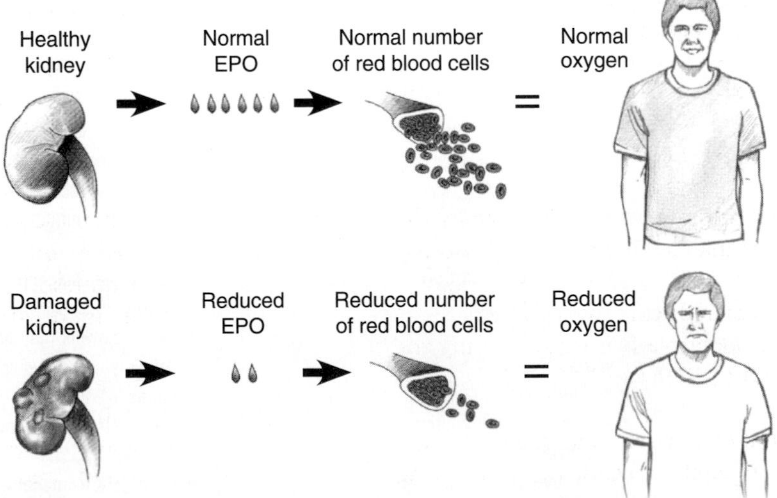

Fig. 3.4 Top: Kidney → normal EPO → normal number RBCs → normal O_2. *Bottom*: Damaged kidney → reduced EPO → fewer RBCs → reduced O_2. *EPO,* Erythropoietin; *RBC,* red blood cell. (From Brugnara, C., & Eckardt, K. U. [2011]. Hematologic aspects of kidney disease. In M. W. Taal [Ed.], *Brenner and Rector's: The kidney* [9th ed., pp. 2081–2120]. St. Louis: Saunders. National Kidney and Urologic Diseases Information Clearinghouse from National Institute of Diabetes and Digestive and Kidney Diseases.)

retention), thereby increasing BP and potassium excretion to maintain homeostasis.

E. Parathyroid glands
   1. Regulates calcium and phosphorus balance levels in blood by increasing or decreasing the manufacture of parathyroid hormone, which influences transference of calcium and phosphorous from the bones.

F. Pituitary gland
   1. Secretes antidiuretic hormone (ADH), which causes the body to retain water by signaling the kidneys to increase the water absorption when filtering the blood.

Electrolyte Imbalance

Clinical Assessment

Refer to Table 3.9.

TABLE 3.9 Electrolyte Imbalances

Abnormalities and Common Causes	Signs and Symptoms	Treatment
Hyponatremia (↓ Na) • Diuretics • GI fluid loss • Hypotonic tube feeding • D5W or hypotonic IV fluids • Diaphoresis	• Anorexia, nausea, vomiting • Weakness • Lethargy • Confusion • Muscle cramps, twitching • Seizures • Na <135 mEq/L	• Restrict fluids (safer). • If IV saline solutions prescribed, administer very slowly; use isotonic saline if fluid restriction not effective.
Hypernatremia (↑ Na) • Water deprivation • Hypertonic tube feeding • Diabetes insipidus • Heatstroke • Hyperventilation • Watery diarrhea • Renal failure • Cushing syndrome	• Thirst • Hyperpyrexia • Sticky mucous membranes • Dry mouth • Hallucinations • Lethargy • Irritability • Seizures • Na >145 mEq/L	• Restrict sodium (Na) in the diet. • Beware of hidden Na in foods and medications. • Increase water intake.
Hypokalemia (↓ K) • Diuretics • Diarrhea • Vomiting • Gastric suction • Steroid administration • Hyperaldosteronism • Amphotericin B • Bulimia • Cushing syndrome	• Fatigue • Anorexia • Nausea, vomiting • Muscle weakness • Decreased GI motility • Dysrhythmias • Paresthesia • Flat T waves on ECG • K <3.5 mEq/L	• Administer potassium (K) supplements orally or IV. • Oral forms of K are unpleasant tasting and are irritating to the GI tract (do not give on empty stomach; dilute). • Never give IV bolus; must be well diluted. • Assess renal status (i.e., urinary output) before administering. • Encourage foods high in K (e.g., bananas, oranges, cantaloupes, avocados, spinach, potatoes).
Hyperkalemia (↑ K) • Hemolyzed serum sample produces pseudohyperkalemia • Oliguria • Acidosis • Renal failure • Addison disease • Multiple blood transfusions	• Muscle weakness • Bradycardia • Dysrhythmias • Flaccid paralysis • Intestinal colic • Tall T waves on ECG • K >5.0 mEq/L	• Eliminate parenteral K from IV infusions and medications. • Administer 50% glucose with regular insulin. • Administer cation exchange resin (Kayexalate). • Monitor ECG. • Administer calcium (Ca) gluconate to protect the heart. • IV loop diuretics may be prescribed. • Renal dialysis may be required.
Hypocalcemia (↓ Ca) • Renal failure • Hypoparathyroidism • Malabsorption • Pancreatitis • Alkalosis	• Diarrhea • Numbness • Tingling of extremities • Convulsions • Positive Trousseau sign • Positive sign • Ca <8.5 mEq/L • At risk for tetany	• Administer Ca supplements orally 30 min before meals. • Administer Ca IV slowly; infiltration can cause tissue necrosis. • Increase Ca intake (e.g., dairy products, greens).

Continued

Hypercalcemia (↑ Ca) • Hyperparathyroidism • Malignant bone disease • Prolonged immobilization • Excess Ca supplementation	• Muscle weakness • Constipation • Anorexia • Nausea, vomiting • Polyuria • Polydipsia • Neurosis • Dysrhythmias • Ca >10.5 mEq/L	• Eliminate parenteral Ca. • Administer agents such as calcitonin to reduce Ca. • Avoid CA-based antacids. • Renal dialysis may be required.
Hypomagnesemia (↓ Mg) • Alcoholism • Malabsorption • Diabetic ketoacidosis • Prolonged gastric suction • Diuretics	• Anorexia, distention • Neuromuscular irritability • Depression • Disorientation • Mg <1.5 mEq/L	• Administer MgSO4 IV. • Encourage foods high in magnesium (Mg; e.g., meats, nuts, legumes, fish, and vegetables).
Hypermagnesemia (↑Mg) • Renal failure • Adrenal insufficiency • Excess replacement	• Flushing • Hypotension • Drowsiness, lethargy • Hypoactive reflexes • Depressed respirations • Bradycardia • Mg >2.5 mEq/L	• Avoid Mg-based antacids and laxatives. • Restrict dietary intake of foods high in Mg.
Hypophosphatemia (↓ pH) • Refeeding after starvation • Alcohol withdrawal • Diabetic ketoacidosis • Respiratory alkalosis	• Paresthesias • Muscle weakness • Muscle pain • Mental changes • Cardiomyopathy • Respiratory failure • pH <2.0 mEq/L	• Correct underlying cause. • Administer oral replacement of phosphates with vitamin D.
Hyperphosphatemia (↑ pH) • Renal failure • Excess intake of phosphorus	• Short-term: tetany symptoms • Long-term: phosphorus precipitation in nonosseous sites • pH >4.5 mEq/L	• Administer aluminum hydroxide with meals to bind phosphorus. • Dialysis may be required if renal failure is underlying cause.

ECG, Electrocardiogram; *GI*, gastrointestinal; *IV*, intravenous.

Clinical Judgment Measures

Refer to Table 3.9.

> **HESI HINT** Potassium imbalances are potentially life threatening and must be corrected immediately. A low magnesium level often accompanies a low potassium, especially with the use of diuretics. Magnesium must be corrected to normalize potassium.

Intravenous Therapy

Description: IV solutions are used to supply electrolytes, nutrients, and water (Table 3.10).

Administration of IV Therapy

A. The purpose and duration of the IV therapy are determined by the underlying condition/situation. This also determines the type of equipment, such as vascular access device, including IV tubing and the size of the catheter.
B. Types of vascular devices for IV administration
   1. Peripheral
   2. Central
C. Gloves must be worn during venipunctures and when discontinuing an IV line.
D. Assess the IV and insertion site frequently (minimum of every 2 hours) for the prescribed rate of infusion and for patency.
E. Intermittent IV therapy may be given through a saline lock; flushing per facility policy.
F. IV tubing and dressing should be changed according to facility policy.
G. When the IV catheter is discontinued, apply pressure to the site for 1 to 3 minutes for peripheral lines and 5 to 10 minutes for central lines after the catheter is removed (central lines are only removed by provider orders, and nurses must be educated on removal to prevent air embolism), and inspect the tip of the catheter to ensure it is intact; then document.

> **HESI HINT** For central line removal (central lines are only removed by provider orders and nurses must be educated on removal to prevent air embolism), inspect the tip of the catheter to ensure it is intact; then document.

TABLE 3.10 **Types of IV Solutions**

Isotonic	Hypotonic	Hypertonic

• Have an osmolality close to the extracellular fluid (ECF).
• Do not cause red blood cells to swell or shrink
• Indicated for intravascular dehydration
• Isotonic solutions
• → Normal saline (0.9% NS)
• → Lactated Ringer's solution (LR)
• → 5% dextrose in water (D5W is on the low end of isotonic; some sources classify it as hypotonic)
• Used to treat intravascular dehydration (not enough fluid in vascular system)
• Common type of dehydration
• Examples: dehydration caused by running, labor, fever, etc.
	• Have an osmolality lower than the ECF.
	• Cause fluid to move from ECF to intracellular fluid (ICF).
	• Indicated for cellular dehydration.
	• Used in the management of the patient who is both volume depleted and hyperosmolar (e.g., in cases of hypernatremia or hyperglycemia).
	• Hypotonic solutions
	  • → 0.5% normal saline (HNS or 0.45% NS)
	  • → 2.5% dextrose in 0.45% saline ($D_{2.5}$ 45% NS)
	  • → 0.33 NaCl allows kidneys to retain needed amounts water
	  • → 0.225% NaCl most hypotonic fluid available
	  • → 2.5 dextrose in water (D2.5W) to treat dehydration and decrease sodium and potassium levels
	• Used to treat intracellular dehydration (cells have too many osmoles, need to drive fluid into the cells).
	• Not a common occurrence.
	• Examples: dehydration caused by prolonged dehydration (may also see in clients who are on total parenteral nutrition for prolonged periods)
		• Have an osmolality higher than the ECF.
		• Indicated for intravascular dehydration with interstitial or cellular over-hydration.
		• To be used with extreme caution.
		• High concentrations of dextrose are given for caloric replacement such as intravenous (IV) hyperalimentation into a central vein for rapid dilution.
		• Hypertonic saline solutions are available but used only when serum osmolality is dangerously low.
		• Hypertonic solutions
		• → 5% dextrose in lactated Ringer's (D5LR)
		• → 5% dextrose in 0.45% saline
		• → 5% dextrose in 0.9% saline (D5NS)
		• → 3% Na
		• → 5% NaCl
		• → 10% dextrose in water (D10W)
		• → 20% dextrose in water (20W) acts as osmotic diuretic
		• → 50% dextrose in water (50% DW)
		• Used to treat intravascular dehydration with cellular or interstitial over-hydration.
		• Examples: dehydration resulting from surgery; blood loss causes intravascular dehydration, but the tissue cuts inflame and pull fluid into the area, causing interstitial over-hydration; may also see with ascites and third-spacing

Flow Rate Calculation

Several formulas exist for calculating IV flow rates.
Infusion pumps are used when measurement of exact flow is necessary.
Using the following steps for IV calculation will ensure proper calculation:

1. mL/h: Total mL fluid to be given/Total hours to be administered = mL/h (rate for IV infusions on a pump)
2. gtts/min: Total mL fluid to be given/Total minutes to be administered × gtts/mL = gtts/min (rate for IV infusions by gravity)

Complications Associated With IV Administration

Occlusion/catheter damage (Table 3.11)

A. Infection/phlebitis (Table 3.12)

> **HESI HINT** If an IV catheter is suspected as the causative factor of sepsis, the catheter should be removed and blood cultures drawn and sent to the laboratory.

B. Dislodgment/migration/incorrect placement (Table 3.13)

C. Skin erosion/hematomas/scar tissue formation over port/infiltration/extravasation (Table 3.14)

D. Pneumothorax/hemothorax/air emboli/hydrothorax (Table 3.15)

> **HESI HINT** Flushing a saline lock: Attach NS prefilled Luer **lock** syringe by twisting the syringe to the positive pressure cap. Inject 3 to 5 mL of solution using turbulent stop-start technique. **Flush** until visibly clear. Do not bottom out syringe (leave 0.2 to 0.5 mL in the syringe).

Acid–Base Balance

Description: An acid–base balance must be maintained in the body because alterations can result in alkalosis or acidosis.

A. Maintaining the acid–base balance is imperative and involves three systems:
   1. Chemical buffer system
   2. Kidneys
   3. Lungs

B. Acid–base balance is determined by the hydrogen ion concentration in body fluids.
   1. Normal range is 7.35 to 7.45 expressed as the pH (Fig. 3.5).
   2. A pH level below 7.35 indicates acidosis.
   3. A pH level above 7.45 indicates alkalosis.
   4. Measurement is made by examining ABGs (Table 3.16).

Chemical Buffer System

Chemical buffers act quickly to prevent major changes in body fluid pH by removing or releasing hydrogen ions. The buffer systems in the human body are extremely efficient, and

TABLE 3.11 **Occlusion/Catheter Damage**

Assess for:	Peripheral	Central	Interventions
Leaks around the insertion site	X	X	Discontinue infusion; either restart peripheral intravenous (IV) or notify physician about central line.
Pinholes, leaks, and tears		X	Discontinue infusion; then notify physician about central line.
Blood return	X	X	Gently flush and attempt to draw back blood.
Inability to infuse fluid	X	X	Starting from the insertion site, double-check for kinks in tubing or catheter.
Needleless adapter placement, if a port or IV catheter tip lodged against the venous wall	X	X	Reposition the client's extremity for peripheral catheter; for central catheter, reposition the client.
Pain in shoulder, neck, or arm		X	Discontinue the infusion and notify physician about central line.
Neck or shoulder edema		X	Discontinue the infusion and notify physician about central line.
Suture damage		X	Secure with a sterile transparent, self-adhesive dressing and notify physician.
			Do not use syringes less than a 10 mL to irrigate because the PSI would be too high and possibly damage the catheter.
			Do not irrigate forcefully.

TABLE 3.12 **Infection/Phlebitis**

Assess for:	Peripheral	Central	Interventions
Insertion site for redness, drainage, edema, or tenderness	X	X	Peripheral IVs → Use aseptic and antiseptic techniques when starting an IV line and when caring for IV site.
			Central IVs → Use sterile technique when inserting and changing central dressings.
Temperature	X	X	Monitor temperature for fever.
Laboratory work		X	Monitor white blood cell (WBC) with differential count/for central lines twice weekly.
IV fluids		X	Ensure parental IV fluids bags are changed out every 24 h or according to institution's policy.
IV tubing	X	X	Change IV tubing according to institution's policy.
IV dressings	X	X	Change IV dressings according to institution's policy; avoid getting dressing wet and/or soiled.

TABLE 3.13 **Dislodgement/Migration/Incorrect Placement**

Assessment:	Site: Peripheral	Site: Central	Usual Interventions
Length of catheter	X	X	Provide tubing long enough for client movement.
Edema, drainage, and coiling of catheter	X	X	Anchor the catheter to the client.
Neck distention or distended neck veins	X	X	Measure and record length of catheter.
Client complaints of gurgling sounds	X	X	Discontinue the infusion and notify physician about probable dislodged intravenous (IV) line.
Change in patency of catheter	X	X	
Chest radiograph	X	X	
Cardiac dysrhythmias	X	X	
Hypotension			

TABLE 3.14 **Skin Erosion/Hematomas/Scar Tissue Formation Over Port/Infiltration/ Extravasation**

Assess for:	Peripheral	Central	Interventions
Loss of tissue or separation at exit site	X	X	Dilute medications adequately.
Drainage at exit site	X	X	Follow institutional protocol for administration of vesicant drugs.
Erythema and edema at exit site	X	X	Change intravenous (IV) line within the time frame outlined in institutional protocol.
Spongy feeling at exit site	X	X	
Labored breathing	X	X	Provide gentle skin care at exit/insertion site.
Complaints of pain	X	X	Avoid selecting site over a joint.
			Anchor the catheter well.

TABLE 3.15 Pneumothorax/Hemothorax/Air Emboli/Hydrothorax

Assess for:	Peripheral	Central	Interventions
Subcutaneous emphysema	X	X	Use clot filters when infusing blood and blood products.
Chest pain	X	X	Avoid using veins in the lower extremities.
Dyspnea and hypoxia	X	X	Prevent fluid containers from becoming empty.
Tachycardia	X	X	Check valves and micropore filters on vented Y-type infusions or piggyback infusions, which allow solutions to run simultaneously. Air may be introduced into the line if the containers become empty.
Hypotension	X	X	
Confusion	X	X	
Nausea	X	X	*If air embolism is suspected, place patient in left lateral Trendelenburg position.*

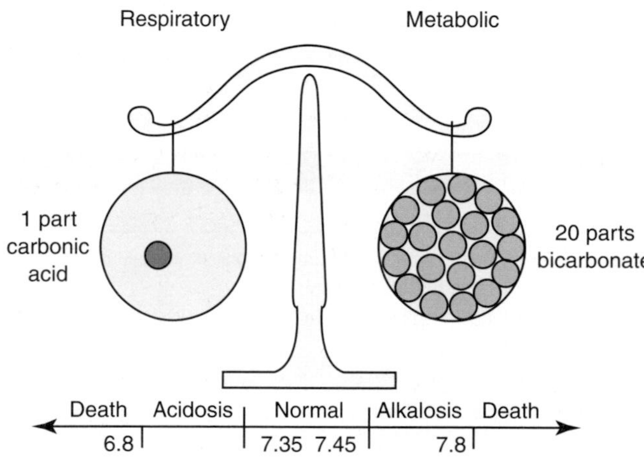

Fig. 3.5 **Relationship of Sodium Bicarbonate to Carbonic Acid.** (From Potter, P. A., & Perry, A. G. [2009]. *Fundamentals of nursing* [7th ed.]. St. Louis: Mosby.)

TABLE 3.16 Arterial Blood Gas Comparisons

Acid–Base Conditions	pH	PCO_2 (mm Hg)	HCO_3 (mEq/L)
Normal	7.35–7.45	35–45	21–28
Respiratory acidosis	↓	↑	Normal
Respiratory alkalosis	↑	↓	Normal
Metabolic acidosis	↓	Normal	↓
Metabolic alkalosis	↑	Normal	↑

different systems work at different rates taking seconds for the chemical buffers in the blood to make adjustments to pH.

The respiratory tract can adjust the blood pH upward in minutes by exhaling CO_2 from the body.

The renal system can also adjust blood pH through the excretion of hydrogen ions (H^+) and the conservation of bicarbonate, but this process takes hours to days to have an effect.

The buffer systems functioning in blood plasma include plasma proteins, phosphate, and bicarbonate and carbonic acid buffers.

The kidneys help control acid–base balance by excreting hydrogen ions and generating bicarbonate that helps maintain blood plasma pH within a normal range. Protein buffer systems work predominantly inside cells.

A. The main chemical buffer is the bicarbonate–carbonic acid (HCO_3-H_2CO_3) system.

B. The bicarbonate-carbonic acid buffer works in a fashion similar to phosphate buffers. The bicarbonate is regulated in the blood by sodium, as are the phosphate ions. When sodium bicarbonate ($NaHCO_3$) comes into contact with a strong acid, such as HCl, carbonic acid (H_2CO_3), which is a weak acid, and NaCl are formed. When carbonic acid comes into contact with a strong base, such as NaOH, bicarbonate and water are formed.

$$NaHCO_3 + HCl \rightarrow H_2CO_3 + NaCl$$
$$\text{(Sodium bicarbonate)} + \text{(strong acid)} \rightarrow \text{(weak acid)} + \text{(salt)}$$
$$H_2CO_3 + NaOH \rightarrow HCO_{3-} + H_2O$$
$$\text{(weak acid)} + \text{(strong base)} \rightarrow \text{(bicarbonate)} + \text{(water)}$$

1. With 20 times more bicarbonate than carbonic acid, this capture system is most efficient at buffering changes that would make the blood more acidic. This is useful because most of the body's metabolic wastes, such as lactic acid and ketones, are acids. Carbonic acid levels in the blood are controlled by the expiration of CO_2 through the lungs.
2. Excess CO_2 in the body alters the ratio and creates an imbalance. Other chemical buffers involve:
   a. Phosphate
   b. Protein
   c. Hemoglobin
   d. Plasma

Lungs

A. Control CO_2 content through respirations (carbonic acid content).

B. Control, to a small extent, water balance ($CO_2 + H_2O = H_2CO_3$).

C. Release excess CO_2 by increasing respiratory rate.

D. Retain CO_2 by decreasing respiratory rate.

Kidneys

A. Regulate bicarbonate levels by retaining and reabsorbing bicarbonate as needed.
B. Provide a very slow compensatory mechanism (can require hours or days).
C. Cannot help with compensation when metabolic acidosis is created by renal failure.

DETERMINING ACID–BASE DISORDERS

A. In uncompensated acid-base disturbances:
B. Arrows are used to indicate whether the pH, PCO_2, or HCO_3 is high (↑), low (↓), or within normal limits (WNL) (← →).
C. When pH is high (↑), alkalosis is present.
D. In respiratory disorders, the HCO_3 is normal, and the arrows for pH and Pco_2 point in opposite directions. The tables should demonstrate the arrows.
E. In metabolic disorders, the PCO_2 is normal, and the arrows for pH and HCO_3 point in the same direction or are equal (Table 3.17).
F. The body will begin to compensate in acid–base disorders to bring the pH back within the normal range of 7.35 to 7.45 (Tables 3.18 and 3.19).
G. Example: for a client with a pH of 7.29 (↓), a PCO_2 of 50 (↑), and an HCO_3 of 28 (← →):
   1. Determine the pH: acidosis.
   2. Determine the PCO_2: respiratory.
   3. Determine HCO_3: not metabolic.
   4. Respiratory acidosis is the disorder (Table 3.20).

TABLE 3.17 Analysis of Arterial Blood Gases

Component	Description	Values
pH	• Measures hydrogen ion (H+) concentration • ↑ in ions (acidosis) reflects in pH • ↓ in ions (alkalosis) reflects in pH	• 7.35–7.45 • <7.35 • >7.45
Pco_2	• Partial pressure of CO_2 in arteries • Respiratory component of acid-base regulation • Hypercapnia/hypoventilation (respiratory acidosis) • Hypocapnia/hyperventilation (respiratory alkalosis)	• 35–45 mm Hg • >45 mm Hg • <35 mm Hg
HCO_3	• Measures serum bicarbonate • May reflect primary metabolic disorder or compensatory mechanism to respiratory acidosis • Metabolic acidosis • Metabolic alkalosis	• Normal 21–28 mEq/L • <21 mEq/L • >28 mEq/L

TABLE 3.18 Determining Respiratory vs. Metabolic and Acidosis vs. Alkalosis

	(7.35–7.45)	(35–45 mm Hg)	(21–28 mEq/L)
R	(+) pH	(–) $PaCO_2$	Alkalosis
O	(–) pH	(+) $PaCO_2$	Acidosis
M	(+) pH	(+) HCO_3	Alkalosis
E	(–) pH	(–) HCO_3	Acidosis

TABLE 3.19 Determining Compensated or Partial Compensated or Uncompensated

pH →	$PaCO_2$ →	HCO_3 →	Compensation
Normal	*Abnormal*	*Abnormal*	FULLY
Abnormal	*Abnormal*	*Abnormal*	PARTIAL
Abnormal	Normal	*Abnormal*	UNCOMPENSATED
Abnormal	*Abnormal*	Normal	UNCOMPENSATED

TABLE 3.20 Potential Causes of Acid–Base Conditions

Condition	Primary Cause	Contributing Causes
Respiratory acidosis	• Hypoventilation	• COPD (primary cause) • Pulmonary disease • Drugs • Obesity • Mechanical asphyxia • Sleep apnea
Metabolic acidosis	• Addition of large amounts of fixed acids to body fluids	• Lactic acidosis (circulatory failure) • Ketoacidosis (diabetes, starvation) • Phosphates and sulfates (renal disease) • Acid ingestion (salicylates) • Secondary to respiratory alkalosis • Adrenal insufficiency
Respiratory alkalosis	• Hyperventilation	• Overventilation on a ventilator • Response to acidosis • Bacteremia • Thyrotoxicosis • Fever • Hepatic failure • Response to hypoxia • Hysteria
Metabolic alkalosis	• Retention of base or removal of acid from body fluids	• Excessive gastric drainage • Vomiting • Potassium depletion (diuretic therapy) • Burns • Excessive NaHCO3 administration

5. Determine state of compensation: The client's ABG reflects an uncompensated state → indicating more interventions need to be implemented (Biga et al., 2020).

HESI HINT The acronym "ROME" can help you remember: **R**espiratory, **O**pposite, **M**etabolic, **E**qual.

REVIEW OF FLUID AND ELECTROLYTE BALANCE

1. List four common causes of fluid volume deficit.
2. List four common causes of fluid volume overload.
3. Identify two examples of isotonic IV fluids.
4. List three systems that maintain acid–base balance.
5. Cite the normal ABGs for the following:
   A. pH
   B. P_{CO_2}
   C. HCO_3
6. Determine the following acid–base disorders:
   A. pH 7.50, P_{CO_2} 30, HCO_3 28
   B. pH 7.30, P_{CO_2} 42, HCO_3 20
   C. pH 7.48, P_{CO_2} 42, HCO_3 32
   D. pH 7.29, P_{CO_2} 55, HCO_3 28

See Answer Key at the end of this text for suggested responses.

ELECTROCARDIOGRAM

Description: The visual representation of the electrical activity of the heart reflected by changes in the electrical potential at the skin surface, which is a record of the heart's electrical events that precede them (Fig. 3.6).

A. The visual representation of an ECG can be recorded as a tracing on a strip of graph paper or seen on an oscilloscope.

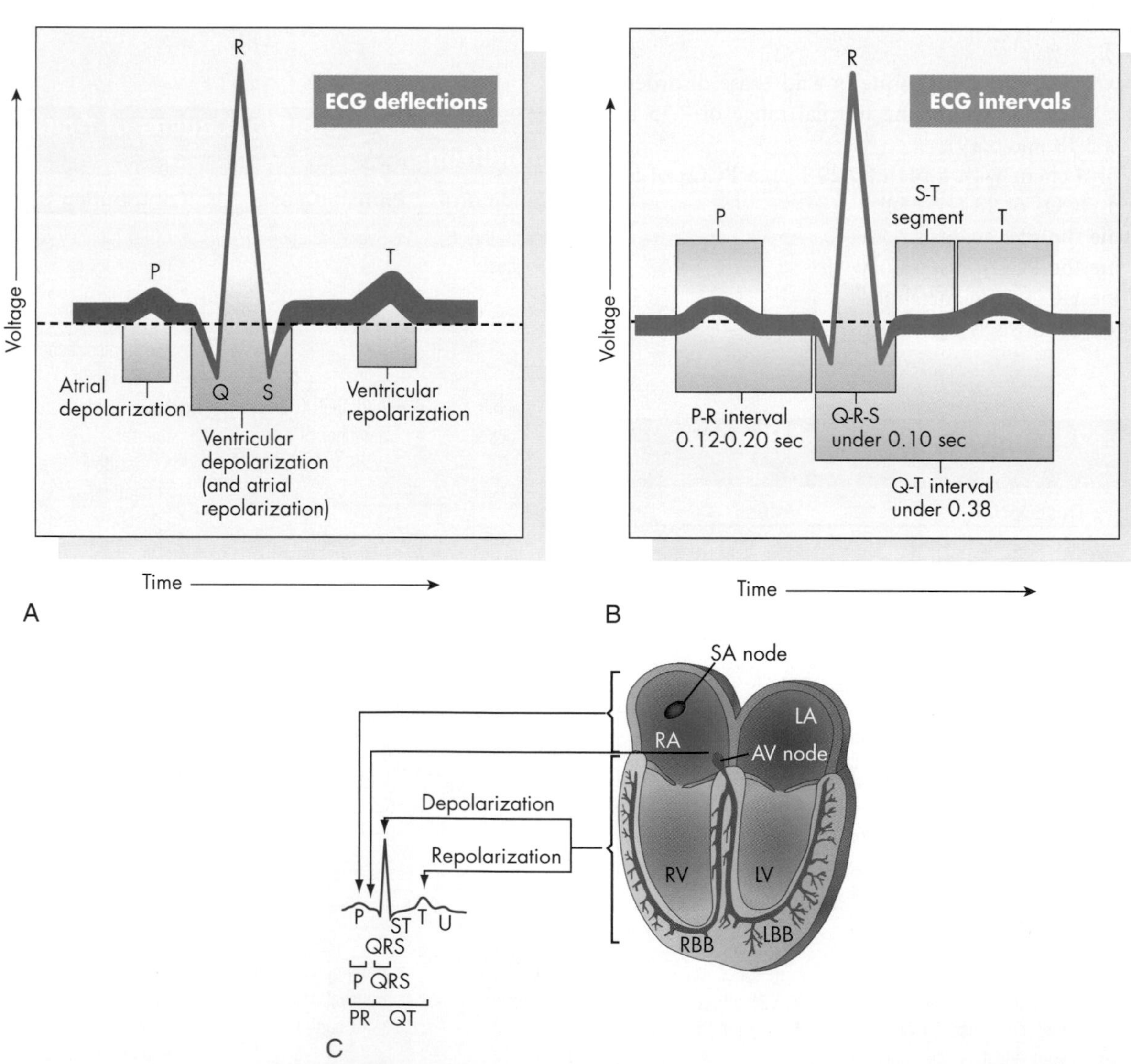

Fig. 3.6 Electrocardiogram (ECG) and Cardiac Electrical Activity (A) Normal electrical conductivity of the heart (B) Normal electrical intervals for atrial and ventricular conductivity (C) Schematic of atrial and ventrical electrical conductivity of the heart. (From Ignatavicius, D. D., & Workman, M. L. [2020]. *Medical surgical nursing: Patient-centered collaborative care* [10th ed.]. St. Louis: Saunders. A and B, From Patton, K. T., & Thibodeau, G. A. [2020]. *Anatomy and physiology.* St. Louis: Mosby.)

B. The following conditions can interfere with normal heart functioning:
   1. Disturbances of rate or rhythm
   2. Disorders of conductivity
   3. Enlarged heart chambers
   4. Presence of MI
   5. Fluid and electrolyte imbalances

C. Each ECG should include identifying information:
   1. Patient's name and identification number
   2. Location, time, and date of recording
   3. Age, gender, and current cardiac and noncardiac medications
   4. Height, weight, and BP
   5. Clinical diagnosis and current clinical status
   6. Any unusual position of the client during the recording
   7. If present, thoracic deformities, respiratory distress, and muscle tremor

HESI HINT Blood flow through the heart:

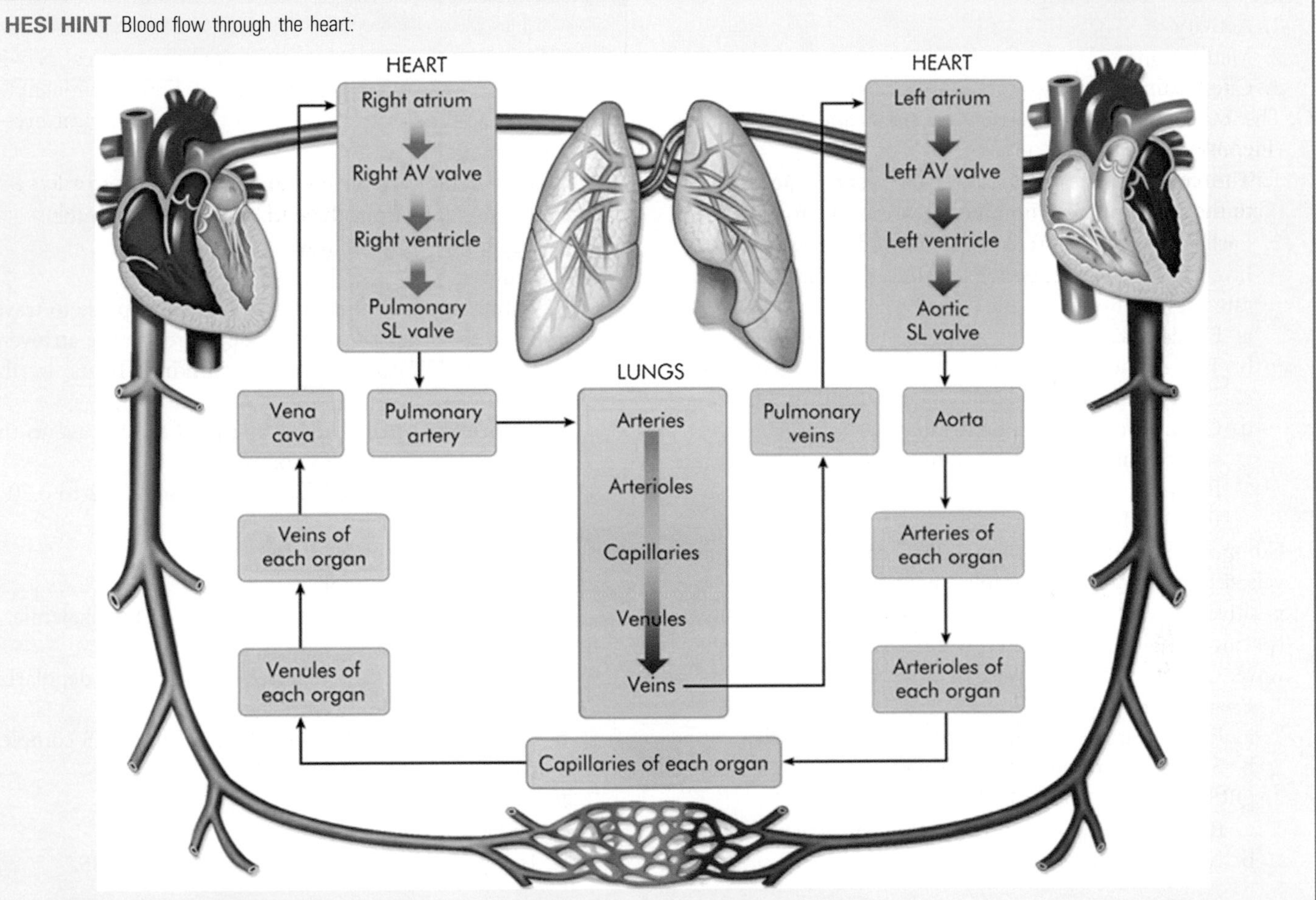

Right-sided heart failure → edema of periorbital, extremities, ascites

Left-sided heart failure leads to congestive heart failure → pulmonary edema/muffled heart sounds (From Patton, K. T., Thibodeau, G. A. [2022]. *Anatomy and physiology* [11th ed.]. St. Louis: Mosby.)

Superior/inferior VENA CAVA (unoxygenated) → Right ATRIUM → (Tricuspid Valve) → Right VENTRICLE → (Pulmonic Valve) Pulmonary Artery → LUNGS (gas exchanged at alveoli—oxygenated) → Left ATRIUM → (Mitral Valve) → Left VENTRICLE → (Aortic Valve) → Aorta

Review the three structures that control the one-way flow of blood through the heart:

Atrioventricular valves
Tricuspid (right side)
Mitral (left side)
Semilunar valves
Pulmonic (in pulmonary artery)
Aortic (in aorta)
Chordae tendineae
Papillary muscles

D. The standard ECG is the 12-lead ECG.
E. Bedside monitoring through telemetry is more commonly seen in the clinical setting.
   1. Telemetry uses three or five leads transmitted to an oscilloscope.
   2. Graphic information is printed either on request or at any time the set parameters are transcended.
F. A portable continuous monitor (Holter monitor) can be placed on the client to provide a magnetic tape recording. While wearing a Holter monitor, the client is instructed to keep a diary concerning:
   1. Activity
   2. Medications
   3. Chest pains
G. The ECG graph paper consists of small and large squares (Fig. 3.7).
   1. The small squares represent 0.04 second each; five of these small squares combine to form one large square.
   2. Each large square represents 0.20 second (0.04 second × 5). Five large squares represent 1 second. Calculation of heart rate uses the 6-second rule (Box 3.5):
      a. Easiest means of calculating the heart rate.
      b. This cannot be used when the heart rate is irregular.
      c. Thirty large squares equal one 6-second time interval.
      d. Count the number of RR intervals in the 30 large squares and multiply by 10 to determine the heart rate for 1 minute (the R is the high peak on the strip; Fig. 3.8, Box 3.5).
H. Composition of the ECG: normal **ECG** contains waves, intervals, segments, and one complex, as defined below. Wave: A positive or negative deflection from baseline that indicates a specific electrical event. The waves on an **ECG** include the P wave, Q wave, R wave, S wave, T wave, and U wave.
   1. P wave: atrial systole
      a. Represents depolarization of the atrial muscle.
      b. Should be rounded and without peaking or notching
   2. QRS complex: ventricular systole
      a. Represents depolarization of the ventricular muscle.
      b. Normally follows the P wave.
      c. Is measured from the beginning of the QRS to the end of the QRS (normal <0.12 second).
      d. T wave: ventricular diastole
         1. Represents repolarization of the ventricular muscle.
         2. Follows the QRS complex.
         3. Usually is slightly rounded, without peaking or notching.

> **HESI HINT** The T wave represents repolarization of the ventricle, so this is a critical time in the heartbeat. This action represents a resting and regrouping stage so that the next heartbeat can occur. If defibrillation occurs during this phase, the heart can be thrust into a life-threatening dysrhythmia.

   3. ST segment
      a. Represents early ventricular repolarization.
      b. Is measured from the end of the S wave to the beginning of the T wave.
   4. PR interval
      a. Represents the time required for the impulse to travel from the atria (sinoatrial node), through the atrioventricular (AV) node, to the Purkinje fibers in the ventricles.
      b. Is measured from the beginning of the P wave to the beginning of the QRS complex.
      c. Represents AV nodal function (normal 0.12 to 0.20 second).
   5. U wave
      a. Is not always present.
      b. Is most prominent in the presence of hypokalemia.
   6. QT interval
      a. Represents the time required to completely depolarize and repolarize the ventricles.
      b. Is measured from the beginning of the QRS complex to the end of the T wave.
   7. RR interval
      a. Reflects the regularity of the heart rhythm.
      b. Is measured from one QRS to the next QRS.

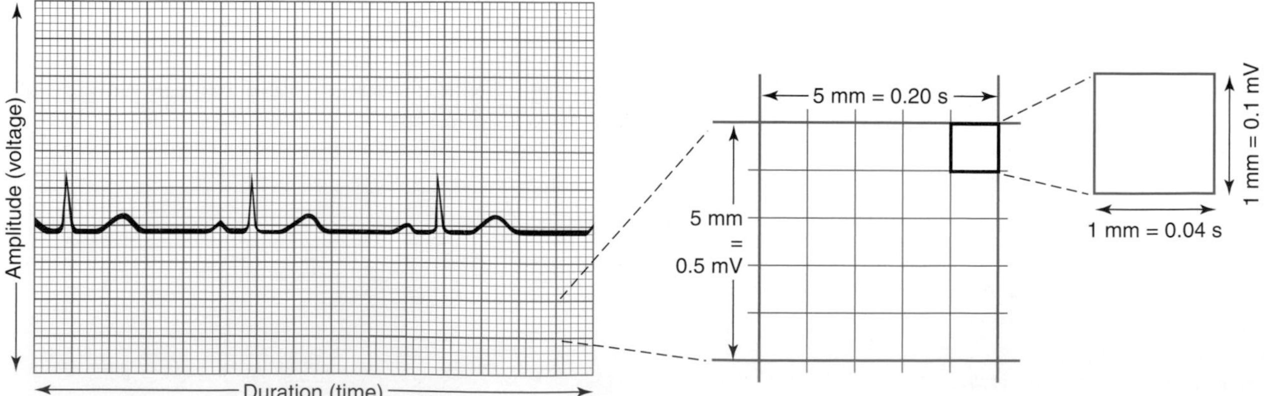

Fig. 3.7 Composition of Electrocardiogram (ECG) Paper. The ECG's waveforms are measured in amplitude (voltage) and duration (time). (From Ignatavicius, D. D., & Workman, M. L. [2020]. *Medical-surgical nursing: Patient-centered collaborative care* [10th ed.]. St. Louis: Saunders.)

BOX 3.5 Methods of Estimating Heart Rate Using an Electrocardiogram Tracing

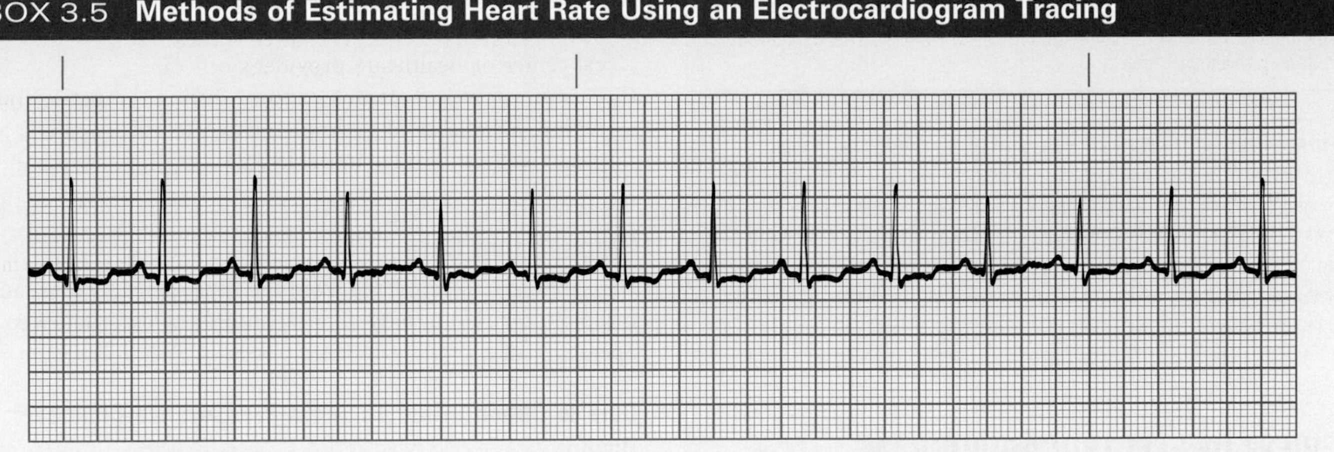

1. Measure the interval between consecutive QRS complexes, determine the number of small squares, and divide 1500 by that number. This method is used only when the heart rhythm is regular.
2. Measure the interval between consecutive QRS complexes, determine the number of large squares, and divide 300 by that number. This method is used only when the heart rhythm is regular.
3. Determine the number of RR intervals within 6 s and multiply by 10. The electrocardiogram paper is conveniently marked at the top with slashes that represent 3-s intervals. This method can be used when the rhythm is irregular. If the rhythm is extremely irregular, an interval of 30 to 60 s should be used.
4. Count the number of big blocks between the same point in any two successive QRS complexes (usually R wave to R wave) and divide into 300 because there are 300 big blocks in 1 min. It is easiest to use a QRS that falls on a dark line. If little blocks are left over when counting big blocks, count each little block as 0.2, add this to the number of big blocks, and then divide by 300.
5. The memory method relies on memorization of the following sequence: 300, 150, 100, 75, 60, 50, 43, 37, 33, 30. Find a QRS complex that falls on the dark line representing 0.2 s or a big block, and count backward to the next QRS complex. Each dark line is a memorized number. This is the method most widely used in hospitals for calculating heart rates for regular rhythms.
6. Calculation of heart rate. In this example, the heart rate using the big block method is 300 divided by four big blocks (between QRS complexes), or 75 beats/min. The memory method is also demonstrated with a heart rate of 75 beats/min.

Figure from Ignatavicius, D. D., & Workman, M. L. (2013). *Medical-surgical nursing: Patient-centered collaborative care* (7th ed.). St. Louis: Saunders. Data from Monahan, F. D., Sands, J. K., Neighbors, M., Marek, J. F., & Green-Nigro, C. J.. (2007). *Phipps' medical-surgical nursing: Health and illness perspectives* (8th ed.). St. Louis:Mosby; Ignatavicius, D. D., & Workman, M. L. (2013). *Medical-surgical nursing: Patient-centered collaborative care* (7th ed.). St. Louis: Saunders.

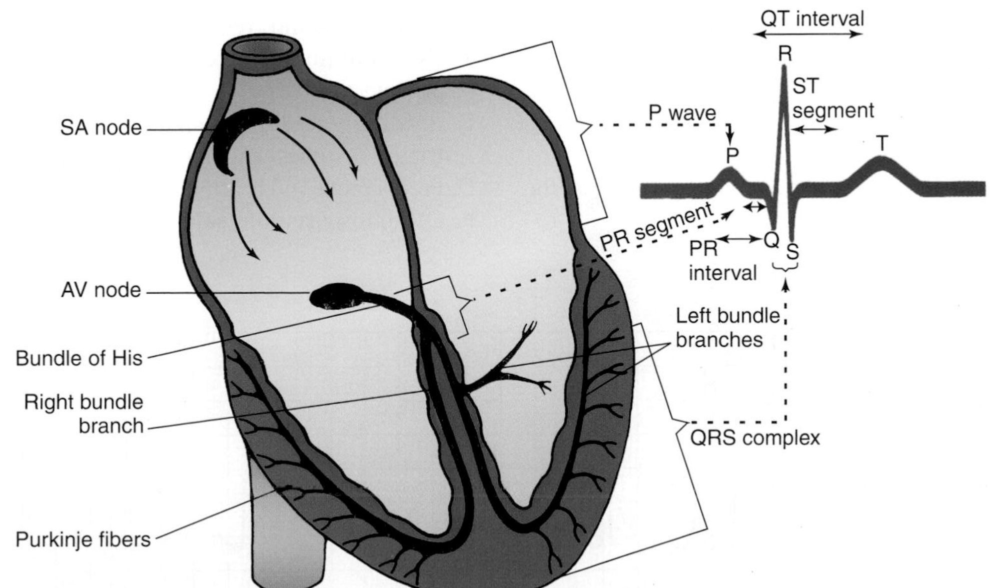

Fig. 3.8 The Cardiac Conduction System. (From Ignatavicius, D. D., & Workman, M. L. [2020]. *Medical-surgical nursing: Patient-centered collaborative care* [10th ed.]. St. Louis: Saunders.)

> **HESI HINT** Observe the patient for tolerance of the current rhythm. This information is the most important data the nurse can collect on a patient with an arrhythmia.

> **HESI HINT** NGN-NCLEX-RN questions are likely to relate to early recognition of abnormalities and associated clinical actions. Remember to monitor the patient as well as the machine! Feel the pulse! Listen to the heart. Evaluate the blood pressure. If the ECG monitor shows a severe dysrhythmia but the client is sitting up quietly watching television without any sign of distress, assess to determine whether the leads are attached properly.

REVIEW OF ELECTROCARDIOGRAM

1. Identify the waveforms found in a normal ECG.
2. In an ECG reading, which wave represents depolarization of the atrium?
3. In an ECG reading, what complex represents depolarization of the ventricle?
4. What does the PR interval represent?
5. If the U wave is most prominent, what condition might the nurse suspect?
6. Describe the calculation of the heart rate using an ECG rhythm strip.
7. What is the most important assessment data for the nurse to obtain in a client with an arrhythmia?
8. Calculate the rate of this rhythm strip.

See Answer Key at the end of this text for suggested responses.

PERIOPERATIVE CARE

Description: The perioperative period includes client care before surgery (preoperative), during surgery (intraoperative), and after surgery (postoperative).

A. The nurse's role is to
   1. Educate and advocate
   2. Reduce anxiety
   3. Promote an uncomplicated perioperative period for the client and family

B. Surgery is performed under aseptic conditions in either a hospital or an alternative hospital setting (ambulatory surgical center or healthcare provider's office).

C. Patient safety is a serious concern during the perioperative period. Steps should be implemented to ensure safety. Surgical risk factors refer to Table 3.21.

Preoperative Care

Description: Care provided from the time the client and family make the decision to have surgery until the client is taken to the operative suite

Data to Obtain When Taking a Preoperative Clinical History

A. Age
B. Allergies to medications, foods, and topical antiseptics (iodine, betadine, hibiclens)
C. Current medications: prescriptions, over-the-counter, and herbal preparations (Box 3.6)
D. History of medical and surgical problems of the patient and immediate family members
E. Previous surgical experiences
F. Previous experience with anesthesia
G. Tobacco, alcohol, and drug abuse
H. Understanding of surgical procedure and risks involved
I. Coping resources
J. Cultural and ethnic factors that may affect surgery (Box 3.6)

Key Components of Preoperative Teaching Plans

A. Regulations concerning valuables, jewelry, dentures, and hearing aids.
B. Food and fluid restrictions such as nothing by mouth (NPO) timing or exceptions per prescription by healthcare provider.
C. Invasive procedures such as urinary catheters, IVs, nasogastric (NG) tubes, enemas, and vaginal preparations.
D. Preoperative medications
E. OR, transportation, skin preparation, postanesthesia

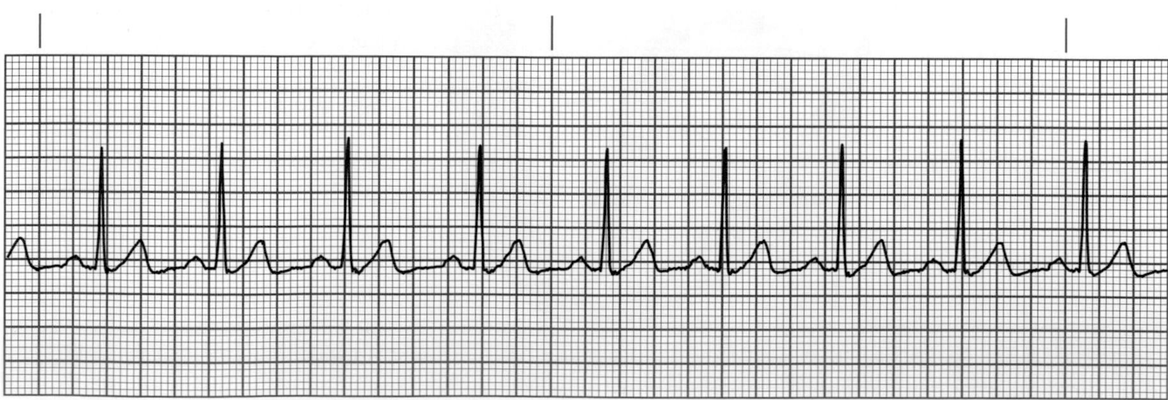

(From Ignatavicius, D. D., & Workman, M. L. [2013]. *Medical-surgical clinical: Patient-centered collaborative care* [7th ed.]. St. Louis: Saunders.)

TABLE 3.21 Surgical Risk Factors

Age	The **very young** and **very old** are greater surgical risks than children and adults.
Nutrition	**Obesity** and **malnutrition** increase surgical risk.
Fluid and Electrolyte	**Dehydration** and **hypovolemia** increase surgical risk because of imbalances in **calcium**, **magnesium**, **potassium**, and **phosphorus**.
General Health: Any infection or pathology increases surgical risk.	1. **Cardiac conditions:** Angina, MIs, hypertension, heart failure; well-controlled cardiac problems pose little risk. 2. **Blood coagulation disorders** can lead to severe bleeding, hemorrhage, and shock. 3. **Upper respiratory tract infections** (surgery is usually delayed when the client has an upper respiratory infection) and **COPD** are exacerbated by general anesthesia and adversely affect pulmonary function. 4. **Renal disease**, such as a renal insufficiency, impairs fluid and electrolyte regulation. 5. **Uncontrolled diabetes mellitus** predisposes clients to wound infection and delayed healing. 6. **Liver disease** impairs the liver's ability to detoxify medications used during surgery to produce prothrombin or to metabolize nutrients for wound healing. 7. **Obesity** exacerbates risk.
Medications (prescribed and OTCs)	1. **Anticoagulants** (increase blood coagulation time) 2. **Tranquilizers** (may cause hypotension) 3. **Heroin** (decreases CNS response) 4. **Antibiotics** (may be incompatible with anesthetics) 5. **Diuretics** (may precipitate electrolyte imbalance) 6. **Steroids** 7. Over-the-counter **herbal preparations** 8. **Vitamin E**

BOX 3.6 Factors Affecting Patterns of Disease

Ethnic group (may be less relevant in multiethnic cultures)
Gender
Socioeconomic factors and lifestyle considerations
Lifestyle decisions
Geographic location

Age (place in the life cycle; i.e., infant, adult, older adult).
Data from Copstead, L.-E., & Banasik, J. (2014). *Pathophysiology* (5th ed.). St. Louis: Saunders.

F. Postoperative procedures:
   1. Respiratory care, such as ventilator, incentive spirometer, deep breather, splinting.
   2. Activity, such as range of motion, leg exercises, early ambulation, turning.
   3. Pain control, such as IM medications, patient-controlled analgesia (PCA)
   4. Dietary restrictions
   5. ICU or postanesthesia care unit (PACU) orientation (recovery room).

Preoperative Checklist Information

A. Informed consent, surgical consent, signed by the surgeon and the client, and witnessed by the nurse. Consent to treatment must be obtained before administration of any narcotics or other medications affecting the client's cognition. (Follow facility policy for consent validity).
B. Site is marked by the person performing surgery. Before the incision is initiated, all team members confirm identity, procedure, site of surgery, and consents.
C. History and physical examination (by healthcare provider) are noted in chart with validity per facility policy.
D. Preop lab or diagnostic tests completed as ordered.
E. Identification band is on client and allergies are noted.
F. Contact lenses, glasses, dentures, partial plates, wigs, jewelry, artificial eyes, prostheses, makeup, and nail polish have been removed per facility policy or as prescribed by healthcare provider.
G. Client has voided or been catheterized.
H. Client is in hospital gown.
I. Vital signs: BP, temperature, pulse, and respirations have been taken.
J. Premedications, including antibiotics, have been given; types and times have been noted.
K. Skin preparation has been performed (if prescribed by healthcare provider or physician):
   Based on facility policy
L. Vital signs completed.
M. Signature of nurse certifies completion of list.

HESI HINT Marking the operative site is required for procedures involving right/left distinctions, multiple structures (fingers, toes), and levels (spinal procedures). Site marking should be done with the involvement of the client.

Intraoperative Care

Description: From the time the client is received in the operative suite until admission to the PACU, an OR nurse is in charge of care.
A. Maintain quiet during induction.

B. Maintain safety:
   1. Conduct client identification: right client, right procedure, and right anatomic site.
   2. Ensure that sponge, needle, and instrument counts are accurate. Counts are to be done and verified and documented by two personnel before, during, before closing incision(s), and end of the surgery.
   3. Position client during procedure to prevent injury.
   4. Strictly adhere to asepsis during all intraoperative procedures.
   5. Ensure adequate functioning suction setups are in place.
   6. Take responsibility for correct labeling, handling, and deposition of any and all specimens.

C. Monitor physical status.
   1. If excessive blood loss occurs, calculate effect on client.
   2. Report changes in pulse, temperature, respirations, and BP to surgeon, in conjunction with anesthesiologist/certified registered nurse anesthetist (CRNA).
   3. Positioning the patient is a critical part of every procedure and usually follows administration of the anesthetic.

D. Provide psychological support:
   1. Provide emotional support to client and family immediately before, during, and after surgery.
   2. Arrange with physician to provide information to the family if surgery is prolonged or complications or unexpected findings occur.
   3. Communicate emotional state of client to other healthcare team members.

Postoperative Care

Description: From admission to discharge or until client has recovered

A. Initially, the patient may go PACU.

B. On arrival, the client is assessed for vital signs (BP, pulse, respirations, temperature), level of consciousness, skin color and condition, dressing location and condition, IV fluids, drainage tubes, position, and O_2 saturation levels.

C. When client has been stabilized, and it has been prescribed by the healthcare provider, the client is then discharged or transferred to the general clinical unit or the ICU.

D. Immediate postoperative clinical care should include:
   1. Monitoring for signs of shock and hemorrhage: hypotension, narrow pulse pressure, rapid weak pulse, cold moist skin, increased capillary filling time, and decreased urine output (Table 3.22)
   2. Positioning client on side (if not contraindicated) to prevent aspiration and to allow client to cough out airway; side rails should be up at all times
   3. Providing warmth with heated blanket
   4. Managing nausea and vomiting with antiemetic drugs and NG suctioning
   5. Managing pain with IV analgesics (Table 3.26).
   6. Checking with anesthesiologist about intraoperative medications before administering pain medications
   7. Determining intraoperative irrigations and instillations with drains to help evaluate amount of drainage on dressing and in drainage collection devices

TABLE 3.22 Common Postoperative Complications

Postoperative Complication	Occurrence	Interventions for Prevention
Urinary retention	8–12 h postoperatively	• Monitor hydration status and encourage oral intake if allowed. • Offer bedpan or assist to commode.
Pulmonary problems • Atelectasis • Pneumonia • Embolus	1–2 days postoperatively	• Assist client to turn, cough, deep breathe every 2 h. • Keep client hydrated. • Enable early ambulation. • Provide early incentive spirometer.
Wound-healing problems	5–6 days postoperatively	• Teach splinting of incision when client coughs. • Monitor for signs of infection, malnutrition, and dehydration. • Provide high-protein diet.
Urinary tract infections	5–8 days postoperatively	• Oral fluid intake. • Emptying of bladder every 4–6 h. • Monitor intake and output. • Avoid catheterization if possible.
Thrombophlebitis	6–14 days postoperatively	• Leg exercises every 8 hr while in bed. • Early ambulation. • Apply antiembolic (TED) stockings or sequential compression devices as prescribed; remove TEDs every 8 h and reapply. • Avoid pressure that may obstruct venous flow; do not raise knee gatch on bed; do not place pillows beneath knees; client should avoid crossing legs at knees. • Low-dose heparin may be used prophylactically.
Decreased gastrointestinal peristalsis • Constipation • Paralytic ileus	2–4 days postoperatively	• Nasogastric tubing to decompress gastrointestinal tract. • Client to limit use of narcotic analgesics, which decrease peristalsis. • Encourage early ambulation.

8. Most PACU settings use a scoring system to determine whether the client meets the criteria to be discharged from the PACU.
9. Handoff report should be in an SBAR* format:

HESI HINT Wound dehiscence is separation of the wound edges; it is more likely to occur with vertical incisions. Wound dehiscence usually occurs after the early postoperative period, when the client's own granulation tissue is "taking over" the wound, after absorption of the sutures has begun. Evisceration of the wound is protrusion of intestinal contents (in an abdominal wound) and is more likely in clients who are older, diabetic, obese, or malnourished, and who have prolonged paralytic ileus. Good.

HESI HINT NGN-NCLEX-RN items may focus on the nurse's role in terms of the entire perioperative process.

Example: A 43-year-old mother of two teenage daughters enters the hospital to have her gallbladder removed in a same-day surgery using an endoscope instead of an incision. What clinical needs will dominate each phase of her short hospital stay?

Preparation phase: education about postoperative care, including NPO, assistance with meeting family needs

Operative phase: assessment, management of the operative suite

Postanesthesia phase: pain management, postanesthesia precautions

Postoperative phase: prevention of complications, assessment for pain management, and teaching about dietary restrictions and activity levels

HESI HINT NGN-NCLEX-RN items may focus on delivery of safe effective care.

Time Out, and Hand-Off (SBAR) communication are all best practices implemented to prevent serious medical error during the perioperative period. **Time Out** occurs before making the incision, and the entire surgical team pauses as the surgical site listed on the consent is read aloud. The entire team confirms that this information is correct. The **Hand-Off** (SBAR) communication is the transfer of relevant patient information during the perioperative period, which is standardized and must include an opportunity to ask and to respond to questions.

REVIEW OF PERIOPERATIVE CARE

1. List five variables that increase surgical risk.
2. Why is a client with liver disease at increased risk for operative complications?
3. Preoperative teaching should include demonstration and explanation of expected postoperative client activities. What activities should be included?
4. What items should the nurse assist the client in removing before surgery?
5. How is the client positioned in the immediate postoperative period, and why?
6. List three nursing judgment measures that prevent postoperative wound dehiscence and evisceration.
7. Identify three nursing judgment measures that prevent postoperative urinary tract infections.
8. Identify nursing judgment measures that prevent postoperative paralytic ileus.
9. List four nursing judgment measures that prevent postoperative thrombophlebitis.
10. During the intraoperative period, what activities should the OR nurse perform to ensure safety during surgery?
11. How is handoff given?

See Answer Key at the end of this text for suggested responses.

HIV INFECTION

Description: Infection with human immunodeficiency virus (HIV). The infection is a blood-borne pathogen. Exposure to this blood pathogen is generally acquired through contact of infected blood or blood products, unprotected sex with an infected individual, or fetal exposure from an infected mother through placental transmission or exposure of maternal bodily fluids during birth. In the United States, according to the Centers for Disease Control (CDC) an estimated 1.2 million people in the United States had HIV at the end of 2018, the most recent year for which this information is available. Of those people, about 14%, or 1 in 7, did not know they had HIV. HIV is a virus that attacks the body's immune system. If HIV is not treated, it can lead to acquired immunodeficiency syndrome (AIDS) (see Box 3.5).

Unfortunately, HIV cannot be cured; however, with proper medication people with HIV can have a productive and long life. Additionally, as long as the person with HIV is compliant their partners can be protected from HIV infection. By taking antiretroviral therapy or ART, people with HIV can live longer and prevent transmitting HIV to their sexual partners. In addition, there are effective methods to prevent getting HIV through sex or drug use, including pre-exposure prophylaxis (PrEP) and post-exposure prophylaxis (PEP).

A. Since HIV is caused by a retrovirus, it is the retrovirus that destroys CD4 cells or T helper cells which assist the immune system to stay healthy. It is the CD4 cells that keep people healthy and protect them from disease.
B. Once the retrovirus enters the cell it begins to copy $CD4^+$ T-cells, which are the major catalysts for cellular and humoral immune responses against exogenous antigens. $CD4^+$ T-cells remain stable by homeostatic mechanisms. HIV binds to the CD4 molecule and replicates on the surface of helper T-cells. This causes the destruction of $CD4^+$ T-cells, which leads to a decrease in the population of T-cells.
C. The destruction of the CD4 T-cell causes depletion in the number of CD4 T-cells and a loss of the body's ability to fight infection. Individuals with fewer than 200 cells/mm3, which

* The SBAR (**Situation-Background-Assessment-Recommendation**) technique provides a framework for communication between members of the healthcare team about a patient's condition. S = Situation (a concise statement of the problem), B = Background (pertinent and brief information related to the situation), **A = Assessment** (analysis and considerations of options—what you found/think), **R = Recommendation** (action requested / recommendation).

TABLE 3.23 **Stages of HIV**

Stage	Description and Symptoms
Primary infection (acute HIV infection or acute HIV syndrome) CD4 T-cell counts of at least 800 cells/mm^3	• Flu-like symptoms, fever, malaise • Mononucleosis-like illness, lymphadenopathy, fever, malaise, rash • Symptoms usually occur within 3 weeks of initial exposure to HIV, after which the person becomes asymptomatic
HIV asymptomatic (CDC Category A) CD4 T-cell counts more than 500 cells/mm^3	• No clinical problems • Characterized by continuous viral replication • Can last for many years (10 years or longer)
HIV symptomatic (CDC Category B) CD4 T-cell counts between 200 and 499 cells/mm^3	• Persistent generalized lymphadenopathy • Persistent fever • Weight loss, diarrhea • Peripheral neuropathy • Herpes zoster • Candidiasis • Cervical dysplasia • Hairy leukoplakia, oral
Acquired immunodeficiency syndrome (CDC Category C) CD4 T-cell counts less than 200 cells/mm^3	• Occurs when a variety of bacteria, parasites, or viruses overwhelm the body's immune system • Once classified as Category C, the patient remains classified as Category C; this has implications for entitlements (e.g., health benefits, housing, food stamps).

CDC, Centers for Disease Control; *HIV,* human immunodeficiency virus.

is one indication for the diagnosis of AIDS, are at risk for opportunistic infections. In adults, a normal CD4 cell count ranges from **500 to 1200 cells/mm^3** (0.64 to 1.18 $\times$ 10^9/L). Normal value ranges may vary slightly among different laboratories. Some labs use different measurements or test different samples (Diao et al., 2020).

D. Individuals experiencing an acute infection includes fever, lymphadenopathy, and sore throat (Table 3.23), which are also symptoms of acute HIV and referral for testing is suggested.

Complications

HIV infection weakens your immune system, making you much more likely to develop many infections and certain types of cancers.

Infections Common to HIV/AIDS

- Pneumocystis pneumonia (PCP). This fungal infection can cause severe illness. Although it has declined significantly with current treatments for HIV/AIDS, in the United States PCP is still the most common cause of pneumonia in people infected with HIV.
- Candidiasis (thrush). Candidiasis is a common HIV-related infection. It causes inflammation and a thick, white coating on your mouth, tongue, esophagus, or vagina.
- Tuberculosis (TB). In resource-limited nations, TB is the most common opportunistic infection associated with HIV. It's a leading cause of death among people with AIDS.
- Cytomegalovirus (CMV). This common herpes virus is transmitted in body fluids such as saliva, blood, urine, semen, and breast milk. A healthy immune system inactivates the virus, and it remains dormant in your body. If your immune system weakens, the virus resurfaces—causing damage to your eyes, digestive tract, lungs, or other organs.
- Cryptococcal meningitis. Meningitis is an inflammation of the membranes and fluid surrounding your brain and spinal cord (meninges). Cryptococcal meningitis is a common central nervous system infection associated with HIV, caused by a fungus found in soil.
- Toxoplasmosis. This potentially deadly infection is caused by Toxoplasma gondii, a parasite spread primarily by cats. Infected cats pass the parasites in their stools, which may then spread to other animals and humans. Toxoplasmosis can cause heart disease, and seizures occur when it spreads to the brain.

Cancers Common to HIV/AIDS

- Lymphoma. This cancer starts in the white blood cells. The most common early sign is painless swelling of the lymph nodes in your neck, armpit or groin.
- Kaposi's sarcoma. A tumor of the blood vessel walls, Kaposi's sarcoma usually appears as pink, red, or purple lesions on the skin and mouth. In people with darker skin, the lesions may look dark brown or black. Kaposi's sarcoma can also affect the internal organs, including the digestive tract and lungs.

Other Complications

- Wasting syndrome. Untreated HIV/AIDS can cause significant weight loss, often accompanied by diarrhea, chronic weakness, and fever.
- Neurological complications. HIV can cause neurological symptoms such as confusion, forgetfulness, depression, anxiety, and difficulty walking. HIV-associated neurocognitive disorders (HANDs) can range from mild symptoms

of behavioral changes and reduced mental functioning to severe dementia causing weakness and inability to function.

- Kidney disease. HIV-associated nephropathy (HIVAN) is an inflammation of the tiny filters in your kidneys that remove excess fluid and wastes from your blood and pass them to your urine. It most often affects black or Hispanic people.
- Liver disease. Liver disease is also a major complication, especially in people who also have hepatitis B or hepatitis C.

E. Initially, an individual commonly experiences an acute infection that includes fever, lymphadenopathy, and sore throat (see Table 3.23), which are also symptoms of acute HIV. Healthcare providers can refer clients and recommend access to laboratory-based follow-up or immediate testing with point-of-care tests performed on finger-stick whole blood or oral secretions or immediate HIV repeat testing with an additional HIV point-of-care test.

F. No HIV test can detect HIV immediately after infection. If there has been an exposure to HIV in the last 72 hours, discuss PEP.

G. The time between when a person gets HIV and when a test can accurately detect it is called the **window period**. The window period varies from person to person and also depends on the type of HIV test.

H. Initial symptoms may occur 2 to 4 weeks post–first exposure to HIV, after which the person becomes asymptomatic. Persons infected with HIV can transmit the virus to others any time after infection has occurred, whether they are symptomatic or asymptomatic. CDC tracks HIV diagnoses among racial and ethnic groups such as American Indian/Alaska Native, Asian, Black/African American, Hispanic/Latino, Native Hawaiian and other Pacific Islander, White, and multiracial people. The CDC site that is most helpful is https://www.cdc.gov/hiv/statistics/overview/index.html

I. Nucleic Acid Test (NAT)—A NAT can usually tell you if you have HIV infection 10 to 33 days after exposure.

J. Antigen/Antibody Test—An antigen/antibody test performed by a laboratory on blood from a vein can usually detect HIV infection 18 to 45 days after exposure. Antigen/antibody tests done with blood from a finger prick take longer to detect HIV (18 to 90 days after an exposure).

K. Antibody Test—An antibody test can take 23 to 90 days to detect HIV infection after an exposure. Most rapid tests and self-tests are antibody tests. In general, antibody tests that use blood from a vein detect HIV sooner after infection than tests done with blood from a finger prick or with oral fluid.

L. Current CDC definition of acquired immunodeficiency syndrome (AIDS; end-stage infection). According to the **CDC definition**, a patient has **AIDS** if they are infected with HIV and have a CD4+ T-cell count below 200 cells/μL, a CD4+ T-cell percentage of total lymphocytes of less than 14%, or one of the **defining** illnesses.

A high viral load is generally considered about 100,000 copies, but you could have 1 million or more. The **virus** is at work making copies of itself, and the disease may progress quickly. A lower HIV **viral load** is below 10,000 copies (HIV testing Overview, HIV.Gov 2020)

When people with HIV don't get treatment, they typically progress through three stages. But HIV medicine can slow or prevent progression of the disease. With the advancements in treatment, progression to Stage 3 is less common today than in the early days of HIV. **Untreated, HIV** typically turns into **AIDS** in about 8 to 10 years. When **AIDS** occurs, your immune system has been severely damaged. You'll be more likely to develop opportunistic infections or opportunistic cancers—diseases that wouldn't usually cause illness in a person with a healthy immune system.

N. Risk groups for acquiring HIV include the following:
1. Have sex with many partners (men or women).
2. Have unsafe sex with an infected person.
3. Share needles to take drugs or steroids.
4. Have unprotected sex for drugs or money.
5. *Have another sexually transmitted infection (STI).*

To help prevent the spread of HIV:

- *Use treatment as prevention (TasP).* If you're living with HIV, taking HIV medication can keep your partner from becoming infected with the virus. If you make sure your viral load stays undetectable—a blood test doesn't show any virus—you won't transmit the virus to anyone else. Using TasP means taking your medication exactly as prescribed and getting regular checkups.
- *Use post-exposure prophylaxis (PEP) if you've been exposed to HIV.* If you think you've been exposed through sex, needles, or in the workplace, contact your doctor or go to the emergency department. Taking PEP as soon as possible within the first 72 hours can greatly reduce your risk of becoming infected with HIV. You will need to take medication for 28 days.
- *Use a new condom every time you have sex.* Use a new condom every time you have anal or vaginal sex. Women can use a female condom. If using a lubricant, make sure it's water-based. Oil-based lubricants can weaken condoms and cause them to break. During oral sex use a nonlubricated, cut-open condom or a dental dam—a piece of medical-grade latex.
- *Consider preexposure prophylaxis (PrEP).* The combination drugs emtricitabine plus tenofovir (Truvada) and emtricitabine plus tenofovir alafenamide (Descovy) can reduce the risk of sexually transmitted HIV infection in people at very high risk. PrEP can reduce your risk of getting HIV from sex by more than 90% and from injection drug use by more than 70%, according to the CDC and Prevention. Descovy hasn't been studied in people who have receptive vaginal sex.

Clinical Assessment

A. Obtain prescription for and review laboratory testing. CDC recommends that everyone between the ages of 13 and 64 get tested for HIV at least once. People at higher risk should get tested more often.

1. All pregnant women should be tested to begin treatment as early as possible to reduce the risk of transmitting HIV to the child.
2. Refer to the CDC for current testing guidelines: https://www.cdc.gov/hiv/guidelines/testing.html
3. HIV treatment should be initiated as quickly as possible after diagnosis.

> **HESI HINT** An individual exposed to HIV may remain asymptomatic for many years dependent on various factors and if he or she is actively under a medical regimen of antiretroviral therapy (ART). The stages of HIV infection are presented in Box 3.8.
>
> Clients usually are not admitted to the hospital for treatment until their HIV status has progressed to an "AIDS" diagnosis.
>
> From CDC. About HIV. Retrieved from: https://www.cdc.gov/hiv/basics/whatishiv.html

A. Clinical Symptoms
1. Extreme fatigue
2. Loss of appetite and unexplained weight loss of more than 10 pounds in 2 months
3. Swollen glands
4. Leg weakness or pain
5. Unexplained fever for more than 1 week
6. Night sweats
7. Unexplained diarrhea
8. Dry cough; may represent PCP
9. White spots in the mouth and throat; may represent candidiasis
10. Painful blisters; may represent shingles
11. Painless, purple-blue lesions on the skin
12. Confusion, disorientation
13. In women, recurrent vaginal infections that are resistant to treatment

B. Opportunistic infections

Refer to Table 3.24. See "What is HIV": https://www.cdc.gov/hiv/basics/whatishiv.html and Box 3.7.

> **HESI HINT** HIV clients with tuberculosis require respiratory isolation.
>
> Tuberculosis can be transmitted in virtually any setting. Clinicians should be aware that transmission has been documented in healthcare settings where healthcare workers and patients come in contact with persons with infectious tuberculosis (TB) who:
> - Have unsuspected TB disease,
> - Have not received adequate or appropriate treatment, or
> - Have not been separated from others.
>
> Tuberculosis Infection Control, CDC, 2021.

Clinical Assessment and Interventions

A. Assess respiratory functioning frequently.
B. Avoid known sources of infection.
C. Use strict asepsis for all invasive procedures.
D. Obtain vital signs frequently.
E. Plan activities to allow for rest periods.
F. Elevate HOB.
G. Refer client to nutritionist.
H. Offer small, frequent feedings.
I. Weigh daily.
J. Encourage client to avoid fatty foods.
K. Monitor for skin breakdown and offer good skin care.
L. Use safety precautions for clients with neurologic symptoms or loss of vision.
M. Orient client who is confused.

> **HESI HINT**
> **Standard Precautions**
> - Wash hands, even if gloves have been worn to give care.
> - Wear examination gloves for touching blood or body fluids or any nonintact body surface.
> - Wear gowns during any procedure that might generate splashes (e.g., changing clients with diarrhea).
> - Use masks and eye protection during activity that might disperse droplets (e.g., suctioning).

TABLE 3.24 Recommendations for HIV Testing and Prevention of HIV (of Adults, Adolescents, and Pregnant Women in Health Care Settings)

Recommendations	Population
Routine HIV screening in healthcare settings	Everyone between the ages of 13 and 64 at least once as part of routine health care
HIV Tests for Screening (Listed Below)	
Antibody tests	Detect the presences of antibodies. Most rapid test and home tests are antibody tests (usually initial HIV test).
Antigen/antibody tests	Detect HIV antibodies and antigens (antigens are produced in a person infected with HIV prior to antibody development). Rapid antigen/antibody tests are available.
Nucleic acid tests (NATs)	Looks for actual virus in the blood (very expensive; not routine). Used for recent high-risk exposure or possibility of early symptoms of HIV.

HIV, Human immunodeficiency virus.
Data from https://www.cdc.gov/hiv/guidelines/testing.html.

BOX 3.7 What Are the Stages of HIV?

When people with human immunodeficiency virus (HIV) don't get treatment, they typically progress through three stages. But HIV medicine can slow or prevent progression of the disease. With the advancements in treatment, progression to Stage 3 is less common today than in the early days of HIV.

Stage 1: Acute HIV Infection

- People have a large amount of HIV in their blood. They are very contagious.
- Some people have flu-like symptoms. This is the body's natural response to infection.
- But some people may not feel sick right away or at all.
- If you have flu-like symptoms and think you may have been exposed to HIV, seek medical care and ask for a test to diagnose acute infection.
- Only antigen/antibody tests or nucleic acid tests (NATs) can diagnose acute infection.

Stage 2: Chronic HIV Infection

- This stage is also called asymptomatic HIV infection or clinical latency.
- HIV is still active but reproduces at very low levels.
- People may not have any symptoms or get sick during this phase.
- Without taking HIV medicine, this period may last a decade or longer, but some may progress faster.
- People can transmit HIV in this phase.
- At the end of this phase, the amount of HIV in the blood (called viral load) goes up and the CD4 cell count goes down. The person may have symptoms as the virus levels increase in the body, and the person moves into Stage 3.
- People who take HIV medicine as prescribed may never move into Stage 3.

Stage 3: Acquired Immunodeficiency Syndrome

- The most severe phase of HIV infection.
- People with AIDS have such badly damaged immune systems that they get an increasing number of severe illnesses, called opportunistic infections.
- People receive an AIDS diagnosis when their CD4 cell count drops below 200 cells/mm, or if they develop certain opportunistic infections.
- People with AIDS can have a high viral load and be very infectious.

AIDS, Acquired immunodeficiency syndrome.
From CDC. About HIV. Retrieved from: https://www.cdc.gov/hiv/basics/whatishiv.html.

BOX 3.8 Benefits of Routine Screening for HIV

Diagnosing human immunodeficiency virus (HIV) quickly and linking people to treatment immediately are crucial to achieving further reduction in new HIV infections.

Primary care providers (PCPs) are the front line for detecting and preventing the spread of HIV. The Centers for Disease Control and Prevention (CDC) is asking PCPs to:

- Conduct routine HIV screening at least once for all their patients
- Conduct more frequent screenings for patients at greater risk for HIV
- Link all patients who test positive for HIV to medical treatment, care, and prevention services

From CDC. Available at: https://www.cdc.gov/hiv/clinicians/screening/benefits.html.

A. Provide emotional, cultural, and spiritual support for the grieving client who is losing all relationships and skills.
B. Provide emotional support for significant others: family, family of choice, partners, and friends.
C. Administer IV fluids for hydration, as prescribed.
D. Administer total parenteral nutrition (TPN) as prescribed.
E. Administer agents that treat specific opportunistic infections and medications for HIV (Table 3.25)
F. See FDA-Approved HIV Medicines: https://hivinfo.nih.gov/understanding-hiv/fact-sheets/fda-approved-hiv-medicines

HESI HINT The CDC does not recommend excluding pregnant healthcare workers from caring for patients with known CMV infection. Healthcare workers should be careful with all patients they encounter. Spread of CMV requires direct contact with virus-containing secretions. Hand washing and using gloves are excellent ways to prevent infection.

PEDIATRIC HIV INFECTION

Description: Infection with HIV in infants and children

A. Sources of infection in pediatric clients
B. The risk of mother-to-child transmission of HIV during pregnancy, delivery, and breastfeeding is as high as 25% to 30% in the absence of treatment. With the implementation of HIV testing, counseling, antiretroviral medication, delivery by cesarean section prior to onset of labor, and discouraging breastfeeding, vertical transmission has decreased to less than 2% in the United States (Nesheim, FitzHarris, Mahle, & Lampe, 2019).
C. For infants acquiring HIV before or around delivery, disease progression occurs rapidly in the first few months of life and often leads to death. Over 80% of HIV-infected infants who are well at 6 weeks progress to become eligible to start ART before 6 months of age. *Early determination of HIV exposure and definitive diagnosis are thus critical. Therefore,*
D. All infants and children should have their *HIV exposure status* established at their first contact with the health system, ideally before 6 weeks of age. To facilitate this, all Maternal, Neonatal and Child service delivery points in health facilities should offer HIV serological testing to mothers and their infants and children. In most cases the HIV status is established by asking about maternal HIV testing in pregnancy, labor, or postpartum period checking the child's and/or mother's health card, offering a rapid antibody test to all infants and/or mothers whose HIV status is unknown, especially where the national HIV prevalence is $> 1\%$.
E. The exact mechanism of mother-to-child transmission of HIV remains unknown. Transmission may occur during intrauterine life, delivery, or breastfeeding. The greatest risk factor for vertical transmission is thought to be advanced maternal

TABLE 3.25 Opportunistic Infections

Pneumocystis carinii Pneumonia	Kaposi Sarcoma	Cryptosporidiosis	Candidiasis of Oral Cavity and Esophagus
• Fever • Dry cough • Dyspnea at rest • Chills	• Purple-blue lesions on skin, often arms and legs • Invasion of gastrointestinal tract, lymphatic system, lungs, and brain	• Severe watery diarrhea (may be 30–40 stools per day) • Abdominal cramps • Nausea • Electrolyte imbalance • Malaise	• Thick white exudate in the mouth • Unusual taste to food • Retrosternal burning • Oral ulcers
Cryptococcal Meningitis	**Cytomegalovirus (CMV) Retinitis**	**CMV Colitis**	**Disseminated CMV**
• Headache • Changes in level of consciousness • Nausea, vomiting • Stiff neck • Blurred vision	• Most common CMV infection in persons with acquired immunodeficiency syndrome • Impaired vision in one or both eyes • Can lead to blindness	• Diarrhea • Malabsorption of nutrients • Weight loss	• Malaise • Fever • Pancytopenia • Weight loss • Positive cultures from blood, urine, or throat
Perirectal Mucocutaneous Herpes Simplex Virus	**Lymphomas of Central Nervous System**	**Tuberculosis (TB)**	**HIV Encephalopathy**
• Severe pain • Bleeding, rectal discharge • Ulceration in the rectal area	• Change in mental status • Apathy • Psychomotor slowing • Seizures	• Pulmonary and extrapulmonary • Lymphatic and hematogenous TB are common • Negative skin testing does not rule out TB	• Memory loss and impaired concentration • Apathy • Depression • Psychomotor slowing (most prominent symptom) • Incontinence • CT scan findings: diffuse atrophy and ventricular enlargement

TABLE 3.26 Routes of Administration for Analgesics

Route	Administration
Oral	• Preferred method of administration • Drug level peak: 1–2 h
Intramuscular	• Acceptable method of managing acute short-term pain • Onset 30 min; peak effect 1–3 h; duration of action: 4 h
Rectal	• Useful for clients with nausea and inability to take analgesics by mouth • Useful for home care and for elderly clients as an alternative to per os (by mouth, PO) and intravenous (IV) administration • Reduced effectiveness with constipation
IV bolus (IV push)	• Provides the most rapid onset (5 min) but has the shortest duration (1 h) • Useful for acute pain, such as a client in labor
Patient-controlled analgesia (PCA)	• Ideal method of pain control; client is able to prevent pain by self-administering smaller doses of the narcotic (usually morphine) as soon as the first sign of discomfort arises • Usually administered IV • A predetermined dose and a set lockout interval (5–20 min) are prescribed by physician; pump is calibrated to deliver the specified dose whenever client hits the button • Lock-out mechanism prevents overdose • Pump can record number of times the client uses the pump and the cumulative dose delivered
Continuous subcutaneous narcotic infusion (CSI)	• Useful for clients who are nil by mouth (NPO) but require prolonged administration of parenteral narcotics • Provides a constant level of analgesia by continuous infusion of a narcotic • Site should be inspected every 8 h and changed at least every 7 days. • Risk for respiratory depression
Continuous epidural analgesia	• Catheter threaded into epidural space with continuous infusion of fentanyl citrate, morphine, or other narcotic analgesics • Risk for respiratory depression
Transdermal patches	• Applied to skin (self-adhesive or with overlay to secure patch) • Also used to deliver hormonal therapy, nitroglycerin, and nicotine • Sites for application and frequency of application are specific to each medication • Document removal of old patch, site, and application date and time of new patch

disease, such as AIDS, likely because of a high maternal HIV viral load. Unfortunately, it has been reported that 30% of pregnant women are not tested for HIV during pregnancy, and another 15% to 20% receive no or minimal prenatal care, thereby allowing for potential newborn transmission. (Peterson & Ramus, 2020; Rahangdale & Cohan, 2008).

F. Viral testing (e.g., PCR) should be conducted at 4 to 6 weeks of age for infants known to be HIV-exposed, or at the earliest possible opportunity for those seen after 4 to 6 weeks of age.

G. Urgent HIV antibody testing should be carried out for any infant or child presenting with signs, symptoms, or medical conditions that indicate HIV.

H. Infants with detectable HIV antibodies should go on for a viral test.

I. Every child should be evaluated for HIV exposures (Rivera & Frye, 2020)

J. Clinical Assessment
  1. Risk groups
    a. Infants born to mothers who are HIV-positive
    b. Hemophiliacs
    c. Infants and children who have received blood transfusions
  2. Clinical Symptoms
    a. Failure to thrive
    b. Lymphadenopathy
    c. Organomegaly
    d. Neuropathy
    e. Cardiomyopathy
    f. Chronic recurrent infections such as thrush
    g. Unexplained fevers

HESI HINT

- Because of the persistence of the maternal HIV antibody, infants younger than 18 months require virologic assays that directly detect HIV in order to diagnose HIV infection.
- Preferred virologic assays include HIV bDNA polymerase chain reaction (PCR) and HIV RNA assays. The HIV PCR DNA qualitative test is usually less expensive.
- Further virologic testing in infants with known perinatal HIV exposure is recommended at 2 weeks, 4 weeks, and 4 months.
- An antibody test to document seroreversion to HIV antibody—negative status in uninfected infants is no longer recommended (Rivera & Frye, 2020).

HESI HINT The focus of NGN-NCLEX-RN questions are likely to be assessment, analysis, synthesis of treatment implications and outcomes, and the impact of clinical assessment of signs of the disease and management of complications associated with HIV.

Clinical Judgment Measures Interventions

A. Avoid exposure to persons with infections.

B. Administer *no* live virus vaccines.

C. Teach the family to
  1. Use gloves when diapering the child.
  2. Clean any soiled surfaces (wearing gloves).
  3. Identify signs of opportunistic infections.

D. Monitor growth parameters.

E. Support use of social services.

F. Support child's attending school as much as child is able.

G. Assist in community and school education programs.

REVIEW OF HIV INFECTION

1. Identify the ways HIV is transmitted.
2. Vertical transmission (from mother to fetus) occurs how often if the mother is not treated during pregnancy?
3. Describe standard precautions.
4. What does the CD4 T-cell count describe?
5. Why does the CD4 T-cell count drop in HIV infections?
6. Describe the ways a pediatric client might acquire HIV infection.

See Answer Key at the end of this text for suggested responses.

PAIN

Pain: In light of research documenting the dramatic rise of opioid addiction and opioid-related deaths, delegates at the 2016 American Medical Association (AMA) meeting voted to stop treating pain as the fifth vital sign because they believe it is likely that the initiative, along with other factors, has exacerbated the opioid crisis (Anson, 2016).

Description: An individual's subjective experience of physical discomfort from illness or injury. Consider multidimensional pain questionnaire used to measure patients' response to postoperative pain therapy is the Overall Benefit of Analgesic Score (OBAS)

A. Client's pain often goes unrecognized and untreated.
  1. Healthcare professionals are increasingly better educated about identifying, assessing, and managing pain.

B. An individual's response to pain is influenced by several factors:
  1. Anxiety: reduction of anxiety can help to control pain.
  2. Past experience with pain: the more pain experienced in childhood, the greater the perception of pain in adulthood.
  3. Culture and religion: cultural and religious practices learned from one's family play an important role in determining how a person experiences and expresses pain.
  4. Gender affects the expression of pain.
  5. Communication, whether it is a language barrier and/or a client who is unable to speak.
  6. Altered level of consciousness.

C. Pain is classified as either acute or chronic.
  1. Acute pain
    a. Is temporary (30 days in relationship to injury; no longer than 6 months)
    b. Occurs after an injury to the body

c. Includes postoperative pain, labor pain, and renal calculus pain
2. Chronic pain (usually lasting beyond 6 months after initial injury)
   a. Nonmalignant (e.g., low back pain, rheumatoid arthritis)
   b. Intermittent (e.g., migraine headaches)
   c. Malignant, associated with neoplastic diseases

Theory of Pain

A. Gate control theory: Pain impulses travel from the periphery to the gray matter in the dorsal horn of the spinal cord along small nerve fibers.
   A "gating" mechanism called the *substantia gelatinosa*, a collection of cells in the gray area (dorsal horns) of the spinal cord. Found at all levels of the cord, it receives direct input from the dorsal (sensory) nerve roots, especially those fibers from pain and thermoreceptors, which will either open to or close off the transmission of pain impulses to the brain.
   1. Stimulation of large, fast-conducting sensory fibers opposes the input from small pain fibers, thus blocking pain transmission.
   2. Modalities used: Stimulation of large fibers by massage, heat, cold, acupuncture, transcutaneous electrical nerve stimulation (TENS).
B. Endorphin/enkephalin theory
   1. Endorphins: naturally occurring compounds that have morphine-like qualities; they modulate pain by preventing the conduction of pain impulses in the CNS.
   2. Enkephalins: specific neurotransmitters that bind with opiate receptors in the dorsal horn of the spinal cord; they modulate pain by closing the gate and stopping the pain impulse.
   3. Modalities used: stimulation of endogenous opiate release through acupuncture, placebos, TENS.

Clinical Assessment

A. Location: Pain may be localized, radiating, or referred.
B. Intensity: Ask client to rate pain before and after an intervention such as medication (use scale such as 0 to 10, with 0 being no pain).
C. Comfort: Often clients can describe what relieves pain better than they can describe the pain itself.
D. Quality: Pain may be sharp, dull, aching, sore, etc.
E. Chronology: Ask client when pain started, what time of day it occurs, how often it appears, how long it lasts, whether it is constant or intermittent, whether the intensity changes.
F. Subjective experience: Determine what decreases or aggravates pain, what other symptoms are associated with pain, what interventions provide relief, what limitations the pain inflicts.

HESI HINT The alphabet mnemonic "PQRST" is an easy tool to use when assessing and documenting a client's experience of pain.

P	Provocative and Palliative or Aggravating Factors	What provokes the painful sensation? What makes it worse or better?
Q	Quality	Type of sensation → dull, aching, sharp, stabbing, burning
R	Region or Location, Radiation	Where is the pain located and does it radiate anywhere?
S	Severity	Ask the client to rate pain on a scale.
T	Timing	How long has it been hurting? How often does it occur? When did it occur?
U	Understanding	Ask the client what he or she thinks may be the cause or the problem causing the pain.

From Ignatavicius, D. D., Workman, L. M., Rebar, C., LaCharity, L. A., & Kumagai, C. K. (2018). *Medical-surgical nursing: Concepts for interprofessional collaborative care* (9th ed.). St. Louis: Saunders.

Clinical Judgment Measures for Pain Management

1. Pharmacologic interventions, Route of administration (Table 3.27)
   a. Non-narcotics, nonsteroidal anti-inflammatory drugs
   b. Act by means of a peripheral mechanism at level of damaged tissue by inhibiting prostaglandin and other chemical mediator syntheses involved in pain
   c. Show antipyretic activity through action on the hypothalamic heat-regulating center to reduce fever
   d. Examples: salicylate—aspirin nonsalicylates, acetaminophen ibuprofen
2. Narcotic mixed agonists/antagonists
   a. Bind to both a receptor that produces pain relief, which is the agonist portion, and to another receptor that does not produce a physiologic effect, which is the antagonist portion. Patients are less likely to have respiratory depression.
   b. May cause withdrawal symptoms if administered after client has been receiving narcotics.
   c. Produce side effects, including drowsiness, occasionally, nausea, and psychomimetic effects, such as hallucinations and euphoria.
   d. Examples: butorphanol nalbuphine
3. Narcotics
   a. Act as opioids, binding with specific opiate receptors throughout the CNS to reduce pain perception.
   b. Cause such side effects such as nausea and vomiting, constipation, respiratory depression, and CNS depression.
   c. Examples: hydromorphone morphine sulfate (see Table 3.27)

HESI HINT For narcotic-induced respiratory depression, naloxone may be administered as prescribed by the healthcare provider.

TABLE 3.27 Onset of Commonly Administrated Narcotics

Medication	Mode	Onset	Comments
Codeine	PO	30–45 min	• Do not administer discolored injection solutions
	IM or SC	10–30 min	• May also be prescribed as an antitussive or antidiarrheal
Hydromorphone	PO	30 min	• Fast-acting, potent narcotic
	IM	15 min	• More likely to cause appetite loss than other narcotics
	IV	10–15 min	
Morphine sulfate	PO	60–90 min	• Drug of choice in relieving pain associated with myocardial infarction
	IM	10–30 min	• May cause transient decrease in blood pressure
	IV	10 min	• Drug of choice for use with chronic cancer pain
Fentanyl citrate	IM	7–15 min	• Synthetic narcotic
	IV	Within 5 min	• Acts quicker; less duration
	Intradermal	Within 12 h	
	Intrabuccal	5–15 min	
	Intrathecal	Immediate	

IM, Intramuscular; *IV*, intravenous, *PO*, per os (by mouth); *SC*, subcutaneous.

A. Adjuvants to analgesics
   1. Are given in combination with an analgesic to potentiate or enhance the analgesic's effectiveness.
   2. Are helpful in controlling discomfort associated with pain, such as nausea, anxiety, and depression (e.g., promethazine).

HESI HINT Use noninvasive methods for pain management when possible:
Relaxation exercises
Distraction
Imagery
Biofeedback
Interpersonal skills
Physical care: altering positions, touch, hot and cold applications

Clinical Assessment of Pain Relief Techniques

A. Pain (see Table 3.27).
B. Response to pharmacologic intervention: tolerance to pharmacologic interventions may occur—that is, the client physiologically requires increasingly larger doses to provide the same effect.
   1. The first sign of tolerance is a decreased duration of a drug's effectiveness.
   2. The need for increased doses can be the result of increased pain rather than tolerance (e.g., clients with advanced cancer) (Table 3.28).

HESI HINT Narcotic analgesics are preferred for pain relief because they bind to the various opiate receptor sites in the CNS. Morphine is often the preferred narcotic (*remember*, it causes respiratory depression).
Another agonist is methadone. Narcotic antagonists block the attachment of narcotics such as naloxone to the receptors. Once naloxone has been given, additional narcotics cannot be given until the naloxone effects have passed.

REVIEW OF PAIN

1. What modalities are associated with the gate control pain theory?
2. How does past experience with pain influence current pain experience?
3. What modalities are thought to increase the production of endogenous opiates?

TABLE 3.28 Pain Relief Techniques

Noninvasive
Cutaneous stimulation that is useful alone or in combination with other pain management techniques
- Heat and cold applications decrease pain and muscle spasm.
- Transcutaneous electrical nerve stimulation (TENS) provides continuous mild electrical current to the skin via electrodes.
- Massage provides a simple, inexpensive, and effective method of pain relief.
- Distraction diverts client's attention from the pain; useful during short periods of pain or during painful procedures such as intravenous venipunctures.
- Relaxation can be used as a distraction and to facilitate sedation or sleep; it rarely decreases pain sensation.
- Biofeedback techniques enable control of autonomic responses (tachycardia, muscle tension) to pain through electrical feedback.

Invasive
Any procedure that invades the body and is used to relieve pain
- Nerve blocks involve injection of anesthetic into or near a nerve to decrease pain pathways (e.g., deadening area for dental work, regional anesthesia used in obstetrics).
- Neurosurgical procedures include surgical or chemical (alcohol) interruption of nerve pathways; it is commonly used in clients with cancer who have severe pain.
- Acupuncture is the insertion of needles at various points in the body to relieve pain.

4. What six factors should the nurse include when assessing the pain experience?
5. What mechanism is involved in the reduction of pain through the administration of nonsteroidal anti-inflammatory drugs (NSAIDs)?
6. If narcotic agonist/antagonist drugs are administered to a client already taking narcotic drugs, what may be the result?
7. List four side effects of narcotic medications.
8. What is the antidote for narcotic-induced respiratory depression?
9. What is the first sign of tolerance to pain analgesics?
10. Which route of administration for pain medications has the quickest onset and the shortest duration?
11. List the six modalities that are considered noninvasive, nonpharmacologic pain relief measures.

See Answer Key at the end of this text for suggested responses.

DEATH AND GRIEF

Description: Death completes the life cycle. Grief is the process an individual goes through to deal with loss. How each person deals with these situations depends on the individual. An individual's past experiences, coping skills, and what other stresses he or she may have going on in his or her life can largely affect how the person responds and reacts to these situations.

Clinical Assessment

Types of Death

There are five modes of **death** (natural, accident, suicide, homicide, and undetermined).

A. Stages of preparing for an expected death may not be sequential. An individual may fluctuate between the stages. An individual may not experience every stage.
   1. Denial
      a. Coping style used to protect self/ego.
      b. Noncompliance, refusal to seek treatment, ignoring of symptoms.
      c. Changing the subject when speaking about illness.
      d. Stating, "Not me, it must be a mistake."
   2. Anger
      a. Often directing it at family or healthcare team members
      b. Stating, "Why me? It's not fair."
   3. Bargaining
      a. Making a deal with God to prolong life.
      b. Usually not sharing this with anyone, keeping it a very private experience.
   4. Depression
      a. Results from the losses experienced because of health status and hospitalization.
      b. Anticipating the loss of life.
   5. Acceptance
      a. Accepting of the inevitable
      b. Beginning to separate emotionally

B. Stages of dealing with loss (grief)
   1. Shock, disbelief, rejection, or denial
      a. Anger and crying
      b. Conflicting emotions
      c. Anger toward the deceased
      d. Guilt
      e. Preoccupation with loss
   2. Resolution
      a. Process taking up to 1 year or more
      b. Renewed interest in activities

C. Complicated grief
   1. Unresolved grief
      a. Determine level of dysfunction
   2. Physical symptoms similar to those of the deceased
   3. Clinical depression
   4. Social isolation
   5. Failure to acknowledge loss

Clinical Judgment Measures

A. Encourage client to express anger in a supportive, nonthreatening environment.
B. Discourage rumination.
C. Assist client in giving up idealized perception of deceased; point out misrepresentations.
D. Encourage interaction with others.
E. Assist client with identification of support systems.
F. Consult spiritual leader as indicated by client need and preference.
G. Assist client toward a comfortable, peaceful death.

> **HESI HINT** Do not take away the coping style used in a crisis state. Denial is a very useful and needed tool for some at the initial stage. Support, do not challenge, unless it hinders or blocks treatment, endangering the patient.

REVIEW OF DEATH AND GRIEF

1. Identify the five stages of grief associated with dying.
2. A client has been told of a positive breast biopsy report. She asks no questions and leaves the healthcare provider's office. She is overheard telling her husband, "The doctor didn't find a thing." What coping style is operating at this stage of grief?
3. Your client, an incest survivor, is speaking of her deceased father, the perpetrator. "He was a wonderful man, so good and kind. Everyone thought so." What would be the most useful intervention at this time?
4. Your client feels responsible for his sister's death because he took her to the hospital where she died. "If I hadn't taken her there, they couldn't have killed her." It has been 1 month since her death. Is this response indicative of a normal or a complicated grief reaction?
5. Mrs. Green lost her husband 3 years ago. She has not disturbed any of his belongings and continues to set a place at the table for him nightly. Is this response indicative of a normal or a complicated grief reaction?

See Answer Key at the end of this text for suggested responses.

NEXT-GENERATION NCLEX EXAMINATION-STYLE QUESTION: BOWTIE QUESTIONS

Case Study #1

Medical Record

Mrs. Nicholas, 65-year-old female, brought into emergency department for difficulty breathing new onset. Grandson visiting and is positive for COVID-19. She has been living independently and providing all selfcare.

Orders

Start IV: normal saline at 50cc/ hr.

Obtain stat laboratory specimens: (e.g. CBC, SMA-12, arterial blood gases)

Evaluate for stroke

Mrs. Nicholas is now on oxygen, saturations are 82%. Her rapid test is COVID positive.

Instructions

Complete the diagram by selecting from the choices below to specify which potential condition the client is most likely experiencing, 2 actions to take, and 2 parameters the nurse would monitor to assess the client's progress.

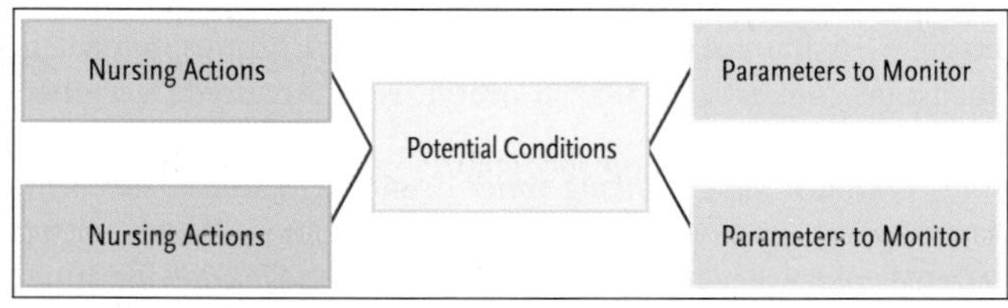

Actions to Take	Potential Conditions	Parameters to Monitor
Administer oxygen to increase saturation	Allergic response	Pain Level
Check musculoskeletal integrity	Hypoxemia	Lab values
Initiate fall precautions	Hypertension	Pulse oximetry
Evaluate for agitation /restlessness	Infection	Nutritional status
Assess for hyperactive bowel sounds		Check for bleeding

Case Study #2

Medical Record

Jamie Medina, 45-year-old LGBTQ, pronoun She/Her/Hers, brought into emergency department for malnutrition, weakness, confusion, and depression. Daughter found her on the floor at home and called an ambulance for concern due to her confusion. Jaime has been living independently and providing all self-care. Jaime has a past history of being HIV positive with a T-cell count $>$ 200 over 2 months ago.

Orders

IV Fluids, Laboratory Data, Stroke Evaluation

Instructions

Complete the diagram by selecting from the choices below to specify which potential condition the client is most likely experiencing, 2 actions to take, and 2 parameters the nurse would monitor to assess the client's progress.

Nursing Actions

Nursing Actions

Potential Conditions

Parameters to Monitor

Parameters to Monitor

Actions to Take	Potential Conditions	Parameters to Monitor
Evaluate for infection	Infection	Monitor EKG
Evaluate pulses	Hypercapnea	Lab values T-cell count
Initiate fall precautions	Hypotension	Pulse oximetry
Evaluate for agitation /restlessness	Constipation	Nutritional status
Evaluate for stroke		Record temperature every 4 hr.

For more review, go to http://evolve.elsevier.com/HESI/RN for HESI's online study examinations.

Answers highlighted in Answer Key at the end of this text

BIBLIOGRAPHY

American Heart Association. (2020). CPR & First Aid Emergency Cardiovascular Care. Algorithms. Retrieved from: https://cpr.heart.org/en/resuscitation-science/cpr-and-ecc-guidelines/algorithms.

Anson, P. (2016). *AMA drops the pain as the fifth vital sign.* https://www.painnewsnetwork.org/stories/2016/6/16/ama-drops-pain-as-vital-sign (accessed December 6, 2021).

Biga, L., Dawson, S., Harwell, A., Hopkins, R., Kaufmann, J., LeMaster, M., et al. (n.d.). 26.4 acid-base balance. *Anatomy physiology.* Retrieved from https://open.oregonstate.education/aandp/chapter/26-4-acid-base-balance/ (accessed October 12, 2021).

Center for Disease Control (CDC). (n.d.). Chapter 7: Tuberculosis infection control. https://www.cdc.gov/tb/education/corecurr/pdf/chapter7.pdf (accessed October 12, 2021).

Centers for Disease Control and Prevention. (2021, June 24). *Statistics overview.* https://www.cdc.gov/hiv/statistics/overview/index.html (accessed October 12, 2021).

Centers for Disease Control and Prevention. (2021, March 15). *Benefits of routine screening.* https://www.cdc.gov/hiv/clinicians/screening/benefits.html (accessed October 12, 2021).

Centers for Disease Control and Prevention. (2021, October 1). *Basic statistics.* https://www.cdc.gov/hiv/basics/statistics.html (accessed October 12, 2021).

Collet, J. P., Thiele, H., Barbato, E., Barthélémy, O., Bauersachs, J., et al., ESC Scientific Document Group. (2021). 2020 ESC Guidelines for the management of acute coronary syndromes in patients presenting without persistent ST-segment elevation. *European Heart Journal, 42*(14), 1289–1367. https://doi.org/10.1093/eurheartj/ehaa575.

cpr.heart.org. (n.d.). *What is CPR.* https://cpr.heart.org/en/resources/what-is-cpr (accessed October 12, 2021).

Diamond, M. (2021, July 25). Acute respiratory distress syndrome (nursing). *StatPearls.* https://www.ncbi.nlm.nih.gov/books/NBK568726/ (accessed October 12, 2021).

Diao, B., Wang, C., Tan, Y., Chen, X., Liu, Y., Ning, L., et al. (2020). Reduction and functional exhaustion of T cells in patients with Coronavirus Disease 2019 (COVID-19). *Frontiers in Immunology, 11*, 827. https://doi.org/10.3389/fimmu.2020.00827.

Gaieski, D. F., & Mikkelsen, M. E. (2021). Definition, classification, etiology, and pathophysiology of shock in adults-up to date. *Scribd.* https://www.scribd.com/document/483466837/Definition-classification-etiology-and-pathophysiology-of-shock-in-adults-UpToDate (accessed October 12, 2021).

Giddens, J. F. (2021). *Concepts for nursing practice* (p. 2021). St. Louis, MO: Elsevier.

Hammer, J. (2013). Acute respiratory failure in children. *Paediatric Respiratory Reviews, 14*(2), 64–69.

HIV.gov. (2021, April 8). HIV testing overview. *HIV.gov.* https://www.hiv.gov/hiv-basics/hiv-testing/learn-about-hiv-testing/hiv-testing-overview (accessed October 12, 2021).

Ignatavicius, D. D., Workman, L., Rebar, C., & Heimgartner, N. M. (2021). *Medical-surgical nursing: Concepts for interprofessional collaborative care* (10th ed.). St. Louis: Saunders.

Marcel, M., & Levi, M. D. (2021, July 19). *Disseminated intravascular coagulation (DIC) treatment & management: Approach considerations, management of underlying disease, administration of blood components and coagulation factors.* Disseminated Intravascular Coagulation (DIC) Treatment & Management: Approach Considerations, Management of Underlying Disease, Administration of Blood Components and Coagulation Factors. https://emedicine.medscape.com/article/199627-treatment (accessed October 12, 2021).

Marcel, Gloria, J., Paulina, & Krista. (2021, October 3). Fluid volume deficit (dehydration) nursing care plans. *Nurseslabs.* https://nurseslabs.com/deficient-fluid-volume/ (accessed October 12, 2021).

Merchant, R. M., Topjian, A. A., Panchal, A. R., Cheng, A., Aziz, K., Berg, K. M., et al., on behalf of the Adult Basic and Advanced Life Support, Pediatric Basic and Advanced Life Support, Neonatal Life Support, Resuscitation Education Science, and Systems of Care Writing Groups. (2020). Part 1: Executive summary: 2020 American Heart Association Guidelines for Cardiopulmonary Resuscitation and Emergency Cardiovascular Care. *Circulation, 142*(Suppl. 2), S337–S357. https://doi.org/10.1161/CIR.0000000000000918.

Monira, T., & Elbaih, A. H. (2017). Pathophysiology and management of different types of shock. *Narayana Medical Journal, 6*, 14–39. https://doi.org/10.5455/nmj./00000120.

Mount Sinai Health System. (n.d.). T-Cell count. https://www.mountsinai.org/health-library/tests/t-cell-count (accessed October 12, 2021).

Nesheim, S. R., FitzHarris, L. F., Mahle Gray, K., & Lampe, M. A. (2019). Epidemiology of perinatal HIV transmission in the United States in the era of its elimination. *The Pediatric Infectious Disease Journal, 38*(6), 611–616. https://doi.org/10.1097/INF.0000000000002290.

Papageorgiou, C., Jourdi, G., Adjambri, E., Walborn, A., Patel, P., Fareed, J., et al. (2018). Disseminated intravascular coagulation: An update on pathogenesis, diagnosis, and therapeutic strategies. *Clinical and Applied Thrombosis/Hemostasis, 24*(Suppl. 9), 8S–28S. https://doi.org/10.1177/1076029618806424.

Peterson, A., & Ramus, R. (2020). *HIV in pregnancy.* https://emedicine.medscape.com/article/1385488-overview#a2 (accessed December 6, 2021).

Provan, F. (n.d.). *How drinking water & staying hydrated can help to boost your immune system.* zazen Alkaline Water. https://zazenalkalinewater.com.au/blogs/water-101/boost-your-immune-system (accessed October 12, 2021).

Rahangdale, L., & Cohan, D. (2008). Rapid human immunodeficiency virus testing on labor and delivery. *Obstetrics & Gynecology, 112*(1), 159–163 [Medline].

Rivera, D., & Frye, R. (2020). *Pediatric HIV infection: practice essentials.* https://www.ncbi.nlm.nih.gov/books/NBK304129/ (accessed December 6, 2021).

Shelley, C., & Springer, J. D. (2021, July 19). Pediatric respiratory failure clinical presentation. History, physical examination. *Medscape.* https://emedicine.medscape.com/article/908172-clinical (accessed October 12, 2021).

Shelley, C., & Springer, J. D. (2021, July 19). Pediatric respiratory failure. Practice essentials, background, pathophysiology. *Medscape.* https://emedicine.medscape.com/article/908172-overview. (accessed October 12, 2021).

Singh, G., Gladdy, G., Chandy, T. T., & Sen, N. (2014). Incidence and outcome of acute lung injury and acute respiratory distress syndrome in the surgical intensive care unit. *Indian Journal of Critical Care Medicine, 18*(10), 659.

Sodium, Electrolytes, and Fluid Balance. (2020, August 13). https://med.libretexts.org/@go/page/8178.

Topjian, A., Raymond, T., Atkins, D., Duff, J., Joyner, B., Lasa, J., et al., on behalf of the Pediatric Basic and Advanced Life Support Collaborators. (2021). Part 4: Pediatric Basic and Advanced Life Support 2020 American Heart Association Guidelines for Cardiopulmonary Resuscitation and Emergency Cardiovascular Care. *Pediatrics, 147*(Suppl. 1), e202003850. https://doi.org/10.1542/peds.2020-038505D.

U.S. Department of Health and Human Services. (n.d.). *FDA-approved HIV medicines.* National Institutes of Health. https://hivinfo.nih.gov/understanding-hiv/fact-sheets/fda-approved-hiv-medicines (accessed October 12, 2021).

Vo, P., & Kharasch, V. S. (2014). Respiratory failure. *Pediatrics in Review, 35*(11), 476–486. https://doi.org/10.1542/pir.35-11-476.

Yu, A. S. L., Chertow, G. M., Luyckx, V. A., Marsden, P. A., Skorecki, K., & Taal, M. W. (2020). *Brenner & Rector's the kidney: Volume two.* Philadelphia: Elsevier.

Zieliński, J., & Przybylski, J. (2012). How much water is lost during breathing? *Pneumonologia i Alergologia Polska, 80*(4), 339–342. Polish. PMID 22714078.

4

Medical-Surgical Nursing

COMMUNICATION

Communication was one of the top root causes of sentinel events reported to The Joint Commission from 2011 through 2013. Additionally, ineffective handoff communication has been a primary contributing factor in many studies of causes leading to medical errors (Nether, 2018; Blazin et al., 2020).

> **HESI HINT** Therapeutic communication is necessary to elicit important information from clients and their families in all nursing interventions and settings. It is important in crisis intervention to ascertain cultural awareness/cultural influences on health; to note and address religious and spiritual influences on health; to assess family dynamics; and to detect sensory alterations, such as hearing loss or speech deficits.

Nurses coordinate client care through communication. Effective communication allows nurses to not only relay empathy and knowledge to clients, it also serves to prevent adverse effects clients may experience and promote quality outcomes. As the nurse communicates with the client, a partnership develops to promote client health and well-being.

Characteristics of Communication

Professional communication is the assimilation of nursing skills and knowledge integrated with dignity and respect for all human beings, incorporating the assumptions and values of the profession while maintaining accountability and self-awareness.

A. Collegial
B. Collaborative
C. Interdisciplinary/interprofessional

> **HESI HINT** The SBAR format is used in many institutions during communication processes with other nurses, health care providers, physical therapists, social workers, pharmacists, laboratory technicians, etc. SBAR stands for **S**ituation, **B**ackground, **A**ssessment, and **R**ecommendations.

D. Confidential
   1. Health Insurance Portability and Accountability Act (HIPAA)
   2. Ethical

> **HESI HINT** Nonverbal communication may be more important than verbal communication. Body language, use of personal space, and verbal/oral messages should be congruent. Tone of voice and facial expression are part of body language. An example of positive body language is leaning in toward a client while talking. Recognition of cultural differences regarding personal space is an important component of communication. Most Americans maintain half a meter (1.7 or 1½ feet) distance between people when talking. Body language and verbal/oral communication should also be congruent; state messages in a positive manner even when providing negative feedback.

Types of Communication

A. Oral/verbal communication
B. Body language communication
   1. Eye contact
   2. Shifting away from nurse or family member
   3. Grimacing
   4. Angry or fearful expression
C. Written communication
D. Technology
   1. Electronic medical records
   2. Bar coding

> **HESI HINT** Clear verbal communication and accurate written records are critical during care transitions. Care transitions include such times as changes of shift, when the client moves from unit to unit, or when the client moves to a new care setting.

A. Basic communication standards can be applied to all clients.
   1. Establish trust.
   2. Offer self; be empathetic.
   3. Demonstrate a nonjudgmental attitude (examine your bias in order to remain nonjudgmental).
   4. Use active listening.
   5. Identify the client's communication deficits and make adjustments to meet the client's abilities.
   6. Accept and support the client's feelings.
   7. Clarify and validate the client's statements.
   8. Provide a matter-of-fact approach.

Multiple factors affect client responses to nurses, including pain, anxiety, life-altering changes, physiologic needs, temperature changes (from client's room to perioperative area or postanesthesia care unit [PACU]), new nurses, difficulty tracking time, various and different stimuli encountered in a hospital or setting that is unusual or unfamiliar to the client.

> **HESI HINT** Therapeutic communication is necessary in eliciting important information from clients and their families in all nursing interventions

and settings, including crisis intervention, cultural awareness/cultural influences on health, religious and spiritual influences on health, family dynamics, and sensory alterations.

Communication Strategies

A. Assess client for hearing deficits or hearing loss.
B. Determine whether client understands questions.
C. Take time to ask yes/no questions if the client is having difficulty communicating.
D. Observe client's nonverbal communication cues (grimacing indicating pain, fear in a child).
E. When possible, provide continuity of care by assigning the same nurse.
F. Encourage presence of family members to reassure client.

HEALTH PROMOTION AND DISEASE PREVENTION

Health

A frequently used definition for health is "the state of complete physical, mental, and social well-being; not merely the absence of disease or infirmity" (World Health Organization). Health promotion actions work toward the goal of developing client attitudes and behaviors that maintain health or enhance well-being. Disease prevention actions work toward the goal of safeguarding clients from real or potential health risks. There are three levels of prevention:

A. Primary prevention is intended to reduce health risks and increase healthy behaviors. Examples: providing immunizations, teaching nutrition classes, and requiring smoke-free zones.
B. Secondary prevention is intended to detect disease (through screening) and treat the disease as early as possible. Examples: a colonoscopy allows colon cancer to be detected so that an intervention can be initiated as early as possible.
C. Tertiary prevention is intended to prevent disability and complications and to provide for a peaceful death. Tertiary prevention includes rehabilitation. Examples: rehabilitation after a stroke or hip replacement surgery. In addition, tertiary prevention includes hospice care.

Healthy Behaviors

Healthy behaviors are associated with longer, more productive lives. Lifestyle choices affect health. Unhealthy behaviors are risk factors for developing disease. It is difficult to change health behavior, especially when the behavior is ingrained in a person's lifestyle patterns. The nurse's role in helping the client to make positive changes includes the following:

A. Identifying unhealthy behaviors as an initial step in health promotion/disease prevention.
B. Asking questions that uncover and define the client's motivation.
C. Delineating behaviors and health status indicators that are outcomes of behavior change.

HESI HINT Changing unhealthy behaviors can modify or even prevent some chronic illnesses. Nurses play a major role in helping clients manage their chronic illnesses and disabilities through behavioral changes. Health teaching and counseling often are the role of the nurse in helping the client focus on improving health habits.

D. Areas of behavioral change include
   1. Physical activity
   2. Nutrition
   3. Stress
   4. Use of tobacco or marijuana
   5. Use of alcohol
   6. Spiritual perspective
   7. Coping skills
   8. Support systems

HESI HINT According to the American Lung Association, smoke is harmful to lung health. Burning wood, tobacco, or marijuana releases toxins and carcinogens.

TEACHING/LEARNING

Nurses possess specific professional knowledge, skills, and values that make them well suited to teach clients and families how to care for their health. Teaching is a deliberate process whereby the nurse implements a series of actions to bring about learning in the client.

Learning is the act of acquiring new, reinforced, or modified knowledge, behaviors, skills, or values. Only the learner can achieve learning. The teaching—learning process is an interactive, individualized interaction between the nurse and the client.

HESI HINT To develop a collaborative learning environment between the nurse and the client, nurses must be acutely aware of their own beliefs and values about the teaching—learning process, including client empowerment.

The teaching—learning process has four steps: assessment, planning, implementation, and evaluation. The process is iterative, where reassessment continually follows evaluation.

A. Assessment: Systematically assess the client's learning needs that relate to the health behaviors and health problems.
   1. Assess learning needs from three domains.
      a. Knowledge
      b. Skills
      c. Values

2. Identify the client characteristics.
   a. Nonmodifiable; for example: age, cultural background, cognitive abilities
   b. Modifiable; for example: knowledge base, and use of community resources
3. Examine the client's readiness to learn.
   a. Motivation to learn
   b. Attitudes and beliefs
4. Recognize potential barriers to client learning.
   a. Involve family members/significant others.
   b. Home environment
   c. Community environment

B. Planning: Demonstrates plan to measure client's achievement toward improving knowledge or health behaviors
1. Collaborate with client about learning needs.
2. Determine client's priorities regarding learning needs.
3. Write behavioral goals/objectives that reflect changes in the client's behavior that are observable or measurable.

C. Implementation: Carry out the teaching strategies with the client.
1. Identify teaching strategies to use; for example, group or videos.
2. Actively involve the client in the learning activities.
3. Include family members/significant others.

D. Review outcomes after implementing a plan.
1. Determine the effectiveness of teaching strategies.
2. Determine whether goals/objectives were met.
3. Alter strategies if goals are not met.

SPIRITUAL ASSESSMENT

During times of illness, religious and/or spiritual practices may be a source of comfort for the client. While obtaining a spiritual assessment, you can discover information about the client's preference for a personal clergy member or the hospital chaplain. A spiritual assessment tool may assist the nurse to integrate a spiritual assessment into the client's plan of care. FICA is an acronym for Faith and Belief: Importance, Community, and Address in care (Pulchaski, 2013, 2021).

Sometimes a simple question can be used to obtain a spiritual history. Ask the client, "Do you have any spiritual needs or concerns related to your health?"

FICA: Taking a Spiritual History

Faith, Belief, Meaning: Do you consider yourself spiritual or religious? Do you have spiritual beliefs that help you cope with stress? If the client says no, ask, "What gives your life meaning?"

Importance: Have your beliefs influenced how you take care of yourself? How does faith or beliefs have a significance in your life? Have your beliefs influenced how you take care of yourself in this illness/situation?

Community: Are you part of a spiritual or religious community? Is this of support to you and, if so, how? Is there a group of people (communities such as friends, church, temple, synagogue, mosque, or support group)?

Address in care: How would you like your nurse to address these issues in your health care?

When nurses empathize with clients, they recognize the concept of humanity in each of us. A client may or may not be open to praying with a nurse. A nurse should be honest in letting a client know that the nurse is not comfortable praying with the client. If comfortable, the nurse can tell the client, "I'll stay with you while you pray but I would rather not join in praying." Remember that prayer may help the client with feelings of loneliness or isolation. Prayer traditions vary for clients.

CULTURAL DIVERSITY

Nurses frequently provide care for clients of different cultural backgrounds. Nurses need to be cognizant of their own cultural biases because everyone has biases. How nurses communicate with clients may be influenced by bias and may create a barrier between client and nurse. Therefore, nurses must learn to accept that differences exist and to accept those cultural differences. Whenever possible, if cultural traditions do not pose a harm to clients, these requests should be incorporated into client treatment plan.

Obtain a cultural and spiritual assessment and include cultural and spiritual preferences in the plan of care when appropriate and feasible. Nurses are expected to provide care for all clients. It is important to note that clients are culturally diverse, regardless of their ethnicity, race, or socioeconomic status, and to note that in every culture subgroups may form. However, culturally diverse clients may be distinguished from mainstream culture by ethnicity, social class, and/or language.

HESI HINT Since the 2000 census, there has been a notable change in the cultural, ethnic, and racial alignment of the United States. Culture influences how clients seek medical attention or treat themselves.

COMPLEMENTARY AND ALTERNATIVE INTERVENTIONS

HESI HINT Reasons why clients use herbal medications:
- Cultural influence
- Perception that supplements are safer and "healthier" than conventional drugs
- Sense of control over one's care
- Emotional comfort from taking action
- Limited access to professional care
- Lack of health insurance
- Convenience
- Media hype and aggressive marketing
- Recommendation from family and friends

The National Academy of Medicine (formally The Institute of Medicine [IOM]) was actively involved in studying "innovative" treatments such as acupuncture, yoga, and the therapeutic use of animals. Acupuncture and massage have also been successfully implemented to decrease pain or decrease the need for pain medication (Stussman et al., 2020). In the treatment for posttraumatic stress disorder (PTSD), for example, the use of eye movement desensitization reprocessing (EMDR) emphasizes the focus on mental images and muscle tension, creating positive images and thoughts while following particular eye movements that create different scenarios for the reality of the traumatic event.

For example, conventional medicine treats premenstrual syndrome (PMS) with selective serotonin reuptake inhibitors (SSRIs) such as fluoxetine, paroxetine, sertraline, and citalopram or a tricyclic antidepressant related to SSRI such as clomipramine (Boyles & Baxter, 2021). A simpler but almost as effective method can be a large block of chocolate! Chocolate has been found to increase serotonin and has been dubbed "the Prozac of plants" by *Forbes* magazine (Farrar & Farrar, 2020).

Acupressure and herbal medicines are among the traditional medical practices used by Asian clients to reestablish the balance between yin and yang. In some Asian countries, healers use a process of "coining," in which a coin is heated and vigorously rubbed on the body to draw illness out of the body. The resulting welts can mistakenly be attributed to child abuse if this practice is not understood. Traditional healers, such as Buddhist monks, acupuncturists, and herbalists, also may be consulted when someone is ill (Arnold, 2019; Stussman et al., 2020).

A Japanese technique used to promote healing, reduce stress, and induce relaxation is called reiki. The process for administering reiki is by "laying on hands," and it is based on the idea that an unseen "life force energy" flows through us and is what causes us to be alive. It is believed that when a person's "life force energy" is low, then the person is more apt to become ill or feel stress. When the life force energy is high, an individual is believed to be more prone to being happy and healthy.

Smell connects to the part of the brain that controls the autonomic nervous system. Aromatherapy is the introduction of essential oils, such as sweet orange to grapefruit scents, which are effective in managing the odor of dressing changes in some hospice settings. It is believed that essential oils stimulate the release of neurotransmitters in the brain. The type of essential oil may induce pain reduction, induce sedation, or stimulate clients to a sense of well-being (Clark, 2021). Many clients also use herbal medications that they used in their country of origin or that they learned about from family traditions. To maintain client safety, nurses need to be aware of those herbal medications, their mechanisms of action, side effects, and food or drug interactions. See Fig. 4.1 and Table 4.1 (Farrar & Farrar, 2020).

Essential Oil	Disorder Treated
True lavender	Anxiety
True lavender	Breast tenderness
Juniper	Fluid retention
Juniper	Breast tenderness
Clary sage	Low-back pain
Geranium	Mood swings
Geranium	Nervous tension

Fig. 4.1 Examples of Essential Oils. (Clark, C. [2021]. Aromatherapy: Essential oils and nursing: explore this option for enhancing well-being. *American Nurse Journal, 16*[8].)

RESPIRATORY SYSTEM

Pneumonia

Description: Inflammation of the lower respiratory tract

A. Infectious agents can cause pneumonia.
B. Organisms that cause pneumonia reach the lungs by three methods.
   1. Aspiration
   2. Inhalation
   3. Hematogenous spread
C. Pneumonia is generally classified according to causative agent.
   1. Bacterial (gram-positive and gram-negative)
   2. Viral
   3. Fungal (rare)
   4. Chemical

HESI HINT Pneumonia affects people of all ages, especially those 65 or older and infants under age 2 (because their immune systems are still developing).

D. Pneumonia may be community-acquired or medical care–associated pneumonia that encompasses hospital-associated, ventilator-associated, and health care–associated pneumonia.
E. High-risk groups include individuals who are
   1. Debilitated by accumulated lung secretions (e.g., asthma, chronic obstructive pulmonary disease [COPD], sickle cell anemia)
   2. Cigarette smokers
   3. Immobile
   4. Immunosuppressed
   5. Experiencing a depressed gag and/or cough reflex
   6. Sedated
   7. Experiencing neuromuscular disorders
   8. Nasogastric (NG)/orogastric intubation
   9. Hospitalized client

Nursing Assessment

A. Tachypnea: shallow respirations, often with use of accessory muscles

TABLE 4.1 Herbal Medications, Uses, Mechanisms of Action, Side Effects, and Interactions

Herbal Medication	Application	Mechanism of Action	Side Effects	Drug Interaction	Efficacy
Bitter orange	Weight reduction	CNS stimulant catecholaminergic	High BP and tachycardia in healthy adults with a normal BP	It can interact with many drugs	Unproven
Black cohosh	Alleviate hot flashes of menopause	Acts on neurotransmitter systems; binds with serotonin receptor subtypes	No evidence of severe side effects		
Echinacea	Reduction in duration of common cold	Stimulation of immune cell function and cytokine production	Allergic reactions	Potential inhibition of CYP450 isoforms	Proven
Ephedra	Reduction of fatigue	CNS stimulation	Excessive adrenergic stimulation, myocardial infarction, stroke	Numerous	Proven
	Weight reduction	CNS stimulant catecholaminergic	Extensive CNS stimulation Agitation, sleep disturbances, psychosis	Synergistic interaction with methylxanthines Synergistic interaction with monoamine oxidase inhibitors (MAOIs) Inhibition of antihypertensive effects	Proven
Garlic	Reduction of hyperlipidemia	**3-hydroxy-3-methylglutaryl-CoA reductase (HMG-CoA reductase)** inhibitor	Odor, diaphoresis, bleeding	Potentiation of anticoagulant and antiplatelet medications Decreased plasma levels of protease inhibitor drug saquinavir	
Ginger	Treatment of nausea in motion sickness and pregnancy	Serotonin antagonist	No major adverse effects	Potential potentiation of anticoagulant antiplatelet drugs (controversial)	Proven
Ginkgo	Enhancement of mental performance	Vasodilator	No major adverse effects	Synergistic interaction with other stimulants (e.g., caffeine)	Unproven
Ginseng	Treatment of erectile dysfunction	Antiandrogen	No major adverse effects	No consistent reports	Supportive
	Reduction of fatigue	Unknown			Unproven
	Enhancement of mental performance	Unknown			Unproven
Hoodia gordonii Also known as Hoodia, Veldkos, Slimming cactus, *Trichocaulon gordonii, Stapelia gordonii*	Weight reduction	P57, the main ingredient, cannot actively reach the brain to suppress the appetite (not proven effective).	May be mildly toxic (confirmed in mice but not humans) increased HR. Possible hepatotoxic as evidenced by increase in alkaline phosphatase (ALP) in healthy women.		Unproven
Kava	Treatment of anxiety	Modulatory effect at Gamma-aminobutyric acid (GABA) receptors	Hepatotoxicity	Inhibition of CYP4502E1 Potentiation of other sedatives (benzodiazepines) Inhibition of effects of levodopa in Parkinson disease clients	Proven
Red yeast rice	Reduction of hyperlipidemia	Precise mechanism of action unknown Lovastatin is principal active ingredient Seven other HMG-CoA reductase inhibitors (statins)	Unknown adverse effects	Unknown	Partly understood
Saw palmetto	Relief of benign prostate hypertrophy	Antiandrogen	None	No major interactions reported	Unproven

Continued

TABLE 4.1 Herbal Medications, Uses, Mechanisms of Action, Side Effects, and Interactions—cont'd

Herbal Medication	Application	Mechanism of Action	Side Effects	Drug Interaction	Efficacy
Soy	Therapeutic for menopausal vasomotor symptoms Prevention of breast cancer Prevention of osteoporosis	Phytoestrogens help balance wildly fluctuating hormone levels Structurally similar to estradiol (major endogenous estrogen)	Can provoke asthma GI disturbance	Dangerous interaction with MAOI inhibitors leading to serotonin syndrome Inhibition of actions of tamoxifen	Proven
Soy protein	Reduction of hyperlipidemia	Unknown			Proven
St. John's wort	Depression	Inhibition of norepinephrine, dopamine, and serotonin reuptake	Mania in bipolar clients Photosensitivity	Many Serotonin syndrome when combined with SSRIs or tricyclic antidepressants Reduced plasma concentrations of many drugs such as oral contraceptives, statins, warfarin	Proven

BP, Blood pressure; *CNS,* central nervous system; *GI,* gastrointestinal; *SSRIs,* selective serotonin reuptake inhibitors
From Buckle, J. (2003). *Clinical aromatherapy: Essential oils in practice* (2nd ed.). St Louis: Elsevier.

B. Abrupt onset of fever with shaking and chills (not reliable in older adults)
C. Productive cough with pleuritic pain
D. Rapid, bounding pulse
E. In older adults, symptoms include
   1. Confusion
   2. Lethargy/malaise
   3. Anorexia
   4. Rapid respiratory rate
   5. Tachycardia
F. Pain and dullness to percussion over the affected lung area
G. Bronchial breath sounds, crackles
   1. Bronchial breath sounds "E" to "A" changes in lungs (egophony); client says letter "E" while nurse listens to the chest. Pneumonia may cause "E" to sound like letter "A" when heard via stethoscope.
   2. Tactile fremitus: nurse can feel the chest vibrations when client says "99." Increased fremitus is heard because solid tissue conducts sound in the pneumonia client.
H. Chest radiograph indication of infiltrates with consolidation or pleural effusion
I. Elevated white blood cell (WBC) count
J. Arterial blood gas (ABG) indication of hypoxemia
K. On pulse oximetry, a decrease in oxygen (O_2) saturation (should be >90%, ideally >95%)

HESI HINT Increased temperature also increases metabolism and the demand for O_2. Fever can also cause dehydration because of excessive fluid loss due to diaphoresis.

HESI HINT

Clients at High Risk for Pneumonia

- Altered level of consciousness
- Brain injury
- Depressed or absent gag and cough reflexes
- Susceptible to aspirating oropharyngeal secretions, including alcoholics, anesthetized individuals
- Drug overdose
- Stroke victims
- Immunocompromised

Nursing Plans and Interventions

A. Assess sputum for volume, color, consistency, clarity, and distinct odors like *Pseudomonas.*
B. Assist client to cough productively by
   1. Deep breathing every 2 hours (may use incentive spirometer)
   2. Using humidity to loosen secretions (may be oxygenated)
   3. Suctioning the airway, if necessary
   4. Chest physiotherapy
C. Provide fluids up to 3 L/day unless contraindicated (helps liquefy lung secretions).
D. Assess lung sounds before and after coughing.
E. Assess rate, depth, and pattern of respirations regularly (normal adult rate is 16 to 20 breaths/min; assess for accessory muscle).
F. Monitor ABGs (partial pressure of oxygen [Po_2] >80 mm Hg; partial pressure of carbon dioxide [Pco_2] <45 mm Hg).

G. Monitor O_2 saturation with pulse oximetry (ideally >95%).
H. Assess skin color (nail beds, mucous membranes, color for appropriate ethnic population).
I. Assess mental status, restlessness, and irritability.
J. Administer humidified O_2 as prescribed.
K. Monitor temperature regularly.
L. Provide adequate rest periods throughout the day, including uninterrupted sleep.
M. Administer antibiotics as prescribed (Table 4.2).
N. Teach high-risk clients and their families about risk factors and include preventive measures.
O. Encourage at-risk groups to get pneumonia and annual influenza ("flu") vaccinations. Healthy adults develop protection within 2 to 3 weeks after receiving the vaccine (CDC).
P. Promote rest and conserve energy.

HESI HINT Bronchial breath sounds are heard over areas of density or consolidation. Sound waves are easily transmitted over consolidated tissue.

HESI HINT
Hydration
- Thins out the mucus trapped in the bronchioles and alveoli, facilitating expectoration
- Is essential for client experiencing fever
- Is important because 300–400 mL of fluid is lost daily by the lungs through evaporation

HESI HINT Irritability and restlessness are early signs of cerebral hypoxia; the client's brain is not receiving enough O_2.

HESI HINT
Pneumonia Preventives
- Older adults: annual flu vaccinations; pneumococcal vaccination at age 65 or older and younger clients who are at high risk (repeat vaccinations may be recommended. See Centers for Disease Control and Prevention [CDC] guidelines); avoiding sources of infection and indoor pollutants (dust, smoke, and aerosols); no smoking
- Immunosuppressed and debilitated persons: annual flu vaccinations, pneumonia vaccination, avoid infections, sensible nutrition, adequate fluid intake, appropriate balance of rest and activity
- Comatose and immobile persons: elevation of head of bed at least 30 degrees for feeding and for 1 h after feeding; turn frequently
- Clients with functional or anatomic asplenia: flu and pneumonia vaccinations

Chronic Airflow Limitation

Description: Chronic lung disease includes chronic bronchitis, pulmonary emphysema, and asthma (Table 4.3).

A. Emphysema and chronic bronchitis, termed *chronic obstructive pulmonary disease* (COPD), are characterized by bronchospasm and dyspnea. The damage to the lung is not reversible and increases in severity.

HESI HINT Exposure to tobacco smoke is the primary cause of COPD in the United States.

B. Asthma, unlike COPD, is an intermittent disease with reversible airflow obstruction and wheezing.

HESI HINT
1. Compensation occurs over time in clients with chronic lung disease, and ABGs are altered.
2. As COPD worsens, the amount of O_2 in the blood decreases (hypoxemia) and the amount of carbon dioxide (CO_2) in the blood increases (hypercapnia), causing chronic respiratory acidosis (increased arterial P_{CO_2}), which results in kidneys retaining bicarbonate (HCO_3) as compensation.
3. Not all clients with COPD are CO_2 retainers, even when hypoxemia is present, because CO_2 diffuses more easily across lung membranes than O_2.
4. In advanced emphysema, due to the alveoli being affected, hypercarbia is a problem, rather than in bronchitis, where the airways are affected.
5. It is imperative that baseline data be obtained for the client.

Nursing Assessment

A. Changes in breathing pattern (e.g., an increase in rate with a decrease in depth)
B. Overinflation of the lungs causes the rib cage to remain partially expanded (barrel chest)
C. Generalized cyanosis of lips, mucous membranes, face, nail beds ("blue bloater")
D. Cough (dry or productive)
E. Higher CO_2 than average
F. Low O_2, as determined by pulse oximetry (<90% to 92%)
G. Decreased breath sounds
H. Coarse crackles in lung fields that tend to disappear after coughing, wheezing
I. Dyspnea, orthopnea
J. Poor nutrition, weight loss
K. Activity intolerance
L. Anxiety concerning breathing; manifested by
   1. Anger
   2. Fear of being alone
   3. Fear of not being able to catch breath

HESI HINT Productive cough and comfort can be facilitated by semi-Fowler or high-Fowler position, which lessens pressure on the diaphragm by abdominal organs. Gastric distention becomes a problem in these clients because it elevates the diaphragm and inhibits full lung expansion.

TABLE 4.2 Antibiotics

Drugs	Indications	Adverse Reactions	Nursing Implications
		PENICILLINS	
• Procaine penicillin G Benzathine penicillin • Penicillin V	• Anti-infectives • Used primarily for gram-positive infections	• Allergic reactions • Anaphylaxis • Phlebitis at IV site • Diarrhea • GI distress • Superinfection	• Use with caution in clients allergic to cephalosporins. • Monitor for allergic reactions. • Observe all clients for at least 30 min after parenteral administration. • Oral penicillin G should be taken on an empty stomach. • Probenecid decreases renal excretion, thereby resulting in an increased blood level of the drug. • Alters contraceptive effectiveness
		SEMISYNTHETIC	
• Oxacillin sodium • Nafcillin sodium • Cloxacillin sodium • Dicloxacillin sodium	• Anti-infectives • Used primarily for gram-positive infections	• Allergic reactions • Anaphylaxis • Superinfection • See "Penicillins," earlier.	• Cannot be used in clients allergic to penicillin • Caution in clients allergic to cephalosporins • Monitor for superinfection (sore mouth, vaginal discharge, diarrhea, cough). • See "Penicillins," earlier.
		ANTIPSEUDOMONAL PENICILLINS AND COMBINATIONS	
• Ampicillin • Ticarcillin + clavulanate • Piperacillin + tazobactam • Ampicillin + sulbactam	• Anti-infectives • Broad spectrums	• Similar to penicillin • Ampicillin rash	• Contraindicated in clients allergic to penicillin • See "Penicillins," earlier.
		TETRACYCLINES	
• Tetracycline HCl • Doxycycline hyclate • Minocycline	• Anti-infectives	• Hypersensitivity reactions • Photosensitivity	• Decrease the effectiveness of oral contraceptives • Avoid concurrent use of antacids, milk products • Inspect IV site frequently. • Monitor for superinfections. • Avoid exposure to sunlight during use. • Avoid use in pregnant clients and children under 8 years; can cause yellow-brown discoloration of teeth and growth retardation.
		AMINOGLYCOSIDES	
• Gentamicin sulfate • Tobramycin sulfate • Amikacin sulfate Miscellaneous Agents • Vancomycin hydrochloride • Metronidazole	• Anti-infectives • Used with gram-negative bacteria	• Neuromuscular blockade • Nephrotoxicity • Ototoxicity	• Monitor renal function, BUN, creatinine, and I&O. • Monitor for ototoxicity: headache, dizziness, hearing loss, tinnitus. • Monitor for superinfection. • Peak and trough levels required • Monitor vancomycin serum drug concentrations. • Peak and trough levels required
		CEPHALOSPORINS	
First Generation • Cefazolin • Cephalexin *Second Generation* • Cefaclor • Cefamandole • Cefuroxime • Cefoxitin • Cefotetan • Cefprozil *Third Generation* • Cefotaxime • Ceftriaxone • Ceftazidime • Cefdinir • Cefixime • Cefpodoxime • Ceftibuten (Cedax) *Fourth Generation* • Cefepime	• Anti-infectives	• Allergic reactions • Thrombophlebitis • GI distress • Superinfection	• Use with caution in clients allergic to penicillin and cephalosporins. • See "Penicillins," earlier.

Continued

CARBAPENEMS			
• Imipenem • Meropenem • Ertapenem	Gram + and (−) bacteria	Injection site redness	Caution with penicillin and cephalosporin allergy
MONOBACTAM			
• Aztreonam	• *Pseudomonas aeruginosa* + many otherwise resistant organisms • Most effective against gram-negatives	• Phlebitis • Pseudomembranous colitis • CNS changes • EEG changes • Headache, diplopia • Hypotension	• Monitor renal and hepatic function, especially in older adults. • Carefully monitor for diarrhea. • Assess motor sensory function and cardiac rhythm.
MACROLIDES			
• Clarithromycin • Azithromycin • Erythromycin	• Clarithromycin (PO): URI, including streptococci; as adjunct treatment for *H. pylori* • Clarithromycin (IV): gram-negative and gram-positive organisms	• Pseudomembranous colitis • Phlebitis: a vesicant • Superinfections • Dizziness • Dyspnea	• Give clarithromycin XL with food. • Space monoamine oxidase inhibitors (MAOI) 14 days before start and after end of clarithromycin • Report diarrhea, abdominal cramping (all macrolides). • Monitor liver and renal laboratories. • PO clarithromycin give on empty stomach.
FLUOROQUINOLONES			
• Ciprofloxacin • Levofloxacin • Moxifloxacin	• Used to treat respiratory infections, UTIs, skin, bone, and joint infections • Has been used as conjunctive treatment for TB and AIDS	• Superinfections • CNS disturbances • Arroyos and cataracts possible with ciprofloxacin • Ciprofloxacin: a vesicant	• Prompt onset • Crosses placenta and in breast milk • Can lower seizure threshold • Monitor liver, renal, and blood counts. • Safety for children not known • Many drug—drug interactions
LINCOSAMIDES			
• Clindamycin	• Soft tissue infections caused by streptococci, staphylococci, and anaerobes • Infections resistant to penicillins and cephalosporins • Used in penicillin- and erythromycin-sensitive clients	• Agranulocytosis • Pseudomembranous colitis • Superinfections	• Periodic liver, renal, and blood count monitoring • Report diarrhea immediately.
STREPTOGRAMIN			
• Quinupristin/dalfopristin	• Life-threatening VRE	• Arthralgia, myalgia • Severe vesicant • Pseudomembranous colitis • Nausea/vomiting, diarrhea • Rash, pruritus	• Incompatible with any saline solutions or heparin • Functionally related to both macrolides and lincosamides • Monitor total bilirubin. • Many drug—drug interactions
OXAZOLIDINONE			
• Linezolid	• Life-threatening VRE and MRSA	• GI disturbances • Headache • Pancytopenia • Pseudomembranous colitis • Superinfections	• Monitor renal and liver laboratories and blood count. • May exacerbate HTN, especially if client ingests foods with tyramine (MAOI-like properties) • Report diarrhea immediately.

BUN, Blood urea nitrogen; *CNS,* central nervous system; *EEG,* electroencephalograph; *HTN,* hypertension; *IV,* intravenous; *MRSA,* methicillin-resistant *Staphylococcus aureus*; *PCP, Pneumocystis pneumonia*; *TB,* tuberculosis; *URI,* upper respiratory infection; *UTIs,* urinary tract infections; *VRE,* vancomycin-resistant enterococcus.

TABLE 4.3 Chronic Airflow Limitation

Chronic Bronchitis	Emphysema	Asthma
	PATHOPHYSIOLOGY	
• Chronic sputum with cough production on a daily basis for a minimum of 3 months in each of 2 consecutive years • Chronic hypoxemia, cor pulmonale • Increase in mucus, cilia production • Increase in bronchial wall thickness (obstructs airflow) • Reduced responsiveness of respiratory center to hypoxemic stimuli	• Reduced gas exchange surface area • Increased air trapping (increased anterior and posterior (AP) diameter) • Decreased capillary network • Increased work, increased O_2 consumption	• Narrowing or closure of the airway due to a variety of stimulants
	PRECIPITATING FACTORS	
• Higher incidence in smokers	• Cigarette smoking • Environmental and/or occupational exposure • Genetic	• Mucosal edema • $\dot{V}/\dot{Q}$ abnormalities • Increased work of breathing • Beta blockers • Respiratory infection • Allergic reaction • Emotional stress • Exercise • Environmental or occupational exposure • Reflux esophagitis
	ASSESSMENT	
• Generalized cyanosis • "Blue bloaters" • Right-sided HF • Distended neck veins • Crackles • Expiratory wheezes	• "Pink puffers" • Barrel chest • Pursed-lip breathers • Distant, quiet breath sounds • Wheezes • Pulmonary blebs on radiograph	• Dyspnea, wheezing, chest tightness • Assess precipitating factors. • Medication history
	NURSING PLANS AND INTERVENTIONS	
• Lowest FiO_2 possible to prevent CO_2 retention • Monitor for signs and symptoms of fluid overload • Maintain PO_2 between 55 and 60 • Baseline ABGs • Teach pursed-lip breathing and diaphragmatic breathing. • Teach tripod position. • Administer bronchodilators and anti-inflammatory agents.	• Lowest FiO_2 possible to prevent CO_2 retention • Monitor for signs and symptoms of fluid overload. • Maintain PO_2 between 55 and 60. • Baseline ABGs • Teach pursed-lip breathing and diaphragmatic breathing. • Teach tripod position. • Administer bronchodilators and anti-inflammatory agents	• Administer bronchodilators. • Administer fluids and humidification. • Education (causes, medication regimen) • ABGs • Ventilatory patterns • C-PAP and Bi-PAP

ABG, Arterial blood gas; *HF*, heart failure; *PAP*, prostatic acid phosphatase

HESI HINT
Normal ABG Values

Blood Gas	Adult	Child
Blood gas	7.35–7.45	7.36–7.44
PCO_2	35–45 mm Hg	Same as adult
PO_2	80–100 mm Hg	Same as adult
HCO_3^-	21–28 mEq/L	Same as adult

The person works harder to breathe, but the amount of O_2 taken in is not adequate to oxygenate the tissues.

Insufficient oxygenation occurs with chronic bronchitis and leads to generalized cyanosis and often right-sided heart failure (HF; known as cor pulmonale).

HESI HINT Overinflation of the lungs causes the rib cage to remain partially expanded, giving the characteristic appearance of a barrel chest.

HESI HINT Cells of the body depend on O_2 to carry out their functions. Inadequate arterial oxygenation is manifested by cyanosis and slow capillary refill (<3 s). A chronic sign is clubbing of the fingernails, and a **late sign** is clubbing of the fingers.

HESI HINT The key to respiratory status is assessment of breath sounds, as well as visualization of the client. Breath sounds are better described, not named; for example, sounds should be described as crackles, wheezes, or high-pitched whistling sounds rather than rales, rhonchi, etc., which may translate the same outcome findings to each clinical professional.

Nursing Plans and Interventions

A. Teach client to sit upright and bend slightly forward to promote breathing.
   1. In bed: Teach client to sit with arms resting on overbed table (tripod position).
   2. In chair: Teach client to lean forward with elbows resting on knees (tripod position; Fig. 4.2).

B. Teach diaphragmatic and pursed-lip breathing. Teach prolonged expiratory phase to prevent bronchiolar collapse and prevent air trapping.

C. Administer O_2 at 1 to 2 L per nasal cannula (Table 4.4).

D. Pace activities to conserve energy.

E. Maintain adequate dietary intake.
   1. Small, frequent meals
   2. Increase calories and protein, but do not overfeed.
   3. Favorite foods
   4. Dietary supplements
      a. For people continuing to smoke tobacco, additional vitamin C may be necessary.
      b. Magnesium and calcium, because of their role in muscle contraction and relaxation, may be important for people with COPD.
      c. Routine monitoring of magnesium and phosphorus levels is important because of their role related to bone mineral density (BMD; e.g., osteoporosis).

F. Provide an adequate fluid intake (minimum 3 L/day) unless contraindicated.

G. Fluids should be taken between meals (rather than with them) to prevent excess stomach distention and to decrease pressure on the diaphragm.

H. Instruct client in relaxation techniques (teach when not in distress).

I. Teach prevention of secondary infections.

J. Teach about medication regimen (Table 4.5).

K. Smoking cessation is imperative.

L. Encourage health-promoting activities.

HESI HINT
Health Promotion
- Eating consumes energy needed for breathing. Offer mechanically soft diets, which do not require as much chewing and digestion. Assist with feeding if needed.
- Prevent secondary infections; avoid crowds, contact with persons who have infectious diseases, and respiratory irritants (tobacco smoke).
- Teach client to report any change in characteristics of sputum.
- Encourage client to hydrate well (3 L/day) and decrease caffeine due to diuretic effect.
- Obtain immunizations when needed (flu and pneumonia).

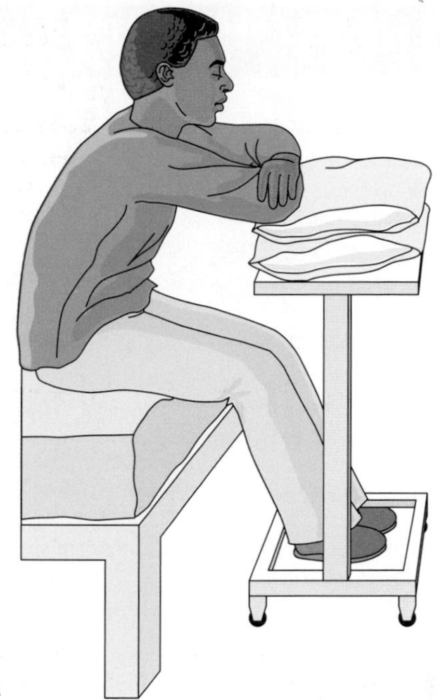

Sitting on the edge of a bed with the arms folded and placed on two or three pillows positioned over a nightstand.

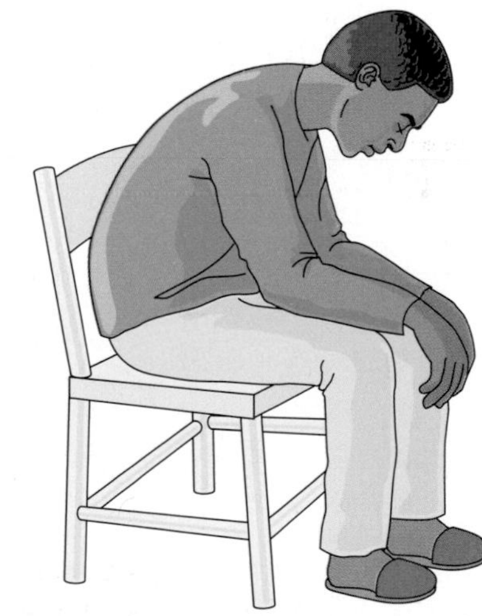

Sitting in a chair with the feet spread shoulder-width apart and leaning forward with the elbows on the knees. Arms and hands are relaxed.

Fig. 4.2 Forward-Leaning Position. (A) The client sits on the edge of the bed with arms folded on a pillow placed on the elevated bedside table. (B) Client in three-point position. The client sits in a chair with the feet approximately 1 foot apart and leans forward with elbows on knees. (From Ignatavicius, D. D., & Workman, M. L. [2013]. *Medical-surgical nursing: Client-centered collaborative care* [7th ed.], St. Louis: Saunders.)

HESI HINT When asked to prioritize nursing actions, use the ABC rule:
- Airway
- Breathing
- Circulation

In cardiopulmonary resuscitation (CPR) circumstances, follow the CAB guidelines.

TABLE 4.4 Nursing Skills: Respiratory Client

Suctioning (Tracheal)
- Suction when adventitious breath sounds are heard, when secretions are present at endotracheal tube, and when gurgling sounds are noted.
- Use aseptic/sterile technique throughout procedure.
- Wear mask and goggles.
- Advance catheter until resistance is felt.
- Apply suction only when withdrawing catheter (gently rotate catheter when withdrawing).
- Never suction for more than 10–15 s, and pass the catheter only three or fewer times.
- Oxygenate with 100% O_2 for 1–2 min before and after suctioning to prevent hypoxia.

Ventilator Setting Maintenance
- Verify that alarms are on.
- Maintain settings and check often to ensure that they are specifically set as prescribed by health care provider.
- Verify functioning of ventilator at least every 4 h.

Oxygen Administration
- Nasal cannula: low O_2 flow for low O_2 concentrations (good for COPD)*
- Simple face mask: low flow, but effectively delivers high O_2 concentrations; cannot deliver <40% O_2
- Nonrebreather mask: low flow, but delivers high O_2 concentrations (60%–90%)
- Partial rebreather mask: low-flow O_2 reservoir bag attached; can deliver high O_2 concentrations
- Venturi mask: high-flow system; can deliver exact O_2 concentration
- C-PAP** and Bi-PAP

Pulse Oximetry
- Easy measurement of O_2 saturation
- Should be >90%, ideally above 95%
- Noninvasive, fastens to finger, toe, or earlobe
- No nail polish
- Must have good peripheral perfusion to be accurate

Tracheostomy Care
- Aseptic technique (remove inner cannula only from stoma)
- Clean nondisposable inner cannula with H_2O_2; rinse with sterile saline in accordance with hospital policy
- 4 × 4 gauze dressing is butterfly folded after inner cannula is inserted.

Respiratory Isolation Technique
- Mask is required for anyone entering room.
- Private room is required with negative air pressure.
- Client must wear mask if leaving room.

Proper Use of an Inhaler with Spacers
- Have client exhale completely.
- Grip mouthpiece (in mouth) only if client has a spacer; otherwise, keep the mouth open to bring in volume of air with misted medication. While inhaling slowly, push down firmly on the inhaler to release the medication.
- Use bronchodilator inhaler before steroid inhaler.
- Wait at least 1 min between puffs (inhaled doses).
- After steroid inhaler use, client must perform oral care to prevent fungal infections.

*COPD**, Chronic obstructive pulmonary disease; *PAP***, prostatic acid phosphatase

HESI HINT Look and listen! If breath sounds are clear but the client is cyanotic and lethargic, adequate oxygenation is not occurring.

HESI HINT Watch for NCLEX-RN questions that deal with O_2 delivery. In adults, O_2 must bubble through some type of water solution so it can be humidified if given at greater than 4 L/min or delivered directly to the trachea. If given at 1–4 L/min or by mask or nasal prongs, the oropharynx and nasal pharynx provide adequate humidification.

Cancer of the Larynx

Description: Neoplasm occurring in the larynx, most commonly squamous cell in origin

A. Prolonged use of combined effects of alcohol and tobacco are directly related to development.
B. Other contributing factors include
   1. Vocal straining
   2. Chronic laryngitis
   3. Family predisposition
   4. Industrial exposure to carcinogens
   5. Nutritional deficiencies: riboflavin
C. Men are affected eight times more often than are women.
D. Diagnosis usually occurs between the ages of 55 and 70.
E. The earliest sign is hoarseness or a change in vocal quality that lasts more than 2 weeks.
F. Medical management includes radiation therapy, often with adjuvant chemotherapy or surgical removal of the larynx (laryngectomy).

Nursing Assessment

A. Magnetic resonance imaging (MRI)
B. Direct laryngoscopy
C. Assessing for hoarseness of longer than 2 weeks (early changes)
D. Assessing for color changes in mouth or tongue

HESI HINT With cancer of the larynx, the tongue and mouth often appear white, gray, dark brown, or black and may appear patchy.

E. Assessing for dysphagia, dyspnea, cough, hemoptysis, weight loss, neck pain radiating to the ear, enlarged cervical nodes, and halitosis (later changes)
F. Radiographs of head, neck, and chest
G. Computed tomography (CT) scan of neck and biopsy

Nursing Plans and Interventions

A. Provide preoperative teaching.
   1. Allow client and family to observe and handle tracheostomy tubes and suctioning equipment.
   2. Explain how and why suctioning will take place after surgery.
   3. Plan for acceptable communication methods after surgery.

TABLE 4.5 Bronchodilators and Corticosteroids

Drugs	Indications	Adverse Reactions	Nursing Implications
Adrenergics and Sympathomimetics			
• Epinephrine • Isoproterenol HCl • Albuterol • Isoetharine • Terbutaline • Salmeterol • Metaproterenol (inhaled) • Levalbuterol	• Bronchodilator	• Anxiety • Increased HR • Nausea, vomiting • Urinary retention	• Check HR. • Monitor for urinary retention, especially in men over 40. • Instruct in proper use of inhaler. • Use bronchodilator inhaler before steroid inhaler. • May cause sleep disturbance.
METHYLXANTHINE			
• Aminophylline (IV) • Theophylline (PO)	• Bronchodilator	• GI distress • Sleeplessness • Cardiac dysrhythmias • Hyperactivity • Tachycardia	• Administer oral forms with food. • Avoid foods containing caffeine. • Check HR. • Instruct in proper use of inhaler. • Monitor therapeutic range. • Crosses placenta.
CORTICOSTEROIDS			
• Prednisone (PO) • Solu-Medrol (IV) • Beclomethasone dipropionate (inhaled) • Budesonide (inhaled) Fluticasone (inhaled) • Triamcinolone (inhaled) • Flunisolide (inhaled) • Mometasone (inhaled)	• Anti-inflammatory	• Cardiac dysrhythmias occur with long-term steroid use	• See "Endocrine System," earlier. • Instruct in proper use of inhaler. • Encourage oral care after use.
ANTICHOLINERGICS			
• Ipratropium • Tiotropium	• Bronchodilator • Control of rhinorrhea	• Dry mouth • Blurred vision • Cough	• Do not exceed 12 doses in 24 h (ipratropium).
COMBINATION PRODUCTS			
• Fluticasone + salmeterol • Ipratropium + albuterol • Budesonide + formoterol	• See individual drugs.	• See individual drugs.	• See individual drugs.
PHOSPHODIESTERASE 4 INHIBITORS			
• Roflumilast	• Reduced lung inflammation in severe COPD	• Insomnia • Weight loss • Depression	• Many drug–drug interactions

COPD, Chronic obstructive pulmonary disease; *HR*, heart rate; *IV*, intravenous; *GI*, gastrointestinal.

4. Consider literacy level.
5. Refer client to speech pathologist.
6. Discuss the planned rehabilitation program.

B. Provide postoperative care.
1. Simplify communications.
2. Use planned alternative communication methods.
3. Keep call bell/light within reach at all times.
4. Ask client yes/no questions whenever possible.
5. Allow client to grieve as related to alteration in body image.

C. Promote respiratory functioning.
1. Assess respiratory rate and characteristics every 1 to 2 hours.
2. Keep bed in semi-Fowler position at all times.
3. Keep laryngeal airway humidified at all times.
4. Auscultate lung sounds every 2 to 4 hours.
5. Clients retain secretions.
6. Suction excess secretions from mouth and tracheostomy as needed immediately after surgery.
7. Provide tracheostomy care every 2 to 4 hours and as needed (PRN).

HESI HINT Tracheostomy care involves cleaning the inner cannula, suctioning, and applying clean dressings.

8. Administer tube feedings as prescribed.
9. Encourage ambulation as early as possible.
10. Referral for speech rehabilitation with artificial larynx or to learn esophageal speech.
11. Humidification of environment

HESI HINT Air entering the lungs is humidified along the nasobronchial tree. This natural humidifying pathway is gone for the client who has had a laryngectomy. If the air is not humidified before entering the lungs, secretions tend to thicken and become crusty.

HESI HINT A laryngectomy tube has a larger lumen and is shorter than the tracheostomy tube. Observe the client for any signs of bleeding or occlusion, which are the greatest immediate postoperative risks (first 24 h).

HESI HINT Always have suction equipment available at the bedside for new and chronic tracheostomy clients.

HESI HINT Fear of choking is very real for laryngectomy clients. They cannot cough as compared to previously because the glottis is no longer present. Teach the glottal stop technique to remove secretions (take a deep breath, occlude the tracheostomy tube momentarily, cough, and simultaneously remove the finger from the tube).

Pulmonary Tuberculosis

Description: Communicable lung disease caused by an infection by *Mycobacterium tuberculosis* bacteria

A. Transmission is by airborne droplets.
B. After initial exposure, the bacteria encapsulate (form a tuberculoma).
C. Bacteria remain dormant until a later time, when clinical symptoms appear.

Nursing Assessment

A. It is often asymptomatic.
B. Symptoms include
   1. Fever with night sweats
   2. Anorexia, weight loss
   3. Malaise, fatigue
   4. Cough, hemoptysis
   5. Dyspnea, pleuritic chest pain with inspiration
   6. Cavitation or calcification as evidenced on chest radiograph
   7. Positive sputum culture is positive for *M. tuberculosis*
   8. Recurring upper respiratory infections (URIs)

HESI HINT Tuberculin skin test (TST) (also called the Mantoux test): A positive tuberculosis (TB) skin test in a healthy client is exhibited by an induration 10 mm or greater in diameter 48–72 h after the skin test. Anyone who has received a bacillus Calmette-Guérin (BCG) vaccine will have a positive skin test and must be evaluated with an initial chest radiograph. A health history with signs and symptoms form may be filled out annually until signs and symptoms arise; then another radiograph is required. Chest x-rays are required on new employment; employer may require an x-ray every 5 years depending on exposure risk.

CDC guidelines indicate that the QuantiFERON-TB Gold test, a new blood test, is more reliable for TB skin testing. Nucleic acid amplification (NAA) testing may be recommended when a client has signs and symptoms of TB.

TST in clients who have received BCG vaccination may cause a false-positive reaction to the TST, which may complicate decisions about prescribing treatment.

Nursing Plans and Interventions

A. Provide client teaching.
   1. Cough into tissues and dispose of immediately into biohazardous waste bags.
      a. Take all medications as prescribed daily for a minimum of 9 to 12 months. It is essential that the client take the medications as prescribed for the entire time. Skipping doses or prematurely terminating the drug therapy can result in a public health hazard.
   2. Wash hands using proper handwashing technique.
   3. Report symptoms of deteriorating condition, especially hemorrhage.
B. Collect sputum cultures as needed; client may return to work after three negative cultures.
C. Place client in respiratory isolation while hospitalized.
D. Administer anti-TB medications as prescribed (Table 4.6).
E. Refer client and high-risk persons to local or state health department for testing and prophylactic treatment.
F. Promote adequate nutrition.

Lung Cancer

Description: Neoplasm occurring in the lung

A. Lung cancer is the leading cause of cancer-related death in the United States.
B. Cigarette smoking is responsible for 80% to 90% of all lung cancers.
C. Exposure to occupational hazards such as asbestos and radioactive dust poses significant risk.
D. Lung cancer tends to appear years after exposure; it is most commonly seen in persons after ages 50 or 60.
E. Lung cancer has a poor prognosis.

Nursing Assessment

A. Persistent dry, hacking cough early, with cough turning productive as disease progresses
B. Hoarseness
C. Dyspnea
D. Hemoptysis; rust-colored or purulent sputum
E. Pain in the chest area
F. Diminished breath sounds, occasional wheezing
G. Abnormal chest radiograph
H. Positive sputum for cytology and for pleural fluid

TABLE 4.6 **Drug Therapy for Tuberculosis**

Drug	Mechanisms of Action	Side Effects	Comments
		FIRST-LINE DRUGS	
• Isoniazid (INH)	• Interferes with DNA metabolism of tubercle bacillus	• Nausea, vomiting, abdominal pain • Rare: neurotoxicity, optic neuritis, and hepatotoxicity • Peripheral neuritis	• Metabolism primarily by liver and excretion by kidneys; pyridoxine (vitamin B_6) administration during high-dose therapy as prophylactic measure; use as single prophylactic agent for active TB in individuals whose PPD converts to positive; ability to cross blood–brain barrier • Drug interaction with alcohol, Antabuse, and phenytoin
• Rifampin	• Has broad-spectrum effects, inhibits RNA polymerase of tubercle bacillus	• Hepatitis, febrile reaction, GI disturbance, peripheral neuropathy, hypersensitivity • Orange body secretions	• Used in conjunction with at least one other antitubercular agent; low incidence of side effects; suppression of effect of birth control pills; possible orange urine • Increases metabolism of digoxin and oral hypoglycemics
• Ethambutol	• Inhibits RNA synthesis and is bacteriostatic for the tubercle bacillus	• Skin rash, GI disturbance, malaise, peripheral neuritis, optic neuritis	• Side effects uncommon and reversible with discontinuation of drug; most common use as substitute drug when toxicity occurs with isoniazid or rifampin
• Pyrazinamide	• Bactericidal effect (exact mechanism is unknown)	• Fever, skin rash, hyperuricemia, jaundice (rare) • Hepatotoxicity, arthralgias, GI distress	• High rate of effectiveness when used with streptomycin or capreomycin
• Rifapentine	• Inhibits DNA-dependent RNA polymerase	• Red discoloration of body fluids and tissues	• Many drug interactions • Always use in conjunction with at least one other antituberculosis drug.
		SECOND-LINE DRUGS	
• Ethionamide	• Inhibits protein synthesis	• GI disturbance, hepatotoxicity, hypersensitivity • Peripheral neuritis	• Valuable for treatment of resistant organisms; contraindicated in pregnancy. • Give with meals; avoid alcohol. • If neuropathy exists, give pyridoxine.
• Capreomycin	• Inhibits protein synthesis and is bactericidal	• Ototoxicity, nephrotoxicity	• Cautious use in older adults. • Undergo periodic hearing evaluation.
• Kanamycin and amikacin	• Interferes with protein synthesis	• Ototoxicity, nephrotoxicity	• Use in select cases for treatment of resistant strains. • Evaluate hearing after starting medication.
• Paraaminosalicylic acid (PAS)	• Interferes with metabolism of tubercle bacillus	• GI disturbance (common), hypersensitivity, hepatotoxicity	• Interferes with absorption of rifampin; used uncommonly. • Give with meals.
• Streptomycin	• Inhibits protein synthesis and is bactericidal	• Ototoxicity (eighth cranial nerve), nephrotoxicity, hypersensitivity	• Cautious use in older adults, those with renal disease, and pregnant women; must be given parenterally.
• Levofloxacin and moxifloxacin	• Inhibits DNA gyrase	• Increased risk of tendinitis	• Many drug–drug interactions.
		SECOND-LINE DRUGS	
• Cycloserine	• Inhibits cell wall synthesis	• Personality changes, psychosis, rash	• Contraindicated in individuals with histories of psychosis; used in treatment of resistant strains.

GI, Gastrointestinal.

Nursing Plans and Interventions

A. Nursing interventions are similar to those implemented for the client with COPD.
B. Place client in semi-Fowler position.
C. Teach pursed-lip breathing to improve gas exchange.
D. Teach relaxation techniques; client often becomes anxious about breathing difficulty.
E. Administer O_2 as indicated by pulse oximetry or ABGs.

F. Take measures to allay anxiety.
   1. Keep client and family informed of impending tests and procedures.
   2. Give client as much control as possible over personal care.
   3. Encourage client and family to verbalize concerns.
G. Decrease pain to manageable level by administering analgesics as needed (within safety range for respiratory difficulty).
H. Surgery
   1. Thoracotomy for clients who have a resectable tumor. (Unfortunately, detection commonly occurs so late that the tumor is no longer localized and is not amenable to resection.)
   2. Pneumonectomy (removal of entire lung)
      a. Position client on operative side or back.
      b. Chest tubes are not usually used.
   3. Lobectomy and segmental resection
      a. Position client on back.
      b. Chest tubes are usually inserted (Fig. 4.3).
      c. Check to ensure chest tubing is not kinked or obstructed.

HESI HINT Some tumors are so large that they fill entire lobes of the lungs. When removed, large spaces are left. Chest tubes are not usually prescribed with these clients because it is helpful if the mediastinal cavity, where the lung used to be, is allowed to fill with fluid. This fluid helps to prevent the shift of the remaining chest organs to fill the empty space.

   4. Chest tubes
      a. Keep all tubing coiled loosely below chest level, ensure connections are tight and taped.
      b. Keep water seal and suction control chamber at the appropriate water levels.
      c. Monitor the fluid drainage and mark the time of measurement and the fluid level.
      d. Observe for air bubbling in the water seal chamber and fluctuations (tidaling).
      e. Monitor the client's clinical status.
      f. Check the position of the chest drainage system.
      g. Encourage the client to breathe deeply periodically.
      h. Do not empty collection container of the chest tube. Replace unit when full.
      i. Do not strip or milk chest tubes.
      j. Chest tubes are not routinely clamped. If the drainage system breaks, place the distal end of the chest tubing connection in a sterile water container at a 2-cm level as an emergency water seal.
      k. Maintain dry occlusive dressing.

HESI HINT If the chest tube becomes disconnected, do not clamp! Immediately place the end of the tube in a container of sterile saline or clean water until a new drainage system can be connected.

If the chest tube is inadvertently dislodged from the client, the nurse should cover with a dry sterile dressing taped on three sides. If an air leak is noted, tape the dressing on three sides only; this allows air to escape and prevents the formation of a tension pneumothorax. Notify the health care provider.

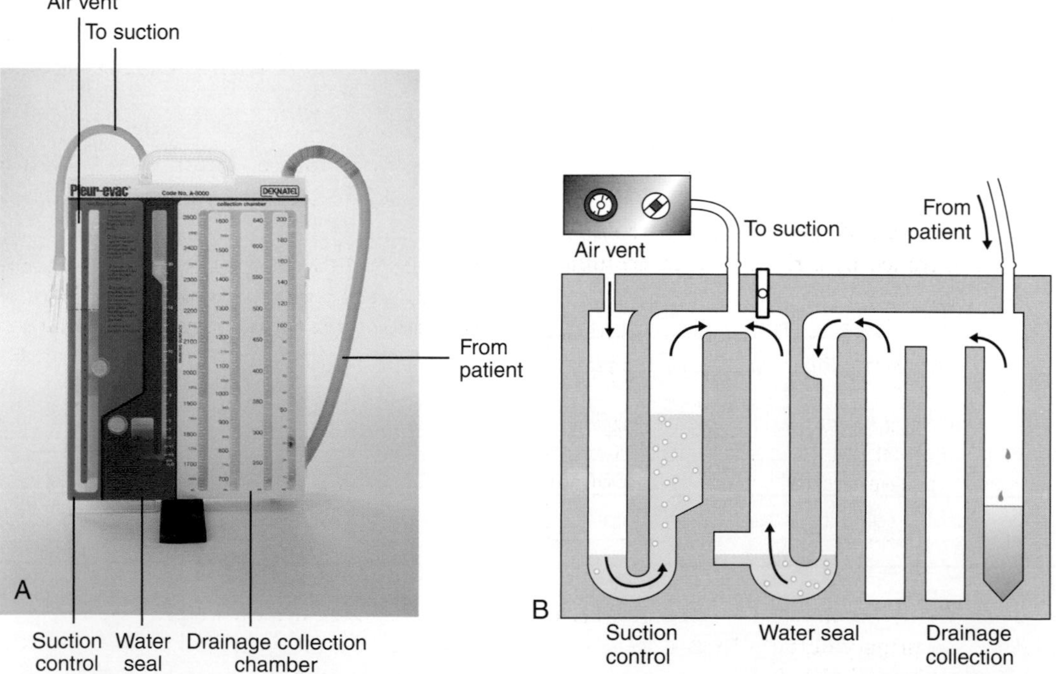

Fig. 4.3 Chest Tubes. Chest tubes are used to remove or drain blood or air from the intrapleural space, to expand the lung after surgery, or to restore subatmospheric pressure to the thoracic cavity. Many brands of commercial chest drainage systems are available; all are based upon the traditional three-bottle water seal system. (A) The Pleur-evac drainage system, a commercial three-chamber chest drainage device. (B) Schematic of the drainage device. (Ignatavicius, D. D., Workman, M. L., & Rebar, C. [2020]. *Medical-surgical nursing: Concepts for interprofessional collaborative care* [10th ed.]. St. Louis: Elsevier.)

HESI HINT
NCLEX-RN Content on Chest Tubes
Fluctuations (tidaling) in the fluid will occur if there is no external suction. These fluctuating movements are a good indicator that the system is intact; they should move upward with each inspiration and downward with each expiration. If fluctuations cease, check for kinked tubing, accumulation of fluid in the tubing, occlusions, or change in the client's position, because expanding lung tissue may be occluding the tube opening. When a chest tube is connected to suction, continuous bubbling is an indication of an air leak between the drain and the client.

I. Chemotherapy
   1. Attend to immunosuppression factor. (See "Hematology and Oncology," later in this chapter.)
   2. Administer antiemetics before administration of chemotherapy.
   3. Take precautions in administrating antineoplastics. (See "Hematology and Oncology" later in this chapter.)
   4. Targeted therapy is used for non—small cell cancer and for treatment of late-stage lung cancer. These drugs are not used alone as therapy for lung cancer.

J. Radiation therapy
   1. Provide skin care according to health care provider's request.
   2. Instruct the client not to wash off the lines drawn by the radiologist.
   3. Instruct client to wear soft cotton garments only.
   4. Avoid use of powders and creams on radiation site unless specified by the radiologist.

REVIEW OF RESPIRATORY SYSTEM

1. List four common symptoms of pneumonia the nurse might note on physical examination.
2. State four nursing interventions for assisting the client to cough productively.
3. What symptoms of pneumonia might the nurse expect to see in an older client?
4. How does the nurse prevent hypoxia during suctioning?
5. During mechanical ventilation, what are three major nursing interventions?
6. When examining a client with emphysema, what physical findings is the nurse likely to see?
7. What is the most common risk factor associated with lung cancer?
8. Describe why preoperative nursing care is important to include for a client undergoing a laryngectomy.
9. List five nursing interventions after chest tube insertion.
10. What immediate action should the nurse take when a chest tube becomes disconnected from a bottle or suction apparatus? What should the nurse do if a chest tube is inadvertently removed from the client?
11. What instructions should be given to a client after radiation therapy?
12. What precautions are required for clients with TB when placed on respiratory isolation?
13. List four components for teaching clients with tuberculosis.

See Answer Key at the end of this text for suggested responses.

RENAL SYSTEM

Acute Kidney Injury

Description: A potentially reversible disorder, it is a rapid loss of kidney function accompanied by a rise in serum creatinine and/or a reduction in urine output.

HESI HINT Normally, kidneys excrete approximately 1 mL of urine per kg of body weight per hour.
For adults, total daily urine output ranges between 1500 and 2000 mL depending on the amount and type of fluid intake, amount of perspiration, environmental or ambient temperature, and the presence of vomiting or diarrhea.

A. Acute kidney failure (AKI) occurs when metabolites accumulate in the body and urinary output changes.
B. There are three major types of AKI (Table 4.7).
C. There are three phases of AKI.
   1. Oliguric phase: less than 0.5 mL/kg/h in children, and less than 400 mL daily in adults
   2. Diuretic phase: daily urine output above 400 mL
   3. Recovery phase: return of glomerular filtration rate (GFR) 70% to 80% of normal values

HESI HINT GFR is a test used to check how well the kidneys are working. Specifically, it estimates how much blood passes through the glomeruli each minute. Glomeruli are the tiny filters in the kidneys that filter waste from the blood.

Nursing Assessment

A. History of taking nephrotoxic drugs (salicylates, antibiotics, nonsteroidal anti-inflammatory drugs [NSAIDs], angiotensin-converting enzyme [ACE] inhibitors, angiotensin receptor blocker [ARBs])
B. Alterations in urinary output
C. Edema, weight gain (ask if waistbands have suddenly become too tight)
D. Change in mental status
E. Hematuria
F. Dry mucous membranes
G. Drowsiness, headache, muscle twitching, seizures

TABLE 4.7 Acute Renal Failure

Types	Description	Causative Factors
• Prerenal	• Interference with renal perfusion	• Hemorrhage • Hypovolemia • Decreased cardiac output • Decreased renal perfusion
• Intrarenal	• Damage to renal parenchyma	• Prolonged prerenal state • Nephrotoxins • Intratubular obstruction • Infections (glomerulonephritis) • Renal injury • Vascular lesions • Acute pyelonephritis
• Postrenal	• Obstruction in the urinary tract anywhere from the tubules to the urethral meatus	• Calculi • Prostatic hypertrophy • Tumors

HESI HINT Electrolytes are profoundly affected by kidney problems (a favorite NCLEX-RN topic). There must be a balance between extracellular fluid and intracellular fluid to maintain homeostasis. A change in the number of ions or in the amount of fluid will cause a shift in one direction or the other. Sodium and chloride are the primary extracellular ions. Potassium and phosphate are the primary intracellular ions.

H. Diagnostic findings in the oliguric phase
   1. Increased blood urea nitrogen (BUN) and creatinine
   2. Increased potassium (hyperkalemia)
   3. Decreased sodium (hyponatremia)
   4. Decreased pH (acidosis)
   5. Fluid overload (hypervolemic)
   6. High urine specific gravity (>1.020 g/mL)
I. Diagnostic findings in the diuretic phase
   1. Decreased fluid volume (hypovolemia)
   2. Decreased potassium (hypokalemia)
   3. Further decrease in sodium (hyponatremia)
   4. Low urine specific gravity (<1.020 g/mL)
J. Diagnostic laboratory work returns to normal range in recovery phase.

HESI HINT In some cases, persons in AKI may not experience the oliguric phase but may progress directly to the diuretic phase, during which the urine output may be as much as 10 L/day.

HESI HINT Clients at risk for developing AKI in the acute care setting are those with chronic kidney disease (CKD), older age, massive trauma, major surgical procedures, extensive burns, cardiac failure, sepsis, or obstetric complications.

Nursing Plans and Interventions

A. Monitor intake and output (I&O) accurately: fluid restriction during the oliguric phase (600 mL plus previous 24-hour fluid loss)
B. Weigh daily: in oliguric phase, client may gain up to 1 lb/day.
C. Document and report any change in fluid volume status.
D. Nutritional therapy
E. Adequate protein intake (0.6 to 2 g/kg/day) depending on degree of catabolism
F. Monitor laboratory values of both serum and urine to assess electrolyte status, especially hyperkalemia indicated by serum potassium levels over 5 mEq/L and electrocardiogram (ECG) changes.
G. Potassium restriction and measures to lower potassium (if elevated). Sodium polystyrene (Kayexalate) may be prescribed if potassium is too elevated.
H. Restrict sodium.
I. Assess level of consciousness for subtle changes.
J. Prevent cross-infection.

HESI HINT Body weight is a good indicator of fluid retention and renal status. Obtain accurate weights of all clients with renal failure; obtain weight on the same scale at the same time every day.

HESI HINT
Fluid Volume Alterations
Watch for signs of hyperkalemia: dizziness, weakness, cardiac irregularities, muscle cramps, diarrhea, and nausea.

Potassium has a critical safe range (3.5–5.0 mEq/L). Out of range (below or above) affects the heart and any imbalance must be corrected by medications or dietary modification. Limit high-potassium foods (apricots, bananas, orange juice, cantaloupe, strawberries, avocados, spinach, fish) and salt substitutes, which are high in potassium.

Clients with renal failure retain sodium. With water retention, the sodium becomes diluted and serum levels may appear near normal. With excessive water retention, the sodium levels appear decreased (dilution). Limit fluid and sodium intake in AKI clients.

Monitor cardiac rate and rhythm (acute cardiac dysrhythmias are usually related to hyperkalemia).

K. Monitor drug levels and interactions.

HESI HINT During oliguric phase, minimize protein breakdown and prevent rise in BUN by limiting protein intake. When the BUN and creatinine return to normal, acute renal failure (ARF) is determined to be resolved.

Chronic Renal Failure: End-Stage Renal Disease

Description: Progressive, irreversible damage to the nephrons and glomeruli, resulting in uremia
A. Causes of chronic renal failure (CRF) are multitudinous.
B. As renal function diminishes, dialysis becomes necessary.
C. Transplantation is an alternative to dialysis for some clients.

Nursing Assessment

A. History of high medication usage
B. Family history of renal disease
C. Increased blood pressure (BP), uncontrolled BP, and/or chronic hypertension (HTN)
D. Diabetes
E. Edema, pulmonary edema
F. Decreasing urinary function
  1. Hematuria
  2. Proteinuria
  3. Cloudy urine
  4. Oliguric (100 to 400 mL/day)
  5. Anuric (<100 mL/day)

> **HESI HINT** Accumulation of waste products from protein metabolism is the primary cause of uremia. Protein must be restricted in CRF clients. However, if protein intake is inadequate, a negative nitrogen balance occurs, causing muscle wasting. The GFR is most often used as an indicator of the level of protein consumption.

G. Dialysis (Table 4.8)

> **HESI HINT**
> **Dialysis Covered by Medicare**
> - All persons in the United States are eligible for Medicare as of their first day of dialysis under special end-stage renal disease (ESRD) funding.
> - Medicare health card will indicate ESRD.
> - Transplantation is covered by Medicare procedure; coverage terminates 6 months postoperative if dialysis is no longer required.

H. Previous kidney transplant
I. Laboratory information
  1. Azotemia
  2. Increased creatinine and BUN
  3. Decreased calcium
  4. Elevated phosphorus, magnesium, potassium, and sodium
  5. Anemia

> **HESI HINT** Be familiar with the normal laboratory ranges and clinical manifestations of out-of-range values for phosphorus, magnesium, potassium, and sodium.

Nursing Plans and Interventions

A. Monitor serum electrolyte levels.
B. Weigh daily.
C. Monitor strict I&O.
D. Check for jugular vein distention and other signs of fluid overload.
E. Monitor for peripheral edema and pulmonary edema.
F. Provide low-protein, low-sodium, low-potassium, low-phosphate diet.

> **HESI HINT** Protein intake is restricted until blood chemistry shows ability to handle the protein catabolites, urea and creatinine. Ensure high caloric intake so protein is spared for its own work; give hard candy, jellybeans, or flavored carbohydrate powders.

> **HESI HINT** Frequent monitoring of laboratory parameters, especially serum albumin, prealbumin (may be a better indicator of recent or current nutritional status than albumin), and ferritin are necessary to evaluate nutritional status. All clients with CKD should be referred to a dietitian for nutritional education and guidance.

G. Administer phosphate binders with food because client is unable to excrete phosphates (no magnesium-based antacids). Timing is important!
H. Encourage client's protein intake to be of high biologic value (eggs, milk, meat) because the client is on a low-protein diet.
I. Teach client fluid allowance is 500 to 600 mL greater than the previous day's 24-hour output.
J. Alternate periods of rest with periods of activity.
K. Encourage strict adherence to medication regimen; teach client to obtain health care provider's permission before taking any over-the-counter medications.
L. Administer prescribed sodium polystyrene sulfonate (Kayexalate) for acute hyperkalemia.
M. Observe for complications.
  1. Anemia (administer anti-anemic drug; Table 4.9)
  2. Renal osteodystrophy (abnormal calcium metabolism causes bone pathology)
  3. Severe, resistant hypertension
  4. Infection
  5. Metabolic acidosis
N. Living related or cadaver renal transplant (Table 4.10)
  1. Monitor for rejection.
  2. Monitor for infection.
  3. Teach client to maintain immunosuppressive drug therapy meticulously.

Urinary Tract Infections

Description: Infection or inflammation at any site in the urinary tract (kidney, pyelonephritis; urethra, urethritis; bladder, cystitis; prostate, prostatitis)

A. Normally, the entire urinary tract is sterile.
B. The most common infectious agent is *Escherichia coli.*
C. Persons at highest risk for acquiring urinary tract infections (UTIs)
  1. Clients diagnosed with diabetes
  2. Pregnant women
  3. Men with prostatic hypertrophy
  4. Immunosuppressed persons
  5. Catheterized clients
  6. Anyone with urinary retention, either short term or long term
  7. Older women (bladder prolapse)

TABLE 4.8 Renal Dialysis

Types of Dialysis	Description	Nursing Implications
• Hemodialysis	• Requires venous access (AV shunt, fistula, or graft) • Treatment is 3–8 h in length, 3 times per week • Correction of fluid and electrolyte imbalance is rapid • Potential blood loss • Does not result in protein loss	• Heparinization is required. • Requires expensive equipment. • Rapid shifts of fluid and electrolytes can lead to disequilibrium syndrome (an unpleasant sensation and a potentially dangerous situation). • Potential hepatitis B and C • Do *not* take BP or perform venipunctures on the arm with the AV shunt, fistula, or graft. • Assess access site for thrill and bruit.
• Continuous arteriovenous hemofiltration (CAVH)	• Requires vascular access: usually femoral or subclavian catheters • Slow process • Correction of fluid and electrolyte imbalance is slow • Does not cause blood loss • Does not result in protein loss	• Requires heparinization of filter tubing. • Filters are costly. • Equipment is simple to use but requires specialized training to monitor. • Limited to special care units; not for home use. • Filter may rupture, causing blood loss.
• Peritoneal	• Surgical placement of abdominal catheter is required (Tenckhoff, Gore-Tex, column disk) • Slow process; up to 8–10 h for repeated cycles • Correction of fluid and electrolyte imbalance is slow • Does not cause blood loss • Protein is lost in dialysate.	• Heparinization is not required. • Fairly expensive. • Simple to perform. • Easy to use at home. • Dialysate is similar to IV fluid and is prescribed for the individual client's electrolyte needs. • Potential complications: • Bowel or bladder perforation • Exit-site and tunnel infection • Peritonitis

AV, Atrioventricular; *BP*, blood pressure; *IV*, intravenous.

TABLE 4.9 Antianemic: Biologic Response Modifier

Drugs	Indications	Adverse Reactions	Nursing Interventions
• Erythropoietin	• Anemia due to decreased production of erythropoietin in ESRD • Stimulates RBC production, increases Hgb, reticulocyte count, and Hct	• Use with caution in older adults because of increased risk for thrombosis. • Hypertension, seizures, depletion of body iron stores	• Monitor Hct weekly; report levels over 30%–33% and increases of more than 4 points in less than 2 weeks. • Monitor serum iron and ferritin levels. • Monitor BP and potassium levels. • Explain pelvic and limb pain should dissipate after 12 h. • Do not shake vial; shaking may inactivate the glycoprotein. • Discard unused contents; does not contain preservatives.

D. Diagnosis
  1. Clean-catch midstream urine collection for culture to identify specific causative organism
  2. Intravenous pyelogram (IVP) to determine kidney functioning
  3. Cystogram to determine bladder functioning
  4. Cystoscopy to determine bladder or urethral abnormalities

F. Disorientation or confusion in older adults may be a sign of UTI.

Nursing Assessment

A. Signs of infection, including fever and chills
B. Urinary frequency, urgency, or dysuria
C. Hematuria
D. Pain at the costovertebral angle
E. Elevated serum WBCs (>10,000)

Nursing Plans and Interventions

A. Administer antibiotics specific to infectious agent.
B. Instruct client in the appropriate medication regimen.
C. Instruct client to complete full medication regimen.
D. Encourage fluid intake of 3000 mL of fluid/day.
E. Maintain I&O.
F. Administer mild analgesics (phenazopyridine [Pyridium], acetaminophen, or aspirin).
G. Encourage client to void every 2 to 3 hours to prevent residual urine from stagnating in bladder.
H. Avoid unnecessary catheterization.

TABLE 4.10 Postoperative Care: Kidney Surgery

Assessment	Nursing Interventions	Rationale
• Respiratory status	• Auscultate lung sounds to detect "wet" sounds indicating infection. • Demonstrate method of splinting incision for comfort when coughing and deep breathing.	• Flank incision causes pain with both inspiration and expiration. Therefore, client avoids deep breathing and coughing; this can lead to respiratory difficulties, including pneumonia.
• Circulatory status	• Check vital signs to detect early signs of bleeding, shock. • Monitor skin color and temperature (pallor and cold skin are signs of shock). • Monitor urinary output (decreases with circulatory collapse). • Monitor surgical site for frank bleeding.	• The kidney is highly vascular. • Bleeding is a constant threat. • Circulatory collapse will occur with hemorrhage and can occur very quickly.
• Pain relief status	• Administer narcotic analgesics as needed to relieve pain.	• Relief of pain will improve the client's cooperation with deep-breathing exercises. • Relief of pain will improve client's cooperation with early ambulation.
• Urinary status	• Check urinary output and drainage from all tubes inserted during the surgery. • Maintain accurate I&O.	• Mechanical drainage of bladder will be implemented after surgery.

I. Remove indwelling catheters within 24 to 48 hours of insertion during hospitalizations.
J. Routine perineal hygiene especially with use of bedpan or if fecal incontinence is present.

HESI HINT The key to resolving UTIs with most antibiotics is to keep the blood level of the antibiotic constant. It is important to tell the client to take the antibiotics around the clock and not to skip doses so that a consistent blood level can be maintained for optimal effectiveness.

K. Develop and implement a teaching plan.
  1. Take entire prescription as directed.
  2. Consume oral fluids up to 3 L/day (water, juices); should not consume *citrus* juices.
  3. Shower rather than bathe as a preventive measure. If bathing is necessary, never take a bubble or oil bath and avoid feminine hygiene sprays.
  4. Cleanse from front to back after toileting (women and girls).
  5. Avoid urinary tract irritants: alcohol, sodas, citrus juices, spices.
  6. Void immediately after intercourse (women).
  7. Void every 2 to 3 hours during the day.
  8. Wear cotton undergarments and loose clothing to help decrease perineal moisture.
  9. Practice good handwashing technique.
  10. Obtain follow-up care.

Urinary Tract Obstruction

Description: Partial or complete blockage of the flow of urine at any point in the urinary system

A. Urinary tract obstruction may be caused by
  1. Foreign body (calculi)
  2. Tumors
  3. Strictures
  4. Functional (e.g., neurogenic bladder)

B. When urinary tract obstruction occurs, urine is retained above the point of obstruction.
  1. Hydrostatic pressure builds, causing dilation of the organs above the obstruction.
  2. If hydrostatic pressure continues to build, hydronephrosis develops, and it can lead to renal failure.

Nursing Assessment

A. Pain
  1. May experience renal colic
  2. Radiating down the thigh and to the genitalia

B. Symptoms of obstruction
  1. Fever, chills
  2. Nausea, vomiting, diarrhea
  3. Abdominal distention

HESI HINT Location of the pain can help to determine the location of the stone.
- Flank pain usually means the stone is in the kidney or upper ureter. If the pain radiates to the abdomen or scrotum, the stone is likely to be in the ureter or bladder.
- Excruciating spastic-type pain is called *colic.*
- During kidney stone attacks, it is preferable to administer pain medications at regularly scheduled intervals rather than PRN to prevent spasm and optimize comfort.

C. Change in voiding pattern
  1. Dysuria, hematuria
  2. Urgency, frequency, hesitancy, nocturia, dribbling
  3. Difficulty in starting a stream
  4. Incontinence

D. Clients with the following conditions are at risk for developing calculi:
   1. Strictures
   2. Prostatic hypertrophy
   3. Neoplasms
   4. Congenital malformations
   5. History of calculi
   6. Family history of calculi

Nursing Plans and Interventions

A. Administer narcotic analgesics to control pain and alpha-adrenergic blockers to relax smooth muscle in the ureter to facilitate stone passage.
B. Apply moist heat to the painful area unless prescribed otherwise.
C. Encourage high oral fluid intake to help dislodge the stone.
D. Administer intravenous (IV) antibiotics if infection is present.
E. Strain all urine!
F. Send any stones found when straining to the laboratory for analysis.
G. Accurately document I&O.
H. Endourologic procedures
   1. Cystoscopy
   2. Cystolitholapaxy
   3. Ureteroscopy
   4. Percutaneous nephrolithotomy
I. Lithotripsy
   1. Ultrasonic
   2. Electrohydraulic
   3. Laser
   4. Extracorporeal shockwave
J. Surgical therapy
   1. Nephrolithotomy
   2. Pyelolithotomy
   3. Ureterolithotomy
   4. Cystotomy

> **HESI HINT** Percutaneous nephrostomy: a needle or catheter is inserted through the skin into the calyx of the kidney. The stone may be dissolved by percutaneous irrigation with a liquid that dissolves the stone or by ultrasonic sound waves (lithotripsy) that can be directed through the needle or catheter to break up the stone, which then can be eliminated through the urinary tract.

K. Develop and implement a teaching plan to include
   1. Pursue follow-up care, because stones tend to recur.
   2. Maintain a high fluid intake of 3 to 4 L/day.
   3. Follow prescribed diet (based on composition of stone).
   4. Avoid long periods of remaining in supine position.

Benign Prostatic Hyperplasia

Description: Enlargement or hypertrophy of the prostate (sometimes called *hypertrophy of the prostate*)

A. Benign prostatic hyperplasia (BPH) tends to occur in men over 40 years of age.
B. Intervention is required when symptoms of obstruction occur.
C. There are three treatment approaches: active surveillance (watchful waiting), drug therapy with 5-alpha-reductase inhibitors such as finasteride (Proscar) and alpha-adrenergic receptor blockers (tamsulosin), or surgery.
D. The most common treatment is transurethral resection of the prostate gland (TURP). The prostate is removed by endoscopy (no surgical incision is made), allowing for a shorter hospital stay.

Nursing Assessment

A. Increased frequency of voiding, with a decrease in amount of each voiding
B. Nocturia
C. Hesitancy
D. Terminal dribbling
E. Decrease in size and force of stream
F. Acute urinary retention
G. Bladder distention
H. Recurrent UTIs

Nursing Plans and Interventions

A. Preoperative teaching: include information concerning pain from bladder spasms that occurs postoperatively.
B. Maintain patent urinary drainage system (large three-way indwelling catheter with a 30-mL balloon) to decrease the spasms.
C. Provide pain relief as prescribed: analgesics, narcotics, and antispasmodics.
D. Minimize catheter manipulation by taping catheter to abdomen or leg or use a leg strap.
E. Maintain gentle traction on urinary catheter.
F. Check the urinary drainage system for clots.
G. Irrigate bladder as prescribed (may be continuous or rarely intermittent). Bladder spasms frequently occur after TURP. The catheter may cause a continuous sensation of bladder fullness. The client should not try to void around the catheter because bladder spasms may occur. Client can request medication to reduce or prevent spasms.

> **HESI HINT** Instillation of hypertonic or hypotonic solution into a body cavity will cause a shift in cellular fluid. Use only sterile saline for bladder irrigation after TURP because the irrigation must be isotonic to prevent fluid and electrolyte imbalance.
> Clients with indwelling urinary catheters require perineal care *and* actual catheter care twice per day.

H. Observe the color and content of urinary output.

1. Normal drainage after prostate surgery is reddish pink, clearing to light pink within 24 hours after surgery. Some small to medium-sized blood clots may be present.
2. Monitor for bright-red bleeding with large clots and increased viscosity.

I. Monitor vital signs frequently for indication of hemorrhagic or hypovolemic shock (circulatory collapse).

J. Monitor hemoglobin (Hgb) and hematocrit (Hct) for pattern of decreasing values that indicates bleeding.

K. After catheter is removed
1. Monitor amount and number of times client voids.
2. Encourage fluids.
3. Have the client use urine cups to provide a specimen with each voiding.
4. Observe for hematuria after each voiding (urine should progress to clear yellow color by the fourth day).
5. Inform client that burning on urination and urinary frequency are usually experienced during the first post-operative week.
6. Generally, the client is not impotent after surgery, but sterility may occur.
7. Instruct client to report any frank bleeding to physician immediately.
8. Monitor for signs of urethral stricture: straining, dysuria, weak urinary stream.
9. Administer antispasmodics as ordered.
10. Ambulate first postop day, if possible.

L. Instruct client to increase fluid intake to 3000 mL/day.

M. Prepare client for discharge with instructions to
1. Continue to drink 12 to 14 glasses of water a day.
2. Avoid constipation, straining.
3. Avoid strenuous activity, lifting, intercourse, and engaging in sports during the first 3 to 4 weeks after surgery.
4. Schedule a follow-up appointment.

HESI HINT Inform the client before discharge that some bleeding is expected after TURP. Large amounts of blood or frank bright bleeding should be reported. However, it is normal for the client to pass small amounts of blood, as well as small clots, during the healing process. He should rest quietly and continue drinking large amounts of fluid.

REVIEW OF RENAL SYSTEM

1. Differentiate between ARF and CRF.
2. During the oliguric phase of renal failure, protein should be severely restricted. What is the rationale for this restriction?
3. Identify two nursing interventions for the client on hemodialysis.
4. A client in renal failure asks why antacids are being given. How should the nurse reply?
5. List four essential elements of a teaching plan for clients with frequent UTIs.
6. What are the most important nursing interventions for clients with possible renal calculi?
7. What discharge instructions should be given to a client who has had urinary calculi?
8. After TURP, hematuria should subside by what postoperative day?
9. After the urinary catheter is removed in the TURP client, what are three priority nursing actions?
10. After kidney surgery, what are the primary assessments the nurse should make?

See Answer Key at the end of this text for suggested responses.

CARDIOVASCULAR SYSTEM

HESI HINT What is the relationship of the kidneys to the cardiovascular system?
- The kidneys filter about 1 L of blood per minute.
- If cardiac output is decreased, the amount of blood going through the kidneys is decreased; urinary output is decreased. Therefore, a decreased urinary output may be an indication of cardiac problems.
- When the kidneys produce and excrete 0.5 mL of urine/kg of body weight or average 30 mL/h output, the blood supply is considered to be minimally adequate to perfuse the vital organs.

Angina

Description: Chest discomfort or pain that occurs when myocardial O_2 demands exceed supply

Common Causes

A. Atherosclerotic heart disease

B. Hypertension

C. Coronary artery spasm

D. Hypertrophic cardiomyopathy

E. Any activity that increases the heart's O_2 demand; physical exertion, cold temperatures

Nursing Assessment

A. Pain
1. Mild to severe intensity, described as heavy, squeezing, pressing, burning, choking, aching, and feeling of apprehension
2. Substernal, radiating to left arm and/or shoulder, jaw, right shoulder
3. Transient or prolonged, with gradual or sudden onset; typically of short duration

4. Often precipitated by exercise, exposure to cold, a heavy meal, mental tension, sexual intercourse
5. Relieved by rest and/or nitroglycerin

B. Dyspnea, tachycardia, palpitations
C. Nausea, vomiting
D. Fatigue
E. Diaphoresis, pallor, weakness
F. Syncope
G. Dysrhythmias
H. Diagnostic information
   1. ECG: Is generally at client baseline unless taken during anginal attack, when ST-segment depression and T-wave inversion may occur
   2. Exercise stress test: Shows ST-segment depression and hypotension
   3. Stress echocardiogram: Looks for changes in wall motion (indicated in women)
   4. Coronary angiogram: Detects coronary artery spasms
   5. Cardiac catheterization: Detects arterial blockage
I. Risk factors
   1. Nonmodifiable
      a. Heredity
      b. Gender: male > female until menopause, then equal risk
      c. Ethnic background: African American
      d. Age
   2. Modifiable
      a. Hyperlipidemia
      b. Total serum cholesterol above 300 mg/dL: four times greater risk for developing coronary artery disease (CAD) than those with levels less than 200 mg/dL (desirable level)
      c. Low-density lipoprotein (LDL), "bad cholesterol": A molecule of LDL is approximately 50% cholesterol by weight (<100 mg/dL desirable).
      d. High-density lipoprotein (HDL), "good cholesterol": HDL is inversely related to the risk for developing CAD (>60 mg/dL is desirable). In fact, HDL may serve to remove cholesterol from tissues.
      e. Hypertension
      f. Cigarette smoking
      g. Obesity
      h. Physical inactivity
      i. Metabolic syndrome
      j. Stress
      k. Elevated homocysteine level
      l. Substance abuse

Nursing Plans and Interventions

A. Monitor medications and instruct client in proper administration.
B. Determine factors precipitating pain and assist client and family in adjusting lifestyle to decrease these factors.
C. Teach risk factors and identify client's own risk factors.
D. During an attack
   1. Provide immediate rest.
   2. Take vital signs.
   3. Record an ECG.
   4. Administer no more than three nitroglycerin tablets, 5 minutes apart (Table 4.11).
   5. Seek emergency treatment if no relief has occurred after taking nitroglycerin.
E. Physical activity
   1. Teach avoidance of isometric activity.
   2. Implement an exercise program.
   3. Teach that sexual activity may be resumed after exercise is tolerated, usually when able to climb two flights of stairs without exertion. Nitroglycerin can be taken prophylactically before intercourse.
F. Provide nutritional information about modifying fats (saturated) and sodium. Antilipemic medications may be prescribed to lower cholesterol levels (Table 4.12).
G. Medical interventions include
   1. Percutaneous transluminal coronary angioplasty (PTCA), also known as *percutaneous coronary intervention (PCI)*. A balloon catheter is repeatedly inflated to split or fracture plaque, and the arterial wall is stretched, enlarging the diameter of the vessel and pulverizing plaque.
   2. Arthrectomy: A catheter with a collection chamber is used to remove plaque from a coronary artery by shaving, cutting, or grinding.
   3. Coronary artery bypass graft (CABG)
   4. Coronary laser therapy
   5. Coronary artery stent or drug-eluting stents

Myocardial Infarction (MI)

Description: Myocardial infarction (MI) is the disruption in or deficiency of coronary artery blood supply, resulting in necrosis of myocardial tissue.

Causes of MI

A. Thrombus or clotting
B. Shock or hemorrhage

Nursing Assessment

A. Sudden onset of pain in the lower sternal region (substernal)
   1. Severity increases until it becomes nearly unbearable.
   2. Heavy and viselike pain often radiates to the shoulders and down the arms and/or to the neck, jaw, and back. Common locations for pain are substernal, retrosternal, or epigastric areas. Pain of MI differs from angina pain in its sudden onset.
      a. Women may also present with shortness of breath or fatigue.
      b. Pain differs from anginal pain in its onset.
   3. Pain is not relieved by rest.
   4. Nausea and vomiting
   5. Anxiety, feeling of impending doom/death
   6. Pain is not relieved by nitroglycerin.
   7. Pain may persist for hours or days.
   8. Client may not have pain (silent MI), especially those with diabetic neuropathy.
B. Rapid, irregular, and thready pulse
C. Decreased level of consciousness indicating decreased cerebral perfusion

TABLE 4.11 Antianginals

Drugs	Indications/Actions	Adverse Reactions	Nursing Implications
Nitrates • Nitroglycerin (NTG) • Isosorbide dinitrate • Isosorbide mononitrate	• Anginal prophylaxis • Acute attack • Reduces vascular resistance	• Headache • Flushing • Dizziness • Weakness • Hypotension • Nausea	• Monitor relief. • Have client rest. • Monitor vital signs. • Store medication in original container. • Protect from light.
BETA BLOCKERS			
• Propranolol HCl Atenolol • Nadolol • Metoprolol	• Anginal prophylaxis • Reduces O_2 demand	• Fatigue • Lethargy • Hallucinations • Impotence • Bradycardia • Hypotension • HF • Wheezing	• Monitor apical HR. • Assess for decreased BP. • Do not stop medication abruptly. • Clients with HF, bronchitis, asthma, COPD, or renal or hepatic insufficiency have increased likelihood of incurring adverse reactions.
CALCIUM CHANNEL BLOCKERS			
• Verapamil • Nifedipine HCl Diltiazem HCl	• Anginal prophylaxis • Inhibits influx of calcium ions • Decreases sinoatrial node automaticity and AV node conduction	• Dizziness • Hypotension • Fatigue • Headache • Syncope • Peripheral edema • Hypokalemia • Dysrhythmia • HF • Gastric distress	• Clients with HF and older adults have an increased likelihood of incurring adverse reactions. • Assess for decreased BP. • Monitor serum potassium. • Swallow pills whole. • Store at room temperature. • Do not stop abruptly. • Take 1 h before meals or 2 h after meals.
OTHER			
• Ranolazine	• Anginal prophylaxis • Inhibits influx of sodium ions	• Dysrhythmia • Constipation	• Many drug–drug interactions. • Contraindication in all levels of hepatic cirrhosis.

AV, Atrioventricular; *BP,* blood pressure; *COPD,* chronic obstructive pulmonary disease; *HR,* heart rate; *HF,* heart failure.

D. Left heart shift sometimes occurring after MI
E. Cardiac dysrhythmias, occurring in about 90% of MI clients
F. Cardiogenic shock or fluid retention
G. Serum cardiac markers
   1. Cardiac-specific troponin is a myocardial muscle protein released into circulation after MI or injury with greater sensitivity and specificity for myocardial injury than creatine kinase-muscle/brain (CK-MB).
   2. Creatine kinase (CK), intracellular enzymes that are released into circulation after an MI, can also be elevated after other intracoronary procedures.
      a. Rise 3 to 12 hours after an MI
      b. Peak within up to 24 hours
      c. Return to normal within 2 to 3 days
   3. CK-MB band is specific to myocardial cells and can help quantify myocardial damage.
      a. Cardiac-specific troponin T (cTnT) and cardiac-specific troponin I (cTnI)
      b. Increase 3 to 12 hours after the onset of MI
      c. Peak at 10 to 24 hours
      d. Return to baseline over 5 to 14 days
H. Narrowed pulse pressure; for example, 90/80 mm Hg
I. Bowel sounds are absent or high pitched, indicating possibility of mesenteric artery thrombosis, which acts as an intestinal obstruction. (See "Gastrointestinal System," later in this chapter.)
J. HF indicated by crackles in the lungs sounds
K. ECG changes occur as early as 2 hours after MI or as late as 72 hours after MI (Table 4.13)
L. Nausea, vomiting, gastric discomfort, indigestion
M. Anxiety, restlessness, feeling of impending doom or death
N. Cool, pale, diaphoretic skin
O. Dizziness, fatigue, syncope

> **HESI HINT** Women more commonly experience dyspnea, unusual fatigue, and sleep disturbances.

Nursing Plans and Interventions

A. Administer medications as prescribed.
   1. For pain and to increase O_2 perfusion, IV morphine sulfate acts as a peripheral vasodilator and decreases venous return

TABLE 4.12 Antilipemics

Drugs	Indications	Adverse Reactions	Nursing Implications
BILE SEQUESTRANTS			
• Colestipol HCl Colesevelam • Cholestyramine	• Treat type IIA hyperlipidemia (hypercholesterolemia) when dietary changes fail	• Abdominal pain, nausea and vomiting, distention, flatulence, belching, constipation • Reduced absorption of lipid-soluble vitamins: A, D, E, and K • Alteration in absorption of other oral medications	• Teach client to mix powder forms with adequate amounts of liquid or fruits high in moisture content such as applesauce to prevent accidental inhalation or esophageal distress. • Monitor PTs. • Assess for visual changes and rickets • Administer other oral medications 1 h before or 6 h after giving bile sequestrants.
HMG-COA REDUCTASE INHIBITORS (STATINS)			
• Atorvastatin • Fluvastatin • Pravastatin • Simvastatin • Lovastatin • Pitavastatin • Rosuvastatin		• Side effects similar to bile sequestrants • May elevate liver enzymes • Hepatitis or pancreatitis • Rhabdomyolysis	• Obtain liver enzymes baseline and monitor every 6 months. • Monitor creatine phosphokinase (CPK) levels. • Review specific drug—food interactions; avoid grapefruit juice. • Timing with or without food varies with drug. • Instruct client to report any muscle tenderness. • Monitor dose limits when interacting medications prescribed.
FIBRIC ACID DERIVATIVES			

• Gemfibrate
• Fenofibrate
• Fenofibric acid
• Clofibrate
	• Used with diet changes to lower elevated cholesterol and triglycerides	• Abdominal and epigastric pain; diarrhea—most common
		• Flatulence, nausea, and vomiting
		• Heartburn
		• Dyspepsia
		• Gallstones
		• Tricor: weakness, fatigue, headache
		• Myopathy
			• Obtain baseline laboratories: liver function, Complete blood count (CBC), and electrolytes; monitor every 3–6 months.
			• Administer
			  • Lopid: 30 min before breakfast and dinner
			  • Tricor: with meals

WATER-SOLUBLE VITAMINS			
• Niacin • Nicotinic acid	• Large doses decrease lipoprotein and triglyceride synthesis and increase HDL	• Flushing of face and neck • Pruritus • Headache • Orthostatic hypotension • (ER form): Hepatotoxicity • Hyperglycemia • Hyperuricemia • Upper GI distress	• Give with milk or food to avoid GI irritation. • Client to change positions slowly. • Instruct client taking extended-release (ER) form to report darkened urine, light-colored stools, anorexia, yellowing of eyes or skin, severe stomach pain.

GI, Gastrointestinal; *HDL,* high-density lipoprotein.

TABLE 4.13 Postmyocardial Infarction Cardiac Enzyme Elevations

Enzyme/Marker	Onset	Peak	Return to Normal
CK-MB (recognized indicator of MI by most clinicians)	4.8 h	12–24 h	48–72 h
Myoglobin	1–4 h (elevate before CK-MB)	12 h	24 h
Cardiac troponins	As early as 1 h postinjury	10–24 h	5–14 days

2. Other medications often prescribed include (see Table 4.11):
   a. Nitrates (e.g., nitroglycerin)
   b. ACE inhibitors
   c. Beta blockers
   d. Calcium channel blockers (when beta blockers are contraindicated)
   e. Aspirin
   f. Antiplatelet aggregates

B. Obtain vital signs, including ECG rhythm strip regularly, per agency policy.
C. Administer O_2 at 2 to 6 L per nasal cannula.
D. Obtain cardiac enzymes as prescribed.
E. Provide a quiet, restful environment.
F. Assess breath sounds for rales (indicating pulmonary edema).
G. Maintain patent IV line for administration of emergency medications.

H. Monitor fluid balance.
I. Keep in semi-Fowler position to assist with breathing.
J. Maintain bed rest for 12 hours.
K. Encourage client to resume activity gradually.
L. Encourage verbalization of fears.
M. Provide information about the disease process and cardiac rehabilitation.
N. Consider medical interventions (see HESI Hint regarding angina):
   1. Thrombolytic agents, within 1 to 4 hours of MI, but not more than 12 hours after MI (Table 4.14)
   2. Intraaortic balloon pump (IABP) to improve myocardial perfusion
   3. Surgical reperfusion with CABG
   4. PCI with stenting.

> **HESI HINT** Remember MONA when administering medications and treatments in the client with MI. MONA: **m**orphine, **o**xygen, **n**itroglycerin, **a**spirin.

Hypertension

Description: Persistent seated BP levels equal to or greater than 140/90 mm Hg

A. Essential (primary) hypertension has no known cause (idiopathic).
B. Secondary hypertension develops in response to an identifiable mechanism or another disease.

> **HESI HINT** BP is created by the difference in the pressure of the blood as it leaves the heart and the resistance it meets flowing out to the tissues. Diet and exercise, smoking cessation, weight control, and stress management can control many factors that influence the resistance blood meets as it flows from the heart.

Nursing Assessment

A. BP equal to or greater than 140/90 mm Hg on two separate occasions
   1. Obtain BP while client is lying down, sitting, and standing.
   2. Compare readings taken lying down, sitting, and standing. A difference of more than 10 mm Hg of either systolic or diastolic indicates postural hypotension. Take pressure in both arms.
B. Genetic risk factors (nonmodifiable)
   Positive family history for hypertension

TABLE 4.14 Fibrinolytic Agents

Drugs	Indications	Adverse Reactions	Nursing Implications
• Streptokinase	• DVT • Pulmonary embolism • Arterial thrombosis and embolism • Coronary thrombosis • Dissolving clots in arteriovenous cannula	• Anaphylactic response ranging from breathing difficulties to bronchospasm, periorbital swelling, or angioneurotic edema • Increased risk for bleeding • Hemorrhagic infarction at site of myocardial damage • Reperfusion dysrhythmias	• Assess for bleeding at puncture site; apply pressure to control bleeding. • Assess for allergic reactions and dysrhythmias during intracoronary perfusion. • Immobilize client's leg for 24 h after femoral coronary cannulation and perfusion; assess pedal pulses for adequate circulation. • Monitor client's thrombin time after therapy. Do *not* administer heparin or oral anticoagulants until thrombin time is less than twice that of control. • Do *not* shake vial when reconstituting; roll and tilt vial gently to mix.
• Tenecteplase • Reteplase	• Acute management of coronary thrombosis	• Do not give if history of uncontrolled hypertension. • Can cause hypotension	• Obtain baseline studies before administration: PT, PTT, CBC, fibrinogen level, renal studies, cardiac enzymes. • Check for abnormal pulse, neurologic vital signs, and presence of skin lesions, which may indicate coagulation defects. • Avoid needle punctures because of the possibility of bleeding; apply pressure for 10 min to venous puncture sites and for 30 min to arterial puncture sites; follow with pressure dressing. • Be prepared to treat reperfusion dysrhythmias.
• Urokinase	• Pulmonary embolism • Coronary thrombosis • IV catheter clearance	• Is nonantigenic and does not cause allergic reactions; otherwise has the same adverse reactions as those cited for streptokinase.	• Infuse heparin and an oral anticoagulant after urokinase therapy to prevent rethrombosis. • Is much more expensive than streptokinase, but does not cause allergic reactions found with streptokinase therapy. • Reconstitute immediately before use.
• Alteplase • Anistreplase	• DVT • Pulmonary embolism • Coronary thrombosis	• Interacts with heparin, oral anticoagulants, and antiplatelet drugs to increase the risk for bleeding.	• Alters coagulation only at the thrombus, *not* systemically (bleeding complications associated with streptokinase and urokinase are reduced with t-PA therapy). • Because t-PA is a human protein, allergic response is unlikely to occur. • Half-life is 3–7 min; use immediately.

DVT, Deep vein thrombosis; *IV,* intravenous; *PT,* prothrombin time; *PTT,* partial thromboplastin time.

1. Gender (Men have a greater risk for being hypertensive at an earlier age than women.)
2. Age (Risk increases with increasing age.)
3. Ethnicity (African Americans are at greater risk than Whites.)

C. Lifestyle and habits that increase risk for becoming hypertensive (modifiable)
1. Use of alcohol, tobacco, and caffeine
2. Sedentary lifestyle, obesity
3. Nutrition history of high salt and fat intake
4. Use of oral contraceptives or estrogens
5. Stress

D. Associated physical problems
1. Renal failure
2. Impaired renal function
3. Respiratory problems, especially COPD
4. Cardiac problems, especially valvular disorders
5. Dyslipidemia
6. Diabetes

E. Pharmacologic history
1. Steroids (increase BP)
2. Estrogens (increase BP)

F. Assess for headache, edema, nocturia, nosebleeds, and vision changes (may be asymptomatic).

G. Assess level of stress and source of stress (related to job, economics, family).

H. Assess personality type (i.e., determine whether client exhibits perfectionist behavior).

> **HESI HINT** Remember the risk factors for hypertension; heredity, race, age, alcohol abuse, increased salt intake, obesity, and use of oral contraceptives.

Nursing Plans and Interventions

A. Develop a teaching plan to include
1. Information about disease process
   a. Risk factors
   b. Causes
   c. Long-term complications
   d. Lifestyle modifications
   e. Relationship of treatment to prevention of complications
2. Information about treatment plan
   a. How to take own BP
   b. Reasons for each medication (Tables 4.15 and 4.16)
   c. How and when to take each medication
   d. Necessity of consistency in medication regimen
   e. Need for ongoing assessment while taking antihypertensives

> **HESI HINT** The number-one cause of a stroke in hypertensive clients is noncompliance with medication regimen. Hypertension is often symptomless, and antihypertensive medications are expensive and have side effects. Studies have shown that the more clients know about their antihypertensive medications, the more likely they are to take them; teaching is important!

   f. Need to monitor serum electrolytes every 90 to 120 days for duration of treatment
   g. Need to monitor renal functioning (BUN and creatinine) every 90 to 120 days for duration of treatment
   h. Need to monitor BP and pulse rate, usually weekly

B. Encourage client to implement nonpharmacologic measures to assist with BP control, such as
1. Stress reduction
2. Weight loss
3. Tobacco cessation
4. Exercise

C. Determine medication side effects experienced by client (see Table 4.16).
1. Impotence
2. Insomnia

D. Provide nutrition guidance, including a sample meal plan and how to dine out (low-salt, low-fat, low-cholesterol diet).

Peripheral Vascular Disease

Description: Circulatory problems that can be due to arterial or venous pathology

Nursing Assessment

A. The signs, symptoms, and treatment of peripheral vascular disease (PVD) can vary widely, depending on the source of pathology. Therefore, careful assessment is very important.

B. Predisposing factors
1. Arterial
   a. Arteriosclerosis (95% of all cases are caused by atherosclerosis)
   b. Advanced age
2. Venous
   a. History of deep vein thrombosis (DVT)
   b. Valvular incompetence

C. Associated diseases
1. Arterial
   a. Raynaud disease (nonatherosclerotic, triggered by extreme heat or cold, spasms of the arteries)
   b. Buerger disease (occlusive inflammatory disease, strongly associated with smoking)
   c. Diabetes
   d. Acute occlusion (emboli/thrombi)
2. Venous
   a. Varicose veins
   b. Thrombophlebitis
   c. Venous stasis ulcers

D. Skin
1. Arterial
   a. Smooth skin
   b. Shiny skin

TABLE 4.15 **Diuretics**

Drugs	Indications	Adverse Reactions	Nursing Implications
		THIAZIDES	

• Chlorthalidone
• Hydrochlorothiazide
• Indapamide
• Metolazone
	• To decrease fluid volume
	• To increase excretion of water, sodium, potassium, and chloride
	• Inexpensive
	• Effective
	• Useful in severe hypertension
	• Effective orally
	• Enhances other antihypertensives
		• Hypokalemia symptoms include
		  • Dry mouth
		  • Thirst
		  • Weakness
		  • Drowsiness
		  • Lethargy
		  • Muscle aches
		  • Tachycardia
		  • Hyperuricemia
		  • Glucose intolerance
		  • Hypercholesterolemia
		  • Sexual dysfunction
			• Observe for postural hypotension; can be potentiated by
			  • Alcohol
			  • Barbiturates
			  • Narcotics
			• Caution with
			  • Renal failure
			  • Gout
			  • Client taking lithium
			• Hypokalemia increases risk for digitalis toxicity.
			• Administer potassium supplements.
			• Encourage intake of potassium-rich foods.

		LOOP	
• Furosemide • Torsemide • Bumetanide	• Rapid action • Potent for use when thiazides fail • Cause volume depletion	• Hypokalemia • Hyperuricemia • Glucose intolerance • Hypercholesterolemia • Hypertriglyceridemia • Sexual dysfunction • Weakness	• Volume depletion and electrolyte depletion are rapid. • All nursing implications cited for thiazides.
		POTASSIUM-SPARING	
• Spironolactone • Amiloride • Triamterene • Eplerenone	• Volume depletion without significant potassium loss	• Hyperkalemia • Gynecomastia • Sexual dysfunction	• Watch for hyperkalemia and renal failure in those treated with ACE inhibitors or NSAIDs. • Watch for increase in serum lithium levels. • Give after meals to decrease GI distress.
		COMBINATION THIAZIDE AND POTASSIUM-SPARING	
• HCTZ and Triamterene • HCTZ + Amiloride HCTZ + Spironolactone	• Decreases fluid volume while minimizing potassium loss	• Side effects of individual drug offset or minimized by its partner	• Caution client previously on a loop or thiazide alone not to overdo potassium foods now because of potassium-sparing component in new drug. • Follow scheduling doses to avoid sleep disruption.

ACE, Angiotensin-converting enzyme; *NSAIDs*, nonsteroidal anti-inflammatory drugs.

c. Loss of hair
d. Thickened nails
e. Dry, thin skin
2. Venous
a. Brown pigment around ankles

E. Color
1. Arterial
a. Pallor on elevation
b. Rubor when dependent
2. Venous—cyanotic when dependent

F. Temperature
1. Arterial
a. Cool
2. Venous
a. Warm

G. Pulses
1. Arterial
a. Decreased or absent
2. Venous
a. Normal

H. Pain
1. Arterial
a. Sharp
b. Increases with walking and elevation
c. Intermittent claudication: classic presenting symptom; occurs in skeletal muscles during exercise; is relieved by rest
d. Rest pain: occurs when the extremities are horizontal; may be relieved by dependent position; often appears when collateral circulation fails to develop

TABLE 4.16 Antihypertensives

Drugs	Indications	Adverse Reactions	Nursing Implications
ALPHA-ADRENERGIC BLOCKERS			
• Prazosin HCl • Terazosin • Phentolamine mesylate • Doxazosin	• Used as peripheral vasodilator that acts directly on the blood vessels • Used in extreme hypertension of pheochromocytoma	• Orthostatic hypotension • Weakness • Palpitations	• Use cautiously in older clients. • Occasional vomiting and diarrhea • Warn clients of possible: • Drowsiness • Lack of energy • Weakness
COMBINED ALPHA/BETA BLOCKERS			

• Labetalol
• Carvedilol
	• Produces decrease in BP without reflex tachycardia or bradycardia	• HF
		• Ventricular dysrhythmias
		• Blood dyscrasias
		• Bronchospasm
		• Orthostatic hypotension
			• Contraindicated with
			  • HF
			  • Heart block
			  • COPD
			  • Asthma

BETA BLOCKERS			
• Metoprolol tartrate • Nadolol • Propranolol HCl • Timolol maleate • Atenolol • Bisoprolol • Metoprolol	• Blocks the sympathetic nervous system, especially to the heart • Produces a slower HR • Lowers BP • Reduces O_2 consumption during myocardial contraction	• Bradycardia • Fatigue • Insomnia • Bizarre dreams • Sexual dysfunction • Hypertriglyceridemia • Decreased HDL • Depression	• Check apical or radial pulse daily. • Monitor for GI distress. • Do not discontinue abruptly. • Watch for shortness of breath; give cautiously with bronchospasm. • Do not vary how taken (with or without food). • Do not vary time taken. • May mask symptoms of hypoglycemia or may prolong a hypoglycemic reaction • Contraindicated in asthma
CENTRAL-ACTING INHIBITORS			
• Clonidine • Guanabenz acetate • Guanfacine • Methyldopa	• Decreases BP by stimulating central alpha receptors, resulting in decreased sympathetic outflow from the brain	• Drowsiness • Dry mouth • Fatigue • Sexual dysfunction	• Watch for rebound hypertension if abruptly discontinued. • Use caution to make position changes slowly, avoid standing still and taking hot baths and showers.
VASODILATORS			
• Hydralazine HCl • Minoxidil	• Decreases BP by decreasing peripheral resistance	• Headache • Tachycardia • Fluid retention (HF, pulmonary edema) • Postural hypotension	• Monitor BP, pulse routinely. • Observe for peripheral edema. • Monitor I&O. • Weigh daily.
ANGIOTENSIN II RECEPTOR ANTAGONISTS			
• Losartan • Valsartan • Irbesartan • Azilsartan • Candesartan • Eprosartan • Olmesartan • Telmisartan	• Blocks the vasoconstrictor and aldosterone-producing effects of angiotensin II at various sites (vascular smooth muscle and adrenal glands)	• Hypotension • Fatigue • Hepatitis • Renal failure • Hyperkalemia (rare)	• Monitor liver enzymes, electrolytes. • Monitor for angioedema in those with history of it when on ACE inhibitors previously.
ANGIOTENSIN-CONVERTING ENZYME (ACE) INHIBITORS			
• Captopril • Enalapril maleate • Lisinopril • Ramipril • Benazepril • Quinapril • Fosinopril • Moexipril • Trandolapril	• Decreases BP by suppressing renin-angiotensin aldosterone system and inhibiting conversion of angiotensin I into angiotensin II • Useful with clients diagnosed with diabetes	• Proteinuria • Neutropenia • Skin rash • Cough	• Observe for ARF (reversible). • Routine renal function tests. • Remain in bed 3 h after first dose.

Continued

CALCIUM CHANNEL BLOCKERS			
• Diltiazem • Nifedipine • Verapamil HCl • Nisoldipine • Felodipine • Nicardipine • Amlodipine	• Inhibits calcium ion influx during cardiac depolarization • Decreases SA/AV node conduction	• Headache • Hypotension • Dizziness • Edema • Nausea • Constipation • Tachycardia • HF • Dry cough	• Check BP and pulse routinely. • Limit caffeine consumption. • Take medications before meals. • Avoid grapefruit juice with these drugs; it increases serum levels, causing hypotension. • High-fat meals elevate serum levels.

ARF, Acute renal failure; *BP,* blood pressure; *GI,* gastrointestinal; *HDL,* high-density lipoprotein; *HF,* heart failure; *HR,* heart rate; *COPD,* chronic obstructive pulmonary disease.

2. Venous
   a. Persistent, aching, full feeling, dull sensation
   b. Relieved when horizontal (elevate and use compression stockings)
   c. Nocturnal cramps

I. Ulcers
1. Arterial
   a. Usually very painful; however, occasionally may not be painful
   b. Occur on lateral lower legs, toes, heels
   c. Demarcated edges
   d. Small, but deep
   e. Circular in shape
   f. Necrotic
   g. Not edematous
2. Venous
   a. Slightly painful (dull ache or heaviness)
   b. Occur on medial legs, ankles
   c. Uneven edges
   d. Superficial, but large
   e. Marked edema
   f. Highly exudative

Treatment

A. Noninvasive treatment
1. Arterial
   a. Elimination of smoking
   b. Topical antibiotic
   c. Saline dressing
   d. Bed rest, immobilization
   e. Fibrinolytic agents if clots are the problem (not used for Raynaud or Buerger disease; see Table 4.14)
2. Venous
   a. Systemic antibiotics
   b. Compression dressing (snug) or alginate dressing if ulcerated
   c. Limb elevation
   d. For thrombosis: fibrinolytic agents (see Table 4.14) and anticoagulants (Table 4.17)

B. Surgery
1. Arterial
   a. Embolectomy: removal of clot
   b. Endarterectomy: removal of clot and stripping of plaque
   c. Arterial bypass: Teflon or Dacron graft or autograft
   d. Percutaneous transluminal angioplasty (PTA): compression of plaque
   e. Amputation: removal of extremity
2. Venous
   a. Vein ligation
   b. Thrombectomy
   c. Debridement

Nursing Plans and Interventions

A. Monitor extremities at designated intervals.
1. Color
2. Temperature
3. Sensation and pulse quality in extremities

B. Schedule activities within client's tolerance level.
C. Encourage rest at the first sign of pain.
D. Encourage client to keep extremities elevated (if venous) when sitting and to change position often.
E. Encourage client to avoid crossing legs and to wear nonrestrictive clothing.
F. Encourage client to keep the extremities warm by wearing extra clothing, such as socks and slippers, and not to use external heat sources such as electric heating pads.
G. Teach methods of preventing further injury.
1. Change position frequently.
2. Wear nonrestrictive clothing (no knee-high hose).
3. Avoid crossing legs or keeping legs in a dependent position.
4. Wear support hose or antiembolism stockings.
5. Wear shoes when ambulating.
6. Obtain proper foot and nail care.

HESI HINT Decreased blood flow results in diminished sensation in the lower extremities. Any heat source can cause severe burns before the client realizes damage is being done.

H. Discourage cigarette smoking (causes vasoconstriction and spasm of arteries).

TABLE 4.17 Anticoagulants

Drugs	Indications	Adverse Reactions	Nursing Implications
• Heparin sodium	• Administered parenterally (SQ or IV) as an antagonist to thrombin and to prevent the conversion of fibrinogen to fibrin	• Hemorrhage • Agranulocytosis • Leukopenia • Hepatitis • Heparin-induced thrombocytopenia	• Assess PTT, Hgb, Hct, platelets. • Assess stools for occult blood. • Avoid IM injection. • Notify anyone performing diagnostic testing of medication. • *Antagonist:* protamine sulfate
• Warfarin sodium	• Blocks the formation of prothrombin from vitamin K	• Hemorrhage • Agranulocytosis • Leukopenia • Hepatitis	• See "Heparin sodium," earlier. • Given orally. • Assess PT. • Avoid sudden change in intake of foods high in vitamin K. • *Antagonist:* vitamin K.
Antiplatelet Agents Ticlopidine Dipyridamole Clopidogrel Prasugrel Ticagrelor	• Short-term use after cardiac interventions • Reduce risk for thrombolytic stroke for those intolerant to aspirin • Prevention of thrombolytic disorders	• Neutropenia • Thrombocytopenia • Agranulocytosis • Leukopenia • Hemorrhage • GI irritation, bleeding • Pancytopenia	• Give PO or with food to decrease gastric irritation with ticlopidine (Ticlid). • Advise not to take antacids within 2 h of taking ticlopidine. • Monitor CBC every 2 weeks for 3 months, and thereafter if signs of infection develop. • Monitor for signs of bleeding. • Give 1 h AC (Persantine); (Plavix) no regard for meals
Low-Molecular–Weight Heparins • Enoxaparin • Tinzaparin • Dalteparin	• Prevention of thrombolytic formation (deep vein)	• Hemorrhage • GI irritation, bleeding • Thrombocytopenia	• Monitor for signs of bleeding. • Give subcutaneously. • Monitor CBC. • Use soft toothbrush; avoid cuts.
Factor Xa Inhibitor • Fondaparinux	• Prevention of thrombolytic formation (deep vein)	• Hemorrhage • GI irritation, bleeding	• Monitor for signs of bleeding. • Give subcutaneously. • Monitor CBC. • Use soft toothbrush; avoid cuts.
Group IIa-IIIb Inhibitor (Platelet Antiaggregant) • Eptifibatide • Tirofiban • Abciximab	• Acute coronary syndrome (unstable angina or non–Q wave MI) • Used in combination with heparin, aspirin, and, in selected situations, Ticlid and Plavix	• Bleeding, most frequent • Hypotension • Thrombocytopenia • Acute toxicity: decreased muscle tone, dyspnea, loss of righting reflex	• Check drug–drug interactions before giving other medications. • Obtain baseline PT/aPTT, Hgb, Hct, and platelet count, and monitor. • Dose adjusted by weight for older adults • Same client teaching as with heparin; review activities to avoid. • Watch for bleeding. • Quickly reversible, so emergency procedures may still be performed shortly after discontinuing infusion.

New Oral Anticoagulants (NOAC) • Dabigatran • Rivaroxaban • Apixaban	For all three: • Prevention of VTE in orthopedic surgery • Prevention of stroke and systemic embolism in clients with atrial fibrillation	• >50% in anticoagulant plasma when used with ketoconazole • Quinidine • Verapamil • <50% in anticoagulant plasma concentrations when used with carbamazepine, rifampin, St John's wort • > risk of bleeding with acetylsalicylic acid (aspirin) (ASA), NSAID, platelet aggregation inhibitors, anticoagulants, thrombolytics • >50% in anticoagulant plasma when used with clarithromycin, ketoconazole, ritonavir • <50% in anticoagulant plasma concentrations when used with carbamazepine, phenytoin, phenobarbital, rifampin, St John's wort • > risk of bleeding with ASA, NSAID, platelet aggregation inhibitors, anticoagulants, thrombolytics • >50% in anticoagulant plasma when used with ketoconazole, itraconazole, ritonavir • <50% in anticoagulant plasma concentrations when used with carbamazepine, phenobarbital, phenytoin rifampin, St John's wort • > risk of bleeding with ASA, NSAID, platelet aggregation inhibitors, anticoagulants, thrombolytics	For all three: • Maintain prescribed length of administration (can be ≥28 for hip surgery) • And ≥10 days for knee surgery • Presence of conditions predisposing to bleeding risks • Avoid concomitant use with other anticoagulants • Renal impairment • Use with care in ages >80; <60 kg; serum creatinine >133 μmol/L
• Rivaroxaban	• Oral anticoagulant	• Increases the risk of bleeding and can cause serious or fatal bleeding. • Cease use at once if there is easy bruising, unusual bleeding (nose, mouth, vagina, or rectum); bleeding from wounds or injection; any bleeding that will not stop; heavy menstrual periods. • Clients with atrial fibrillation are at increased risk of forming blood clots in the heart. Do not stop taking without contacting the health care provider. • Increased risk of bleeding when taken in conjunction with aspirin or aspirin-containing products, NSAIDS, warfarin, sodium, any medicine that contains heparin, clopidogrel, or other medications used to prevent or treat blood clots.	• Give orally. Does not require monitoring like warfarin
• Dabigatran	• Oral anticoagulant	• Contraindicated in concomitant use with dronedarone. • May have an effect on some pathology tests. • There is an increased risk of bleeding especially for clients 75 years old or older, having moderate kidney impairment (creatinine 3050 mL/min); use with clients with congenital or acquired coagulation disorders, thrombocytopenia or functional platelet defects, active ulcerative GI disease, recent biopsy or major trauma, recent intracranial hemorrhage; brain, spinal, or ophthalmic surgery, or bacterial endocarditis. Must not be used with clients with prosthetic heart valves. • Medication must be stored and dispensed in the original packaging (blister pack or bottle) because of the increased risk of exposure to moisture or humidity causing breakdown and loss of potency.	• Give orally. Does not require monitoring like warfarin.

IV, intravenous; *PTT,* partial thromboplastin time; *PT,* prothrombin time; *GI,* gastrointestinal; *NSAIDs,* nonsteroidal anti-inflammatory drugs.

I. Provide preoperative and postoperative care if surgery is required.
   1. Preoperative: Maintain affected extremity in a level position (if venous) or in a slightly dependent position (if arterial; 15 degrees), at room temperature, and protect from trauma.
   2. Postoperative: Assess surgical site frequently for hemorrhage and check distal peripheral pulses.
   3. Anticoagulants may be continued after surgery to prevent thrombosis of affected artery and to diminish development of thrombi at the initiating site.

Abdominal Aortic Aneurysm

Description: Dilatation of the abdominal aorta caused by an alteration in the integrity of its wall

A. The most common cause of abdominal aortic aneurysm (AAA) is atherosclerosis. It is a late manifestation of syphilis.
B. Without treatment, rupture and death will occur.
C. AAA is often asymptomatic.
D. The most common symptom is abdominal pain or low back pain, with the complaint that the client can feel his or her heart beating.
E. Those taking antihypertensive drugs are at risk for developing AAA.

> **HESI HINT** A client is admitted with severe chest pain and states that he feels a terrible tearing sensation in his chest. He is diagnosed with a dissecting aortic aneurysm. What assessments should the nurse obtain in the first few hours?
> - Vital signs every hour
> - Neurologic vital signs
> - Respiratory status
> - Urinary output
> - Peripheral pulses

Nursing Assessment

A. Bruit (swooshing sound heard over a constricted artery when auscultated) heard over abdominal aorta, pulsation in upper abdomen
B. Abdominal or lower back pain
C. May feel heartbeat in abdomen, or feel an abdominal mass
D. Abdominal radiograph (aortogram, angiogram, abdominal ultrasound) to confirm diagnosis if aneurysm is calcified
E. Symptoms of rupture: hypovolemic or cardiogenic shock with sudden, severe abdominal pain

Nursing Plans and Interventions

A. Assess all peripheral pulses and vital signs regularly.
   1. Radial
   2. Femoral
   3. Popliteal
   4. Posterior tibial
   5. Dorsalis pedis
B. Observe for signs of occlusion after graft.
   1. Change in pulses
   2. Severe pain
   3. Cool to cold extremities below graft
   4. White or blue extremities
C. Observe renal functioning for signs of kidney damage (artery clamped during surgery may result in kidney damage).
   1. Output of less than 30 mL/h
   2. Amber urine
   3. Elevated BUN and creatinine (early signs of renal failure)

> **HESI HINT** During aortic aneurysm repair, the large arteries are clamped for a certain period, and kidney damage can result. Monitor daily BUN and creatinine levels. Normal BUN is 10–20 mg/dL, and normal creatinine is 0.6–1.2 mg/dL. The ratio of BUN to creatinine is 20:1. When this ratio increases or decreases, suspect renal problems.

D. Observe for postoperative ileus.
   1. NG tube to low continuous suction for 1 to 2 days postoperative (may help to prevent ileus)
   2. Bowel sounds checked every shift

Thrombophlebitis

Description: Inflammation of the venous walls with the formation of a clot; also known as *venous thrombosis*, *phlebothrombosis*, or *DVT*

Nursing Assessment

A. Calf tenderness, redness or pain, calf pain with dorsiflexion of the foot
B. Functional impairment of extremity
C. Edema and warmth in extremity
D. Asymmetry
   1. Inspect legs from groin to feet
   2. Measure diameters of calves
E. Tender areas on affected extremity with very gentle palpation
F. Occlusion with diagnostic testing
   1. Venogram
   2. Doppler ultrasound
   3. Fibrinogen scanning
G. Risk factors
   1. Prolonged, strict bed rest
   2. General surgery
   3. Leg trauma
   4. Previous venous insufficiency
   5. Obesity
   6. Oral contraceptives
   7. Pregnancy
   8. Malignancy

HESI HINT Heparin prevents conversion of fibrinogen to fibrin and prothrombin to thrombin, thereby inhibiting clot formation. Because the clotting mechanism is prolonged, do not cause tissue trauma, which may lead to bleeding when giving heparin subcutaneously. Do not massage area or aspirate; give in the abdomen between the pelvic bones, 2 inches from umbilicus; rotate sites.

Nursing Plans and Interventions

A. Administer anticoagulant therapy as prescribed (see Table 4.17).

HESI HINT

Heparin
Antagonist: protamine sulfate
Laboratory: PTT or aPTT determines efficacy
Keep 1.5–2.5 times normal control

Warfarin (Coumadin)
Antagonist: vitamin K
Laboratory: PT determines efficacy
Keep 1.5–2.5 times normal control
International normalized ratio (INR): desirable therapeutic level usually 2:3 (reflects how long it takes a blood sample to clot)

1. Observe for side effects, especially bleeding.
2. Teach client the side effects of medications included in treatment regimen.
3. Monitor laboratory data to determine the efficacy of medications included in treatment regimen.
4. Note on all laboratory requests that client is receiving anticoagulants.
5. Partial thromboplastin time (PTT) determines efficacy of heparin.
6. Prothrombin time (PT) or INR determines efficacy of Coumadin.
7. Maintain pressure on venipuncture sites to minimize hematoma formation.
8. Notify physician of any unusual bleeding.
   a. Abnormal vaginal bleeding
   b. Nosebleeds
   c. Melena
   d. Hematuria
   e. Gums
   f. Hemoptysis
9. Advise client to use soft toothbrush, floss with waxed floss.
10. Advise client to wear medical alert symbol.
11. Advise client to avoid alcoholic beverages.
12. Advise client to avoid safety razors if taking warfarin (Coumadin).
13. Advise client to avoid aspirin, aspirin products, and NSAIDs.
14. Advise client to wear anti-embolic stockings and to elevate extremity and use shock blocks at foot of bed.
15. Advise bed rest; strict, if prescribed, means no out-of-bed bathroom privileges! Advise client to avoid straining.
16. Monitor for decreasing symptomatology.
   a. Pain
   b. Edema
17. Monitor for pulmonary embolus (chest pain, shortness of breath).
18. Teach client that there is increased risk for DVT formation in the future.
19. Dietary precautions if taking warfarin (Coumadin).

HESI HINT Clients may ingest foods high in vitamin K to maintain therapeutic blood levels based on their dietary intake.

Dysrhythmias

Description: Disturbance in heart rate (HR) (beats per minute) or heart rhythm

A. Dysrhythmias are caused by a disturbance in the electrical conduction of the heart, not by abnormal heart structure.
B. Client is often asymptomatic until cardiac output is altered.
C. Common causes of dysrhythmias
   1. Drugs (e.g., digoxin, quinidine, caffeine, nicotine, alcohol), illicit drugs
   2. Acid–base and electrolyte imbalances (potassium, calcium, and magnesium)
   3. Marked thermal changes
   4. Disease and trauma
   5. Stress

Nursing Assessment

A. Change in pulse rate or rhythm
   1. Tachycardia: fast rates (>100 bpm)
   2. Bradycardia: slow rates (<60 bpm)
   3. Irregular rhythm
   4. Pulselessness
B. ECG changes
C. Complaints of
   1. Palpitations
   2. Syncope
   3. Pain
   4. Dyspnea
D. Diaphoresis
E. Hypotension
F. Electrolyte imbalances

Selected Dysrhythmias

A. Atrial fibrillation (Fig. 4.4A)
   1. Description
      a. Chaotic activity in the atrioventricular (AV) node
      b. No true P waves visible
      c. Irregular ventricular rhythm
   2. Assessment and treatment
      a. Anticoagulant therapy due to risk for stroke
      b. Antidysrhythmic drugs

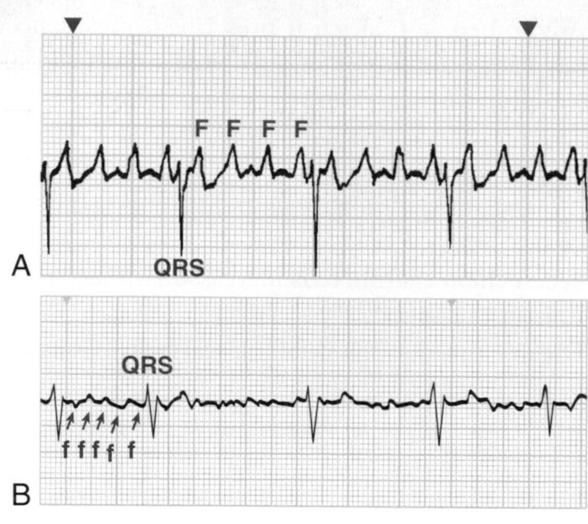

Fig. 4.4 (A) Atrial flutter with a 4:1 conduction (four flutter *[F]* waves to each QRS complex). (B) Atrial fibrillation. Note the chaotic fibrillatory *(f)* waves between the QRS complexes. Note: Recorded from lead V_1. (A, From Urden, L., Stacy, K., & Lough, M. [2013] *Priorities in critical care nursing* [6th ed.]. St. Louis: Elsevier/Mosby; B, From Sole, M., Klein, D., & Moseley, M. [2013]. *Introduction to critical care nursing* [6th ed.]. St. Louis: Elsevier/Saunders.)

c. Cardioversion to treat atrial dysrhythmias
d. Cardiac catheter ablation

B. Atrial flutter (see Fig. 4.4*A*)
1. Description
a. Saw-toothed waveform
b. Fluttering in chest
c. Ventricular rhythm stays regular
2. Assessment and treatment
a. Cardioversion to treat atrial dysrhythmia
b. Antidysrhythmic drugs
c. Radiofrequency catheter ablation

C. Ventricular tachycardia
1. Description
a. Wide, bizarre QRS
2. Assessment and treatment
a. Pulse
b. Impaired cardiac output
c. Synchronized cardioversion if pulse present (if no pulse, treat as ventricular fibrillation)
d. Antidysrhythmic drugs

D. Ventricular fibrillation
1. Description
a. Cardiac emergency
b. Irregular undulations of varying amplitudes, from coarse to fine
c. No cardiac output (no pulse or BP)
2. Assessment and treatment
a. CPR
b. Defibrillation as quickly as possible
c. Antidysrhythmic drugs

Nursing Plans and Interventions

A. Determine medications client is currently taking.
B. Determine serum drug levels, especially digitalis.
C. Determine serum electrolyte levels, especially potassium and magnesium.
D. Obtain ECG reading on admission and monitor continuously.
E. Holter monitoring, either event monitor or loop recorder.

HESI HINT A Holter monitor offers continuous observation of the client's HR. To make assessment of the rhythm strips most meaningful, teach the client to keep a record/report.
- Medication times and doses
- Chest pain episodes: type and duration
- Valsalva maneuver (straining at stool, sneezing, coughing)
- Sexual activity
- Exercise and other activities

F. Approach client in a calm, reassuring manner.
G. Monitor client's activity and observe for any symptoms occurring during activity.
H. Ensure proper administration of medications and monitor for side effects (Table 4.18).
I. Be prepared for emergency measures, such as cardioversion or defibrillation.

HESI HINT Cardioversion is the delivery of synchronized electrical shocks to the myocardium.

J. Be prepared for pacemaker insertion.
1. Temporary pacemaker: used temporarily in emergency situations. A pacing wire is threaded into the right ventricle via the superior vena cava, or an epicardial wire is put in place (through the client's chest incision) during cardiac surgery.
2. Permanent internal pacemaker with pulse generator implanted in the abdomen or shoulder: may be single or dual chambered. Programmable pacemakers can be reprogrammed by placing a magnetic device over the generator.
3. Instruct the client to
a. Report pulse rate lower than the set rate of the pacemaker.
b. Avoid leaning over an automobile with the engine running.
c. Stand 4 to 5 feet away from high-output generators and electromagnetic sources, such as operating radar detectors.
d. Avoid MRI diagnostic testing.
e. For airport travel, notify Transportation Security Administration (TSA) of the presence of a pacemaker. Handheld screening rod should not be placed directly over the pacemaker.

TABLE 4.18 **Antidysrhythmics**

Drugs	Indications	Adverse Reactions	Nursing Implications
		CLASS I (A, B, C)	
• Quinidine • Disopyramide phosphate • Procainamide • Moricizine • Lidocaine HCl • Mexiletine • Tocainide HCl • Phenytoin sodium • Propafenone • Flecainide acetate	• Premature beats • Atrial flutter, fibrillation • Contraindicated in heart block • Ventricular dysrhythmias • Unlabeled use: digitalis for induced dysrhythmias • Ventricular dysrhythmias	• Diarrhea • Hypotension • ECG changes • Cinchonism • Interacts with many common drugs • Hypotension • CNS effects • Seizures • GI distress • Bradycardia • Dizziness • Slurred speech • Ventricular dysrhythmias	• Instruct client to monitor pulse rate and rhythm. • Monitor ECG. • Monitor for tinnitus and visual disturbances. • Lidocaine administered IV bolus and by infusion. • Monitor for confusion, drowsiness, slurred speech, seizures with lidocaine. • Administer oral drugs with food. • May cause digoxin toxicity.
		CLASS II	
• Propranolol HCl • Metoprolol • Atenolol	• Supraventricular and ventricular tachydysrhythmias	• Hypotension • Bradycardia • Bronchospasm	• Monitor vital signs. • Contraindicated in asthma.
		CLASS III (INOTROPICS)	
• Amiodarone HCl • Sotalol • Dofetilide • Dronedarone • Ibutilide	• Ventricular dysrhythmias	• Dysrhythmias • Hypertension or hypotension • Muscle weakness, tremors • Photophobia	• Amiodarone is now one of the first-choice drugs. • Monitor vital signs, ECG. • Instruct client taking amiodarone to wear sunglasses and sunscreens when outside.
		CLASS IV	
• Verapamil HCl • Diltiazem	• Supraventricular dysrhythmias	• Hypotension • Bradycardia • Constipation	• Monitor BP and pulse. • Instruct client to change positions slowly.
Miscellaneous Agents			
• Atropine sulfate	• Bradycardia	• Chest pain • Urinary retention • Dry mouth	• Monitor HR and rhythm. • Assess for chest pain. • Assess for urinary retention. • Avoid use with glaucoma.
• Digoxin	• Supraventricular dysrhythmias • Atrial fibrillation	• Bradycardia • Dysrhythmias • Anorexia, nausea, vomiting, diarrhea, visual disturbances	• Monitor pulse rate and rhythm. • Check apical pulse for one full minute before administering; hold if BP is less than 60 bpm and notify health care provider. • Instruct client to report signs of toxicity. • Hypokalemia increases the risk for toxicity. • Causes hypercalcemia.
• Epinephrine	• Cardiac arrest	• Tachycardia • Hypertension	• Impaired renal function can cause toxicity; monitor BUN and creatinine. • Monitor pulse return in asystole. • Monitor vital signs.

ADDITIONAL DRUGS THAT PROMOTE CARDIOVASCULAR PERFUSION IN THE FAILING HEART

Drugs	Indications	Adverse Reactions	Nursing Implications
		VASOPRESSORS	
• Norepinephrine bitartrate	• Dilated coronary arteries and causes peripheral vasoconstriction for emergency hypotensive states not caused by blood loss, vascular thrombosis, or anesthesia using cyclopropane or halothane	• Can cause *severe* tissue necrosis, sloughing, and gangrene if infiltrates (blanching along vein pathway is preliminary sign of extravasation)	• Rapidly inactivated by various body enzymes; need to ensure IV patency. • Use cautiously in previously hypertensive clients. • Check BP every 2–5 min. • Use large veins to avoid complications of prolonged vasoconstriction. • Pressor effects potentiated by many drugs; check drug–drug interactions. • Have phentolamine (Regitine) diluted per protocol for local injection if infiltrates.

Continued

CARDIOTONIC/VASODILATOR (HUMAN B-TYPE NATRIURETIC PEPTIDE: HBNP)			
• Nesiritide	• Treatment of acutely decompensated HF in clients who have dyspnea at rest or with minimal activity • Reduces PCWP and reduces dyspnea	• Hypotension is primary side effect and can be dose limiting • Dysrhythmias • Headache, dizziness, insomnia, tremors, paresthesias • Abdominal pain, nausea and vomiting	• Many drug–drug interactions. • Monitor BP and telemetry. • As diuresis occurs, monitor electrolytes, especially potassium. • Watch for overresponse to treatment in older adults.

BP, Blood pressure; *CNS,* central nervous system; *ECG,* electrocardiogram; *GI,* gastrointestinal; *HR,* heart rate; *IV,* intravenous; *PCWP,* pulmonary capillary wedge pressure.

HESI HINT Difference in synchronous and asynchronous pacemakers include the following:
- Synchronous, or demand: Pacemaker fires only when the client's HR falls below a rate set on the generator.
- Asynchronous, or fixed: Pacemaker fires at a constant rate.
- Implantable cardioverter-defibrillator (ICD); device defibrillates to detect life-threatening ventricular arrhythmias. May have dual function as a pacemaker.

K. Recognize and treat symptomatic premature ventricular contractions (PVCs) as prescribed (Fig. 4.5). A PVC is a contraction originating in an ectopic focus in the ventricles. It is the premature occurrence of a QRS complex that is wide and distorted in shape (report and treat PVCs).
   1. If they occur more often than once in 10 beats
   2. If they occur in groups of two or three; three consecutive PVCs is ventricular tachycardia.
   3. If they occur near the T wave (R-on-T phenomenon)
   4. If they take on multiple configurations

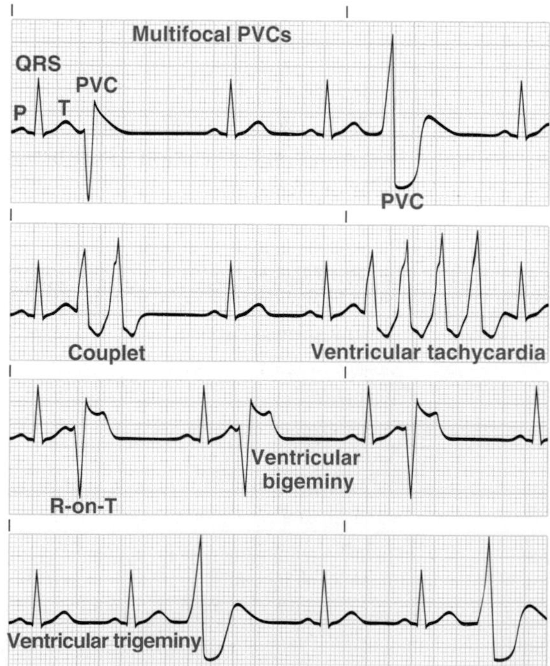

Fig. 4.5 **Various Forms of Premature Ventricular Contractions.** Note: Recorded from lead II. *PVC,* Premature ventricular contraction. (From Sole, M., Klein, D., & Moseley, M. [2021]. *Introduction to critical care nursing* [8th ed.]. St. Louis: Elsevier/Saunders.)

Heart Failure

Description: Inability of the heart to pump enough blood to meet the tissue's O_2 demands

A. Primary underlying conditions causing HF
   1. Ischemic heart disease
   2. MI
   3. Cardiomyopathy
   4. Valvular heart disease
   5. Hypertension

Nursing Assessment

A. Observe for symptoms associated with left-sided or right-sided failure.
   1. Left-sided HF: pulmonary edema (left ventricular failure)
      a. Description: Results in pulmonary congestion due to the inability of the left ventricle to pump blood to the periphery
      b. Symptoms
         1) Dyspnea
         2) Orthopnea
         3) Crackles
         4) Cough
         5) Fatigue
         6) Tachycardia
         7) Anxiety
         8) Restlessness
         9) Confusion
         10) Paroxysmal nocturnal dyspnea
   2. Right-sided HF: Peripheral edema (right ventricular failure)
      a. Description: Results in peripheral congestion due to the inability of the right ventricle to pump blood out to the lungs; often results from left-sided failure or pulmonary disease
      b. Symptoms
         1) Peripheral edema
         2) Weight gain
         3) Distended neck veins
         4) Anorexia, nausea
         5) Nocturia
         6) Weakness
         7) Hepatomegaly
         8) Ascites

B. Enlargement of ventricles as indicated by chest radiograph
C. Brain natriuretic peptide (BPN) test measures levels of protein in heart and blood vessels. High BPN levels occur with HF.
D. N-terminal probrain natriuretic peptide (NT-proBNP) is used for diagnosis of impaired left ventricular ejection fraction (LVEF) after MI.

HESI HINT Restricting sodium reduces salt and water retention, thereby reducing vascular volume and preload.

Nursing Plans and Interventions

A. Monitor vital signs at least every 4 hours for changes.
B. Monitor apical HR with vital signs to detect dysrhythmias, or abnormal heart sounds such as S3 or S4.
C. Assess for hypoxia.
   1. Restlessness
   2. Tachycardia
   3. Angina
D. Auscultate lungs for indication of pulmonary edema (wet sounds or crackles).
E. Administer O_2 as needed.
F. Elevate head of bed to assist with breathing.
G. Observe for signs of edema.
   1. Weigh daily.
   2. Monitor I&O.
   3. Measure abdominal girth; observe ankles and fingers.
H. Limit sodium intake.
I. Elevate lower extremities while sitting.
J. Check apical HR before administration of digitalis; withhold medication and call physician if rate is less than 60 bpm (Table 4.19).
K. Administer diuretics in the morning if possible (see Table 4.15).
L. Provide periods of rest after periods of activity.

Inflammatory and Infectious Heart Disease

Description: Inflammatory and infectious process involving the endocardium and pericardium

A. Endocarditis is an inflammatory disease involving the inner surface of the heart, including the valves. Organisms travel through the blood to the heart, where vegetation adheres to the valve surface or endocardium and can break off and become emboli.
B. Causes of endocarditis
   1. Rheumatic heart disease
   2. Congenital heart disease
   3. IV drug abuse
   4. Cardiac surgery
   5. Immunosuppression
   6. Dental procedures
   7. Invasive procedures
C. Pericarditis is an inflammation of the outer lining of the heart.
D. Causes of pericarditis
   1. MI
   2. Trauma
   3. Neoplasm
   4. Connective-tissue disease
   5. Heart surgery
   6. Idiopathic
   7. Infections

Nursing Assessment

A. Endocarditis
   1. Fever
   2. Chills, malaise, night sweats, fatigue
   3. Murmurs
   4. Symptoms of HF
   5. Atrial embolization
B. Pericarditis
   1. Pain: sudden, sharp, severe
      a. Substernal, radiating to the back or arm
      b. Aggravated by coughing, inhalation, deep breathing
      c. Relieved by leaning forward

TABLE 4.19 Digitalis Preparations

Drugs	Indications	Adverse Reactions	Nursing Implications
• Digoxin	• HF • Increases the contractility of cardiac muscle • Slows HR and conduction	• Severe: AV block • Headache • Dysrhythmias • Nausea • Vomiting • Blurred vision • Yellow-green halos • Hypotension • Fatigue	• Monitor serum electrolytes; hypokalemia increases risk for digoxin toxicity. • Monitor serum digitalis levels if any side effects are present. • Check apical pulse before administration; call health care provider if rate is < 60 bpm. • Teach client to take radial pulse before administration and call health care provider if <60 bpm in adults. • Therapeutic range: 0.5–2 mg.
• Digoxin-immune Fab	• Antidote for digitalis toxicity • Binds with digoxin to prevent binding at the site of action	• Decreased cardiac output • Atrial tachydysrhythmias • Use with caution in children and older adults.	• Use with 0.22-mcm filter. • Place client on continuous cardiac monitor. • Have resuscitation equipment at bedside before giving first dose.

HF, Heart failure; *HR*, heart rate; *IV*, intravenous

2. Pericardial friction rub heard best at left lower sternal border
3. Fever

HESI HINT Infective endocarditis damage to heart valves occurs with the growth of vegetative lesions on valve leaflets. These lesions pose a risk for embolization, erosion, or perforation of the valve leaflets or abscesses within adjacent myocardial tissue. Valvular stenosis or regurgitation (insufficiency), most commonly of the mitral valve, can occur, depending on the type of damage inflicted by the lesions, and can lead to symptoms of left- or right-sided HF (see "Valvular Heart Disease," later, and "Heart Failure," earlier).

HESI HINT The presence of a friction rub is an indication of pericarditis (inflammation of the lining of the heart). ST-segment elevation and T-wave inversion are also signs of pericarditis.

HESI HINT

Acute and Subacute Infective Endocarditis

There are two types of infective endocarditis: acute, which often affects individuals with previously normal hearts and healthy valves and carries a high mortality rate, and subacute, which typically affects individuals with preexisting conditions, such as rheumatic heart disease, mitral valve prolapse, or immunosuppression. IV drug abusers are at risk for both acute and subacute bacterial endocarditis. When this population develops subacute infective endocarditis, the valves on the right side of the heart (tricuspid and pulmonic) are typically affected because of the introduction of common pathogens that colonize the skin (*Staphylococcus epidermis* or *Candida* spp.) into the venous system.

Nursing Plans and Interventions

A. Endocarditis
   1. Monitor hemodynamic status (vital signs, level of consciousness, urinary output).
   2. Administer antibiotics IV for 4 to 6 weeks. The American Heart Association recommends administration of antibiotics before dental or genitourinary procedures in high-risk clients.
   3. Clients may be instructed in IV therapy for home health care.
   4. Teach clients about anticoagulant therapy if prescribed.
   5. Encourage client to maintain good hygiene.
   6. Instruct client to inform dentist and other health care providers of history.

B. Pericarditis
   1. Provide rest and maintain position of comfort.
   2. Administer analgesics and anti-inflammatory drugs.

Valvular Heart Disease

Description: Heart valves that are unable to open fully (stenosis) or close fully (insufficiency or regurgitation)

A. Valve dysfunction most commonly occurs on the left side of the heart; the mitral valve is most commonly involved, followed by the aortic valve.

HESI HINT In mitral valve stenosis, blood is regurgitated back into the left atrium from the left ventricle. In the early period, there may be no symptoms, but as the disease progresses, the client will exhibit excessive fatigue, dyspnea on exertion, orthopnea, dry cough, hemoptysis, or pulmonary edema. There will be a rumbling apical diastolic murmur, and atrial fibrillation is common.

B. Common causes of valvular disease
   1. Rheumatic fever
   2. Congenital heart diseases
   3. Syphilis
   4. Endocarditis
   5. Hypertension

C. Prevention of rheumatic heart disease would reduce the incidence of valvular heart disease.

Nursing Assessment

A. Pericardial effusion with possible tamponade that requires pericardiocentesis
B. Fatigue
C. Dyspnea, orthopnea
D. Hemoptysis and pulmonary edema
E. Murmurs
F. Irregular cardiac rhythm
G. Angina

Nursing Plans and Interventions

A. See "Heart Failure," earlier.
B. Monitor client for atrial fibrillation with thrombus formation.
C. Teach the necessity for prophylactic antibiotic therapy before any invasive procedure, such as dental procedures, that is likely to produce gingival or mucosal bleeding: bronchoscopy, esophageal dilation, upper endoscopy, colonoscopy, sigmoidoscopy, or cystoscopy.
D. Prepare the client for surgical repair or replacement of heart valves.
E. Instruct clients receiving mechanical valve replacement of the need for lifelong anticoagulant therapy to prevent thrombus formation. Tissue (biologic) valves and autografts do not require lifelong anticoagulant therapy.

REVIEW OF CARDIOVASCULAR SYSTEM

1. How do clients experiencing angina describe that pain?
2. Develop a teaching plan for a client prescribed nitroglycerin.
3. List the parameters of BP for diagnosing hypertension.
4. Differentiate between essential and secondary hypertension.
5. Develop a teaching plan for a client taking antihypertensive medications.
6. Describe intermittent claudication.
7. Describe the nurse's discharge instructions to a client with venous PVD.
8. What is often the underlying cause of an AAA?
9. What laboratory values should be monitored daily in a client with thrombophlebitis who is undergoing anticoagulant therapy?
10. When do PVCs present a grave danger?
11. Differentiate between the symptoms of left-sided cardiac failure and right-sided cardiac failure.
12. List three symptoms of digitalis toxicity.
13. What condition increases the likelihood that digitalis toxicity will occur?
14. What lifestyle changes can the client who is at risk for hypertension initiate to reduce the likelihood of becoming hypertensive?
15. What immediate actions should the nurse implement when a client is having an MI?
16. What symptoms should the nurse expect to find in a client with hypokalemia?
17. Bradycardia is defined as an HR below _____ bpm. Tachycardia is defined as an HR above _____ bpm.
18. What precautions should clients with valve disease take before invasive procedures or dental work?

See Answer Key at the end of this text for suggested responses.

GASTROINTESTINAL SYSTEM

Hiatal Hernia and Gastroesophageal Reflux Disease (GERD)

A. Hiatal hernia is a herniation of the esophagogastric junction and a portion of the stomach into the chest through the esophageal hiatus of the diaphragm.
   1. Sliding hernia is the most common type, accounting for 75% to 90% of adult hiatal hernias.

B. Gastroesophageal reflux disease (GERD) is the result of an incompetent lower esophageal sphincter that allows regurgitation of acidic gastric contents into the esophagus.
   1. Multiple factors determine whether GERD is present.
      a. Efficiency of anti-reflux mechanism
      b. Volume of gastric contents
      c. Potency of refluxed material
      d. Efficiency of esophageal clearance
      e. Resistance of the esophageal tissue to injury and the ability to repair tissue
   2. The client must have several episodes of reflux for GERD to be present.

Nursing Assessment

A. Heartburn after eating that radiates to arms and shoulders
B. Feeling of fullness and discomfort after eating
C. Positive diagnosis determined by fluoroscopy, barium swallow, or gastroscopy

Nursing Plans and Interventions

A. Determine an eating pattern that alleviates symptoms.
   1. Encourage small, frequent meals.
   2. Encourage elimination of foods that are determined to aggravate symptoms (these foods are client specific but can include caffeine, catsup, strawberries, and chocolate).
   3. Encourage client to sit up while eating and remain in an upright position for at least 1 hour after eating.
   4. Encourage client to stop eating 3 hours before bedtime.
   5. Elevate the head of the bed on 6- to 8-inch blocks.
   6. Teach about commonly prescribed medications (H2 antagonists, antacids).

> **HESI HINT** A Fowler or semi-Fowler position is beneficial in reducing the amount of regurgitation, as well as in preventing the encroachment of the stomach tissue upward through the opening in the diaphragm.

B. Teaching plan for client and family should include the following:
   1. Differentiate between the symptoms of hiatal hernia and those of MI.
   2. Be alert to the possibility of aspiration.
   3. Give information about drugs used for treatment (Table 4.20).

Peptic Ulcer Disease

Description: Ulceration that penetrates the mucosal wall of the gastrointestinal (GI) tract

A. Gastric ulcers tend to occur in the lesser curvature of the stomach.
B. Duodenal ulcers occur in the duodenum, which is the most common location of peptic ulcer disease (PUD).
C. Esophageal ulcers occur in the esophagus.
D. The cause of some PUD is unknown. A significant number of gastric ulcers are caused by a bacterium, *Helicobacter pylori,* and can be successfully treated by drug therapy. Risk factors for the development of peptic ulcers include
   1. Drugs (NSAIDs, corticosteroids)
   2. Alcohol
   3. Cigarette smoking
   4. Acute medical crisis or trauma
   5. Familial tendency
   6. Blood type O

TABLE 4.20 Antiulcer Drugs

Drugs	Indications	Adverse Reactions	Nursing Implications
ANTACIDS			
• Aluminum hydroxide/ magnesium hydroxide	• Treatment of peptic ulcers • Work by neutralizing or reducing acidity of stomach contents • Differences in absorption rate	• Constipation • Diarrhea • Drug interactions	• Need to take several times a day. • Administer after meals. • Assess for history of renal diseases when client is taking magnesium products; electrolyte readjustment occurs and can result in renal insufficiency and calcinosis.
HISTAMINE-2 ANTAGONISTS			
• Ranitidine HCl • Cimetidine • Famotidine • Nizatidine	• Treatment of peptic ulcers • Prophylactic treatment for clients at risk for developing ulcers (those on steroids or highly stressed)	• Multiple drug interactions	• Cigarette smoking interferes with drug action. • Expensive
MUCOSAL HEALING AGENTS			

• Sucralfate	• Treatment of peptic ulcers	• Constipation
		• Drug interaction with
		  • Tetracycline
		  • Phenytoin sodium
		  • Digoxin
		  • Cimetidine
			• Medication to be taken at least 1 h before meals.
			• Antacids interfere with absorption.

PROTON PUMP INHIBITORS			
• Lansoprazole • Pantoprazole (available PO and IV) • Esomeprazole • Omeprazole • Rabeprazole • Dexlansoprazole	• Treatment of erosive esophagitis associated with GERD	• Constipation • Heartburn • Anxiety • Diarrhea • Abdominal pain, hepatocellular damage, pancreatitis, gastroenteritis • Tinnitus, vertigo, confusion, headache • Blurred vision, hypokinesia • Chest pain, dyspnea	• Taken before meals • Do not crush or chew pantoprazole IV. • Resume oral therapy as soon as feasible. • Long-lasting effects of drug may inhibit absorption of other drugs. • Not removed by hemodialysis • Monitor for indications of adverse reactions.
ADDITIONAL DRUGS			
• Prokinetic agents • Antiemetics • Cough suppressants • Stool softeners	• Treatment of slow peristalsis and increased intraabdominal pressure in clients with GERD	• Diarrhea	• Monitor for indications of adverse reactions

GERD, Gastroesophageal reflux disease; *IV,* intravenous.

E. Symptoms common to all types of ulcers include the following:
 1. Belching
 2. Bloating
 3. Epigastric pain radiating to the back (not associated with the type of food eaten) and relieved by antacids. Peptic ulcer pain is relieved with food.

Nursing Assessment

A. Determine how food intake affects pain.
B. Take history of antacid, histamine antagonist, or proton pump inhibitor use.
C. Determine presence of melena (black, tarry stools).
D. Determine presence and location of peptic ulcer as determined by
 1. Esophagogastroduodenoscopy (EGD)
 2. Barium swallow
 3. Gastric analysis indicating increased levels of stomach acid
E. Potential complications
 1. Hemorrhage
 2. Perforation (which always requires surgery)
 3. Obstruction

Nursing Plans and Interventions

A. Determine symptom onset and how symptoms are relieved.
B. Monitor color, quantity, consistency of stools and emesis; test for occult blood.
C. Administer medications as prescribed, usually 1 to 2 hours after meals and at bedtime (see Table 4.20).
D. Administer mucosal healing agents at least 1 hour before meals, as prescribed (see Table 4.20).
E. Encourage small, frequent meals; no bedtime snacks; and avoidance of beverages containing caffeine.

F. Prepare client for surgery if uncontrolled bleeding, obstruction, or perforation occurs.
   1. Gastric resection
   2. Vagotomy
   3. Pyloroplasty
G. Teach client that dumping syndrome may occur postoperatively.
   1. Secondary to rapid entry of hypertonic food into jejunum (pulls water out of bloodstream)
   2. Occurs 5 to 30 minutes after eating
   3. Characterized by vertigo, syncope, sweating, pallor, tachycardia, and/or hypotension
   4. Minimized by small, frequent meals: high-protein, high-fat, low-carbohydrate diet
   5. Exacerbated by consuming liquids with meals; helped by lying down after eating
   6. Can also be observed in clients on hypertonic tube feeding
H. Teach client to avoid medications that increase the risk for developing peptic ulcers.
   1. Salicylates
   2. NSAIDs such as ibuprofen
   3. Corticosteroids in high doses
   4. Anticoagulants
I. Teach client the importance of informing all health care personnel of ulcer history.
J. Teach client symptoms of GI bleeding.
   1. Dark, tarry stools
   2. Coffee-ground emesis
   3. Bright-red rectal bleeding
   4. Fatigue
   5. Pallor
   6. Severe abdominal pain, which should be reported immediately (could denote perforation)
K. Teach client importance of smoking cessation and stress management.

> **HESI HINT** Stress can cause or exacerbate ulcers. Teach stress-reduction methods and encourage those with a family history of ulcers to obtain medical surveillance for ulcer formation.

> **HESI HINT** Clinical manifestations of GI bleeding include the following:
> - Pallor: conjunctival, mucous membranes, nail beds
> - Dark, tarry stools
> - Bright-red or coffee-ground emesis
> - Abdominal mass or bruit
> - Decreased BP, rapid pulse, cool extremities (shock), increased respirations

Inflammatory Bowel Diseases

Description: Consists of Crohn disease and ulcerative colitis

Crohn Disease (Regional Enteritis)

Description: Subacute, chronic inflammation extending throughout all layers of intestinal mucosa (most commonly found in terminal ileum), which has a cobblestone appearance of the GI mucosa, with periods of remission interspersed with periods of exacerbation. Crohn disease occurs during the teenage years and early adulthood, but has a second peak in the sixth decade. Capsule endoscopy has shown greater sensitivity than radiography when diagnosing Crohn disease. There is speculation that Crohn disease could be caused by a combination of environmental factors and genetic predisposition, but as of now, there is no cure, so treatment relies on medications to treat the acute inflammation and maintain a remission. Surgery is reserved for clients who are unresponsive to medications or who develop life-threatening complications. In a total proctocolectomy (the colon and rectum are removed and the anus is closed), the terminal ileum is brought through the abdominal wall, and a permanent ileostomy is formed.

Nursing Assessment

A. Abdominal pain (unrelieved by defecation), right lower quadrant
B. Diarrhea, steatorrhea (the excretion of abnormal quantities of fat with the feces owing to reduced absorption of fat by the intestine), and weight loss, with client becoming emaciated
C. Constant fluid loss
D. Low-grade fever
E. Perforation of the intestine occurring due to severe inflammation; constitutes a medical emergency
F. Anorexia related to pain after eating
G. Weight loss, anemia, malnutrition

Nursing Plans and Interventions

A. Determine bowel elimination pattern and control diarrhea with diet and medication as indicated.
B. Provide a nutritious, well-balanced, low-residue, low-fat, high-protein, high-calorie diet, with no dairy products.
C. Administer vitamin supplements and iron.
D. Advise client to avoid foods that are known to cause diarrhea, such as milk products and spicy foods.
E. Advise client to avoid smoking, caffeinated beverages, pepper, and alcohol.
F. Provide complete bowel rest with IV total parenteral nutrition (TPN) if necessary.
G. Administer medications as prescribed: aminosalicylates, antimicrobials, corticosteroids, immunosuppressants, and biologic therapy as necessary for acute symptoms and chronic treatment.
H. Monitor I&O and serum electrolytes.
I. Weigh at least twice a week.
J. Provide emotional support and encourage use of support groups such as the Crohn's and Colitis Foundation of America.
K. Encourage client to talk with the enterostomal therapists before surgery.
L. If ileostomy is performed, teach stoma care (see "Stoma Care," later).

HESI HINT The GI tract usually accounts for only 100–200 mL of fluid loss per day, although it filters up to 8 L/day. Large fluid losses can occur if vomiting or diarrhea exists.

Ulcerative Colitis

Description: Disease that affects the superficial mucosa of the large intestines and rectum, causing the bowel to eventually narrow, shorten, and thicken due to muscular hypertrophy. Sigmoidoscopy and colonoscopy allow direct examination of the large intestinal mucosa and are used for diagnosis of ulcerative colitis.

Nursing Assessment

A. Diarrhea
B. Abdominal pain and cramping
C. Intermittent tenesmus (anal contractions) and rectal bleeding
D. Liquid stools containing blood, mucus, and pus (may pass 10 to 20 liquid stools per day)
E. Weakness and fatigue
F. Anemia

Nursing Plans and Interventions

A. Determine bowel elimination pattern, and control diarrhea with diet and medication as indicated.
B. Provide a nutritious, well-balanced, low-residue, low-fat, high-protein, high-calorie diet, with no dairy products.
C. Administer vitamin supplements and iron.
D. Advise client to avoid foods that are known to cause diarrhea, such as milk products and spicy foods.
E. Advise client to avoid smoking, caffeinated beverages, pepper, and alcohol.
F. Provide complete bowel rest with IV hyperalimentation if necessary.
G. Administer medications as prescribed, often corticosteroids, antidiarrheals, sulfasalazine (Azulfidine), mesalamine (various brands), and infliximab (Remicade) or other biologic treatments, if there is no response to previous medications.
H. Monitor I&O and serum electrolytes.
I. Weigh at least twice a week.
J. Provide emotional support and encourage use of support groups such as the local Ileitis and Colitis Foundation.
K. Encourage client to talk with the enterostomal therapists before surgery.
L. If ileostomy is performed, teach stoma care (see "Stoma Care," later).

HESI HINT Opiate drugs tend to depress gastric motility. However, they should be given with caution. The nurse should assess for abdominal distention, abdominal pain, abdominal rigidity, signs and symptoms of shock-increased HR, and decreased BP, indicating possible perforation/GI bleed.

Diverticular Diseases

Description: Manifested in two clinical forms: diverticulosis and diverticulitis

A. Diverticulosis: bulging pouches in the GI wall (diverticula), which push the mucosa lining through the surrounding muscle
B. Diverticulitis: inflamed diverticula, which may cause obstruction, infection, and hemorrhage

HESI HINT Diverticulosis is the presence of pouches in the wall of the intestine. There is usually no discomfort, and the problem goes unnoticed unless seen on radiologic examination (usually prompted by some other condition). In contrast, diverticulitis is an inflammation of the diverticula (pouches), which can lead to perforation of the bowel.

Nursing Assessment

A. Left lower quadrant pain
B. Increased flatus
C. Rectal bleeding
D. Signs of intestinal obstruction
   1. Constipation alternating with diarrhea
   2. Abdominal distention
   3. Anorexia
   4. Low-grade fever
E. Barium enema or colonoscopy positive for diverticular disease: obstruction, ileus, or perforation confirmed by abdominal radiograph (barium not used during acute phase of illness)

Nursing Plans and Interventions

A. Provide a well-balanced, high-fiber diet unless inflammation is present, in which case client is NPO, followed by low-residue bland foods.

HESI HINT A client admitted with complaints of severe lower abdominal pain, cramping, and diarrhea is diagnosed as having diverticulitis. What are the nutritional needs of this client throughout recovery?

- Acute phase: NPO, graduating to liquids
- Recovery phase: no fiber or foods that irritate the bowel
- Maintenance phase: high-fiber diet with bulk-forming laxatives to prevent pooling of foods in the pouches where they can become inflamed; avoidance of small, poorly digested foods such as popcorn, nuts, seeds, etc.

B. Include bulk-forming laxatives such as Metamucil in daily regimen.
C. Increase fluid intake to 3 L/day.
D. Monitor I&O and bowel elimination; avoid constipation (administer stool softener or bulk laxatives).
E. Observe for complications.
   1. Obstruction
   2. Peritonitis or other infections

3. Hemorrhage (treatment for ruptured diverticula is a temporary colostomy and is maintained for approximately 3 months to allow the bowel to rest)
4. Infection

Intestinal Obstruction

Description: Partial or complete blockage of intestinal flow (fluids, feces, gas) that occurs mostly in the small intestines

A. Mechanical causes of intestinal obstruction
   1. Adhesions (most common cause)
   2. Hernia (strangulates the gut)
   3. Volvulus (twisting of the gut)
   4. Intussusception (telescoping of the gut within itself)
   5. Tumors; develop slowly; usually a mass of feces becomes lodged against the tumor
B. Neurogenic causes of intestinal obstruction
   1. Paralytic ileus (usually occurs in postoperative clients)
   2. Spinal cord lesion
C. Vascular cause of intestinal obstruction
   1. Mesenteric artery occlusion (leads to gut infarct)

HESI HINT
Bowel Obstructions
- Mechanical: due to disorders outside the bowel (hernia, adhesions) caused by disorders within the bowel (tumors, diverticulitis) or by blockage of the lumen in the intestine (intussusception, gallstone)
- Nonmechanical: due to paralytic ileus, which does not involve any actual physical obstruction but results from inability of the bowel itself to function

Nursing Assessment

A. Sudden onset of abdominal pain, tenderness, or guarding
B. History of abdominal surgeries
C. History of obstruction
D. Distention
E. Increased peristalsis when obstruction first occurs, then peristalsis becoming absent when paralytic ileus occurs
F. Bowel sounds that are high pitched with early mechanical obstruction and diminish to absent with neurogenic or late mechanical obstruction

Nursing Plans and Interventions

A. Maintain client NPO, with IV fluids and electrolyte therapy.
B. Monitor I&O; an indwelling urinary catheter maintains strict output.
C. Implement NG intubation.
   1. Attach to low suction (intermittent; 80 mm Hg).
   2. Document output every 8 hours.
   3. Irrigate with normal saline if policy dictates.
D. NG tube (passed through the nose into the stomach; Miller—Abbott tube is used for decompression; it is passed through the nose and the stomach into the small intestines then connected to suction; placement is usually performed by the health care provider).
   1. NG tube
      a. Measure correct length of tubing to be inserted by measuring from the tip of the client's nose to the client's earlobe to the xiphoid process.
   2. Advance decompression tube every 1 to 2 hours.
   3. Do not secure to nose until tube reaches specified position.
   4. Reposition client every 2 hours to assist with placement of the tube.
   5. Connect tube to suction.
   6. Irrigate NG tube with normal saline; irrigate Miller-Abbott tube with air only.
   7. Note amount, color, consistency, and any unusual odor of drainage.
   8. Assess for signs of dehydration (skin turgor, amount and color of urine).
   9. Monitor electrolyte values.

HESI HINT A client admitted with complaints of constipation, thready stools, and rectal bleeding over the past few months is diagnosed with a rectal mass. What are the nursing priorities for this client?
- NPO
- NG tube (possibly an intestinal tube such as a Miller-Abbott)
- IV fluids
- Surgical preparations of bowel (if obstruction is complete)
- Foods and fluids are restricted for 8–10 h before surgery if possible.
- If the client has a bowel obstruction or perforation, bowel cleansing is contraindicated.
- Oral erythromycin and neomycin are given to further decrease the amount of colonic and rectal bacteria.
- If possible, all clients who require surgery for obstruction undergo NG intubation and suction before surgery. However, in cases of complete obstruction, surgery should proceed without delay.
- Teaching (preoperative nutrition, etc.)

E. Document pain; medicate as prescribed.
F. Assess abdomen regularly for distention, rigidity, and change in status of bowel sounds.
G. If conservative medical interventions fail, surgery will be required to remove obstruction.

Colorectal Cancer

Description: Tumors occurring in the colon

A. Cancer of the colon is the fourth most common cancer in the United States.
B. This is the second-leading cause of cancer-related deaths in the United States.
C. Approximately 45% of cancerous tumors of the colon occur in the rectal or sigmoid area, 25% in the cecum and ascending colon, and 30% in the remainder of colon.
D. The highest incidence occurs in persons older than 50 years of age.
E. A diet of high-fiber, low-fat foods, including cruciferous vegetables, may be a factor in the prevention of colon cancer.

> **HESI HINT** The diet recommended by the American Cancer Society to prevent bowel cancer includes the following:
> - Eat more cruciferous vegetables (those from the cabbage family, such as broccoli, cauliflower, Brussels sprouts, cabbage, and kale).
> - Increase fiber intake.
> - Maintain average body weight.
> - Eat less animal fat.

F. Early detection is important.

> **HESI HINT** American Cancer Society recommendations for early detection of colon cancer include the following:
> - A digital rectal examination (DRE) every year after 40.
> - A stool blood test every year after 50.
> - A colonoscopy or sigmoidoscopy examination every 10 years after the age of 50 in average-risk clients, or more often based on the advice of a physician.

G. Usual treatment is surgical removal of the tumor, with adjuvant radiation or antineoplastic chemotherapy.
H. Diagnosis is made by digital examination, flexible fiberoptic sigmoidoscopy with biopsy, colonoscopy, and barium enema.
I. Carcinoembryonic antigen (CEA) serum level is used to evaluate effectiveness of chemotherapy.

Nursing Assessment

A. Rectal bleeding
B. Change in bowel habits
C. Sense of incomplete evacuation, tenesmus
D. Abdominal pain, nausea, vomiting
E. Weight loss, cachexia
F. Abdominal distention or ascites
G. Family history of cancer, particularly cancer of the colon
H. History of polyps

Nursing Plans and Interventions

A. Prepare client for surgery.
B. Prepare client for bowel preparation, which may include laxatives and gut lavage with polyethylene glycol.
C. If colostomy has been performed, teach stoma care. (See "Stoma Care," later in this chapter.)
D. Provide high-calorie, high-protein diet.
E. Promote prevention of constipation with high-fiber diet.

> **HESI HINT** An early sign of colon cancer is rectal bleeding. Encourage clients 50 years of age or older and those with increased risk factors to be screened yearly with fecal occult blood testing. Routine colonoscopy at 50 is also recommended.

F. General information
   1. The more distal the stoma is, the greater chance for continence. Greatest chance for continence is with a stoma created from the sigmoid colon on the left side of the abdomen.
   2. An ileostomy drains liquid material; peristomal skin is prone to breakdown by enzymes.
   3. The lower the stoma's location is in the GI tract, the more solid, or formed, is the effluence (stoma drainage).
   4. Consultation with an enterostomal therapist is essential.

G. Preoperative care
   1. Client and family must be informed about what to expect postoperatively
      a. Proposed location of the stoma
      b. Approximate size
      c. What it will look like (provide picture, if indicated)
   2. The family should be included in teaching, but it should be emphasized that the client is ultimately responsible for his or her own care.

H. Pouch care
   1. Ostomates often wear pouches.
   2. The adhesive-backed opening, designed to cover the stoma, should provide about ⅛-inch clearance from the stoma.
   3. A rubber band or clip is used to secure the bottom of the pouch and prevent leakage.
   4. A simple squirt bottle is used to remove effluence from the sides of the bag. Pouch system is changed every 3 to 7 days.
   5. Clients should maintain an extra supply of pouches so that they never run out and should change the pouch when bowel is inactive.
   6. Pouch should be emptied when one-third to one-half full.

I. Irrigation
   1. Those with descending-colon colostomies can irrigate to provide control over effluence.
      a. Clients should irrigate at approximately the same time daily.
      b. Clients should use warm water (cold or hot water causes cramping).
      c. Clients should wash around stoma with lukewarm water and a mild soap.
      d. Commercial skin barriers may be purchased for home use.
   2. Odor control
      a. Commercial preparations are available.
      b. Foods in diet that cause offensive odors can be eliminated.

J. Diet
   1. Ileostomy
      a. Clients should chew food thoroughly.
      b. High-fiber foods (popcorn, peanuts, unpeeled vegetables) can cause severe diarrhea and may have to be eliminated.

2. Colostomy
    a. Client should resume the regular diet gradually. Foods that were a problem preoperatively should be tried cautiously.

Cirrhosis

Description: Degeneration of liver tissue, causing enlargement, fibrosis, and scarring

A. Causes of cirrhosis include the following:
   1. Chronic alcohol ingestion (Laënnec cirrhosis)
   2. Viral hepatitis
   3. Exposure to hepatotoxins (including medications)
   4. Infections
   5. Congenital abnormalities
   6. Chronic biliary tree obstruction
   7. Chronic severe right-sided HF
   8. Idiopathy

B. Initially, hepatomegaly occurs; later, the liver becomes hard and nodular.

Nursing Assessment

A. History of alcohol, prescriptive and street drug use
B. Work history of exposure to toxic chemicals (pesticides, fumes, etc.)
C. Medication history of long-term use of hepatotoxic drugs
D. Family health history of liver abnormalities
E. Physical findings
   1. Weakness, malaise
   2. Anorexia, weight loss
   3. Palpable liver (early); abdominal girth increases as liver enlarges
   4. Jaundice
   5. Fetor hepaticus (fruity or musty breath)

> **HESI HINT**
> **Clinical Manifestations of Jaundice**
> - Yellow skin, sclera, or mucous membranes (bilirubin in skin)
> - Dark-colored urine (bilirubin in urine)
> - Chalky or clay-colored stools (absence of bilirubin in stools)

> **HESI HINT** Fetor hepaticus is a distinctive breath odor of chronic liver disease. It is characterized by a fruity or musty odor that results from the damaged liver's inability to metabolize and detoxify mercaptan, which is produced by the bacterial degradation of methionine, a sulfurous amino acid.

   6. Asterixis (hand-flapping tremor that often accompanies metabolic disorders)
   7. Mental and behavioral changes
   8. Bruising, erythema
   9. Dry skin, spider angiomas
   10. Gynecomastia (breast development), testicular atrophy
   11. Ascites, peripheral neuropathy
   12. Hematemesis
   13. Palmar erythema (redness in palms of the hands)

> **HESI HINT** For treatment of ascites, paracentesis and peritoneovenous shunts (LeVeen and Denver shunts) may be indicated.

> **HESI HINT** Esophageal varices may rupture and cause hemorrhage. Immediate management includes insertion of an esophagogastric balloon tamponade (a Blakemore-Sengstaken or Minnesota tube). Other therapies include vasopressors, vitamin K, coagulation factors, and blood transfusions.

F. Clotting defects noted in laboratory findings include
   1. Elevated bilirubin, aspartate aminotransferase (AST), alanine aminotransferase (ALT), alkaline phosphatase, PT, and ammonia
   2. Decreased Hgb, Hct, electrolytes, potassium, sodium, and albumin

> **HESI HINT** Ammonia is not broken down as usual in the damaged liver; therefore, the serum ammonia level rises.
> The metabolism of drugs is slowed down, so they remain in the system longer.

G. Complications include
   1. Ascites, edema
   2. Portal hypertension
   3. Esophageal varices
   4. Encephalopathy
   5. Respiratory distress
   6. Coagulation defects

Nursing Plans and Interventions

A. Eliminate causative agent (alcohol, hepatotoxin).
B. Administer vitamin supplements (A, B complex, C, K), and teach client and family the need for continuing these supplements.
C. Observe mental status frequently (at least every 2 hours); note any subtle changes.
D. Avoid initiating bleeding and observe for bleeding tendencies.
   1. Avoid injections whenever possible.
   2. Use small-bore needles for IV insertion.
   3. Maintain pressure to venipuncture sites for at least 5 minutes.
   4. Use electric razor.
   5. Provide a soft-bristle toothbrush and encourage careful mouth care.
   6. Check stools and emesis for frank or occult blood.
   7. Prevent straining at stool.
      a. Administer stool softeners as prescribed.
      b. Provide high-fiber diet.

TABLE 4.21 Ammonia Detoxicants/ Stimulant Laxative

Drug	Implications	Adverse Reactions	Nursing Implications
• Lactulose • Rifaximin	• Encephalopathy • Used to decrease ammonia levels and bowel pH	• Diarrhea	• Instruct client regarding need for medication. • Observe for diarrhea. • Monitor ammonia levels.

E. Provide special skin care.
   1. Avoid soap, rubbing alcohol, and perfumed products (these are drying to the skin).
   2. Apply moisturizing lotion or baby oil frequently.
   3. Observe skin for any lesions, including scratch marks.
   4. Turn frequently and provide lotion to exposed skin.

F. Monitor fluid and electrolyte status daily.
   1. I&O (accurate output measurement may require ~~Foley~~ a catheter)
   2. Observe for edema, pulmonary edema.
   3. Measure abdominal girth (determines increase or decrease of ascites).
   4. Weigh daily (determines increase or decrease of edema and ascites).
   5. Restrict fluids to 1500 mL/day (may help to reduce edema and ascites).

G. Monitor dietary intake carefully, especially protein intake. Restrict protein if client has hepatic coma; otherwise, encourage foods with high biologic protein.

H. Explain dietary restrictions: low sodium, low potassium, low fat, high carbohydrate.

I. If encephalopathy is present, lactulose is used to decrease ammonia levels (Table 4.21).

J. If esophageal varices are present, esophagogastric balloon tamponade (Sengstaken-Blakemore tube), sclerotherapy, and/or portal systemic shunts may be used for treatment.

Hepatitis

Description: Widespread inflammation of liver cells, usually caused by a virus (Table 4.22)

Nursing Assessment

A. Known exposure to hepatitis

B. Individuals at risk for contracting hepatitis
   1. Homosexual males engaging in unprotected sex
   2. IV drug users (disease transmitted by dirty needles)
   3. Those who received tattoos or body piercing that could have been applied using dirty needles.
   4. Those living in crowded conditions
   5. Health care workers who do not use personal protective equipment (PPE) properly are at high risk

C. Monitor clients with the following symptoms:
   1. Fatigue, malaise, weakness
   2. Anorexia, nausea, and vomiting
   3. Jaundice, dark urine, clay-colored stools

TABLE 4.22 Comparison of Three Types of Hepatitis

Characteristics	Hepatitis A (Infectious Hepatitis)	Hepatitis B (Serum Hepatitis)	Hepatitis C (Non-A, Non-B Hepatitis)
• Source of infection	• Contaminated food • Contaminated water or shellfish	• Contaminated blood products • Contaminated needles or surgical instruments • Mother to child at birth	• Contaminated blood products • Contaminated needles; IV drug use • Dialysis
• Route of infection	• Oral • Fecal • Parenteral • Person to person	• Parenteral • Oral • Fecal • Direct contact • Breast milk • Sexual contact	• Parenteral • Sexual contact
• Incubation period	• 15–50 days	• 14–180 days	• Average: 14–180 days
• Onset	• Abrupt	• Insidious	• Insidious
• Seasonal variation	• Autumn • Winter	• All year	• All year
• Age group affected	• Children • Young adults	• Any age	• Any age
• Vaccine	• Yes	• Yes	• No
• Inoculation	• Yes	• Yes	• Yes
• Potential for chronic liver disease	• No	• Yes	• Yes
• Immunity	• Yes	• Yes	• No

IV, Intravenous.

4. Myalgia (muscle aches), joint pain
5. Dull headaches, irritability, depression
6. Abdominal tenderness in right upper quadrant
7. Fever (with hepatitis A)
8. Elevations of liver enzymes (ALT, AST, alkaline phosphatase), bilirubin

Nursing Plans and Interventions

A. Assess client's response to activity, and plan periods of rest after periods of activity.
B. Assist client with care as needed; encourage client to get help with daily activities at home (caring for children, preparing meals, etc.).
C. Provide high-calorie, high-carbohydrate diet with moderate fats and proteins.
   1. Serve small, frequent meals.
   2. Provide vitamin supplements.
   3. Provide foods the client prefers.
D. Administer medications, interferon, nucleoside and nucleotide analogs, protease.

HESI HINT For clients who are anorexic or nauseated
- Remove strong odors immediately; they can be offensive and increase nausea.
- Encourage client to sit up for meals; this can decrease the propensity to vomit.
- Serve small, frequent meals.
- Give antiemetic before eating.

E. Teach client importance of adhering to personal hygiene, using individual drinking and eating utensils, toothbrushes, and razors. Prevention of spread to others must be emphasized.
F. Teach client to avoid hepatotoxic substances such as alcohol, aspirin, acetaminophen, and sedatives.

HESI HINT Liver tissue is destroyed by hepatitis. Rest and adequate nutrition are necessary for regeneration of the liver tissue being destroyed by the disease. Many drugs are metabolized in the liver, so drug therapy must be scrutinized carefully. Caution the client that recovery takes many months, and previously taken medications and/or over-the-counter drugs should not be resumed without the health care provider's directions.

Pancreatitis

Description: Nonbacterial inflammation of the pancreas

A. Acute pancreatitis occurs when there is digestion of the pancreas by its own enzymes, primarily trypsin.
B. Alcohol ingestion and biliary tract disease are major causes of acute pancreatitis.
C. Chronic pancreatitis is a progressive, destructive disease that causes permanent dysfunction.
D. Long-term alcohol use is the major factor in chronic pancreatitis.
E. Alcohol consumption should be stopped when acute pancreatitis is suspected, and consumption completely avoided in chronic pancreatitis.

Nursing Assessment

A. Acute pancreatitis
   1. Severe mid-epigastric pain radiating to back; usually related to excess alcohol ingestion or a fatty meal
   2. Abdominal guarding; rigid, board-like abdomen, and abdominal pain
   3. Nausea and vomiting
   4. Elevated temperature, tachycardia, decreased BP
   5. Bluish discoloration of flanks (Grey Turner sign) or periumbilical area (Cullen sign)
   6. Elevated amylase, lipase, triglycerides, and glucose levels
   7. Low serum calcium levels
B. Chronic pancreatitis
   1. Continuous burning or gnawing abdominal pain
   2. Recurring attacks of severe upper abdominal and back pain
   3. Ascites
   4. Steatorrhea, diarrhea
   5. Weight loss
   6. Jaundice, dark urine
   7. Signs and symptoms of diabetes mellitus (DM)

Nursing Plans and Interventions

A. Acute pancreatitis
   1. Maintain NPO status.
   2. Maintain NG tube to suction; TPN may be prescribed.
   3. Administer hydromorphone (Dilaudid) or fentanyl (Sublimaze) as needed.
   4. Administer antacids, histamine H2 receptor-blocking drugs, anticholinergics, proton pump inhibitors.
   5. Assist client to assume position of comfort on side with legs drawn up to chest.
   6. Teach client to avoid alcohol, caffeine, and fatty and spicy foods.
   7. If severe, blood sugar monitoring and regular insulin coverage may be needed temporarily.
   8. Monitor for neuromuscular manifestations of hypocalcemia (e.g., tetany, muscle twitching, cramping, grimacing, seizure, altered deep tendon reflexes (DTRs), and spasm).
   9. Place in semi-Fowler position to decrease pressure on the diaphragm.
   10. Encourage client to cough and deep breathe, and/or use incentive spirometry.
   11. Monitor ECG for dysrhythmias related to electrolyte imbalances.

HESI HINT Acute pancreatic pain is located retroperitoneally. Any enlargement of the pancreas causes the peritoneum to stretch tightly. Therefore, sitting up or leaning forward reduces the pain.

B. Chronic pancreatitis
   1. Administer analgesics such as hydromorphone (Dilaudid), fentanyl (Sublimaze), and morphine (narcotic tolerance and dependency may be a problem).
   2. Administer pancreatic enzymes such as pancreatin (Creon) or pancrelipase (Viokase) with meals or snacks. Powdered forms should be mixed with fruit juice or applesauce (mixing with proteins should be avoided).
   3. Monitor client's stools for number and consistency to determine effectiveness of enzyme replacement.
   4. Teach client about consuming a bland, low-fat diet and to avoid rich foods, alcohol, and caffeine.
   5. Monitor for signs and symptoms of DM.

Cholecystitis and Cholelithiasis

Description: Cholecystitis: acute inflammation of the gallbladder; cholelithiasis: formation or presence of stones in the gallbladder

A. Incidence of these diseases is greater in females who are multiparous and overweight.
B. Treatment for cholecystitis consists of IV hydration, administration of antibiotics, and pain control with morphine or NSAIDs; anticholinergics are administered to decrease smooth muscle spasms.
C. Treatment for cholelithiasis consists of nonsurgical removal of stones.
   1. Dissolution therapy (administration of bile salts; used rarely)
   2. Endoscopic retrograde cholangiopancreatography (ERCP)

> **HESI HINT** The scope is placed in the gallbladder, and the stones are crushed and left to pass on their own. These clients may be prone to pancreatitis.

   3. Lithotripsy (not covered by many insurance carriers, thereby limiting its use)

D. Cholecystectomy is performed if stones are not removed non-surgically and inflammation is absent. It may be done through laparoscope.

Nursing Assessment

A. Pain, anorexia, vomiting, or flatulence precipitated by ingestion of fried, spicy, or fatty foods
B. Fever, elevated WBCs, and other signs of infection (cholecystitis)
C. Abdominal tenderness
D. Jaundice and clay-colored stools (blockage)
E. Elevated liver enzymes, bilirubin, and WBCs

Nursing Plans and Interventions

A. Administer analgesic for pain as needed.
B. Maintain NPO status.
C. Maintain NG tube to suction if indicated.
D. Administer IV antibiotics for cholecystitis and administer antibiotics prophylactically for cholelithiasis.
E. Monitor I&O.
F. Monitor electrolyte status regularly.
G. Teach client to avoid fried, spicy, and fatty foods and to reduce caloric intake if indicated.

> **HESI HINT**
> - Low-fat diet
> - Decompression of the stomach via NG tube
> - Medications for pain and clotting if required

H. Provide preoperative and postoperative care if surgery is indicated
I. Monitor T-tube drainage.

REVIEW OF GASTROINTESTINAL SYSTEM

1. List four nursing interventions for the client with a hiatal hernia.
2. List three categories of medications used in the treatment of PUD.
3. List the symptoms of upper and lower GI bleeding.
4. What bowel sound disruptions occur with an intestinal obstruction?
5. List four nursing interventions for postoperative care of a client with a colostomy.
6. List the common clinical manifestations of jaundice.
7. What are the common food intolerances for clients with cholelithiasis?
8. List five symptoms indicative of colon cancer.
9. In a client with cirrhosis, it is imperative to prevent further bleeding and observe for bleeding tendencies. List six relevant nursing interventions.
10. What is the main side effect of lactulose, which is used to reduce ammonia levels in clients with cirrhosis?
11. List four groups who have a high risk for contracting hepatitis.
12. How should the nurse administer pancreatic enzymes?

See Answer Key at the end of this text for suggested responses.

ENDOCRINE SYSTEM

Hyperthyroidism (Graves Disease, Goiter)

Description: Excessive activity of thyroid gland, resulting in an elevated level of circulating thyroid hormones. Possibly long-term or lifelong treatment.

A. Hyperthyroidism can result from a primary disease state; from the use of replacement hormone therapy; or from excess thyroid-stimulating hormone (TSH) being produced by an anterior pituitary tumor.
B. Graves disease is thought to be an autoimmune process and accounts for most cases.
C. Diagnosis is made on the basis of serum hormone levels.
D. Common treatment for hyperthyroidism—goal is to create a euthyroid state
   1. Thyroid ablation by medication
   2. Radioactive iodine therapy
   3. Thyroidectomy
   4. Adenectomy of portion of anterior pituitary where TSH-producing tumor is located
E. All treatments make the client hypothyroid, requiring hormone replacement.

Nursing Assessment

A. Enlarged thyroid gland
B. Acceleration of body processes
   1. Weight loss
   2. Increased appetite
   3. Diarrhea
   4. Heat intolerance
   5. Tachycardia, palpitations, increased systolic BP
   6. Diaphoresis, wet or moist skin
   7. Nervousness, insomnia
C. Exophthalmos (Fig. 4.6)
D. T_3 elevated above 220 ng/dL

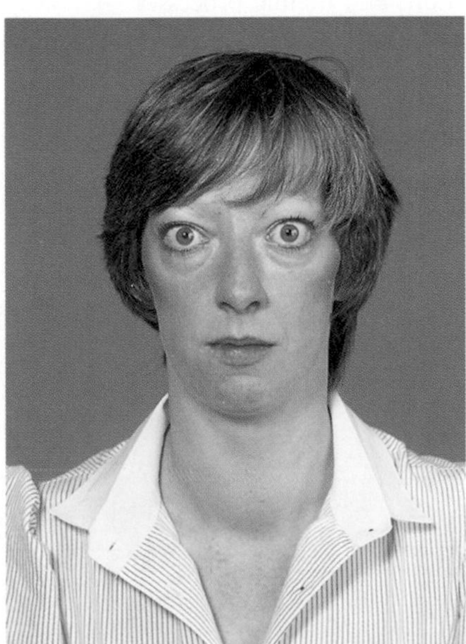

Fig. 4.6 Graves Disease. This woman has a diffuse goiter and exophthalmos. (From Forbes, C. D., & Jackson, W. F. [2003]. *Colour atlas and text of clinical medicine* [3rd ed.]. London: Mosby.)

E. T_4 elevated above 12 mcg/dL
F. Low level of TSH indicates primary disease; elevated T_4 level suppresses thyroid-releasing hormone (TRH), which suppresses TSH secretion. If source is anterior pituitary, both will be elevated.
G. Radioactive iodine uptake (^{131}I) (indicates presence of goiter)
H. Thyroid scan (indicating presence of goiter)

Nursing Plans and Interventions

A. Provide a calm, restful atmosphere.
B. Observe for signs of thyroid storm (sudden over secretion of thyroid hormone; is life threatening).

> **HESI HINT** Thyroid storm is a life-threatening event that occurs with uncontrolled hyperthyroidism due to Graves disease. Other causes include childbirth, congestive heart failure (CHF), diabetic ketoacidosis (DKA), infection, pulmonary embolism, emotional distress, trauma, and surgery. Symptoms include fever, tachycardia, agitation, anxiety, and hypertension. Primary nursing interventions include maintaining an airway and adequate aeration.
>
> Propylthiouracil (PTU) and methimazole (Tapazole) are antithyroid drugs used to treat thyroid storm. Propranolol (Inderal) may be given to decrease excessive sympathetic stimulation.

C. Teach the following:
   1. After treatment, resulting hypothyroidism will require daily hormone replacement.
   2. Client should wear Medic Alert jewelry in case of emergency.
   3. Signs of hormone replacement overdosage are the signs for hyperthyroidism (see "Nursing Assessment" in "Hyperthyroidism," in this chapter).
   4. Signs of hormone replacement underdosage are the signs for hypothyroidism (see "Nursing Assessment" in "Hyperthyroidism," in this chapter).
D. Explain to client the recommended diet: high-calorie, high-protein, low-caffeine, low-fiber diet (if diarrhea is present).
E. Perform eye care for exophthalmos.
   1. Artificial tears to maintain moisture
   2. Sunglasses when in bright light
   3. Annual eye examinations
F. Prepare client for treatment of hyperthyroidism.
   1. Thyroid ablation
      a. PTU and methimazole (Tapazole) act by blocking synthesis of T_3 and T_4.
      b. Dosage is calculated based on body weight and is prescribed over several months.
      c. Client should take medication exactly as prescribed so that the desired effect can be achieved.
      d. The expected effect is to make the client euthyroid, often given to prepare the client for thyroidectomy.
   2. Radiation
      a. ^{131}I is given to destroy thyroid cells.
      b. ^{131}I is very irritating to the GI tract.
      c. Clients commonly vomit (vomitus is radioactive).

d. Place client on radiation precautions. Use time, distance, and shielding as means of protection against radiation (see "Reproductive System," in this chapter).

3. Thyroidectomy

HESI HINT After a thyroidectomy, be prepared for the possibility of laryngeal edema. Put a tracheostomy set at the bedside along with O_2 and a suction machine; calcium gluconate should be easily accessible if parathyroid glands have been accidently removed.

a. Check frequently for bleeding (on the anterior or posterior of the dressing), irregular breathing, neck swelling, frequent swallowing, and sensations of fullness at the incision site.
b. Support the neck when moving client (do not hyperextend).
c. Check for laryngeal edema, laryngeal nerve damage leads to vocal cord paralysis; therefore, observe for hoarseness or inability to speak clearly.
d. Monitor Trousseau and Chvostek signs because removal of the parathyroid(s) may lead to tetany.
e. Keep drainage devices, like Jackson-Pratt drains, compressed and empty.

4. Hypophysectomy (pituitary adenectomy)
   a. Is employed if the client's condition is the result of increased pituitary secretion of adrenocorticotropic hormone (ACTH).
   b. TSH-secreting pituitary tumors are resected using a transnasal approach (transsphenoidal hypophysectomy) via endoscopic transnasal approach.
   c. Monitor for nasal discharge or postnasal drip that may be indicative of cerebrospinal leakage (assess drainage for glucose).

HESI HINT Normal serum calcium is 9.0—10.5 mEq/L. The best indicator of parathyroid problems is a decrease in the client's calcium compared with the preoperative value.

HESI HINT If two or more parathyroid glands have been removed, the chance of tetany increases dramatically.
- Monitor serum calcium levels (9.0—10.5 mg/dL is normal range).
- Check for tingling of toes and fingers and around the mouth.
- Check Chvostek sign (twitching of lip after a tap over the facial nerve at the angle of the jaw means it is positive; Fig. 4.7).
- Check Trousseau sign (carpopedal spasm after BP cuff is inflated above systolic pressure and held for 3 min means it is positive; see Fig. 4.7).

Hypothyroidism (Hashimoto Disease, Myxedema)

Description: Hypofunction of the thyroid gland, with resulting insufficiency of thyroid hormone

A. Early symptoms of hypothyroidism are nonspecific but gradually intensify.
B. Hypothyroidism is treated by hormone replacement.
C. Endemic goiters occur in individuals living in areas where there is a deficit of iodine. Iodized salt has helped to prevent this problem.

HESI HINT Myxedema coma can be precipitated by acute illness, withdrawal of thyroid medication, anesthesia, use of sedatives, or hypoventilation (with the potential for respiratory acidosis and CO_2 narcosis). The airway must be kept patent and ventilator support used as indicated.

Nursing Assessment

A. Fatigue
B. Thin, dry hair; dry skin
C. Thick, brittle nails
D. Constipation
E. Bradycardia, hypotension
F. Goiter
G. Periorbital edema, facial puffiness
H. Cold intolerance
I. Weight gain
J. Dull emotions and mental processes
K. Diagnosis
   1. Low T_3 (below 70)
   2. Low T_4 (below 5)
   3. Presence of T_4 antibody (indicating that T_4 is being destroyed by the body)
L. Husky voice
M. Slow speech

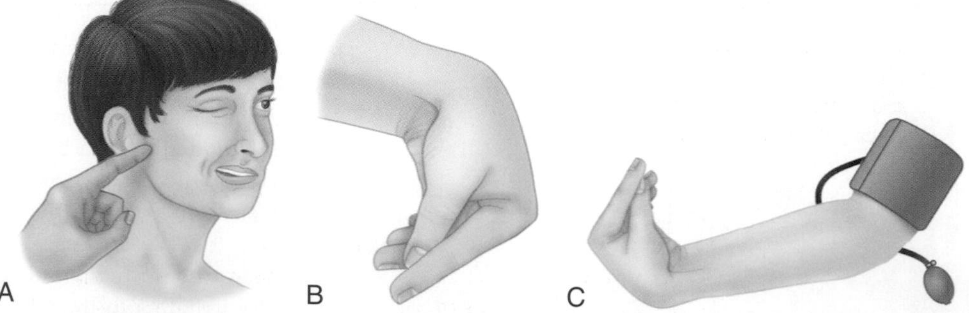

Fig. 4.7 Tests for Hypocalcemia. (A) Chvostek sign is contraction of facial muscles in response to a light tap over the facial nerve in front of the ear. (B) Trousseau sign is a carpal spasm induced by (C), inflating a BP cuff above the systolic pressure for a few minutes. (From Lewis, S. M., Heitkemper, M. M., & Dirksen, S. R. [2019]. *Medical-surgical nursing: Assessment and management of clinical problems* [11th ed.]. London: Mosby.)

TABLE 4.23 **Thyroid Preparations**

Drugs	Indications	Adverse Reactions	Nursing Implications
• Levothyroxine • Liothyronine sodium • Desiccated thyroid	• Action is to increase metabolic rates • Synthetic T_4	• Anxiety • Insomnia • Tremors • Tachycardia • Palpitations • Angina • Dysrhythmias	• Give in early morning before meals. • Check serum hormone levels routinely. • Check BP and pulse regularly. • Weigh daily. • Report side effects to health care provider. • Avoid foods and products containing iodine. • Initiate cautiously in clients with cardiovascular disease.

BP, Blood pressure.

Nursing Plans and Interventions

A. Teach the following:
   1. Medication regimen: daily dose of prescribed hormone
   2. Medication effects and side effects (Table 4.23)
   3. Ongoing follow-up to determine serum hormone levels
   4. Signs and symptoms of myxedema coma (hypoventilation, hypotension, hypothermia, hyponatremia, hypoglycemia, lactic acidosis, and respiratory failure)

B. Develop a bowel elimination plan to prevent constipation.
   1. Fluid intake to be 3 L/day
   2. High-fiber diet, including fresh fruits and vegetables
   3. Increased activity
   4. Little or no use of enemas and laxatives

C. Avoid sedating client; it can lead to respiratory difficulties.

Addison Disease (Primary Adrenocortical Deficiency)

Description: Autoimmune process commonly found in conjunction with other endocrine diseases of an autoimmune nature; a primary disorder; hypofunction of the adrenal cortex

A. Sudden withdrawal from corticosteroids may precipitate symptoms of Addison disease (Table 4.24).

B. Addison disease is characterized by lack of cortisol, aldosterone, and androgens.

C. Definitive diagnosis is made using an ACTH stimulation test.

D. If ACTH production by the anterior pituitary has failed, it is considered secondary Addison disease.

HESI HINT Many people take steroids for a variety of conditions. NCLEX-RN questions often focus on the need to teach clients the importance of following the prescribed regimen precisely. They should be cautioned against stopping the medications suddenly and should be informed that it is necessary to taper off the dosage when taking steroids.

Nursing Assessment

A. Fatigue, weakness

B. Weight loss, anorexia, nausea, vomiting

C. Postural hypotension

D. Hypoglycemia

E. Hyponatremia

F. Hyperkalemia

G. Hyperpigmentation of mucous membranes and skin (only if **primary** Addison disease; not seen in **secondary** Addison disease)

H. Signs of shock when in Addison crises

I. Loss of body hair

J. Hypovolemia
   1. Hypotension
   2. Tachycardia
   3. Fever

Nursing Plans and Interventions

A. Take vital signs frequently (every 15 minutes if in crisis).

B. Monitor I&O and weigh daily.

C. Instruct client to rise slowly because of the possibility of postural hypotension.

TABLE 4.24 **Corticosteroids**

Drugs	Indications	Adverse Reactions	Nursing Implications
• Hydrocortisone • Prednisone • Dexamethasone • Methylprednisolone	• Hormone replacement • Severe rheumatoid arthritis • Autoimmune disorders	• Emotional lability • Impaired wound healing • Skin fragility • Abnormal fat deposition • Hyperglycemia • Hirsutism • Moon face • Osteoporosis • All symptoms of Cushing syndrome if overdosage occurs	• Wean slowly (administer a high dose, then taper off); careful monitoring is required during withdrawal. • Monitor serum potassium, glucose (can become diabetic), and sodium. • Weigh daily; report weight gain of more than 5 lb per week. • Administer with antiulcer drugs or food. • Use care to prevent injuries. • Teach symptoms of Cushing syndrome. • Monitor BP and pulse closely.

BP, Blood pressure.

D. During Addison crises, administer IV glucose with parenteral hydrocortisone, a steroid with both mineralocorticoid and glucocorticoid properties; requires large fluid volume replacement.
E. Monitor serum electrolyte levels.
F. Maintain low-stress environment (protect client from noise, light, and temperature extremes because client cannot physiologically cope with stress).
G. Teach the following:
   1. Need for lifelong hormone replacement
   2. Need for close medical supervision
   3. Need for Medic Alert jewelry
   4. Signs and symptoms of overdosage and underdosage of medication
   5. Diet requirements: high sodium, low potassium, and high carbohydrate (complex carbohydrates)
   6. Fluid requirements: intake of at least 3 L of fluid per day
H. Provide ulcer prophylaxis.

> **HESI HINT** *Addison crisis is a medical emergency.* It is brought on by sudden withdrawal of steroids, a stressful event (trauma, severe infection), exposure to cold, overexertion, or decrease in salt intake.
> A. Vascular collapse: Hypotension and tachycardia occur; administer IV fluids at a rapid rate until stabilized.
> B. Hypoglycemia: Administer IV glucose.
> C. Essential to reversing the crisis: Administer parenteral hydrocortisone.
> D. Aldosterone replacement: Administer fludrocortisone acetate (Florinef) PO (available only as oral preparation) with simultaneous administration of salt (sodium chloride) if client has a sodium deficit.

Description: Excess adrenocorticoid activity
I. Cause is usually chronic administration of corticosteroids.
J. Cushing syndrome can also be caused by adrenal, pituitary, or hypothalamus tumors.

Nursing Assessment

A. Physical symptoms include
   1. Moon face
   2. Truncal obesity
   3. Buffalo hump
   4. Abdominal striae
   5. Muscle atrophy
   6. Thinning of the skin
   7. Hirsutism in females
   8. Hyperpigmentation
   9. Amenorrhea
   10. Edema, poor wound healing
   11. Impotence
   12. Bruises easily
B. Hypertension
C. Susceptibility to multiple infections
D. Osteoporosis
E. Peptic ulcer formation
F. Many false positives and false negatives in laboratory testing
G. Laboratory data often include the following findings:
   1. Hyperglycemia
   2. Hypernatremia
   3. Hypokalemia
   4. Decreased eosinophils and lymphocytes
   5. Increased plasma cortisol
   6. Increased urinary 17-hydroxycorticoids

Nursing Plans and Interventions

A. Encourage the client to protect self from exposure to infection.
B. Wash hands; use good handwashing technique.
C. Monitor client for signs of infection
   1. Fever
   2. Oral infection by *Candida* spp.
   3. Vaginal yeast infections
   4. Adventitious lungs sounds
   5. Skin lesions
   6. Elevated WBCs
D. Teach safety measures.
   1. Position bed close to floor, with call light within easy reach.
   2. Encourage use of side rails.
   3. Be sure walkways are unobstructed.
   4. Encourage wearing shoes when ambulating.
E. Provide low-sodium diet; encourage consumption of foods that contain vitamin D and calcium.
F. Provide good skin and perineal care.
G. Discuss possibility of weaning from steroids after surgery. (If weaning is done too quickly, symptoms of Addison disease will occur.)
H. Encourage selection of clothing that minimizes visible aberrations; encourage maintenance of normal physical appearance.
I. Monitor I&O and weigh daily.
J. Provide ulcer prophylaxis.

> **HESI HINT** Teach clients to take steroids with meals to prevent gastric irritation. They should never skip doses. If they have nausea or vomiting for more than 12–24 h, they should contact the physician.

Diabetes Mellitus (DM)

Description: A metabolic disorder characterized by high levels of glucose resulting from defects in insulin secretion, insulin action, or both
A. DM is characterized by hyperglycemia.
B. DM affects the metabolism of protein, carbohydrate, and fat.
C. Four ways to diagnose DM
   1. Fasting plasma glucose (FPG) greater than or equal to 126 mg/dL
   2. Glycosylated Hgb (HbA_{1c}) greater than or equal to 6.5%
   3. Random blood glucose greater than or equal to 200 mg/dL in a client with classic symptoms of hyperglycemia
   4. Oral glucose tolerance test (OGTT) greater than 200
      a. Use plasma glucose, not fingersticks, to diagnose diabetes.
      b. Results should be confirmed on a subsequent visit.

D. The major classifications of diabetes are
  1. Type 1: results from B-cell destruction
  2. Type 2: results from progressive secretory insulin deficit and/or defect in insulin uptake
  3. Other: transplant-related diabetes, cystic fibrosis–related diabetes, iatrogenic-induced (stress, hospital) diabetes, steroid-induced diabetes
  4. Gestational diabetes
  5. Prediabetes: Blood glucose levels when fasting are 100 to 125 mg/dL or HbA_{1C} of 5.7% to 6.4%.
E. Many clients diagnosed with type 2 DM use insulin but retain some degree of pancreatic function.
F. Obesity is a major risk factor in type 2 DM (Table 4.25).

Clinical Characteristics and Treatment of Diabetes Mellitus

A. Type 1
  1. Description: Results from the progressive autoimmune-based destruction of beta cells
    a. Can become hyperglycemic and ketosis-prone relatively easily
    b. Precipitating factors for DKA include infection and inadequate or under-management of glucose.
  2. Clinical characteristics of DKA
    a. Serum glucose of 250 and above
    b. Ketonuria in large amounts
    c. Arterial pH of <7.30 and HCO_3 <15 mEq/L
    d. Nausea, vomiting, dehydration, abdominal pain, Kussmaul's respirations, acetone odor to breath
  3. Treatment
    a. Usually with isotonic IV fluids, 0.9% sodium chloride (NaCl) solution until BP stabilized and urine output 30 to 60 mL/h
    b. Slow infusion by IV pump of regular insulin, too rapid infusion of insulin to lower serum glucose can lead to cerebral edema
    c. Careful replacement of potassium based on laboratory data
B. Type 2
  1. Description: Results from either the inadequate production of insulin by the body or lack of sensitivity to the insulin being produced
    a. Rare development of ketoacidosis
    b. With extreme hyperglycemia, hyperosmolar hyperglycemia nonketotic syndrome (HHNKS) develops.
  2. Clinical characteristics of HHNKS
    a. Hyperglycemia >600 mg/dL
    b. Plasma hyperosmolality
    c. Dehydration
    d. Changed mental status
    e. Absent ketone bodies
  3. Treatment
    a. Usually with isotonic IV fluid replacement and careful monitoring of potassium and glucose levels
    b. IV insulin given until blood glucose stable at 250 mg/dL

Nursing Assessment

Complications of diabetes
A. Integument
  1. Skin infections
  2. Wounds that do not heal
  3. Acanthosis

HESI HINT Why do clients with diabetes have trouble with wound healing? High blood glucose contributes to damage of the smallest vessels, the capillaries. This damage causes permanent capillary scarring, which inhibits the normal activity of the capillary. This phenomenon causes disruption of capillary elasticity and promotes problems such as diabetic retinopathy, poor healing of breaks in the skin, and cardiovascular abnormalities.

TABLE 4.25 Comparison of Type 1 and Type 2 Diabetes Mellitus

Variable	Type 1 DM	Type 2 DM
Prevalence	5% of U.S. population with DM	90%–95% of U.S. population with DM
Pathology	Beta-cell destruction leading to absolute insulin deficiency	Basic defect is insulin resistance and usually have relative rather than absolute insulin deficiency
Onset	Sudden	Gradual, insidious
Signs and symptoms	Polyuria, polydipsia, polyphagia, weight loss	Polydipsia, polyuria, polyphagia, weight loss, fatigue, frequent infections, blurred vision, impotence
Age at onset	Any age but mostly young, under 21	Any age but mostly in adults
Weight	Thin, slender	Overweight, obese
Ketosis	Common	Rare
Pathology	Autoimmune and viral component	Obesity, cardiovascular disease (CVD) an equal comorbidity Genetic predisposition
Lifestyle management	MNT: carbohydrate counting Physical activity	MNT: Heart-healthy, portion-controlled diet Physical activity
Pharmacologic management	Intensive insulin therapy	Typically a stepwise approach Diet, exercise Oral agents Oral agents and insulin Insulin

B. Oral cavity
   1. Periodontal disease
   2. Candidiasis (raised, white patchy areas on mucous membranes)
C. Eyes
   1. Cataracts
   2. Retinopathy
D. Cardiopulmonary system
   1. Angina
   2. Dyspnea
   3. Hypertension
E. Periphery
   1. Hair loss on extremities, indicating poor perfusion
   2. Other signs of poor peripheral circulation
      a. Coolness
      b. Skin shininess and thinness
      c. Weak or absent peripheral pulses
      d. Ulcerations on extremities
      e. Pallor
      f. Thick nails with ridges
F. Kidneys
   1. Edema of face, hands, and feet
   2. Symptoms of UTI
   3. Symptoms of renal failure: edema, anorexia, nausea, fatigue, difficulty in concentrating
   4. Diabetic nephropathy is the primary cause of end-stage renal failure in the United States
G. Neuromusculature
   1. Neuropathies
   2. Symptoms of neuropathies: numbness, tingling, pain, burning
H. GI disturbances
   1. Nighttime diarrhea
   2. Gastroparesis (faulty absorption)
I. Reproductive
   1. Male: impotence
   2. Female: vaginal dryness, frequent vaginal infections
   3. Menstrual irregularities
J. Psychosocial issues
   1. Depression: Persons with DM have a high rate of depression. Depression contributes to poor DM regimen adherence, feelings of helplessness, and poor health outcomes.
   2. Increased risk of developing anorexia nervosa and bulimia nervosa in women with type 1 DM.

HESI HINT
Glycosylated Hgb (HbA_{1c})
- Indicates glucose control over previous 90–120 days (life of red blood cells [RBCs])
- Is a valuable measurement of diabetes control
- Informs diagnosis of diabetes and prediabetes

Nursing Plans and Interventions

A. Determine baseline laboratory data.
   1. Serum glucose
   2. Electrolytes
   3. Creatinine
   4. BUN
   5. Cholesterol, both LDL and HDL
   6. Triglycerides
   7. ABGs as indicated
B. Teach injection technique and/or oral medication(s).
   1. Identify the prescribed dose and type of insulin (Tables 4.26 and 4.27).
   2. For insulin
      a. Lift skin; use 90-degree angle. If client is very thin or using 5/16-inch needle, the nurse may need to use a 45-degree angle.
      b. Do not reuse syringes or needles.
   3. Rotate injection sites.
   4. Usually insulins are premixed; if insulin is not premixed, draw regular insulin into syringe first when mixing insulins.
C. Teach about medical nutrition therapy (MNT).
   1. Work with dietitian to reinforce specific meal plan.
   2. Overall goal is to make healthy nutritional choices and eat a varied diet.
   3. Encourage carbohydrate counting for those on complex insulin regimens.
   4. Teach that meals should be timed according to medication (insulin) peak times.
   5. Teach diet regimen.
      a. 45% to 50% carbohydrates
      b. 15% to 20% protein
      c. 30% or less fat
      d. Foods high in complex carbohydrates, high in fiber, and low in fat, whenever possible
      e. Alcoholic beverages can be included in diet with proper planning
   6. Teach about managing sick days (illness raises blood glucose).
      a. Teach client to keep taking insulin.
      b. Monitor glucose more frequently.
      c. Watch for signs of hyperglycemia.

HESI HINT The body's response to illness and stress is to produce glucose. Therefore, any illness results in hyperglycemia.

D. Teach exercise regimen because exercise decreases blood sugar levels.
   1. Exercise after mealtime; either exercise with someone or let someone know where exercise will take place to ensure safety.
   2. A snack may be needed before or during exercise.

TABLE 4.26 **Oral Hypoglycemics**

Drugs	Indications	Adverse Reactions	Nursing Implications
SULFONYLUREAS			
First Generation • Tolbutamide • Chlorpropamide *Second Generation* • Glyburide • Glipizide • Glimepiride	• Lowers blood sugar by stimulating the release of insulin by the beta cells of the pancreas and causes tissues to take up and store glucose more easily • First generation is low potency and short acting • Second generation is high potency and longer acting	*First Generation* • Hypoglycemia • Nausea, heartburn, constipation, anorexia • Agranulocytosis • Allergic skin reactions *Second Generation* • Weight gain • Hypoglycemia, particularly in older adults	*First Generation* • Responsiveness may decline over time. • Given once daily with first meal. • Monitor blood sugar. • Hard to detect hypoglycemia if older adult or also on beta-blockers. *Second Generation* • Less likely to interact with other medications
BIGUANIDES			
• Metformin	• Lowers serum glucose levels by inhibiting hepatic glucose production and increasing sensitivity of peripheral tissue to insulin	• Abdominal discomfort • Diarrhea • Lactic acidosis	• Many drug–drug interactions. • Extended-release tablets should be taken with the evening meal. • Use cautiously with preexisting renal or liver disease or HF. • Discontinue 48 h before and wait 48 h to restart dosage after diagnostic studies requiring IV iodine contrast media. • Can lead to vitamin B_{12} deficiency
ALPHA-GLUCOSIDASE INHIBITORS			
• Acarbose • Miglitol	• Lowers blood glucose by blunting sugar levels after meals	• Hypoglycemia	• Optimally, must be taken with the *first* bite of each meal. • May be taken with other classes of oral hypoglycemics. • Monitor blood sugar. • Use is controversial in inflammatory bowel disease (IBD) client.
THIAZOLIDINEDIONES			
• Rosiglitazone • Pioglitazone	• Lowers blood sugar by decreasing the insulin resistance of the tissues	• Hypoglycemia • Increased total cholesterol, weight gain • Edema, anemia	• Many drug–drug interactions. • Skip dose if meal skipped. • Monitor liver function. • Caution with use in CAD; may precipitate HF.
MEGLITINIDES			
• Repaglinide • Nateglinide	• Lowers blood sugar by stimulating beta cells in pancreas to release insulin; does this by closing potassium channels and opening calcium channels	• Hypoglycemia • Angina, chest pain • Arthralgia, back pain • Nausea and vomiting, dyspepsia, constipation, or diarrhea	• May be used with metformin. • Give before meals; if a meal is skipped, skip the dose. • Monitor blood sugar.
INCRETIN ENHANCER			
• Linagliptin • Saxagliptin • Sitagliptin	• Lowers blood glucose by inhibiting degradation of incretins, which increases insulin secretion	• Hypoglycemia	• Not considered a first-line agent
COMBINATIONS			
• Glyburide + metformin • Pioglitazone + metformin • Rosiglitazone + glimepiride • Rosiglitazone + metformin • Glipizide + metformin	• Lowers blood sugar by combining the advantages of two classes of hypoglycemics	• Note possible adverse reactions to both classes • Hypoglycemia (severe)	• Note implications of both classes of drugs.

CAD, Coronary artery disease; *HF*, heart failure; *IV*, intravenous.

TABLE 4.27 Types of Insulin and Other Injectable Therapies

Type	Name	Onset	Peak Action	Duration	Nursing Implications
• Rapid-acting	• Human insulin lispro Aspart • Glulisine	• 15–30 min • 15–30 min • 15–30 min	• 30–90 min • 30–90 min • 30–90 min	• 3–5 h • 3–5 h • 3–5 h	• Give within 15 min of a meal.
• Short-acting	• Regular insulin (human)	• 30–60 min	• 2–3 h	• 5–7 h	• Regular insulin may be given IV.
• Intermediate-acting	• Isophane insulin (human)	• 1–2 h	• 4.6 h	• 14.24 h	• Not to be given IV. • Mixtures combine rapid-acting regular insulin with intermediate-acting NPH insulin in a 30% regular with 70% NPH proportion or at 50/50 combination.
• Long-acting	• Glargine • Detemir	• 1 h • 1.1 h	• 14.20 h • 5 h peakless (source: niddk.nih.gov)	• 24 h	• Not to be given IV. • Recommended: give once daily (subcutaneous) at bedtime. • In some cases, given two times a day. • Acts as basal insulin. • Caution: Solution is clear, but bottle is distinctly different shape from regular insulin. • Do not confuse insulins. • Do not shake solution. • Do not mix other insulins with Lantus. • Use cautiously if client is NPO.
• Premix	• Humalog 75/25 • Human 70/30 • NovoLog 70/30 • Humalog 50/50	• 10–30 min • 5–10 min	• Varies 1–4 h	• 10–16 h	• For all premixes: Offer when food readily available • 25% Lispro/75% Humulin N (NPH) • 30% Regular/70% NPH • 30% Aspart/70% NPH

OTHER INJECTABLE THERAPIES

Drugs	Action/Indications	Adverse Reaction	Implications and Precautions
• Exenatide	• Stimulates release of insulin; ↓ glucagon secretion; ↑ satiety; ↓ gastric emptying; may facilitate weight loss (≈3–5 kg) • Indicated for clients with type 2 DM who are not adequately controlled with oral therapy. It is not indicated for clients with type 1 DM.	• Nausea, vomiting, hypoglycemia, diarrhea, headache	• Not a substitute for insulin • Not recommended for ESRD, pancreatitis, severe renal impairment, or severe GI disease • May slow absorption of other drugs
• Pramlintide	• Slows gastric emptying time, suppresses the release of glucagon, and appears to suppress appetite. • Indicated as adjunct treatment in type 1 DM for clients who have not obtained adequate glycemic control with insulin therapy and for clients with type 2 DM who have not obtained adequate glycemic control with insulin with or without oral therapy	• Nausea, vomiting, • Hypoglycemia, diarrhea, headache	• Contraindicated for clients with diabetic gastroparesis. It is also avoided in clients who have exhibited significant hypoglycemic reactions or who are not able to recognize and manage hypoglycemic reactions.

ESRD, End-stage renal disease; *GI*, gastrointestinal; *IV*, intravenous.

TABLE 4.28 **Comparison of Hyperglycemia and Hypoglycemia**

HYPERGLYCEMIA		HYPOGLYCEMIA	
Signs and Symptoms	**Nursing Action**	**Signs and Symptoms**	**Nursing Action**
• Polydipsia • Polyuria • Polyphagia • Blurred vision • Weakness • Weight loss • Syncope	• Encourage water intake. • Check blood glucose frequently. • Assess for ketoacidosis: • Urine ketones • Urine glucose • Administer insulin as directed	• Headache • Nausea • Sweating • Tremors • Lethargy • Hunger • Confusion • Slurred speech • Tingling around mouth • Anxiety, nightmares	• Usually occurs rapidly and is potentially life threatening; treat immediately with complex carbohydrates (CHO). • Example: fast-acting carbohydrates. • One tube glucose gel, 120–180 mL fruit juice or cola, 10–16 jellybeans, 10 gum drops, 3 pieces of hard candy (Jolly Rancher), 5–7 pieces Life Savers–type candy • Check blood glucose (may seize if < 40).

3. Monitor blood glucose before, during, and after exercise when beginning a new regimen.

E. Teach signs and symptoms of hyperglycemia and hypoglycemia (Table 4.28).

HESI HINT If in doubt whether a client is hyperglycemic or hypoglycemic, treat for hypoglycemia.

HESI HINT Teach self-monitoring of blood glucose (SMBG)
- Uses techniques that are specific to each meter
- Frequency of monitoring based on treatment regimen, change in meals, illness, and exercise regimen
- Requires recording results and reporting results to health care provider at time of visit
- Results of monitoring used to assess the efficacy of therapy and to guide adjustments in MNT, exercise, and medications to achieve the best possible blood glucose control

F. Teach about foot care.
1. Feet should be checked daily for changes; signs of injury and breaks in skin should be reported to health care provider.
2. Feet should be washed daily with mild soap and warm water; soaking is to be avoided; feet should be dried well, especially between toes.
3. Feet may be moisturized with a lanolin product, but not between the toes.
4. Well-fitting leather shoes should be worn; going barefoot and wearing sandals are to be avoided.
5. Clean socks should be worn daily.
6. Garters and tight elastic-topped socks should never be worn.
7. A professional should remove corns and calluses.
8. Nails should be cut or filed straight across.
9. Warm socks should be worn if feet are cold.

G. Encourage regular health care follow-ups.
1. Ophthalmologist
2. Podiatrist
3. Annual physical examination

H. Teach that immediate attention should be sought if any sign of infection occurs.

I. Refer client to the American Diabetes Association for additional information.

REVIEW OF ENDOCRINE SYSTEM

1. What diagnostic test is used to determine thyroid activity?
2. What condition results from all treatments for hyperthyroidism?
3. State three symptoms of hyperthyroidism and three symptoms of hypothyroidism.
4. List five important teaching aspects for clients who are beginning corticosteroid therapy.
5. Describe the physical appearance of clients who have Cushing syndrome.
6. Which type of diabetes always requires insulin replacement?
7. Which type of diabetes sometimes requires no medication?
8. List five symptoms of hyperglycemia.
9. List five symptoms of hypoglycemia.
10. Name the necessary elements to include in teaching a client newly diagnosed with diabetes.
11. The nurse is in a situation where there is no premixed insulin. In fewer than 10 steps, describe the method of drawing up a mixed dose of insulin (regular with NPH).
12. Identify the peak action time of the following types of insulin: rapid-acting regular insulin, intermediate-acting insulin, and long-acting insulin.
13. When preparing a client with diabetes for discharge, the nurse teaches the client the relationship between stress, exercise, bedtime snacking, and glucose balance. State the relationships among each of these.

14. When making rounds at night, the nurse notes that a client prescribed insulin is complaining of a headache, slight nausea, and minimal trembling. The client's hand is cool and moist. What is the client most likely experiencing?

15. Identify five foot-care interventions that should be taught to a client with diabetes.

See Answer Key at the end of this text for suggested responses.

MUSCULOSKELETAL SYSTEM

Rheumatoid Arthritis

Description: Chronic, systematic, progressive deterioration of the connective tissue (synovium) of the joints; characterized by inflammation

A. The exact cause is unknown, but it is classified as an immune complex disorder.
B. Joint involvement is bilateral and symmetrical.
C. Severe cases may require joint replacement (see "Joint Replacement," later).

Nursing Assessment

A. Fatigue
B. Generalized weakness
C. Weight loss

> **HESI HINT** A client comes to the clinic complaining of morning stiffness, weight loss, and swelling of both hands and wrists. Rheumatoid arthritis is suspected. Which methods of assessment might the nurse use, and which methods would the nurse not use? Use inspection, palpation, and strength testing. Do not assess range of motion (ROM); this activity promotes pain because ROM is limited.

D. Anorexia
E. Morning stiffness
F. Bilateral inflammation of joints with the following symptoms:
   1. Decreased ROM
   2. Joint pain
   3. Warmth
   4. Edema
   5. Erythema
G. Joint deformity

> **HESI HINT** In the joint, the normal cartilage becomes soft, fissures and pitting occur, and the cartilage thins. Spurs form and inflammation sets in. The result is deformity marked by immobility, pain, and muscle spasm. The prescribed treatment regimen is corticosteroids for the inflammation; splinting, immobilization, and rest for the joint deformity; and NSAIDs for the pain. Synovial tissues line the bones of the joints. Inflammation of this lining causes destruction of tissue and bone. Early detection of rheumatoid arthritis can decrease the amount of bone and joint destruction. Often the disease goes into remission. Decreasing the amount of bone and joint destruction reduces the amount of disability.

H. Diagnosis is confirmed by the following:
   1. Elevated erythrocyte sedimentation rate (ESR)
   2. Positive rheumatoid factor
   3. Presence of antinuclear antibody
   4. Joint-space narrowing indicated by arthroscopic examination (provides joint visualization)
   5. Abnormal synovial fluid (fluid in joint) indicated by arthrocentesis
   6. C-reactive protein indicated by active inflammation

Nursing Plans and Interventions

A. Implement pain relief measures.
   1. Use moist heat.
      a. Warm, moist compresses
      b. Whirlpool baths
      c. Hot shower in the morning
   2. Use diversionary activities.
      a. Imaging
      b. Distraction
      c. Self-hypnosis
      d. Biofeedback
   3. Administer medications and teach client about medications (Table 4.29; see Table 4.24).

TABLE 4.29 Nonsteroidal Anti-inflammatory Drugs

Drugs	Indications	Adverse Reactions	Nursing Implications
• Aspirin • Ibuprofen • Indomethacin • Ketorolac tromethamine • Celecoxib • Etodolac • Diclofenac • Naproxen • Piroxicam	• Used as anti-inflammatory • Antipyretic • Analgesic • Can be used with other agents; only NSAID available for IV administration.	• GI irritation, bleeding • Nausea, vomiting, constipation • Elevated liver enzymes • Prolonged coagulation time • Tinnitus • Thrombocytopenia • Fluid retention • Nephrotoxicity • Blood dyscrasias	• Teach to take with food or milk to reduce GI symptoms. • Teach to watch for signs of bleeding. • Teach to avoid alcohol. • Teach to observe for tinnitus. • Administer corticosteroids for severe rheumatoid arthritis (see Table 4.24). • NSAIDs reduce the effect of ACE inhibitors in hypertensive clients. • Note name similarity of Celebrex with other drugs having one-letter difference in spelling. • Encourage routine appointments to check liver/renal laboratories and CBC.

ACE, Angiotensin-converting enzyme; *GI*, gastrointestinal; *IV*, intravenous; *NSAIDs*, nonsteroidal anti-inflammatory drugs.

B. Provide periods of rest after periods of activity.
   1. Encourage self-care to maximal level.
   2. Allow adequate time for the client to perform activities.
   3. Perform activities during time of day when client feels most energetic.
C. Encourage the client to avoid overexertion and to maintain proper posture and joint position.
   1. Do not exercise painful, swollen joints.
   2. Do not exercise any joint to the point of pain.
   3. Perform exercises slowly and smoothly; avoid jerky movements.
D. Encourage use of assistive devices.
   1. Elevated toilet seat
   2. Shower chair
   3. Cane, walker, and wheelchair
   4. Reachers
   5. Adaptive clothing with Velcro closures
   6. Straight-backed chair with elevated seat
E. Develop a teaching plan to include the following:
   1. Medication regimen
   2. Need for routine follow-up for evaluation of possible side effects
   3. ROM and stretching exercises tailored to specific client needs
   4. Safety tips and precautions about equipment use and environment

Lupus Erythematosus

Description: Systemic inflammatory connective-tissue disorder
A. There are two classifications of lupus erythematosus.
   1. Discoid lupus erythematosus (DLE) affects skin only.
   2. Systemic lupus erythematosus (SLE) can cause major body organs and systems to fail.
B. SLE is more prevalent than DLE.
C. Lupus is an autoimmune disorder.
D. Kidney involvement is the leading cause of death in clients with lupus; it is followed by cardiac involvement as a leading cause of death.

> **HESI HINT** NCLEX-RN questions often focus on the fact that avoiding sunlight is key in the management of lupus erythematosus; this is what differentiates it from other connective-tissue diseases.

E. Factors that trigger lupus
   1. Sunlight
   2. Stress
   3. Pregnancy
   4. Drugs

Nursing Assessment

A. DLE
   1. Dry, scaly rash on face or upper body (butterfly rash)
B. SLE
   1. Joint pain and decreased mobility
   2. Fever
   3. Nephritis
   4. Pleural effusion
   5. Pericarditis
   6. Abdominal pain
   7. Photosensitivity
   8. Hypertension

Nursing Plans and Interventions

A. Instruct client to avoid prolonged exposure to sunlight.
B. Instruct client to clean the skin with mild soap.
C. Monitor and instruct client in administration of steroids.

Osteoarthritis (Formerly Known as Degenerative Joint Disease)

Description: Noninflammatory arthritis
A. Osteoarthritis (OA) is characterized by a degeneration of cartilage, a wear-and-tear process.
B. It usually affects one or two joints.
C. It occurs asymmetrically.
D. Obesity and overuse are predisposing factors.

Nursing Assessment

A. Joint pain that increases with activity and improves with rest
B. Morning stiffness
C. Asymmetry of affected joints
D. Crepitus (grating sound in the joint)
E. Limited movement
F. Visible joint abnormalities indicated on radiographs
G. Joint enlargement and bony nodules

Nursing Plans and Interventions

(See "Rheumatoid Arthritis," earlier.)
A. Instruct in weight-reduction diet.
B. Remind client that excessive use of the involved joint aggravates pain and may accelerate degeneration.
C. Teach the client to
   1. Use correct posture and body mechanics
   2. Sleep with rolled terry cloth towel under cervical spine if neck pain is a problem
   3. Relieve pain in fingers and hands by wearing stretch gloves at night
   4. Keep joints in functional position

Osteoporosis

Description: Metabolic disease in which bone demineralization results in decreased density and subsequent fractures
A. Many fractures in older adults occur as a result of osteoporosis and often occur before the client's falling rather than as the result of a fall.
B. The cause of osteoporosis is unknown.
C. Postmenopausal women are at highest risk.

Nursing Assessment

A. Classic dowager's hump, or kyphosis of the dorsal spine (Fig. 4.8)

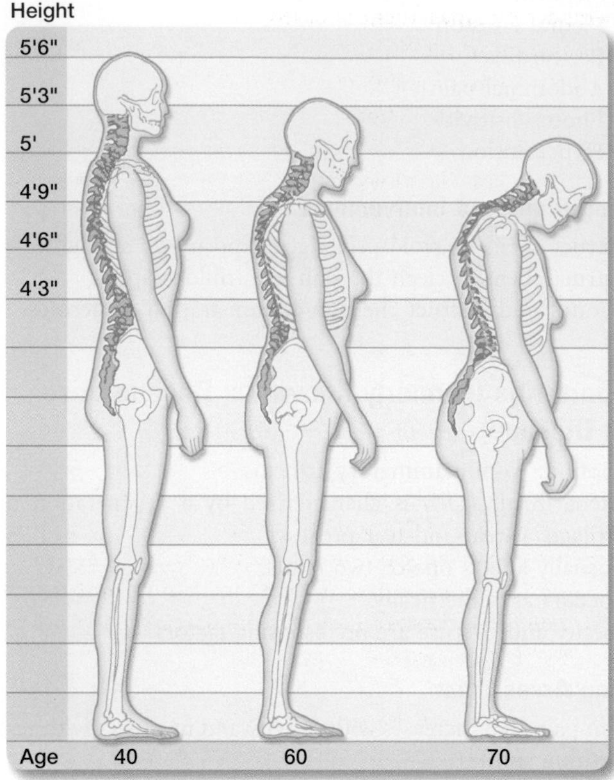

Fig. 4.8 Osteoporotic Changes. A normal spine at 40 years of age, and osteoporotic changes at ages 60 and 70 years. These changes can cause a loss of height and may result in dorsal kyphosis. (Ignatavicius, D. D., Workman, M. L., & Rebar, C. [2020]. *Medical-surgical nursing: Concepts for interprofessional collaborative care* [10th ed.]. St. Louis: Elsevier.)

B. Loss of height, often 2 to 3 inches
C. Back pain, often radiating around the trunk
D. Pathologic fractures, often occurring in the distal end of the radius and the upper third of the femur
E. Compression fracture of spine: assess ability to void and defecate.

> **HESI HINT** Postmenopausal, thin, white women are at highest risk for development of osteoporosis. Encourage exercise, a diet high in calcium, and supplemental calcium. Tums are an excellent source of calcium, but they are also high in sodium, so hypertensive or edematous individuals should seek another source of supplemental calcium. The main cause of fractures in older adults, especially in women, is osteoporosis. The main fracture sites seem to be hip, vertebral bodies, and Colles fracture of the forearm.

Nursing Plans and Interventions

A. Create a hazard-free environment.
B. Keep bed in low position.
C. Encourage client to wear shoes or nonskid slippers when out of bed.
D. Encourage environmental safety.
  1. Provide adequate lighting.
  2. Keep floor clear.
  3. Discourage use of throw rugs.
  4. Clean spills promptly.
  5. Keep side rails up at all times.
E. Provide assistance with ambulation.
  1. Client may need walker or cane.
  2. Client may need standby assistance when initially getting out of bed or chair.
F. Teach regular exercise program.
  1. ROM exercise several times a day
  2. Ambulation several times a day
  3. Use of proper body mechanics
  4. Regular weight-bearing exercises promote bone formation
G. Provide diet that is high in protein, calcium, and vitamin D; discourage use of alcohol and caffeine.
H. Encourage preventive measures for females.
  1. Hormone replacement therapy (HRT) has been used as a primary prevention strategy for reducing bone loss in the postmenopausal woman. However, recent studies demonstrated that HRT may increase a woman's risk of breast cancer, cardiovascular disease, and stroke. If using HRT, the benefits should outweigh the risks.
  2. Take prescribed medications to prevent further loss of BMD.
    a. Bisphosphonates: inhibit osteoclast-mediated bone resorption, thereby increasing BMD. Common side effects are anorexia, weight loss, and gastritis. Instruct the client to take with full glass of water, take 30 minutes before food or other medications, and remain upright for at least 30 minutes after taking.
      1) Alendronate (Fosamax)
      2) Etidronate (Didronel)
      3) Ibandronate (Boniva)
      4) Pamidronate (Aredia)
      5) Risedronate (Actonel)
      6) Tiludronate (Skelid)
    b. Selective estrogen receptor modulator: to mimic the effect of estrogen on bone by reducing bone resorption without stimulating the tissues of the breast or uterus. The most common side effects are leg cramps and hot flashes.
      1) Raloxifene (Evista)
      2) Teriparatide (Forteo)
      3) High calcium and vitamin D intake beginning in early adulthood
      4) Calcium supplementation after menopause (Tums are an excellent source of calcium).
      5) Weight-bearing exercise
I. Dual-energy x-ray absorptiometry (DEXA), which measures bone density in the spine, hips, and forearm, as a baseline after menopause, with frequency as recommended by health care provider
J. Osteopenia is defined as bone loss that is more than normal and has a T-score less than or equal to a range of −1 to −2.5

but is not yet at the level for a diagnosis of osteoporosis. BMD is commonly reported as a "T-score," which is the difference between the client's BMD and the BMD of "young normal adults" of the same gender. The difference between the client's score and the young adult norm is expressed as standard deviation below or above the average.

Fracture

Description: Any break in the continuity of the bone

A. Fractures are described by the type and extent of the break.
B. A direct blow, crushing force, a sudden twisting motion, or a disease such as cancer or osteoporosis causes fractures.
   1. Complete fracture: a break across the entire cross section of the bone
   2. Incomplete fracture: a break across only part of the bone
   3. Closed fracture: no break in the skin
   4. Open fracture: broken bone protrudes through skin or mucous membranes (much more prone to infection)
C. Five types of fractures
   1. Greenstick: one side of a bone is broken; the other side is bent.
   2. Transverse: break occurs straight across the bone shaft
   3. Oblique: break occurs at an angle across the bone
   4. Spiral: break twists around the bone
   5. Comminuted: break has more than three fragments (Table 4.30)

Nursing Assessment

A. Signs and symptoms of fracture include
   1. Pain, swelling, tenderness
   2. Deformity, loss of functional ability
   3. Discoloration, bleeding at the site through an open wound
   4. Crepitus: crackling sound between two broken bones

> **HESI HINT** An intracapsular fracture heals with greater difficulty, and there is a greater likelihood that necrosis will occur because the fracture is cut off from the blood supply.
>
> The risk for the development of a fat embolism, a syndrome in which fat globules migrate into the bloodstream and combine with platelets to form emboli, is greatest in the first 36 h after a fracture. It is more common in clients with multiple fractures, fractures of long bones, and fractures of the pelvis. The initial symptom of a fat embolism is confusion due to hypoxemia (check blood gases for Po_2). Assess for respiratory distress, restlessness, irritability, fever, and petechiae. If an embolus is suspected, notify physician stat, draw blood gases, administer O_2, and assist with endotracheal intubation.
>
> Clients with fractures, edema, or casts on the extremities need frequent neurovascular assessment distal to the injury. Skin color, temperature, sensation, capillary refill, mobility, pain, and pulses should be assessed.
>
> In clients with hip fractures, thromboembolism is the most common complication. Prevention includes passive ROM exercises, use of elastic stockings, elevation of the foot of the bed 25 degrees to increase venous return, and low-dose heparin therapy.

> **HESI HINT** Assess the 5 Ps of neurovascular functioning: **p**ain, **p**aresthesia, **p**ulse, **p**allor, and **p**aralysis.

B. Fracture is evident on radiograph.
C. Therapeutic management is based on
   1. Reduction of the fracture
   2. Maintenance of realignment by immobilization
   3. Restoration of function

> **HESI HINT** NCLEX-RN questions focus on safety precautions. Improper use of assistive devices can be very risky. When using a nonwheeled walker, the client should lift and move the walker forward and then take a step into it. The client should avoid scooting the walker or shuffling forward into it; these movements take more energy and provide less stability than does a single movement.

D. Observe client's use of assistive devices.
   1. Crutches
      a. There should be two to three finger widths between the axilla and the top of the crutch.
      b. A three-point gait is most common. The client advances both crutches and the impaired leg at the same time. The client then swings the uninvolved leg ahead to the crutches.
   2. Cane
      a. It is placed on the unaffected side.
      b. The top of the cane should be at the level of the greater trochanter.
   3. Walker
      a. Strength of upper extremity and unaffected leg is assessed and improved with exercises, if necessary, so that upper body is strong enough to use walker.
      b. Client lifts and advances the walker and steps forward.
E. Many clients now use walkers with wheels. The client should plant the foot of weaker side first then advance the client and the walker using the foot on stronger side.
F. See Chapter 5: Pediatric Nursing for cast care and care of a client in traction.

Joint Replacement

Description: Surgical procedure in which a mechanical device, designed to act as a joint, is used to replace a diseased joint

A. The most commonly replaced joints
   1. Hip
   2. Knee
   3. Shoulder
   4. Finger
B. Prostheses may be ingrown or cemented.
C. Accurate fitting is essential.
D. Client must have healthy bone stock for adequate healing.
E. Joint replacement provides excellent pain relief in 85% to 90% of the clients who have the surgery.
F. Infection is the concern postoperatively.

Nursing Assessment

A. Joint pathology
   1. OA

TABLE 4.30 **Common Types of Fractures**

Description	Illustration	Description	Illustration
Burst: Characterized by multiple pieces of bone; often occurs at bone ends or in vertebrae	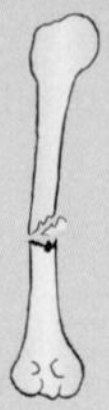	Longitudinal: Fracture line extends in the direction of the bone's longitudinal axis	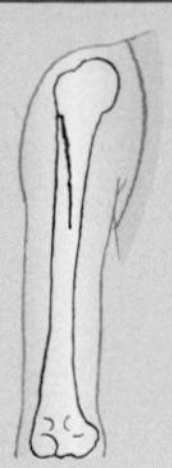
Comminuted: More than one fracture line; more than two bone fragments; fragments may be splintered or crushed.	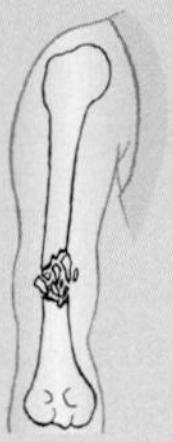	Nondisplaced: Fragments aligned at fracture site	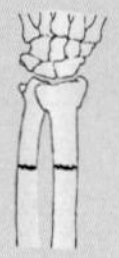
Complete: Break across the entire section of bone, dividing it into distinct fragments; often displaced	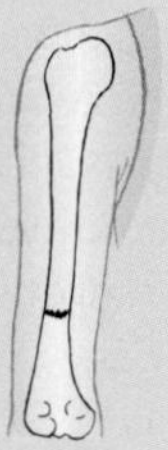	Oblique: Fracture line occurs at approximately 45-degree angle across the longitudinal axis of the bone	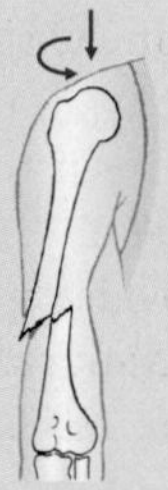
Displaced: Fragments out of normal position at fracture site	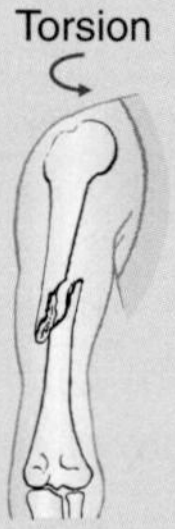 Torsion	Spiral: Fracture line results from twisting force; forms a spiral encircling the bone	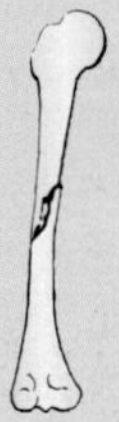
Incomplete: Fracture occurs through only one cortex of the bone; usually nondisplaced.	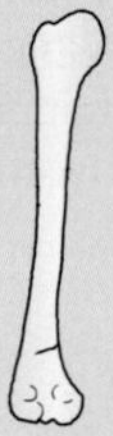	Stellate: Fracture lines radiate from one central point	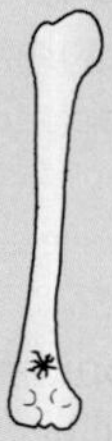
Linear: Fracture line is intact; fracture is caused by minor to moderate force applied directly to the bone.		Traverse: Fracture line occurs at 90-degree angle to longitudinal axis of bone	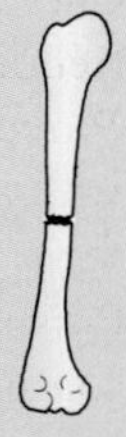
Avulsion: Bone fragments are torn away from the body of the bone at the site of attachment of a ligament or tendon.	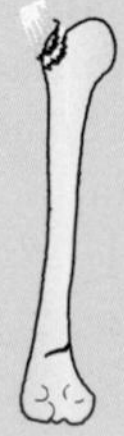	Colles: fracture within the last inch of the distal radius; distal fragment is displaced in a position of dorsal and medial deviation	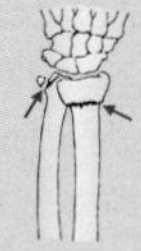

Continued

Compression: Bone buckles and eventually cracks as the result of unusual loading force applied to its longitudinal axis

Greenstick: Incomplete fracture in which one side of the cortex is broken and the other side is flexed but intact

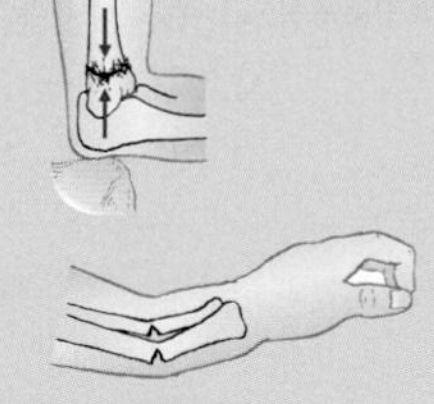

Pott: Fracture of the distal fibula, seriously disrupting the tibiofibular articulation; a piece of the medial malleolus may be chipped off as a result of rupture of the internal lateral ligament

Impacted: Telescoped fracture, with one fragment driven into another

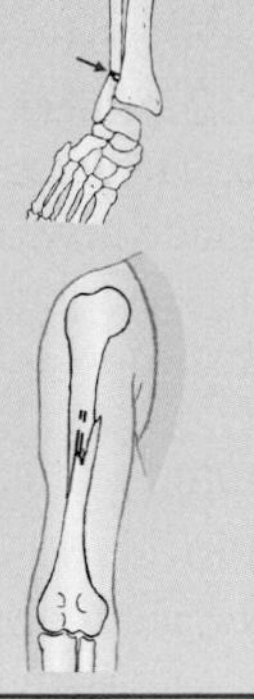

2. Rheumatoid arthritis
3. Fracture

B. Pain not relieved by medication

C. Poor ROM in the affected joint

Nursing Plans and Interventions

A. Provide postoperative care for wound and joint.
   1. Monitor incision site.
      a. Assess for bleeding and drainage.

> **HESI HINT** Orthopedic wounds have a tendency to ooze more than other wounds. A suction drainage device usually accompanies the client to the postoperative floor. Check drainage often.
> a. Assess suture line for erythema and edema.
> b. Assess suction drainage apparatus for proper functioning.
> c. Assess for signs of infection.

> **HESI HINT** NCLEX-RN questions about joint replacement focus on complications. A big problem after joint replacement is infection.

   2. Monitor functioning of extremity.
      a. Check circulation, sensation, and movement of extremity distal to replacement.
      b. Provide proper alignment of affected extremity. (Client will return from the operating room with alignment for the initial postoperative period.)
      c. Provide abductor appliance (hip replacement) or continuous passive motion (CPM) device if indicated.

B. Monitor I&O every shift, including suction drainage.

> **HESI HINT** Fractures of bone predispose the client to anemia, especially if long bones are involved. Check Hct every 3–4 days to monitor erythropoiesis.

C. Encourage fluid intake of 3 L/day.

D. Encourage client to perform self-care activities at maximal level.

E. Coordinate rehabilitation: work closely with health care team to increase client's mobility gradually.
   1. Get client out of bed as soon as possible.
   2. Keep client out of bed as much as possible.
   3. Keep abductor pillow in place while client is in bed (hip replacement).
   4. Use elevated toilet seat and chairs with high seats for those who have had hip or knee replacements (prevents dislocation).
   5. Do not flex hip more than 90 degrees (hip replacement).

> **HESI HINT** After hip replacement, instruct the client not to lift the leg upward from a lying position or to elevate the knee when sitting. This upward motion can pop the prosthesis out of the socket.

F. Provide discharge planning that includes rehabilitation on an outclient basis as prescribed.

> **HESI HINT** Immobile clients are prone to complications: skin integrity problems, formation of urinary calculi (client's milk intake may be limited), and venous thrombosis (client may be on prophylactic anticoagulants).

Amputation

Description: Surgical removal of a diseased part or organ

A. Causes for amputation include the following:
   1. PVD, 80% (75% of these are clients with diabetes)
   2. Trauma
   3. Congenital deformities
   4. Malignant tumors
   5. Infection

B. Amputation necessitates major lifestyle and body image adjustments.

Nursing Assessment

A. Before amputation, symptoms of PVD include
   1. Cool extremity
   2. Absent peripheral pulses
   3. Hair loss on affected extremity
   4. Necrotic tissue or wounds

a. Blue or blue-gray, turning black
b. Drainage possible, with or without odor
5. Leathery skin on affected extremity
6. Decrease of pain sensation in affected extremity
B. Inadequate circulation as determined by
1. Arteriogram
2. Doppler flow studies

Nursing Plans and Interventions

A. Provide wound care.
1. Monitor surgical dressing for drainage.
a. Mark dressing for bleeding, and check marking at least every 8 hours.
b. Measure suction drainage every shift.
2. Change dressing as needed (physician usually performs initial dressing change).
a. Maintain aseptic technique.
b. Observe wound color, warmth, and approximation of the incision.
c. Observe for wound healing.
d. Monitor for signs of infection.
1) Fever
2) Tachycardia
3) Redness of incision area
B. Maintain proper body alignment in and out of bed.
C. Position client to relieve edema and spasms at residual limb (stump) site.
1. Elevate residual limb (stump) for the first 24 hours postoperatively.

> **HESI HINT** The residual limb (stump) should be elevated on one pillow. If the residual limb (stump) is elevated too high, the elevation can cause a contracture.

2. Do not elevate residual limb (stump) after 48 hours postoperatively.
3. Keep residual limb (stump) in extended position and turn client to prone position three times a day to prevent hip flexion contracture.
D. Be aware that phantom pain is real; it will eventually disappear, and it responds to pain medication.
E. Handle affected body part gently and with smooth movements.
F. Provide passive ROM until client is able to perform active ROM. Collaborate with rehabilitation team members for mobility improvement.
G. Encourage independence in self-care, allowing sufficient time for client to complete care and to have input into care.

REVIEW OF MUSCULOSKELETAL SYSTEM

1. Differentiate between rheumatoid arthritis and OA in terms of joint involvement.
2. Identify the categories of drugs commonly used to treat arthritis.
3. Identify pain relief interventions for clients with arthritis.
4. What measures should the nurse encourage female clients to take to prevent osteoporosis?
5. What are the common side effects of salicylates?
6. What is the priority nursing intervention used with clients taking NSAIDs?
7. List three of the most common joints that are replaced.
8. Describe postoperative residual limb (stump) care (after amputation) for the first 48 hours.
9. Describe nursing care for the client who is experiencing phantom pain after amputation.
10. A nurse discovers that a client who is in traction for a long bone fracture has a slight fever, is short of breath, and is restless. What does the client most likely have?
11. What are the immediate nursing actions if fat embolization is suspected in a client with a fracture or other orthopedic condition?
12. List three problems associated with immobility.
13. List three nursing interventions for the prevention of thromboembolism in immobilized clients with musculoskeletal problems.

See Answer Key at the end of this text for suggested responses.

Neurosensory System

Glaucoma

Chronic open-angle glaucoma is also known as simple adult primary glaucoma and as primary open-angle glaucoma.

Description: Condition characterized by increased intraocular pressure (IOP) that involves gradual painless vision loss that can lead to blindness if untreated.

A. Is the second leading cause of blindness in the United States and especially among those over 80 years old.
B. Glaucoma usually occurs bilaterally in those who have a family history of the condition.
C. Aqueous fluid is inadequately drained from the eye.
D. It is generally asymptomatic, especially in early stages.
E. It tends to be diagnosed during routine visual examinations.
F. It cannot be cured but can be treated with success pharmacologically and surgically.

Nursing Assessment

A. Early signs
1. Increase in IOP greater than 22 mm Hg
2. Decreased accommodation or ability to focus

> **HESI HINT** Glaucoma is often painless and symptom free. It is usually detected as part of a regular eye examination.

B. Late signs include
 1. Loss of peripheral vision
 2. Seeing halos around lights
 3. Decreased visual acuity not correctable with glasses
 4. Headache or eye pain that may be so severe as to cause nausea and vomiting (acute closed-angle glaucoma)
C. Diagnostic tests include the following:
 1. Tonometer, used to measure IOP
 2. Electronic tonometer, used to detect drainage of aqueous humor
 3. Gonioscopy, used to obtain a direct visualization of the lens
D. Risk factors include the following:
 1. Family history of glaucoma
 2. Family history of diabetes
 3. History of previous ocular problems
 4. Medication use
  a. Glaucoma is a side effect of many medications (e.g., antihistamines, anticholinergics).
  b. Glaucoma can result from the interaction of medications.

Nursing Plans and Interventions

A. Administer eye drops as prescribed (Table 4.31).

> **HESI HINT** Eye drops are used to cause pupil constriction because movement of the muscles to constrict the pupil also allows aqueous humor to flow out, thereby decreasing the pressure in the eye. Pilocarpine is commonly used. Caution client that vision may be blurred for 1–2 h after administration of pilocarpine and that adaptation to dark environments is difficult because of pupillary constriction (the desired effect of the drug).

B. Orient client to surroundings.
C. Avoid nonverbal communication that requires visual acuity (e.g., facial expressions).
D. Develop a teaching plan that includes the following:
 1. Careful adherence to eye-drop regimen can prevent blindness.
 2. Vision already lost cannot be restored.
 3. Eye drops are needed for the rest of client's life.
 4. Teach proper eye-drop instillation technique. Obtain a return demonstration.
  a. Wash your hands and external eye.
  b. Tilt head back slightly.
  c. Instill drop into lower lid, without touching the lid with the tip of the dropper.
  d. Release the lid and sponge excess fluid from lid and cheek.
  e. Close eye gently and leave closed 3 to 5 minutes.
  f. Apply gentle pressure on inner canthus to decrease systemic absorption.
 5. Safety measures to prevent injuries
  a. Remove throw rugs.
  b. Adjust lighting to meet needs.
 6. Avoid activities that may increase IOP.
  a. Emotional upsets
  b. Exertion: pushing, heavy lifting, shoveling
  c. Coughing severely or excessive sneezing (get medical attention before URI worsens)
  d. Wearing constrictive clothing (tight collar or tie, tight belt, or girdle)
  e. Straining at stool and constipation
   1) Older patients should especially be assessed for constipation that can increase IOP.

Nursing Plans and Interventions: The Nonseeing (Blind) Client

A. On entering room, announce your presence clearly and identify yourself; address client by name.
B. Never touch client unless he or she knows you are there.
C. On admission, orient client thoroughly to surroundings.
 1. Demonstrate use of the call bell.
 2. Walk client around the room and acquaint him or her with all objects: chairs, bed, TV, telephone, etc.
D. Guide client when walking:
 1. Walk ahead of client and place his or her hand in the bend of your elbow.
 2. Describe where you are walking. Note whether passageway is narrowing or you are approaching stairs, curb, or an incline.
E. Always raise side rails for newly sightless persons (e.g., clients wearing postoperative eye patches).
F. Assist with meal enjoyment by describing food and its placement in terms of the face of a clock (e.g., "meat at 6 o'clock").
G. When administering medications, inform client of number of pills, and give only a half glass of water (to avoid spills).

Cataract

Description: Condition characterized by opacity of the lens. Cataracts are the leading cause of blindness in the world. The lens of the eye is responsible for projecting light onto the retina so that images can be discerned. Without the lens, which becomes opaque with cataracts, light cannot be filtered and vision is blurred.
A. Aging accounts for 95% of cataracts (senile).
B. The remaining 5% result from trauma, toxic substances, or systemic diseases or are congenital.
C. Safety precautions may reduce the incidence of traumatic cataracts.
D. Surgical removal is done when vision impairment interferes with daily activities. Intraocular lens implants may be used.
E. Most operations are performed under local anesthesia on an out-client basis.

Nursing Assessment

A. Early signs include
 1. Blurred vision
 2. Decreased color perception
 3. Photophobia

TABLE 4.31 Treatment of Glaucoma

Drugs	Indications	Adverse Reactions	Nursing Implications
		PARASYMPATHOMIMETICS	

• Pilocarpine HCl (multiple brands available); 0.5%–6% is the drug of choice	• Enhances papillary constriction (available in drops, gel, and time-release wafer)	• Bronchospasm
		• Nausea, vomiting, diarrhea
		• Blurred vision, twitching eyelids, eye pain with focusing, reduced visual acuity in dim light
			• Use cautiously with
			  • Pregnancy
			  • Asthma
			  • Hypertension
			• Teach proper drop instillation technique.
			• Need for ongoing use of the drug at prescribed intervals.
			• Blurred vision tends to decrease with regular use of this drug.

		BETA-ADRENERGIC RECEPTOR–BLOCKING AGENTS	

• Timolol maleate optic
• Carteolol
• Levobunolol
• Betaxolol
• Metipranolol
	• Inhibits formation of aqueous humor	• Side effects are insignificant.
		• Hypotension
		• Bradycardia
			• Use cautiously with
			  • Hypersensitivity
			  • Asthma
			  • Second- or third-degree heart block
			  • HF
			  • Congenital glaucoma
			  • Pregnancy
			  • Teach proper drop instillation technique.
			• Need for ongoing use of the drug at prescribed intervals.
			• Blurred vision tends to decrease with regular use of this drug.

		CARBONIC ANHYDRASE INHIBITORS	
• Acetazolamide • Brinzolamide • Dorzolamide	• Reduces aqueous humor production	• Numbness, tingling of hands and feet • Nausea • Malaise • Postural hypotension if taken orally	• Administer orally or IV. • Produces diuresis. • Assess for metabolic acidosis. • Contraindicated in clients with sulfa allergy.
		ALPHA AGONISTS	
• Brimonidine • Iopidine	• Lowers IOP of glaucoma by decreasing fluid produced		Teach to use no more than prescribed. Caution with patients who have history of depression, orthostatic hypotension, or Reynaud.
		PROSTAGLANDIN ANTAGONISTS	
• Latanoprost • Travoprost • Bimatoprost	• Lowers IOP of glaucoma by increasing outflow of aqueous humor	• Local irritation • Foreign-body sensation • Increased brown pigmentation of iris • Increased eyelash growth	

HF, Heart failure; *IOP*, intraocular pressure; *IV*, intravenous.

B. Late signs include
   1. Diplopia
   2. Reduced visual acuity, progressing to blindness
   3. Clouded pupil, progressing to a milky-white appearance

C. Diagnostic tests include use of the following:
   1. Ophthalmoscope
   2. Slit-lamp biomicroscope
   3. Keratometry and A-scan ultrasound

Nursing Plans and Interventions

A. Preoperative: Demonstrate and request a return demonstration of eye medication instillation from client or family member.

B. Develop a postoperative teaching plan that includes
   1. Warning not to rub or put pressure on eye
   2. Teaching that glasses or shaded lens should be worn during waking hours. An eye shield should be worn during sleeping hours.
   3. Teaching to avoid lifting objects over 5 pounds, bending, straining, coughing, or any other activity that can increase IOP
   4. Teaching to use a stool softener to prevent straining at stool
   5. Teaching to avoid lying on operative side
   6. Teaching the need to keep water from getting into eye while showering or washing hair
   7. Teaching to observe and report signs of increased IOP and infection (e.g., pain, changes in vital signs)

> **HESI HINT** When the cataract is removed, the lens is gone, making prevention of falls important. Remember that client safety is always the nurse's priority.

Eye Trauma

Description: Injury to the eye sustained as the result of sharp or blunt trauma, chemicals, or heat

A. Permanent visual impairment can occur.
B. Every eye injury should be considered an emergency.
C. Protective eye shields in hazardous work environments and during athletic sports may prevent injuries.

Nursing Assessment

A. Determine type of injury and symptoms.
B. Diagnostic tests include
   1. Slit-lamp examination
   2. Instillation of fluorescein to detect corneal injury
   3. Testing of visual acuity for medical documentation and legal protection

Nursing Plans and Interventions

A. Position the client according to the type of injury; a sitting position decreases IOP.
B. Remove conjunctival foreign bodies unless embedded.
C. Never attempt to remove a penetrating or embedded object. Do not apply pressure.
D. Apply cold compresses to eye contusion.
E. After chemical injuries, irrigate the eye with copious amounts of water.
F. Administer eye medications as prescribed.
G. Explain that an eye patch may be applied to rest the eye. Reading and watching TV may be restricted for 3 to 5 days.
H. Explain that a sudden increase in eye pain should be reported.

Detached Retina

Description: Hole or tear in, or separation of the sensory retina from, the pigmented epithelium

A. It can be result of increasing age, severe myopia, eye trauma, retinopathy (diabetic), cataract or glaucoma surgery, family or personal history.
B. Resealing is done by surgery.
   1. Cryotherapy (freezing)
   2. Photocoagulation (laser)
   3. Diathermy (heat)
   4. Scleral buckling (most often used)

Nursing Plans and Interventions

A. The client may be on bed rest.
B. Place eye patch over affected eye.
C. Administer medication to inhibit accommodation and constriction; cycloplegics (mydriatics and homatropine) are prescribed to dilate pupil before surgery.
D. Administer medication for postoperative pain.
E. If gas bubble is used (inserted in vitreous), position client so bubble can rise against area to be reattached.
F. Teach the client not to do any heavy lifting or straining with bowel movement, and no vigorous activity for several weeks.

Hearing Loss

Conductive Hearing Loss

Description: Hearing loss in which sound does not travel well to the sound organs of the inner ear. The volume of sound is less, but the sound remains clear. If volume is raised, hearing is normal.

A. Hearing loss is the most common disability in the United States.
B. It usually results from cerumen (wax) impaction or middle ear disorders such as otitis media.

> **HESI HINT** The ear consists of three parts: the external ear, the middle ear, and the inner ear. Inner ear disorders, or disorders of the sensory fibers going to the central nervous system (CNS), often are neurogenic in nature and may not be helped with a hearing aid. External and middle ear problems (conductive) may result from infection, trauma, or wax buildup. These types of disorders are treated more successfully with hearing aids.

Sensorineural Hearing Loss

Description: Form of hearing loss in which sound passes properly through the outer and middle ear but is distorted by a defect in the inner ear or damage to cranial nerve VIII, or both

A. It involves perceptual loss, usually progressive and bilateral.
B. It involves damage to the eighth cranial nerve.
C. It is detected easily by the use of a tuning fork.
D. Common causes
   1. Infections
   2. Ototoxic drugs
   3. Trauma
   4. Neuromas
   5. Noise
   6. Aging process

Nursing Assessment

A. Inability to hear a whisper from 1 to 2 feet away
B. Inability to respond if nurse covers mouth when talking, indicating that client is lip-reading
C. Inability to hear a watch tick 5 inches from ear
D. Shouting in conversation
E. Straining to hear
F. Turning head to favor one ear
G. Answering questions incorrectly or inappropriately
H. Raising volume of radio or TV

Nursing Plans and Interventions

A. The nurse should do the following to enhance therapeutic communication with the hearing impaired:
   1. Before starting conversation, reduce distraction as much as possible.
   2. Turn the TV or radio down or off, close the door, or move to a quieter location.
   3. Devote full attention to the conversation; do not try to do two things at once.
   4. Look and listen during the conversation.
   5. Begin with casual topics and progress to more critical issues slowly.
   6. Do not switch topics abruptly.
   7. If you do not understand, let the client know.
   8. If the client is a lip-reader, face him or her directly.
   9. Speak slowly and distinctly; determine whether you are being understood.
   10. Allow adequate time for the conversation to take place; try to avoid hurried conversations.
   11. Use active-listening techniques.
   12. Speak in a low-pitched voice, slowly and distinctly.
   13. Stand in front of the person, with the light source behind the client.
   14. Use visual aids if available.

> **HESI HINT** NCLEX-RN questions often focus on communicating with older adults who are hearing impaired.

B. Be sure to inform the health care staff of the client's hearing loss.
C. Helpful aids may include a telephone amplifier, earphone attachments for the radio and TV, and lights or buzzers that indicate the doorbell is ringing located in the most commonly used rooms of the house.
D. Maintain proper care of hearing aids and cochlear implants

NEUROLOGIC SYSTEM

Altered State of Consciousness

Nursing Assessment

A. Use agency's neurologic vital signs assessment tool. It will sometimes contain a scale for scoring, such as the Glasgow Coma Scale, which objectively documents the client's level of consciousness (Table 4.32).
   1. Maximum total is 15; minimum is 3.
   2. A score of 7 or less indicates coma.
   3. Clients with low scores (i.e., 3 to 4) have high mortality rates and poor prognosis.
   4. Clients with scores greater than 8 have a good prognosis for recovery.

> **HESI HINT** Use of the Glasgow Coma Scale eliminates ambiguous terms to describe neurologic status, such as *lethargic, stuporous,* or *obtunded.*

TABLE 4.32 Glasgow Coma Scale

Variable	Response	Score
Eye opening	Spontaneously	4
	To verbal command	3
	To pain	2
	No response	1
Motor response	To verbal command	6
	To painful stimuli	5
	• Localizes pain	4
	• Flexes/withdraws	3
	• Flexor posturing (decorticate)	2
	• Extensor posturing (decerebrate)	1
	• No response	
Verbal response	Oriented and converses	5
	Disoriented, converses	4
	Uses inappropriate words	3
	Incomprehensible sounds	2
	No response	1

B. Neurologic vital signs sheet will also address pupil size (with sizing scale), limb movement (with scale), and vital signs (BP, temperature, pulse, respirations).
C. Assess skin integrity and corneal integrity.
D. Check bladder for fullness, auscultate lungs, and monitor cardiac status.
E. Family members and significant others should be assessed for knowledge of client status, coping skills, need for extra support, and the ability to assist or provide care on an ongoing basis.

> **HESI HINT** Nursing care: a client with an altered state of consciousness is fed via enteral routes because the likelihood of aspiration is high with oral feedings. Residual feeding is the amount of previous feeding still in the stomach. The presence of 100 mL of residual in an adult usually indicates poor gastric emptying, and the feeding should be withheld; however, the residual should be returned because it is partially digested.

> **HESI HINT** Paralytic ileus is common in comatose clients. A gastric tube aids in gastric decompression.

> **HESI HINT** Any client on bed rest or immobilized must have ROM exercises often and very frequent position changes. Do not leave the client in any one position for longer than 2 h. Any position that decreases venous return, such as sitting with dependent extremities for long periods, is dangerous.

Nursing Plans and Interventions

A. Maintain adequate respirations, airway, and oxygenation.
   1. Document and report breathing pattern changes.

2. Position client for maximum ventilation: three-quarters prone position or semi-prone position to prevent tongue from obstructing airway and slightly to one side with arms away from chest wall.
3. Insert airway if tongue is obstructing or if client is paralyzed.
4. Prepare for insertion of cuffed endotracheal tube.
5. Keep airway free of secretions with suctioning (see Table 4.4).
6. Monitor arterial Po_2 and Pco_2.
7. Prepare for tracheostomy if ventilator support is needed.
8. Provide chest physiotherapy as prescribed by physician.
9. Hyperventilate with 100% O_2 before and after suctioning.

B. Provide nutritional, fluid, and electrolyte support.
1. Keep client NPO until responsive and provide mouth care every 4 hours.
2. Maintain calorie count.
3. Administer feedings as prescribed (Box 4.1).
4. Monitor I&O.
5. Record client's weight (weigh at same time each day).

C. Prevent complications of immobility.
1. Monitor impairment in skin integrity.
   a. Turn client every 2 hours and assess bony prominences.
   b. Use egg-crate or alternating-pressure mattress or waterbed.
   c. Use minimal amount of linens and underpads.
2. Potential for thrombus formation
   a. Perform passive ROM exercises to lower extremities every 4 hours.
   b. Apply sequential compression device (SCD) or elastic hose (remove and reapply every 8 hours).
   c. Avoid positions that decrease venous return.
   d. Avoid pillows under knees
3. Urinary calculi
   a. Increase fluid intake by mouth (PO) or via gastric tube or intravenously.
   b. Assess urine for high specific gravity (dehydration) and balance between I&O.
4. Contractures and joint immobility
   a. Perform passive ROM every 4 hours.
   b. Sit client up in bed or chair, if possible, or use neuro chair if necessary.
   c. Reposition every 2 hours, maintaining proper body alignment.
   d. Apply splints or other assistive devices to prevent foot drop, wrist drop, or other improper alignment.

D. Monitor and evaluate the vital sign changes indicating changes in condition.
1. Pulse: a pulse rate change to less than 60 or greater than 100 bpm can indicate increased intracranial pressure (ICP). A fast rate (>100 bpm) can indicate infection, thrombus formation, or dehydration.
2. BP: rising BP or widening pulse pressure can indicate increased ICP.
3. Temperature: report any abnormalities; temperature elevation can indicate worsening condition, damage to temperature-regulating area of brain, or infection. If temperature elevates, take quick measures to decrease it, because fever increases cerebral metabolism and can increase cerebral edema.
4. Level-of-consciousness changes: they may range from active to somnolent.
5. Pupillary changes: they may range from prompt to sluggish or may increase in size.

HESI HINT Safety features for immobilized clients include the following:
- Prevent skin breakdown by frequent turning.
- Maintain adequate nutrition.
- Prevent aspiration with slow, small feedings or NG feedings or enteral feedings.
- Monitor neurologic signs to detect the first signs that ICP may be increasing.
- Provide ROM exercises to prevent deformities.
- Prevent respiratory complications; frequent turning and positioning provide optimal drainage.

BOX 4.1 Unconscious Client

Gastric Gavage
- Check bowel sounds and begin feeding when GI peristalsis returns.
- Place client in high-Fowler position.
- Place towel over chest.
- Check gastric tube placement.
- Connect gastrostomy tube to funnel or large syringe.
- Check gastric residual to assess absorption and client tolerance; return residual.
- Pour feeding into tilted funnel and unclamp tubing to allow feeding to flow by gravity.
- Regulate flow by raising or lowering container. Feeding too quickly causes diarrhea, gastric distention, pain. Feeding too slowly causes possible obstruction of flow.
- After feeding, irrigate tube with (tepid) water and clamp tube.
- Apply small dressing over tube opening; coil tube and attach to dressing. May cover with an abdominal binder.
- Keep head of bed elevated 30 degrees or more during feeding and for at least 1 h after feeding.

Bowel Management Program
- Get bowel history from reliable source.
- Establish specific time for evacuation. Regularity is essential.
- An unconscious client can evacuate the bowel after the last tube feeding of day, because the gastrocolic and duodenocolic reflexes are active after "meal."
- Stimulate anorectal reflex by insertion of glycerin suppository 15–30 min before scheduled evacuation time. May need stronger suppository, such as bisacodyl (Dulcolax).
- Ensure adequate fiber in tube feedings and adequate fluid intake of 2–4 L/day.
- May apply a rectal pouch to contain fecal material (ostomy bag with seal over anal opening).

E. Prevent injury and promote safety.
   1. Place bed in low position and keep side rails up at all times.
   2. Pad side rails if client is agitated or if there is a history of seizure activity.
   3. Restrain client if client is trying to remove tubes or attempting to get out of bed.
   4. Touch gently, and talk softly and calmly to the client, remembering that hearing is commonly intact.
   5. Avoid oversedating the client because sedatives and narcotics depress responsiveness and affect pupillary reaction (an important assessment in neurologic vital signs).

HESI HINT Restlessness may indicate a return to consciousness but can also indicate anoxia, distended bladder, covert bleeding, or increasing cerebral anoxia. Do not oversedate, and report any symptoms of restlessness.

   6. During all activities, tell the client what you are doing, regardless of the level of consciousness.

F. Maintain hygiene and cleanliness.
   1. Provide bathing, grooming, and dressing.
   2. Provide oral hygiene.
   3. Wash hair weekly.
   4. Provide nail care within agency guidelines.

G. Observe for bladder elimination problems.
   1. Insert indwelling catheter if prescribed.
   2. Remove indwelling catheter as soon as possible; use adult brief or condom catheter.

H. Document and record bowel movements, and report abnormal patterns of constipation or diarrhea.
   1. Rapid infusion of tube feedings may cause diarrhea; lack of fiber and inadequate fluids may cause constipation.
   2. Initiate bowel program (see Box 4.1).

I. Prevent corneal injury and drying.
   1. Remove contact lenses if present.
   2. Irrigate eyes with sterile prescribed solution and instill ophthalmic ointment in each eye every 8 hours to prevent corneal ulceration.
   3. Close eyelids if blink reflex is absent.

Head Injury

Description: Any traumatic damage to the head

A. Open traumatic brain injury (TBI) occurs when there is a fracture of the skull or penetration of the skull by an object.

B. Closed TBI is the result of blunt trauma (more serious because of chance of increased ICP in closed vault).

C. Increased ICP is the main concern in head injury; it is related to edema, hemorrhage, impaired cerebral autoregulation, and hydrocephalus.

HESI HINT The forces of impact influence the type of TBI. They include acceleration injury, which is caused by the head being in motion, and deceleration injury, which occurs when the head stops suddenly. Helmets are a great preventive measure for motorcyclists and bicyclists (Fig. 4.9).

Nursing Assessment

A. Unconsciousness or disturbances in consciousness

B. Vertigo

C. Confusion, delirium, or disorientation

D. Symptoms of increased ICP
   1. Change in level of responsiveness is the most important indicator of increased ICP.

HESI HINT Even subtle behavior changes, such as restlessness, irritability, or confusion, may indicate increased ICP.

   2. Changes in vital signs
      a. Slowing of respirations or respiratory irregularities

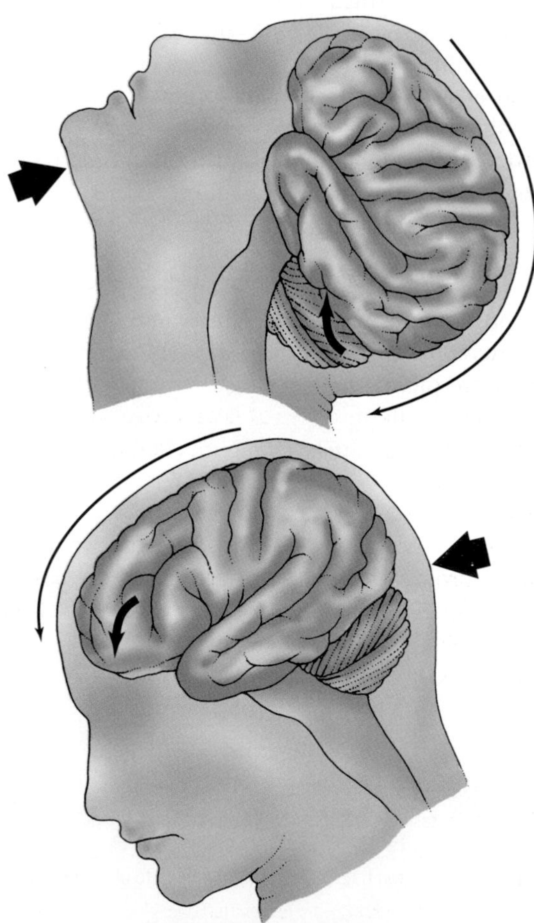

Fig. 4.9 Head movement during acceleration–deceleration injury, which is typically seen in motor vehicle accidents. (Ignatavicius, D. D., Workman, M. L., & Rebar, C. [2020]. *Medical-surgical nursing: Concepts for interprofessional collaborative care* [10th ed.]. St. Louis: Elsevier.)

b. Increase or decrease in pulse
c. Rising BP or widening pulse pressure
d. Temperature rise
1) Headache
2) Vomiting (projectile)
3) Pupillary changes reflecting pressure on optic or oculomotor nerves
a) Decrease or increase in size or unequal size of pupils
b) Lack of conjugate eye movement
c) Papilledema
(1) Seizures
(2) Ataxia
(3) Abnormal posturing (decerebrate or decorticate)
(4) Cerebrospinal fluid (CSF) leakage through nose (rhinorrhea) or through ear (otorrhea).
(5) Hematomas

HESI HINT CSF leakage carries the risk for meningitis and indicates a deteriorating condition. Because of CSF leakage, the usual signs of increased ICP may not occur.

E. CT scan or MRI will show a lesion, such as an epidural or subdural hematoma, requiring surgery.
F. Electroencephalograph (EEG) determines presence of seizure activity.

Nursing Plans and Interventions

A. Maintain adequate ventilation and airway.
1. Monitor P_{O_2} and P_{CO_2} for the development of hypoxia and hypercapnia.
2. Position client semiprone or lateral recumbent to prevent aspiration.
3. Turn from side to side to prevent lung secretion stasis.

B. Keep head of bed elevated 30 to 45 degrees to aid venous return from the neck and to decrease cerebral volume.
C. Obtain neurologic vital signs as prescribed (at least every 1 to 2 hours), and maintain a continuous record of observations and Glasgow Coma Scale ratings.
D. Notify physician at first sign of deterioration or improvement in condition.
E. Avoid activities that increase ICP, such as
1. Change in bed position for caregiving and extreme hip flexion
2. Endotracheal suctioning
3. Compression of jugular veins (keep head straight and not to one side)
4. Coughing, vomiting, or straining of any type (no Valsalva: Increased intrathoracic pressure increases ICP)

F. If temperature increases, take immediate measures to reduce it (aspirin, acetaminophen, cooling blanket) because increased temperature increases cerebral blood flow drastically; avoid shivering.
G. Use intracranial monitoring system when available.
1. A catheter is inserted into the lateral ventricle, a sensor placed on the dura, or a screw into the subarachnoid space attached to a pressure transducer.
2. Elevations of ICP over 20 mm Hg should be reported stat.

H. Administer medications prescribed by physician to reduce ICP.
1. Hyperosmotic agents and diuretics to dehydrate brain and reduce cerebral edema
a. Mannitol (Table 4.33)
b. Urea
2. Steroids
a. Dexamethasone (Decadron)
b. Methylprednisolone sodium succinate (Solu-Medrol) to reduce brain edema
3. Barbiturates
a. To reduce brain metabolism and systemic BP

I. Insert indwelling catheter to prevent restlessness caused by distended bladder and to monitor balance between restricted fluid I&O, especially if placed on osmotic diuretics.

HESI HINT Try not to use restraints; they only increase restlessness. Avoid narcotics because they mask the level of responsiveness.

J. Physician may order passive hyperventilation on ventilator: leads to respiratory alkalosis, which causes cerebral vasoconstriction and decreased cerebral blood flow, and therefore decreased ICP.
K. Continue seizure precautions. Health care provider may order prophylactic phenytoin (Dilantin).

TABLE 4.33 Osmotic Diuretic

Drug	Indications	Adverse Reactions	Nursing Implications
• Mannitol	• Acts on renal tubules by osmosis to prevent water reabsorption • In bloodstream, draws fluid from the extravascular spaces into the plasma	• Disorientation, confusion, and headache • Nausea and vomiting • Convulsions and anaphylactic reactions	• Use for short-term therapy *only*. • Never give to clients with cerebral hemorrhage. • IV infusion is usually adjusted to urine output; filter and watch for crystals. • Never give to clients with no urine output (anuria); if output is <30 mL/h, accumulation can cause pulmonary edema and water intoxication.

IV, Intravenous.

L. Prevent complications of immobility (see "Nursing Plans and Interventions" for "Altered State of Consciousness," earlier).
M. Inform at discharge, if feasible, aftereffects of head injury.
   1. Posttraumatic syndrome: headache, vertigo, emotional instability, inability to concentrate, impaired memory
   2. Posttraumatic epilepsy
   3. Posttraumatic neuroses or psychoses

Spinal Cord Injury

Description: Disruption in nervous system function, which may result in complete or incomplete loss of motor and sensory function. Changes occur in the function of all physiologic systems.

A. Injuries are described by location in the spinal cord. The most common sites are the fifth, sixth, and seventh cervical vertebrae (C5, C6, C7), the twelfth thoracic (T12), and the first lumbar (L1).
B. Damage can range from contusion to complete transection.
C. Permanent impairment cannot be determined until spinal cord edema has subsided, usually by 1 week.

Nursing Assessment

A. Assess breathing pattern and auscultate lungs.

HESI HINT Physical assessment should concentrate on respiratory status, especially in clients with injury at C3 to C5, because the cervical plexus innervates the diaphragm.

B. Check neurologic vital signs frequently, especially sensory and motor functions. Assess cardiovascular status.
C. Assess abdomen: girth, bowel sounds; assess lower abdomen for bladder distention.
D. Assess temperature, remembering that hyperthermia occurs commonly.
E. Assess psychosocial status.
F. Hypotension and bradycardia occur with any injury above T6 because sympathetic outflow is affected.

Nursing Plans and Interventions

A. In acute phase of spinal cord injury
   1. See "Nursing Plans and Interventions" for "Altered State of Consciousness," earlier.
   2. Maintain client in an extended position with cervical collar on during any transfer.
   3. Stabilize the client when transferring between the accident scene and the emergency department. The client will be realigned and stabilized in the emergency room.
   4. Maintain a patent airway (most important).
   5. In cervical injuries, skeletal traction is maintained by use of skull tongs or a halo ring (Crutchfield tongs or a Gardner-Wells fixation device).
   6. High-dose corticosteroids are often given to help control edema during the first 8 to 24 hours.
   7. Use a kinetic therapy treatment table which provides continuous side-to-side motion.
   8. Use Stryker frame or very firm mattress with board underneath.
   9. Assess for respiratory failure, especially in clients with high cervical injuries.
   10. Further loss of sensory or motor function below injury can indicate additional damage to cord due to edema and should be reported immediately.
   11. Evaluate for presence of spinal shock (a complete loss of all reflex, motor, sensory, and autonomic activity below the lesion). This medical emergency occurs immediately after the injury.
       a. Hypotension, bradycardia
       b. Complete paralysis and lack of sensation below lesion
       c. Bladder and bowel distention

HESI HINT It is imperative to reverse spinal shock as quickly as possible. Permanent paralysis can occur if a spinal cord is compressed for 12–24 h.

   12. Evaluate for autonomic dysreflexia (exaggerated autonomic responses to stimuli), which occurs in clients with lesions at or above T6. This medical emergency usually occurs after the period of spinal shock has finished and is usually triggered by a noxious stimulus such as bowel or bladder distention. It may also be triggered by a vaginal examination.
       a. Elevated BP
       b. Pounding headache, sweating, nasal congestion, goose bumps, bradycardia
       c. Bladder and bowel distention
   13. Watch for acute paralytic ileus, lack of gastric activity.
       a. Assess bowel sounds frequently.
       b. Initiate gastric suction to reduce distention, prevent vomiting and aspiration.
       c. Use rectal tube to relieve gaseous distention.
   14. Suction with caution to prevent vagus nerve stimulation, which can cause cardiac arrest.
   15. Administer high-dose corticosteroids intravenously to decrease edema and reduce cord damage.
B. In rehabilitative phase of spinal cord injury
   1. Encourage deep-breathing exercises.
   2. Administer chest physiotherapy.
   3. Provide kinetic bed to promote blood flow to extremities.
   4. Apply anti-embolic stockings or SCDs.
   5. Facilitate ROM exercises.
   6. Mobilize client to chair as soon as possible.
   7. Turn client frequently.
   8. Keep client clean and dry.
   9. Observe for impending skin breakdown.
   10. Teach client importance of impeccable skin care.
   11. Perform intermittent catheterization every 4 hours.
       a. Begin teaching client catheterization technique.
       b. Teach family member if client is unable.

12. Teach bladder-emptying techniques according to level of injury and bladder muscle response.
    a. Upper motor neuron (UMN; i.e., spastic) bladder
    b. Lower motor neuron (LMN; i.e., flaccid) bladder
13. Instruct client in monitoring I&O.
14. Encourage the client to drink fluids that promote acidic urine, including cranberry juice, prune juice, bouillon, tomato juice, and water.

> **HESI HINT** Keeping the bladder emptied assists in avoiding bacterial growth in urine that has stagnated in the bladder.

15. Begin bowel-training program.
16. Talk with client and family about permanence of disability.
17. Encourage rehabilitation facility staff to visit client.
18. Encourage client and family to visit rehabilitation facility.
19. Assist family in finding support group and refer to community resources after dismissal from rehabilitation facility.

Brain Tumor

Description: Neoplasm occurring in the brain

A. Primary tumors can arise in any tissue of the brain.
B. Secondary tumors are a result of metastasis from other areas (most often from the lungs, followed by breast).
C. Without treatment, benign as well as malignant tumors lead to death.

> **HESI HINT** Benign tumors continue to grow and take up space in the confined area of the cranium, causing neural and vascular compromise in the brain, increased ICP, and necrosis of brain tissue. Even benign tumors must be treated because they may have malignant effects.

Nursing Assessment

A. Headache that is more severe on awakening
B. Vomiting not associated with nausea
C. Papilledema with visual changes
D. Behavioral and personality changes
E. Seizures
F. Aphasia, hemiplegia, ataxia
G. Cranial nerve dysfunction
H. Abnormal CT scan/MRI or positron emission tomography scan (looking for metastasis)

Nursing Plans and Interventions

A. Institute nursing plans and interventions that are similar to those implemented for the client with a head injury and increased ICP.
B. Elevate the head of the bed 30 to 40 degrees; maintain head in neutral position.
C. Facilitate radiation therapy.
    1. Provide skin care with non–oil-based soap and water. Avoid putting alcohol, powder, or oils on the skin.
    2. Explain that alopecia is temporary.
    3. Instruct client not to wash off the lines drawn by the radiologist.
D. Administer chemotherapy: medications may be injected intraventricularly or intravenously.
E. Facilitate surgical removal of tumor (craniotomy).
    1. Preoperative (shave head)
    2. Postoperative
        a. Perform frequent neurologic and vital sign assessment.
        b. Position client with head of bed elevated for supratentorial lesions and flat for infratentorial lesions.
        c. Position client on side opposite the operative site.
        d. Monitor dressings for signs of drainage (excess amount of CSF).
        e. Monitor respiratory status to prevent hypoventilation.
        f. Avoid activities that cause increased ICP.
        g. Monitor for seizure activity.
        h. Administer medications (see "Head Injury," earlier).

> **HESI HINT** Corticosteroids to reduce swelling include the following:
> - Agents and osmotic diuretics to reduce secretions (atropine, glycopyrrolate)
> - Agents to reduce seizures (phenytoin)
> - Prophylactic antibiotics

Multiple Sclerosis

Description: Demyelinating disease resulting in the destruction of CNS myelin and consequent disruption in the transmission of nerve impulses

A. Onset is insidious, with 50% of clients still ambulatory 25 years after diagnosis.
B. Diagnosis determined by a combination of data
    1. Presenting symptoms
    2. Increased white matter density seen on CT scan
    3. Presence of plaques seen on MRI
    4. CSF electrophoresis shows presence of oligoclonal (immunoglobulin) bands.
C. Current thinking is that multiple sclerosis (MS) is autoimmune in origin.

Nursing Assessment

A. Nursing history of client to include
    1. History of symptoms
    2. Progression of illness
    3. Types of treatment received and the responses
    4. Additional health problems
    5. Current medications
    6. Client's and family's perception of illness
    7. Community resources used by the client

HESI HINT Symptoms involving motor function usually begin in the upper extremities with weakness progressing to spastic paralysis. Bowel and bladder dysfunction occurs in 90% of cases. MS is more common in women. Progression is not "orderly."

B. Physical assessment to include
   1. Optic neuritis (loss of vision or blind spots)
   2. Visual or swallowing difficulties
   3. Gait disturbances; intention tremors
   4. Unusual fatigue, weakness, and clumsiness
   5. Numbness, particularly on one side of face
   6. Impaired bladder and bowel control
   7. Speech disturbances
   8. Scotomas (white spots in visual field, diplopia)

Nursing Plans and Interventions

A. Allow hospitalized client to keep own routine.
B. Orient client to environment and teach strategies to maximize vision.
C. Encourage self-care and frequent rest periods.
D. With exercise programs, encourage client to work up to the point just short of fatigue.
E. Teach client that, for muscle spasticity, stretch-hold-relax exercises are helpful, as are riding a stationary bicycle and swimming; take precautions against falls.
F. Initially, work with client on a voiding schedule.
G. Teach client that, as incontinence worsens, the female may need to learn clean self-catheterization; the male may need a condom catheter.
H. Encourage adequate fluid intake, high-fiber foods, and a bowel regimen for constipation problems.
I. Encourage the client and the family to verbalize their concerns about ongoing care issues.
J. Encourage client to maintain contact with a support group.
K. Refer client for home health care services.
L. Encourage client to contact the local MS Society for emotional support and direct services.
M. Administer steroid therapy and chemotherapeutic drugs in acute exacerbations to shorten length of attack.
N. ACTH, cortisone, cyclophosphamide (Cytoxan), and other immunosuppressive drugs.

HESI HINT Nursing implications for administration of these drugs should focus on the prevention of infection.

O. Remember that biologic response modifiers such as interferon-beta products (Betaseron, Rebif, and Avonex) have shown recent success for MS relapses.

Myasthenia Gravis

Description: Disorder affecting the neuromuscular transmission of impulses in the voluntary muscles of the body

A. It is considered an autoimmune disease characterized by the presence of acetylcholine receptor (AChR) antibodies, which interfere with neuronal transmission.
B. It usually affects females between ages 10 and 40 and men between ages 50 and 70.

Nursing Assessment

A. Diplopia (double vision), ptosis (eyelid drooping)
B. Masklike affect: sleepy appearance due to facial muscle involvement
C. Weakness of laryngeal and pharyngeal muscles: dysphagia, choking, food aspiration, difficulty speaking
D. Muscle weakness improved by rest, worsened by activity
E. Advanced cases: respiratory failure, bladder and bowel incontinence
F. Myasthenic crisis symptoms (attributed to disease worsening) associated with undermedication. Increase in myasthenic gravis symptoms; more difficulty swallowing, diplopia, ptosis, dyspnea.
G. Cholinergic crisis (attributed to anticholinesterase overdosage): diaphoresis, diarrhea, fasciculations, cramps, marked worsening of symptoms resulting from overmedication

HESI HINT In clients with myasthenia gravis, be alert for changes in respiratory status; the most severe involvement may result in respiratory failure.

Nursing Plans and Interventions

A. If client is hospitalized, have tracheostomy kit available at bedside for possible myasthenic crisis.
B. Teach client the importance of wearing a Medic Alert bracelet.
C. Administer cholinergic drugs as prescribed (Table 4.34).
D. Schedule nursing activities to conserve energy (e.g., complete daily hygiene activities, administration of medications, and treatments all at once), and allow rest periods. Plan activities during high-energy times, often in the early morning.
E. Instruct client to avoid situations that produce fatigue or physical or emotional stress (any type of stress can exacerbate symptoms).
F. Encourage coughing and deep breathing every 4 to 6 hours. (Muscle weakness limits ability to cough up secretions, promotes URI.)
G. If symptoms worsen, identify type of crisis and report immediately: myasthenic or cholinergic.

HESI HINT Myasthenic crisis is associated with a positive edrophonium (Tensilon) test, whereas a cholinergic crisis is associated with a negative test.

TABLE 4.34 Treatment of Myasthenia Gravis

Drug	Indications	Adverse Reactions	Nursing Implications
• Pyridostigmine bromide	• Inhibits the action of cholinesterase at the cholinergic nerve endings • To promote accumulation of acetylcholine at cholinergic receptor sites	• Cholinergic crisis can occur with overdose	• Atropine is an antidote for drug-induced bradycardia • Take drug with milk or food to decrease GI side effects • Dosage regulation required; record keeping, regarding: side effects, drug response • Observe for symptoms of cholinergic crisis • Fasciculations • Abdominal cramps, diarrhea, incontinence of stool or urine • Hypotension, bradycardia, respiratory depression • Lacrimation, blurred vision • Drug therapy is lifelong and requires family teaching and support

GI, Gastrointestinal.

Parkinson Disease

Description: Chronic, progressive, debilitating neurologic disease of the basal ganglia and substantia nigra, affecting motor ability and characterized by tremor at rest, increased muscle tone (rigidity), slowness in the initiation and execution of movement (bradykinesia), and postural instability (difficulties with gait and balance)

Nursing Assessment

A. Rigidity of extremities
B. Masklike facial expressions with associated difficulty in chewing, swallowing, and speaking
C. Drooling
D. Stooped posture and slow, shuffling gait
E. Tremors at rest, "pill-rolling" movement
F. Emotional lability
G. Increased tremors with stress or anxiety

> **HESI HINT** NCLEX-RN questions often focus on the features of Parkinson disease: tremors (a coarse tremor of fingers and thumb on one hand that disappears during sleep and purposeful activity; also called "pill rolling"), rigidity, hypertonicity, and stooped posture. Focus: *safety!*

Nursing Plans and Interventions

A. Schedule activities later in the day to allow sufficient time for client to perform self-care activities without rushing.
B. Encourage activities and exercise. A cane or walker may be needed.
C. Eliminate environmental noise, and encourage the client to speak slowly and clearly, pausing at intervals.
D. Serve a soft diet, which is easy to swallow.
E. Administer antiparkinsonian drugs as prescribed (Table 4.35).

> **HESI HINT** The pathophysiology involves an imbalance between acetylcholine and dopamine, so symptoms can be controlled by administering a dopamine precursor (levodopa).

Guillain–Barré Syndrome

Description: Clinical syndrome of unknown origin involving peripheral and cranial nerves

A. Is usually preceded by a (viral) respiratory or GI infection 1 to 4 weeks before the onset of neurologic deficits
B. Constant monitoring of these clients is required to prevent the life-threatening problem of acute respiratory failure.
C. Full recovery usually occurs within several months to a year after onset of symptoms.
D. About 30% of those diagnosed with Guillain–Barré syndrome are left with a residual disability. Death occurs in 5%.

Nursing Assessment

A. Paresthesia (tingling and numbness)
B. Muscle weakness of legs progressing to the upper extremities, trunk, and face
C. Paralysis of the ocular, facial, and oropharyngeal muscles, causing marked difficulty in talking, chewing, and swallowing. Assess for
   1. Breathlessness while talking
   2. Shallow and irregular breathing
   3. Use of accessory muscles while breathing
   4. Any change in respiratory pattern
   5. Paradoxical inward movement of the upper abdominal wall while in a supine position, indicating weakness and impending paralysis of the diaphragm
D. Increasing pulse rate and disturbances in rhythm
E. Transient hypertension, orthostatic hypotension
F. Possible pain in the back and in calves of legs
G. Weakness or paralysis of the intercostal and diaphragm muscles; may develop quickly

Nursing Plans and Interventions

A. Monitor for respiratory distress and initiate mechanical ventilation if necessary.
B. See "Nursing Plans and Interventions" for "Altered State of Consciousness," earlier.

TABLE 4.35 Antiparkinsonian Drugs

Drugs	Indications	Adverse Reactions	Nursing Implications
ANTICHOLINERGICS (PARASYMPATHOLYTICS [OLDER DRUGS])			
• Atropine sulfate • Benztropine mesylate • Trihexyphenidyl	• Used to treat secondary cholinergic symptoms, such as drooling, sweating, tremors.	• Increased HR • Postural hypotension • Dry mouth • Constipation • Urinary retention • Blurred vision	• Review client's history for glaucoma, urinary obstruction. • Warn to avoid rapid position changes. • Avoid extreme heat. • Provide gum, hard candy, and frequent mouth care. • Contraindicated in narrow-angle glaucoma
DOPAMINE REPLACEMENTS			

• Levodopa
• Levodopa-carbidopa
• *Dopamine-Releasing Agents*
  • Amantadine HCl
• Dopamine-Releasing Agonists
  • Bromocriptine mesylate
  • Pramipexole
  • Ropinirole
	• Stimulates dopamine production or increases sensitivity of dopamine receptors
	• Newer drugs require lower dosage
		• Involuntary movements
		• Nausea
		• Vomiting
			• Explain that drugs may take months to achieve desired effects.
			• Warn to avoid sudden position changes.
			• Avoid foods high in vitamin B_6 (meats, liver, i.e., high-protein foods).
			• If insomnia occurs, suggest taking last dose earlier in day.
			• May initially cause drowsiness; teach to avoid driving until response is determined.

MONOAMINE OXIDASE TYPE B INHIBITOR			
• Selegiline • Rasagiline	• Used with dopamine agonist when client symptoms do not respond	• Confusion, dizziness • Nausea, dry mouth • Insomnia	• Review drug–drug interactions carefully. • Not an option if client is on antidepressants (SSRIs or tricyclics) • Can cause hypertensive crisis
CATECHOL-O-METHYL TRANSFERASE (COMT) INHIBITOR			
• Entacapone • Tolcapone	• Used with levodopa-carbidopa	• May increase levodopa-carbidopa side effects, including dyskinesias	• Levodopa dose may need to be decreased. • Combination product may decrease pill burden.

HR, Heart rate; *SSRIs*, selective serotonin reuptake inhibitors.

Stroke/Brain Attack: Cerebral Vascular Accident

Description: Sudden loss of brain function resulting from a disruption in the blood supply to a part of the brain; classified as thrombotic or hemorrhagic

> **HESI HINT** CNS involvement related to cause of stroke includes the following:
> - Hemorrhagic: caused by a slow or fast hemorrhage into the brain tissue; often related to hypertension
> - Embolic: caused by a clot that has broken away from a vessel and has lodged in one of the arteries of the brain, blocking the blood supply. It is often related to atherosclerosis (so it may occur again).

A. Risk factors include
   1. Hypertension
   2. Previous transient ischemic attacks (TIAs)
   3. Cardiac disease: atherosclerosis, valve disease, history of dysrhythmias (particularly atrial flutter or fibrillation)
   4. Advanced age
   5. Diabetes
   6. Oral contraceptives and HRT
   7. Smoking
   8. Alcohol, more than 2 drinks per day

> **HESI HINT** Atrial flutter and fibrillation produce a high incidence of thrombus formation after dysrhythmia caused by turbulence of blood flow through all valves and heart.

B. Diagnosis is made by observation of clinical signs and is confirmed by
   1. Cranial CT scan
   2. MRI
   3. Doppler flow studies
   4. Ultrasound imaging

C. Presenting symptoms relate to the specific area of the brain that has been damaged (Table 4.36).

D. Generally there is
   1. Motor loss, usually exhibited as hemiparesis or hemiplegia
   2. Communication loss, exhibited as dysarthria, dysphasia, aphasia, or apraxia
   3. Perceptual disturbance that can be visual, spatial, and sensory

TABLE 4.36 Location of Disruption in the Brain

Feature	Left Hemisphere	Right Hemisphere
• Language	• Aphasia • Agraphia	• May be alert and oriented
• Memory	• No deficit	• Disoriented • Cannot recognize faces
• Vision	• Unable to discriminate words and letters • Reading problems • Deficits in right visual field	• Visual/spatial deficits • Neglect of left visual fields • Loss of depth perception
• Behavior	• Slow • Cautious • Anxious when attempting a new task • Depression or catastrophic response to illness • Sense of guilt • Feeling of worthlessness • Worries over future • Quick anger and frustration	• Impulsive • Unaware of neurologic deficits • Confabulates • Euphoric • Constantly smiles • Denies illness • Poor judgment • Overestimates abilities • Impaired sense of humor
• Hearing	• No deficit	• Loses ability to hear tonal variations

4. Impaired mental acuity or psychological changes, such as decreased attention span, memory loss, depression, lability, and hostility

E. Bladder dysfunction may be either incontinence or retention.

F. Rehabilitation is begun as soon as the client is stable.

> **HESI HINT** A woman who had a stroke 2 days earlier has left-sided paralysis. She has begun to regain some movement in her left side. What can the nurse tell the family about the client's recovery period?
>
> "The quicker movement is recovered, the better the prognosis is for full or improved recovery. She will need patience and understanding from her family as she tries to cope with the stroke. Mood swings can be expected during the recovery period, and bouts of depression and tearfulness are likely."

Nursing Assessment

A. Change in level of consciousness
B. Paresthesia, paralysis
C. Aphasia, agraphia
D. Memory loss
E. Vision impairment
F. Bladder and bowel dysfunction
G. Behavioral changes
H. Assessment of client's functional abilities, including
  1. Mobility
  2. Activities of daily living (ADLs)
  3. Elimination
  4. Communication
I. Ability to swallow, eat, and drink without aspiration

> **HESI HINT** Words that describe losses in strokes include the following:
> 1. *Apraxia:* inability to perform purposeful movements in the absence of motor problems
> 2. *Dysarthria:* difficulty articulating
> 3. *Dysphasia:* impairment of speech and verbal comprehension
> 4. *Aphasia:* loss of the ability to speak
> 5. *Agraphia:* loss of the ability to write
> 6. *Alexia:* loss of the ability to read
> 7. *Dysphagia:* dysfunctional swallowing

Nursing Plans and Interventions

A. Control hypertension to help prevent future stroke.
B. Maintain proper body alignment while client is in bed. Use splints or other assistive devices (including bedrolls and pillows) to maintain functional position.
C. Position client to minimize edema, prevent contractures, and maintain skin integrity.
D. Perform full ROM exercises four times a day. Follow up with program initiated by other team members.
E. Encourage client to participate in or manage own personal care.
F. Set realistic goals; add new tasks daily.
G. Teach client that appropriate self-care activities for the hemiparetic person include
  1. Bathing
  2. Brushing teeth
  3. Shaving with electric razor
  4. Eating
  5. Combing hair
H. Encourage client to assist with dressing activities and modify them as necessary (client will wear street clothes during waking hours).
I. Analyze bladder elimination pattern.
  1. Offer bedpan or urinal according to client's particular pattern of elimination.
  2. Reassure client that bladder control tends to be regained quickly.
J. The speech and language therapist initiates follow-up speech program.
  1. Ensure consistency with this program.
  2. Reassure the client that regaining speech is a very slow process.
K. Do not place client in sensory overload; give only one set of instructions at a time.
L. Encourage total family involvement in rehabilitation.
M. Encourage client and family to join a support group.
N. Encourage family members to allow the client to perform self-care activities as outlined by the rehabilitation team.

O. Refer for outclient follow-up or for home health care.
P. Teach that swallowing modifications may include a soft diet (pureed foods, thickened liquids) and head positioning.

HESI HINT Steroids are administered after a stroke to decrease cerebral edema and retard permanent disability. H2 inhibitors are administered to prevent peptic ulcers.

REVIEW OF NEUROLOGIC SYSTEM

1. What are the classifications of the commonly prescribed eye drops for glaucoma?
2. Identify two types of hearing loss.
3. Write four nursing interventions for the care of the blind person and four nursing interventions for the care of the deaf person.
4. In your own words, describe the Glasgow Coma Scale.
5. State four independent nursing interventions to maintain adequate respiration, airway, and oxygenation in the unconscious client.
6. Who is at risk for stroke?
7. Complications of immobility include the potential for thrombus development. State three nursing interventions to prevent thrombi.
8. List four rationales for the appearance of restlessness in the unconscious client.
9. What nursing interventions prevent corneal drying in a comatose client?
10. When can a comatose client on IV hyperalimentation begin to receive tube feedings instead?
11. What is the most important principle in a bowel management program for a client with neurologic deficits?
12. Define stroke.
13. A client with a diagnosis of stroke presents with symptoms of aphasia and right hemiparesis but no memory or hearing deficit. In what hemisphere has the client suffered a lesion?
14. What are the symptoms of spinal shock?
15. What are the symptoms of autonomic dysreflexia?
16. What is the most important indicator of increased ICP?
17. What vital sign changes are indicative of increased ICP?
18. A neighbor calls the neighborhood nurse stating that his very hyperactive dog knocked him hard to the floor. He is wondering what symptoms would indicate the need to visit an emergency department. What should the nurse tell him to do?
19. What activities and situations that increase ICP should be avoided?
20. What is the action of hyperosmotic agents (osmotic diuretics) used to treat ICP?
21. Why should narcotics be avoided in clients with neurologic impairment?
22. Headache and vomiting are symptoms of many disorders. What characteristics of these symptoms would alert the nurse to refer a client to a neurologist?
23. How should the head of the bed be positioned for postcraniotomy clients with infratentorial lesions?
24. Is MS thought to occur because of an autoimmune process?
25. Is paralysis always a consequence of spinal cord injury?
26. What types of drugs are used in the treatment of myasthenia gravis?

See Answer Key at the end of this text for suggested responses.

HEMATOLOGY AND ONCOLOGY

Anemia

Description: Deficiency of erythrocytes (RBCs) reflected as decreased Hct, Hgb, and RBCs

Nursing Assessment

A. Pallor, especially of the ears and nail beds; palmar crease; conjunctiva
B. Fatigue, exercise intolerance, lethargy, orthostatic hypotension
C. Tachycardia, heart murmurs, HF
D. Signs of bleeding, such as hematuria, melena, menorrhagia
E. Dyspnea
F. Irritability, difficulty concentrating
G. Cool skin, cold intolerance
H. Risk factors
  1. Diet lacking in iron, folate, and/or vitamin B_{12}
  2. Family history of genetic diseases such as sickle cell or congenital hemolytic anemia
  3. Medication history of anemia-producing drugs, such as salicylates, thiazides, and diuretics
  4. Exposure to toxic agents, such as lead or insecticides
I. Diagnostic tests indicate abnormally low results
  1. Hgb less than 10 g/dL
  2. Hct less than 36%
  3. RBCs less than 4×10^{12}
  4. Bone marrow aspiration positive for anemia
J. Blood loss either acute or chronic
K. Medical history of kidney disorders

HESI HINT Physical symptoms occur as a compensatory mechanism when the body is trying to make up for a deficit somewhere in the system. For instance, cardiac output increases when Hgb levels drop below 7 g/dL.

Nursing Plans and Interventions

A. Administer blood products as prescribed (see Table 3.7)
B. Alternate periods of activity with periods of rest.

TABLE 4.37 Administration of Iron

Do's	Don'ts
• Use Z-track method of administration. • Use air bubble to avoid withdrawing medication into subcutaneous tissue.	• Do *not* use deltoid muscle. • Do *not* massage injection site.

C. Teach about diet.
   1. Instruct in food selection and preparation to maximize intake of
      a. Iron (red meats, organ meats, whole wheat products, spinach, carrots)
      b. Folic acid (green vegetables, liver, citrus fruits)
      c. Vitamin B_{12} (glandular meats, yeast, green leafy vegetables, milk, and cheese)
   2. Instruct in need for prescribed vitamin supplements.
      a. Take iron on an empty stomach to enhance absorption; 1 hour before meals or 2 hours after meals.
      b. Give vitamin C to enhance absorption of iron.
      c. Administer B_{12} and folic acid orally except to clients with pernicious anemia who should receive B_{12} parenterally.

D. If parenteral iron is required, use Z-track method for administration to prevent staining the skin (Table 4.37).

E. Provide genetic information if client has sickle cell or congenital hemolytic anemia.

F. Teach that sickle cell crisis is precipitated by hypoxia (see Chapter 5: Pediatric Nursing).
   1. Provide pain relief.
   2. Provide adequate hydration.
   3. Teach client to avoid activities that cause hypoxia.
   4. Teach client when to seek medical attention.

G. Teach client that iron (oral) may turn stools black.

H. Give liquid iron through a straw, with oral care afterward, to prevent discoloring of teeth.

I. Teach the client to report any unusual bleeding to health care professional.

HESI HINT Use only normal saline to flush IV tubing or to run with blood. Never add medications to blood products. Two registered nurses should simultaneously check the physician's prescription, the client's identity, and the blood bag label.

Leukemia

Description: Malignant neoplasm of the blood-forming organs

A. Leukemia is characterized by an abnormal overproduction of immature forms of any of the leukocytes. There is an interference with normal blood production that results in decreased numbers of RBCs and platelets.
   1. Anemia results from decreased RBC production and blood loss.
   2. Immunosuppression occurs because of the large number of immature WBCs or profound neutropenia.
   3. Hemorrhage occurs because of thrombocytopenia.
   4. There may be leukemic invasion of other organ systems, such as the liver, spleen, lymph nodes, kidneys, lungs, and brain.

B. The exact cause of leukemia is unknown, but identified precipitating factors include
   1. Genetic abnormalities
   2. Ionizing radiation (therapeutic or atomic)
   3. Viral infections (human T cells, leukemia virus)
   4. Exposure to certain chemicals or drugs (Box 4.2)
      a. Benzene
      b. Alkylating chemotherapeutic agents
      c. Immunosuppressants
      d. Chloramphenicol

C. Incidence is highest in children 3 to 4 years of age; declines until age 35; then a steady increase occurs.

D. Biopsy, bone marrow aspiration, lumbar puncture, and frequent blood counts allow for diagnosis of leukemia.

E. Leukemia is treated with antineoplastic chemotherapy (Table 4.38).

Types of Leukemia

A. Acute myelogenous leukemia (AML)
   1. It involves the inability of leukocytes to mature; those that do are abnormal.
   2. It can occur at any time during the life cycle.
   3. Onset is insidious.
   4. Prognosis is poor: 5-year survival of 20%; overall, 50% for children.
   5. Cause of death tends to be overwhelming infection.

B. Chronic myelogenous leukemia (CML)
   1. It results from abnormal production of granulocytic cells.
   2. It is a biphasic disease.

BOX 4.2 Administration of Antineoplastic Chemotherapeutic Agents

- Follow Occupational Safety and Health Administration (OSHA) guidelines for administration as well as for decontamination of nondisposable areas and equipment and of self.
- Obtain complete and detailed instructions about administration (routine knowledge of procedures for IV administration is not sufficient).
- These drugs are toxic to cancer cells and normal cells in both the client and the caregivers who are infusing the drugs.
- Nurses who are pregnant or are considering becoming pregnant should notify supervisor (many agencies discourage or prohibit such caregivers from administering these drugs).
- Wear gloves when handling drugs.
- Check the drug with another nurse against the health care provider's prescription and the client's record to ensure that it is the correct medication.
- If IV catheter line is used for infusion, verify line placement and patency with another nurse and aspirate a blood return.
- If a vesicant (caustic) drug is administered peripherally, stay with the client throughout administration and check IV placement and patency frequently by aspirating a blood return.
- If a peripheral site is used for infusion, use a new site daily.
- Dispose of all IV equipment in the specially provided waste receptacle so that personnel handling trash do not come into contact with vesicant drugs.

TABLE 4.38 Antineoplastic Chemotherapeutic Agents

Drugs	Indications	Adverse Reactions	Nursing Implications
		ALKYLATING AGENTS	
• Cyclophosphamide Mechlorethamine HCl • Cisplatin • Busulfan • Procarbazine • Imidazole carboxamide	• Hodgkin disease • Leukemia • Neuroblastoma • Retinoblastoma • Multiple myeloma	• Bone marrow suppression • Nausea and vomiting • Cystitis • Stomatitis • Alopecia • Gonadal suppression • Toxic effects occur slowly with high dosage • Toxic to kidneys and ears • Pleural effusion • Seizures	• Use immediately after reconstitution. • Avoid vapors in eyes. • Vesicant; if comes in contact with skin, flush with water. • Check placement of infusing system. • Hydrate well before and during treatment with IV fluids and mannitol. • Monitor renal functioning and watch for signs of cystitis. • Force fluids. • Monitor hearing and vision.
		ANTIMETABOLITES	
• Fluorouracil • Methotrexate sodium; requires leucovorin rescue to prevent toxic effects • Mercaptopurine/6-MP • Cytarabine • Gemcitabine	• Acute lymphocytic leukemia • Acute myelocytic leukemia • Brain tumors • Ovarian, breast, prostatic, testicular cancers	• Nausea and vomiting • Diarrhea • Myelosuppression (bone marrow depression) • Proctitis • Stomatitis • Dermatitis • Renal toxicity • Hepatotoxicity • Anaphylaxis	• Administer antiemetics as needed. • Teach to wear sunscreen when outdoors. • Toxic to liver and kidney; avoid: • Aspirin • Sulfonamide • Tetracycline • Vitamins containing folic acid • Leucovorin is used with methotrexate as antidote for high doses; called "leucovorin rescue." • Give allopurinol concurrently with 6-MP to inhibit uric acid production by cell destruction; it increases drug's potency. • Monitor liver function.
		ANTITUMOR ANTIBIOTICS	
• Dactinomycin • Bleomycin sulfate • Daunorubicin I • Mitomycin • Doxorubicin HCl • Idarubicin	• Sarcoma • Neuroblastoma • Head and neck tumors • Testicular, ovarian, breast cancer • Hodgkin disease • Lymphocytic leukemia • Acute myelocytic leukemia	• Bone marrow suppression • Anorexia • Nausea and vomiting • Alopecia • Cardiac toxicity • Vesicant	• Monitor placement and patency of infusing system. • Monitor for cardiac dysrhythmia. • Inform client that urine turns red. • Administer antiemetics as needed.
		ANGIOGENESIS INHIBITORS	
• Bevacizumab	• Recombinant humanized monoclonal antibody that prevents neoangiogenesis	• Hypertension • Bleeding • Thrombosis	• Report abdominal pain. • Monitor for complications. • May inhibit wound healing.
		ENDOTHELIAL GROWTH FACTOR RECEPTOR INHIBITORS	
• Cetuximab • Panitumumab	• Inhibits cell growth • Increases programmed cellular death	• Severe infusion reactions with airway obstruction • Hypotension • Acne-like rash • Fatigue • GI disturbances	• Monitor for severe infusion reactions. • Use diphenhydramine before administration.
Miscellaneous Antineoplastics			
• Hydroxyurea • Asparaginase	• Urea-derived antineoplastic agent against solid tumors and CML • Anticancer enzyme against ALL	• Drowsiness • Renal dysfunction • Nausea and vomiting, diarrhea • Hepatitis • Myelosuppression	• Comfort measures for stomatitis, GI discomforts. • Monitor for complications. • Maintain adequate hydration.

Continued

PLANT ALKALOIDS			
• Vincristine sulfate • Vinblastine sulfate	• Acute lymphocytic leukemia • Hodgkin disease • Wilms tumor • Sarcoma • Breast cancer • Testicular cancer	• Bone marrow suppression • Neurotoxicity • Weakness • Paresthesia • Jaw pain • Constipation • Stomatitis • Alopecia • Headaches • Minimal nausea and vomiting	• Administer antiemetics as needed. • Monitor for neurotoxicity. • Check placement and patency of infusing system.
MITOTIC INHIBITORS			
• Paclitaxel • Docetaxel	• Breast cancer • Ovarian cancer • Non—small cell lung cancer • Kaposi sarcoma	• Decreased WBCs and RBCs • Alopecia • Nausea and vomiting, diarrhea • Joint, muscle pain	• Monitor for signs and symptoms of infection. • Administer antiemetics and antidiarrheals as needed.
HORMONAL AGENTS (CORTICOSTEROIDS)			
• Prednisone • Dexamethasone	• Leukemia • Hodgkin disease • Breast cancer • Lymphoma • Multiple myeloma • Cerebral edema (due to brain metastasis)	• See "Endocrine System," earlier.	• See "Endocrine System," earlier.
MALE-SPECIFIC HORMONAL AGENTS			
• Flutamide • Leuprolide • Goserelin	• Prostate cancers • Testicular cancers	• Headache, paresthesias, cardiac dysrhythmias, nausea and vomiting, hypoglycemia, neuropathies	• Bone pain and voiding problems • Safety with neuropathies
FEMALE-SPECIFIC HORMONAL AGENTS			
• Tamoxifen citrate • Megestrol • Medroxyprogesterone	• Breast cancer	• Hot flashes • Mild nausea	• Administer antiemetics as needed.
ANDROGENS			
• Testosterone • Fluoxymesterone	• Breast cancer (postmenopausal women)	• Fluid retention • Nausea • Masculinization	• Low-salt diet
TOPOISOMERASE-I INHIBITORS			
• Irinotecan • Topotecan	• Used after failure of initial treatment of ovarian, small-cell lung, and colorectal cancers	• Myelosuppression • Moderate nausea and vomiting • Diarrhea	• Camptosar diarrhea treated with atropine due to physiologic cause • Give antiemetics per protocol.
MONOCLONAL ANTIBODIES			
• Trastuzumab • Rituximab	• Targets specific malignant cells with less damage to healthy cells in non-Hodgkin lymphoma, breast cancer	• Fever, chills, infection • Nausea and vomiting, diarrhea • Bronchospasm, dyspnea, acute respiratory distress syndrome • Hypotension • Ventricular dysfunction, HF	• Premedicate with antiemetics. • Monitor for identified side effects.
BIOLOGIC RESPONSE MODIFIERS			
ANTIANEMIC			
• Epoetin	• Anemia due to CRF, chemotherapy, HIV-related treatments	• Seizures • Hypertension • Pain at injection site	• Do not shake vial; may cause inactivation of medication. • Monitor Hct levels. • Pain at injection site; give slowly (subcutaneous).

Continued

TABLE 4.38 Antineoplastic Chemotherapeutic Agents—cont'd

		GRANULOCYTE-STIMULATING FACTOR	
• Filgrastim	• Improves immune competence by increasing neutrophils	• Medullary bone pain during initial treatment • Pain at injection site	• Monitor WBC/differential; absolute neutrophil count (ANC). • Give SC slowly due to local pain at site. • Assess bone pain and medicate with analgesics.
		THROMBOTIC GROWTH FACTOR	
• Oprelvekin	• Stimulates production of megakaryocytes and platelets	• Dizziness, headache, insomnia, blurred vision, nervousness • Pleural effusion • Vasodilation, cardiac dysrhythmias • Bone pain, myalgia • GI upsets • Fluid retention	• Give slowly to reduce pain at injection site. • Assess for complications related to fluid retention. • Start within 6–24 h of chemotherapy start and continue for 10–21 days. • Monitor CBC: H&H may decrease; monitor platelets.
		INTERFERON-BETA PRODUCTS	
• Interferon beta-1a • Interferon beta-1b	• Relapsing MS • AIDS • Kaposi sarcoma • Malignant melanoma • Hepatitis C	• Seizures, H/A, weakness, insomnia, depression, suicidal ideation • Hypertension, chest pain, vasodilation, edema, palpitations • Dyspnea • Nausea and vomiting, elevated liver function studies, GI disorders • Myalgia, flulike symptoms	• Anticipate discomfort from side effects and initiate relief measures early. • Notify physician if evidence of depression. • Sunscreen and protective clothing are needed because of photosensitivity. • Do not shake or swirl solution; use soon after reconstitution. • Monitor CBC and blood chemistries.
		INTERLEUKINS	
• Aldesleukin	• Metastatic renal cell carcinoma	• Respiratory failure; pulmonary edema • HF, MI, dysrhythmias, stroke • Bowel perforation, hepatomegaly, GI disturbances • Serious electrolyte imbalances • Coagulation disorders • Pancytopenia	• Vigilance in monitoring for serious side effects with stat response.
		INTERFERON-ALFA PRODUCTS	
• Interferon-alfa-2a • Interferon-alfa-2b	• 2a: hairy cell leukemia, Kaposi sarcoma • 2b: chronic hepatitis B and C, Kaposi sarcoma, hairy cell leukemia	• Similar to those of interferon-beta products	• Similar to those of interferon-beta products
		ANTIEMETICS	
• Prochlorperazine • Promethazine HCl	• Nausea and vomiting	• Drowsiness • Dizziness • Extrapyramidal symptoms • Orthostatic hypotension • Blurred vision • Dry mouth	• Dilute oral solution with water or juice. • Determine baseline BP before administration. • Give deep IM. • Monitor BP carefully.
• Metoclopramide HCl • Haloperidol	• Nausea and vomiting	• Drowsiness • Restlessness • Fatigue • Extrapyramidal symptoms	• Caution client of decreased alertness. • Avoid alcohol. • Discontinue if extrapyramidal symptoms occur.
• Diphenhydramine HCl	• Given with Reglan and Haldol to reduce extrapyramidal symptoms	• Sedation • Dizziness • Hypotension • Dry mouth	• Caution client of decreased alertness. • Avoid alcohol. • Discontinue if extrapyramidal symptoms occur.

Continued

ANTIEMETICS			
• Ondansetron HCl	• Prevention of nausea and vomiting associated with cancer • Postoperative nausea and vomiting	• Headache often requiring analgesic for relief	• Administer tablets 30 min before chemotherapy and 1–2 h before radiation therapy. • Dilute IV injection in 50 mL of 5% dextrose or 0.9% NaCl.
• Granisetron	• Nausea and vomiting associated with chemotherapy and abdominal radiation	• Hypertension • CNS stimulation • Elevated liver enzymes	• Assess for extrapyramidal symptoms. • Monitor liver enzymes. • Give only on day of chemotherapy or radiation treatment and 1 h before.

ALL, Acute lymphoblastic anemia; *BP*, blood pressure; *CML*, cell-mediated lympholysis; *CNS*, central nervous system; *CRF*, chronic renal failure; *GI*, gastrointestinal; *HF*, heart failure; *IM*, intramuscular; *IV*, intravenous; *MI*, myocardial Infarction; *RBCs*, red blood cells; *WBCs*, white blood cells.

3. The chronic stage lasts approximately 3 years.
4. The acute phase tends to last 2 to 3 months.
5. It occurs in young to middle-aged adults.
6. Known causes include
   a. Ionizing radiation
   b. Chemical exposure
7. Prognosis is poor: 5-year survival rate of 37%.
8. Treatment is conservative, involving oral antineoplastic agents.
   a. Hydroxyurea (Hydrea, an inhibitor of DNA synthesis)
   b. Interferon (mechanism of action not known)
   c. Imatinib mesylate (Gleevec) targeted therapy if cells are Philadelphia chromosome positive

C. Acute lymphocytic leukemia (ALL)
1. Abnormal leukocytes are found in blood-forming tissue.
2. It occurs in children (is the most common childhood cancer).
3. The prognosis is favorable: 80% of children treated live 5 years or longer.

D. Chronic lymphocytic leukemia (CLL)
1. It involves increased production of leukocytes and lymphocytes and proliferation of cells within the bone marrow, spleen, and liver.
2. It occurs after the age of 35, often in older adults.
3. The 5-year survival rate is 73% overall.
4. Most clients are asymptomatic and are not treated.

Nursing Assessment

A. Tendency to bleed
1. Petechiae
2. Nosebleeds
3. Bleeding gums
4. Ecchymoses
5. Nonhealing skin abrasions

B. Anemia
1. Fatigue
2. Pallor
3. Headache
4. Bone and joint pain
5. Hepatosplenomegaly

C. Infection
1. Fever
2. Tachycardia
3. Lymphadenopathy (swollen lymph nodes)
4. Night sweats
5. Skin infection, poor healing

D. GI distress
1. Anorexia
2. Weight loss
3. Sore throat
4. Abdominal pain
5. Diarrhea
6. Oral lesions, typically thrush

Nursing Plans and Interventions for Immunosuppressed Clients and Clients With Bone Marrow Suppression

A. Monitor WBC count daily and inform physician of count.

B. Routinely assess oral cavity and genital area for signs of yeast infection.

C. Monitor vital signs frequently.
1. Note baseline.
2. Report fever to physician as requested.
   a. Be aware that parameters for reporting tend to be lower than those in postoperative clients.
   b. Usually report temperature elevations of 38.05°C or above.

D. Administer antibiotics as prescribed, maintaining a strict schedule.

E. Notify physician if delay in administration occurs.
1. Obtain trough and peak blood levels of antibiotics.
   a. Trough: Draw blood sample shortly before administration of antibiotic.
   b. Peak: Draw blood sample 30 minutes to 1 hour after administration of drug.
2. Monitor blood levels of antibiotics for therapeutic dose range.

F. Teach client and family the importance of infection control.
1. Wash hands using good handwashing technique.
2. Avoid contact with any infected person.
3. Avoid crowds.

4. Maintain daily hygiene to prevent spread of microorganisms.
5. Avoid eating uncooked foods; they contain bacteria.
6. Avoid water standing in cups, vases, etc. because they are excellent sources of growth for microorganisms (especially mold spores).
7. Neutropenic and reverse isolation precautions PRN.

G. Institute an oral hygiene regimen.
1. Use soft-bristle toothbrush to avoid bleeding.
2. Use salt and soda mouth rinse.
3. Perform oral hygiene after each meal and at bedtime.
4. Lubricate lips with water-soluble gel.
5. Avoid lemon-glycerin swabs; they dry oral mucosa.

H. Encourage coughing and deep breathing to prevent stasis of secretions in lungs.

I. Avoid rectal thermometers and suppositories to prevent bleeding.

J. Monitor fluid status and balance; febrile clients dehydrate rapidly.
1. Monitor I&O.
2. Encourage fluid intake of at least 3 L/day.

K. Encourage mobility to decrease pulmonary stasis.

L. Provide care for invasive catheters and lines (Box 4.3).
1. Use strict aseptic technique for all invasive procedures.
2. Change dressings two or three times per week and when soiled.
3. Use catheter line for piggybacking medication, depending on the purpose of the line and the fluid being infused; no medications can be piggybacked with an infusion of chemotherapeutic agents.
4. Central lines and implanted ports can often be used for collecting blood samples, but regular IV sites cannot.

M. Protect the client from bleeding and injury.
1. Handle the client gently.
2. Avoid needle sticks. Use smallest gauge needle possible and apply pressure for 10 minutes after needle sticks.
3. Encourage use of electric razor only for shaving.
4. Instruct client to avoid blowing or picking nose.
5. Assess for signs of bleeding.
6. Avoid use of salicylates.

Hodgkin Disease

Description: Malignancy of the lymphoid system that initiates in a single lymph node

A. Hodgkin disease is characterized by a generalized painless lymphadenopathy.

B. Incidence is higher in males and young adults.

C. Cause is unknown.

D. Prognosis is good: 5-year survival rate of 90%; however, late recurrences after 5 to 10 years are not uncommon.

E. Diagnosis is made by excision of node for biopsy; characteristic cell is called *Reed-Sternberg.*

F. Determination of stage of disease is done by surgical laparotomy.
1. Stage I: involvement of single lymph node region or a single extralymphatic organ or site
2. Stage II: involvement of two or more lymph nodes on the same side of the diaphragm or localized involvement of an extralymphatic organ or site
3. Stage III: involvement of lymph node areas on both sides of the diaphragm to localized involvement of one extralymphatic organ, the spleen, or both
4. Stage IV: diffuse involvement of one or more extralymphatic organs, with or without lymph node involvement

G. Treatment
1. Radiotherapy
2. Chemotherapy: Adriamycin, Blenoxane, Velban, Dacarbazine (ABVD)
3. Splenectomy

Nursing Assessment

A. Enlarged lymph nodes (one or more), usually cervical lymph nodes

B. Anemia, thrombocytopenia, elevated leukocytes, decreased platelets

C. Fever, increased susceptibility to infections

D. Anorexia, weight loss

E. Malaise, bone pain

F. Night sweats

G. Pruritus

H. Pain in affected lymph node after consuming alcohol

BOX 4.3 Care of Intravenous Lines and Catheters

Types of IV Lines and Catheters	Use and Care of IV Lines and Catheters

• Nontunneled percutaneous central venous catheter (CVC)
• Tunneled catheter (Broviac & Hickman)
• Implant reservoir (Port-A-Cath)
• PICC (peripherally inserted central catheter)
	• Stays in place for extended periods of time
	• Used for clients who require immunosuppressive therapy or are receiving long-term IV therapy
	• Exit sites include
	  • At the upper chest
	  • Femoral area
	  • Antecubital area
	• To prevent an air embolus when a central line is open to air, position client in Trendelenburg position or have client perform a Valsalva maneuver if there is no slide clamp on the line.
	• Maintain a patent IV site by flushing with heparin or saline. (The amount of heparin used depends on size of lumen, length of tubing, whether reservoir exists [e.g., Port-A-Cath].)
	• Immediately after insertion of a central line, the nurse should auscultate breath sounds.
	• After insertion of a central line, a chest radiograph must be taken to determine correct placement and detect pneumothorax (observe for unequal expansion of chest wall).

Nursing Plans and Interventions

A. Protect client from infection, monitor temperature carefully.
B. Observe for signs of anemia.
C. Provide adequate rest.
D. Provide preoperative and postoperative care for laparotomy or splenectomy.
E. Encourage high-nutrient foods.
F. Provide emotional support to client and family.

> **HESI HINT** Hodgkin disease is one of the most curable of all adult malignancies. Emotional support is vital. Career development is often interrupted for treatment. Chemotherapy renders many male clients sterile. May bank sperm before treatment, if desired.

General Oncology Content

A. Oncology terms
   1. Cancer: a disease characterized by uncontrolled growth of abnormal cells
   2. Neoplasm: a new formation
   3. Carcinoma: a malignant tumor arising from epithelial tissue
   4. Sarcoma: a malignant tumor arising from nonepithelial tissue
   5. Differentiation: degree to which neoplastic tissue is different from parent tissue
   6. Metastasis: spread of cancer from the original site to other parts of the body
   7. Adjuvant therapy: therapy supplemental to the primary therapy
   8. Palliative procedure: relieves symptoms without curing the cause
B. Tumors identified by tissue of origin
   1. Adeno: glandular tissue
   2. Angio: blood vessels
   3. Basal cell: epithelium (sun-exposed areas)
   4. Embryonal: gonads
   5. Fibro: fibrous tissue
   6. Lympho: lymphoid tissue
   7. Melano: pigmented cells of epithelium
   8. Myo: muscle tissue
   9. Osteo: bone
   10. Squamous cell: epithelium
C. Seven warning signs of cancer
   1. Change in usual bowel and bladder function
   2. A sore that does not heal
   3. Unusual bleeding or discharge, hematuria, tarry stools, ecchymosis, bleeding mole
   4. Thickening or a lump in the breast or elsewhere
   5. Indigestion or dysphagia
   6. Obvious changes in a wart or mole
   7. Nagging cough or hoarseness

REVIEW OF HEMATOLOGY AND ONCOLOGY

1. List three potential causes of anemia.
2. What is the only IV fluid compatible with blood products?
3. What actions should the nurse take if a hemolytic transfusion reaction occurs?
4. List three interventions for clients with a tendency to bleed.
5. Identify two sites that should be assessed for infection in immunosuppressed clients.
6. Name three food sources of vitamin B_{12}.
7. Describe care of invasive catheters and lines.
8. List three safety precautions for the administration of antineoplastic chemotherapy.
9. Describe the use of leucovorin.
10. Describe the method of collecting the trough and peak blood levels of antibiotics.
11. List four nursing interventions for care of the client with Hodgkin disease.
12. List four topics you would cover when teaching an immunosuppressed client about infection control.

See Answer Key at the end of this text for suggested responses.

REPRODUCTIVE SYSTEM

Benign Tumors of the Uterus (Leiomyomas Fibroids, Myomas, Fibromyomas, Fibromas)

Description: Benign tumors arising from the muscle tissue of the uterus

A. Benign tumors are more common in black women than in white women.
B. Benign tumors are more common in women who have never been pregnant.
C. The most common symptom is abnormal uterine bleeding.
D. They tend to disappear after menopause.
E. They rarely become malignant.
F. Treatment for abnormal uterine bleeding (menorrhagia)
   1. Dilation and curettage (D&C)
      a. Used only in extreme cases of bleeding
      b. For older women when endometrial biopsy and ultrasonography have not provided the necessary diagnostic information
   2. Endometrial ablation
      a. Laser or electrosurgical technique
      b. Successful with many clients with menorrhagia

G. Treatment of uterine fibroids with menorrhagia
  1. Myomectomy (removal of fibroids without removal of the uterus) via laparotomy, laparoscopy, or hysteroscopy
  2. Abdominal or vaginal hysterectomy (see "Nursing Plans and Interventions for Hysterectomy," later)
  3. Hormonal regimens (e.g., synthetic analog of gonadotropin-releasing hormone [GnRH], nafarelin [Synarel], leuprolide [Lupron] to shrink the tumor)
  4. Uterine artery embolization (UAE) of the blood vessels supplying the fibroid tumor
  5. Cryosurgery

Nursing Assessment

A. Menorrhagia (hypermenorrhea: profuse or prolonged menstrual bleeding)
B. Dysmenorrhea (extremely painful menstrual periods)
C. Uterine enlargement
D. Low back pain and pelvic pain

> **HESI HINT** Menorrhagia (profuse or prolonged menstrual bleeding) is the most important factor relating to benign uterine tumors. Assess for signs of anemia.

Nursing Plans and Interventions

A. GnRH
  1. Explain regrowth will occur after the treatment is stopped.
  2. A small loss in bone mass and changes in lipid levels can occur.
  3. Amenorrhea may occur.
  4. Adding raloxifene to GnRH administration has been effective in preventing these effects in premenopausal women.
  5. Women who wish to avoid pregnancy should use a nonhormonal or barrier method of contraception.
  6. Discuss administration methods for GnRH agonists (subcutaneous and intramuscular [IM] injections, intranasal administration, and subcutaneous implantation).

B. UAE
  1. Preoperative teaching: Do not drink alcohol, smoke, take aspirin or anticoagulant medications 24 hours before the procedure.
  2. During procedure: Expect cramping during injection of the polyvinyl alcohol pellets into selected blood vessels.
  3. Postoperatively: Pelvic pain, fever, malaise, and nausea and vomiting may be caused by acute fibroid degeneration.
  4. Pain may be controlled with a patient-controlled analgesia pump.
  5. Postoperative nursing assessments: Check for bleeding in the groin and vital signs, assess pain level, check pedal pulse and neurovascular condition of affected leg.
  6. Discharge teaching
     a. Take prescribed medications as ordered.
     b. Call physician if there are any of the following symptoms: bleeding, pain, swelling or hematoma at the puncture site, fever of 101°F (38.3°C), urinary retention, or abnormal vaginal drainage (foul odor, brown color, tissue).
     c. Eat a normal diet, including fluids and fiber.
     d. Do not use tampons or douche or have vaginal intercourse for at least 4 weeks.
     e. Avoid straining during bowel movements.
     f. Keep follow-up appointment.
  7. An ultrasound or MRI examination may be done after the UAE to determine the effectiveness of the procedure.

Uterine Prolapse, Cystocele, and Rectocele

Description: Uterine prolapse is downward displacement of the uterus. Cystocele is the relaxation of the anterior vaginal wall with prolapse of the bladder. Rectocele is the relaxation of the posterior vaginal wall with prolapse of the rectum.

A. Preventive measures
  1. Postpartum perineal exercises
  2. Spaced pregnancies
  3. Weight control
B. Surgical intervention
  1. Hysterectomy
  2. Anterior and posterior vaginal repair (A&P repair)
C. Nonsurgical intervention (for uterine prolapse)
  1. Kegel exercises
  2. Knee-chest position
  3. Pessary use

> **HESI HINT** What is the anatomic significance of a prolapsed uterus? When the uterus is displaced, it impinges on other structures in the lower abdomen. The bladder, rectum, and small intestine can protrude through the vaginal wall.

Nursing Assessment

A. Predisposing conditions
  1. Multiparity
  2. Pelvic tearing during childbirth
  3. Vaginal muscle weakness associated with aging
  4. Obesity
B. Symptoms associated with uterine prolapse
  1. Dysmenorrhea
  2. Pulling and dragging sensations in pelvis and back
  3. Dyspareunia
  4. Pressure, protrusions
  5. Fatigue
  6. Low backache
  7. Symptoms may be worse after prolonged standing or deep penile penetration during intercourse.
C. Symptoms associated with cystocele
  1. Incontinence or stress incontinence (dribbling with coughing or sneezing or any activity that increases intra-abdominal pressure)
  2. Urinary retention
  3. Bladder infections (cystitis)

D. Symptoms associated with rectocele
  1. Constipation
  2. Hemorrhoids
  3. Sense of pressure or need to defecate

Nursing Plans and Interventions for Hysterectomy

A. Provide preoperative and postoperative care.
B. Administer enema and douche as prescribed preoperatively.
C. Note amount and character of vaginal discharge. Postoperatively, there should be less than one saturated pad in 4 hours.
D. Avoid rectal thermometers or tubes, especially when A&P repair has been performed.
E. Check extremities for warmth and tenderness as indicators of thrombophlebitis.
F. Pain management postoperatively
  1. Assess character of pain and determine appropriate analgesic.
  2. Administer analgesics as needed and determine effectiveness.
G. Encourage ambulation as soon as possible.
H. Monitor urinary output (Foley catheter is usually inserted in surgery).
I. After catheter removal, assess voiding patterns; catheterize every 6 to 8 hours PRN.
J. Observe incision for bleeding.
K. Note abdominal distention; it may be a sign of gas (flatus) or internal bleeding.
L. Gradually increase diet from liquids to general.
M. Provide stool softeners before first bowel movement and thereafter as needed.
N. Instructions to client regarding follow-up care
  1. Limit tampon use.
  2. Avoid douching.
  3. Refrain from intercourse until approved by physician (usually 3 to 6 weeks).
  4. Avoid heavy lifting (6 to 8 lb) or heavy housework for 4 to 6 weeks postoperatively.
O. Maintain adequate fluid intake (3 L/day).
P. Notify physician of complications:
  1. Elevated temperature above 101°F (38.3°C)
  2. Redness, pain, or swelling of suture line
  3. Foul-smelling vaginal drainage
Q. Encourage verbalization of feelings.

Cancer of the Cervix

Description: Of cancers occurring in the cervix, 95% are squamous cell in origin. Some cervical cancers are directly linked to the human papillomavirus (HPV). Young women between the ages of 9 and 30 years of age are encouraged to be immunized with an IM injection of quadrivalent HPV (types 6, 11, 16, 18) recombinant vaccine (Gardasil). All women should be tested for HPV, and women over 21 years of age and those who have engaged in sexual intercourse for at least 3 years should continue to have yearly Papanicolaou (Pap) tests.

A. The Pap test easily detects cancer of the cervix early.
B. The precursor to cancer of the cervix is dysplasia.
C. Cancer of the cervix is subdivided into three stages.
  1. Early dysplasia can be treated in a variety of ways, including the following:
    a. Cryosurgery
    b. Loop electrocautery excision procedure (LEEP)
    c. Laser
    d. Conization
    e. Hysterectomy
  2. Early carcinoma can be treated by
    a. Hysterectomy
    b. Intracavity radiation
  3. Late carcinoma (the tumor size and stage of invasion of surrounding tissues are greater) can be treated by
    a. External beam radiation along with hysterectomy
    b. Antineoplastic chemotherapy; this is of limited use for cancers arising from squamous cells.
    c. Pelvic exenteration

Care of the Client with Radiation Implants

A. Radiation implants are used to treat disease by delivering high-dose radiation seeds directly to the affected tissue.
B. The nurse must take certain precautions for protection of self as well as the client and visitors.
C. Follow specific guidelines provided by the agency. General care guidelines include
  1. Remind the client that she is not radioactive; only the implants contain radioactivity.
  2. Remind the client that her isolation time is limited; isolation is not necessary indefinitely.
D. Assign client to a private room and place a "Caution: Radioactive Material" sign on the door.
E. Do not permit pregnant caretakers or pregnant visitors into the room.
F. Keep a lead-lined container in the room for disposal of the implant should it become dislodged.
G. Client should remain in bed with as little movement as possible.
H. Be aware that all client secretions have the potential of being radioactive.
I. Wear latex gloves when handling potentially contaminated secretions.
J. Wear a dosimeter when providing care to clients with radiation implants.
  1. Badge is not to be worn outdoors.
  2. Health officials check badge at regular intervals.
K. Provide nursing care in an efficient but caring manner.
  1. Plan care to limit overall time in the client's room. Time at the bedside is limited—each contact should last no more than 30 minutes. Staff is rotated to limit their exposure.

2. Staff members should wear a dosimeter during every client contact to monitor radiation exposure.
3. When in the room, stand at the greatest possible distance away from the client to minimize exposure.
4. Stop by frequently to check on the client from the door.
5. Precautions for nurses' exposure include limit time, maintain distance, and wear protective shielding.

L. Keep all supplies and equipment the client might need within reach.

> **HESI HINT** Prevention: American College of Obstetricians and Gynecologists (ACOG) 2021. Recommendations: Pap smears. In women aged 30–65 years, annual cervical cancer screening should not be performed (level A evidence). Clients should be counseled that annual well-woman visits are recommended even if cervical cancer screening is not performed at each visit. Every three years is the recommended time frame for Pap smears. Women ages 30–65 years should have a Pap smear with an HPV test every 5 years. Women over 65 do not need a Pap smear. Pap smears should not be performed for any woman under age 21 regardless of onset of sexual activity.

Ovarian Cancer

Description: Cancer of the ovaries can occur at all ages, including infancy and childhood. Early diagnosis is difficult because no useful screening test exists at present. Malignant germ cell tumors are most common in women between 20 and 40 years of age, and epithelial cancers occur most often in the perimenopausal age groups.

Nursing Assessment

A. It is asymptomatic in early stages.
B. Laparotomy is the primary tool for diagnosis and staging of the disease; ovarian cancer is surgically staged rather than clinically staged.
C. Advanced clinical manifestations include
   1. Pelvic discomfort
   2. Low back pain and leg pain
   3. Weight change
   4. Abdominal pain
   5. Increased abdominal girth
   6. Nausea and vomiting
   7. Constipation
   8. Urinary frequency

Nursing Plans and Interventions

A. Provide the care required after any major abdominal surgery after laparotomy (see "Nursing Plans and Interventions for Hysterectomy," earlier).
B. Provide the care required for a client on chemotherapy (see "Nursing Plans and Interventions for Immunosuppressed Clients," earlier).
C. Teach client and family about disease and follow-up treatment.
D. Offer supportive care to client and family throughout diagnosis and treatment.

> **HESI HINT** The major emphasis in nursing management of cancers of the reproductive tract is early detection.

Breast Cancer

Description: Cancer originating in the breast

A. Breast cancer is the leading cancer in women in the United States.
B. One in eight women will develop breast cancer in her lifetime.
C. Early detection is important to successful treatment.
D. Men can develop breast cancer. They account for less than 1% of reported cases.
E. Risk factors include
   1. Positive family history
   2. Menarche before 12 years of age and menopause after age 50
   3. Nulliparous and those bearing first child after age 30
   4. History of uterine cancer
   5. Daily alcohol intake
   6. Highest incidence: those age 40 to 49 and over 65
F. Breast cancer is generally adenocarcinoma, originating in epithelial cells, and it occurs in the ducts or lobes.
G. Tumors tend to be located in the upper outer quadrant of the breast and more often in the left breast than the right.
H. Early detection is important.
   1. Every woman should be familiar with how their breasts normally look and feel and should immediately report any changes to their health care provider.
   2. Mammography is very helpful in early detection of cancer of the breast.
      a. Baseline mammogram at approximately 35 to 40 years of age
      b. Mammogram every 1 to 2 years for women between ages 40 and 44
      c. Annual mammogram for women between ages 45 and 54
      d. No use of lotions, talc powder, or deodorant under arms before procedure (may mimic calcium deposits on radiograph)
   3. Physical examination by a professional skilled in examination of the breast should be done annually.
I. Tumors less than 4 cm are deemed curable.
J. Larger tumors require much more aggressive treatment (cure is difficult).
K. Definitive diagnosis of cancer of the breast is made by biopsy.
L. Common sites of metastasis (spread) are the axillary, supraclavicular, and mediastinal lymph nodes, followed by metastases to the lungs, liver, brain, and spine.
M. Bone metastasis is extremely painful.
N. Treatment is dependent on the stage of disease.
   1. Mastectomy is commonly performed.

a. Alternatives to mastectomy are lumpectomy/partial mastectomy.
b. Axillary lymph node dissection often performed in conjunction with other surgery
2. Adjuvant treatment consists of radiation (either external beam or implants), antineoplastic chemotherapy, and hormonal therapy.
a. Targeted therapy such as estrogen inhibitors (tamoxifen) or trastuzumab.
b. Aromatase inhibitors

HESI HINT The presence or absence of hormone receptors is paramount in selecting clients for adjuvant therapy.

Nursing Assessment

A. Hard lump (not freely movable and not painful)
B. Dimpling of skin
C. Retraction of nipple
D. Alterations in contour of breast
E. Change in skin color
F. Change in skin texture (peau d'orange)
G. Discharge from nipple
H. Pain and ulcerations (late signs)
I. Diagnostic tests include
1. Mammogram
2. Biopsy and frozen section

Nursing Plans and Interventions

A. Assess lesion
1. Location
2. Size
3. Shape
4. Consistency
5. Fixation to surrounding tissues
6. Lymph node involvement
B. Preoperative
1. Explore client's expectations of surgery and what the surgical site will look like postoperatively.
2. Discuss skin graft if one is possible and cosmetic reconstruction that might be implemented with mastectomy or at a later time.
C. Postoperative
1. Monitor bleeding; check under dressing, wound drainage system, and under client's back (bleeding will run to back).
2. Position arm on operative side on a pillow, slightly elevated.
3. Avoid BP measurements, injections, and venipuncture in arm where surgery occurred.
4. Instruct client to avoid injury such as burns or scrapes to affected arm.
5. Encourage hand activity for the arm on the side where surgery occurred by squeezing a small rubber ball.
6. Encourage client to perform activities that will use arm, like brushing hair.
7. Teach postmastectomy exercises (wall climbing with affected arm and rope turning).
D. Encourage client to verbalize concerns.
1. Cancer
2. Death
3. Loss of breast
E. Encourage client to discuss operation, diagnosis, feelings, concerns, and fears.
F. Be with client when she first looks at the operative site; offer emotional support.
G. Arrange for Reach to Recovery (American Cancer Society); physician prescription required.
H. Recognize the grief process.
1. Allow client to cry, withdraw, etc.
2. Help client to focus on the future while allowing discussions of loss.
I. If reconstruction was not discussed preoperatively, encourage client to discuss or explore these options postoperatively.
J. Discuss use of temporary and permanent prostheses.

Testicular Cancer

Description: Cancer of the testes is the leading cause of death from cancer in males 15 to 35 years of age. If untreated, death usually occurs within 2 to 3 years. If detected and treated early, there is a 90% to 100% chance of cure.

Nursing Assessment

A. Early signs are subtle and usually go unnoticed.
B. There is a feeling of heaviness or dragging sensation in lower abdomen and groin.
C. There is a lump or swelling (painless) on the testicle. Late signs include
1. Low back pain
2. Weight loss
3. Fatigue

Nursing Plans and Interventions

A. Postoperative care after orchidectomy
1. Observe for hemorrhage.
2. Active movement may be contraindicated.
B. Care for clients receiving radiation therapy.
C. Encourage genetic counseling (sperm banking is often recommended before surgery).
D. Counsel that sexual functioning is usually not affected because the remaining testis undergoes hyperplasia, producing sufficient testosterone to maintain sexual functioning. Although ejaculatory ability may be decreased, orgasm is still possible.

HESI HINT Prevention: All males should do testicular self-examination (TSE) regularly at the same time every month after age 14.

Cancer of the Prostate

Description: Prostate cancer rarely occurs before 40 years of age, but it is the second-leading cause of death from cancer in American men. High-risk groups include those with a history of multiple sexual partners, sexually transmitted diseases (STDs), certain viral infections, and family history.

Nursing Assessment

A. Asymptomatic if confined to gland
B. Symptoms of urinary obstruction
C. With metastasis: low back pain, fatigue, aching in legs, and hip pain
D. Elevated prostate-specific antigen (PSA)
   1. PSA test should be conducted before a DRE so that manipulation of the prostate does not give a false-positive reading.
   2. Serial blood screening should be done to observe trends. A rise in PSA or consistently high PSA is more reliable than a single assay.
   3. PSA levels can rise with inflammation, benign hypertrophy, or irritation, as well as in response to cancer.
E. Elevated prostatic acid phosphatase (PAP)
F. DRE revealing palpable nodule
G. Transrectal ultrasound (TRUS) visualizing nonpalpable tumors
H. Definitive diagnosis by biopsy

Nursing Plans and Interventions

A. Teach the importance of early detection.
B. Suggest resources: local and national prostate cancer support groups; information is also available from the American Cancer Society (Man to Man program) and the Urology Care Foundation.
C. Prepare client for radiation therapy
   1. External beam "teletherapy" radiation irradiates the prostate and pelvic region, and conformal techniques allow the delivery of a higher radiation dose without increasing the risk of complications by focusing the radiation and limiting the exposure of adjacent structures.
      a. Explain how treatments help cancer.
         1) Need for repetitive treatments
         2) Attend all sessions for successful outcome.
      b. Expected outcomes
      c. Side effects
         1) Radiation-induced cystitis or proctitis
         2) Dysuria (discomfort with voiding): subsides within 4 to 6 weeks; reduced intake of foods or beverages likely to irritate the bowel or bladder, including caffeine and heavily spiced or fatty foods.
         3) Daytime voiding frequency
         4) Increase in the number of times client awakens to void
         5) Suprapubic discomfort—may irritate the perineal skin; teach client to cleanse the perineal skin with a mild cleanser and lukewarm water, pay special attention to skin folds, and pat dry, wearing loose cotton clothing to help relieve skin irritation.
         6) Fatigue and loss of appetite: six small meals per day, foods that are high in protein and carbohydrates; a multivitamin should be taken daily throughout radiation therapy.
   2. Proton beam radiotherapy combines conformal imaging and charged protons to target more specifically prostate cancer cells while limiting damage to the overlying skin or adjacent structures including the bladder and rectum (see external beam radiation).
   3. Brachytherapy is the internal implantation of radioactive iodine-125 or palladium-103 seeds directly into the prostate, which emit highly localized radiation energy to kill localized cancer cells without excessive harm to nearby healthy cells.
      a. Preparation includes bowel cleansing and administration of prophylactic antibiotics.
      b. A clear liquid diet 12 to 24 hours before the procedure
      c. Rectal pressure or mild discomfort is felt when the ultrasound probe is placed, but pain is not associated with implantation of radioactive seeds.
      d. A catheter is left in place that may be removed on the day of the procedure. Complete a voiding trial with removal of the catheter.
      e. Seed implantation will cause inflammation of the prostate and may cause symptoms including daytime voiding frequency, an increase in nocturia, and difficulty initiating a urinary stream. These manifestations are typically transient and subside as prostatic inflammation diminishes.
      f. Semen may have a brownish color over the first 1 to 2 months after implantation; intercourse should be avoided during this period and childbearing is contraindicated.
      g. Monitor stool for passage of large volumes of bright red blood (rare); advise client about how to manage radiation cystitis and proctitis.
      h. Teach the client and partner the principles of radiation safety.
      i. Avoid close contact with pregnant women and infants; refrain from having children (or adults) sit in their lap for a prolonged period during the first 2 months after therapy.
D. Provide preoperative bowel preparation to prevent fecal contamination of operative site.
   1. Enemas and cathartics
   2. Sulfasalazine (Azulfidine) or neomycin
   3. Clear fluids only the day before surgery to prevent fecal contamination of operative site
E. Provide postoperative care.
   1. Monitor for urine leaks, hemorrhage, and signs of infection.
   2. Provide support dressing or supportive underwear to perineal incision.

3. Use donut cushion to relieve pressure on incision site while sitting.
4. Avoid rectal manipulation (rectal thermometers, rectal tubes, and hard suppositories).
5. Provide low-residue diet until wound healing is advanced.
6. Institute measures to prevent bowel action in the first postoperative week to prevent contamination of incision.

Sexually Transmitted Diseases (STDs)

Description: STDs are diseases that can be transmitted during intimate sexual contact.

A. STDs are the most prevalent communicable diseases in the United States.
B. Most cases of STDs occur in adolescents and young adults.

> **HESI HINT** STDs in infants and children usually indicate sexual abuse and should be reported. The nurse is legally responsible to report suspected cases of child abuse.

Nursing Assessment

See Table 4.39.

> **HESI HINT** Chlamydia is the most commonly reported communicable disease in the United States.

Nursing Plans and Interventions

A. Use a nonjudgmental approach; be straightforward when taking history.
B. Reassure client that all information is strictly confidential. Obtain a complete sexual history, which should include
   1. The client's sexual orientation
   2. Sexual practices
      a. Penile-vaginal
      b. Penile-anal
      c. Penile-oral
      d. Oral-vaginal
      e. Anal-oral
   3. Type of protection (barrier) used
   4. Contraceptive practices
   5. Previous history of STDs
C. Develop teaching plan and include
   1. Signs and symptoms of STDs
   2. Mode of transmission of STDs
   3. Reminder that sexual contact should be avoided with anyone while infected
   4. Assess literacy level of client and if appropriate provide written instructions about treatment; request a return verbalization of these instructions to ensure the client has heard the instructions and understands them.
D. Encourage client to provide information regarding all sexual contacts.
E. Report incidents of STDs to appropriate health agencies and departments.
F. Instruct women of childbearing age about risks to a newborn.
   1. Gonorrheal conjunctivitis
   2. Neonatal herpes
   3. Congenital syphilis
   4. Oral candidiasis

> **HESI HINT**
> **Complications**
> Pelvic inflammatory disease (PID) involves one or more of the pelvic structures. The infection can cause adhesions and eventually result in sterility. Manage the pain associated with PID with analgesics. Bed rest in a semi-Fowler position may increase comfort and promote drainage. Antibiotic treatment is necessary to reduce inflammation and pain and should be effective for *Neisseria gonorrhoeae* and *Chlamydia trachomatis*.

G. Teach safer sex.
   1. Reduce the number of sexual contacts.
   2. Avoid sex with those who have multiple partners.
   3. Examine genital area and avoid sexual contact if anything abnormal is present.
   4. Wash hands and genital area before and after sexual contact.
   5. Use a latex condom as a barrier.
   6. Use water-based lubricants rather than oil-based lubricants.
   7. Use a vaginal spermicidal gel.
   8. Avoid douching before and after sexual contact; douching increases risk for infections because the body's normal defenses are reduced or destroyed.
   9. Seek attention from health care provider immediately if symptoms occur.

> **HESI HINT** A client comes into the clinic with a chancre on his penis. What is the usual treatment?
> IM dose of penicillin (such as benzathine penicillin G, 2.4 million units). Obtain a sexual history, including the names of his sex partners, so that they can receive treatment.

TABLE 4.39 Sexually Transmitted Diseases and Treatment Options

STD	Symptoms	Treatment
	***TREPONEMA PALLIDUM*, SYPHILIS**	
Laboratory diagnosis: VDRL, FTA-ABS	**Primary (local):** up to 90 days postexposure • Chancre (red, painless lesions with indurated border) • Highly infectious **Secondary (systemic):** 6 weeks to 6 months postexposure • Influenza-type symptoms • Generalized rash that affects palms of hands and soles of feet • Lesions contagious **Tertiary:** 10–30 years postexposure • Cardiac and neurologic destruction	• Penicillin G IM (usually 2.4 million units) • If penicillin allergic (adults), alternatives: tetracycline, or doxycycline, or ceftriaxone
	***NEISSERIA GONORRHOEAE*, GONORRHEA**	
Laboratory diagnosis: smears, cultures	• Females: majority are asymptomatic • Males: dysuria, yellowish-green urethral discharge, urinary frequency	• Ceftriaxone sodium plus doxycycline hyclate or azithromycin • Cefixime, plus doxycycline or azithromycin
	***CHLAMYDIA TRACHOMATIS*, CHLAMYDIA**	
Laboratory diagnosis: tissue culture; chlamydiazyme; MicroTrak	• Females: many asymptomatic, but may exhibit dysuria, urgency, vaginal discharge, oral temp >38.3, uterine or adnexal tenderness • Males: leading cause of nongonococcal urethritis	• Doxycycline hyclate or azithromycin • Cefoxitin, Gentamycin
	***TRICHOMONAS VAGINALIS*, TRICHOMONIASIS**	
Laboratory diagnosis: wet slide	• Females: green, yellow, or white frothy foul-smelling vaginal discharge with itching • Males: asymptomatic	• Metronidazole (Flagyl) (male partners to be treated to prevent reinfection)
	***CANDIDA ALBICANS*, CANDIDIASIS**	
Laboratory diagnosis: viral culture	• Females: odorless, white or yellow, cheesy discharge with itching • Males: asymptomatic	• Miconazole nitrate (Monistat) • Clotrimazole (Gyne-Lotrimin) • Nystatin (Mycostatin) • Fluconazole (Diflucan) PO single dose
	HERPES SIMPLEX VIRUS 2, HERPES	
	• Vesicles in clusters that rupture and leave painful erosions that cause painful urination • Characterized by remissions and exacerbations • May be contagious even when asymptomatic	• Acyclovir (Zovirax) partially controls symptoms • Famciclovir • Valacyclovir • Palliative care • Viscous lidocaine topically to ease pain • Keep lesions clean and dry
	HUMAN PAPILLOMAVIRUS (HPV)	
	• Multiple strains (>70), some of which are implicated in cervical cancer • Alarming rate increase in adolescent population • Lesions may be small, wartlike or clustered. • May be flat or raised	• Routine vaccination is recommended for select populations before onset of sexual activity. • Applied medications such as podophyllum resin (contraindicated in pregnancy) • Trichloroacetic acid (TCA) • Laser • Cryotherapy (freezing)
	HUMAN IMMUNODEFICIENCY VIRUS (HIV), AIDS	
	(See Advanced Clinical Concepts)	

FTA-ABS, Fluorescent treponemal antibody absorption; *VDRL*, Venereal Disease Research Laboratory.

REVIEW OF REPRODUCTIVE SYSTEM

1. What are the indications for a hysterectomy in a client who has fibromas?
2. List the symptoms and conditions associated with a cystocele.
3. What are the most important nursing interventions for the postoperative client who has had a hysterectomy with an A&P repair?
4. Describe the priority nursing care for a client who has had radiation implants.
5. What screening tool is used to detect cervical cancer? What are the American Cancer Society's recommendations for the Pap smear screening for females under age 21?
6. What are the most important tools for early detection of breast cancer? How often should these tools be used?
7. Describe three nursing interventions to help decrease edema postmastectomy.
8. Name three priorities to include in a discharge plan for a client who has had a mastectomy.
9. What is the most common cause of nongonococcal urethritis?
10. What is the causative organism of syphilis?
11. Malodorous, frothy, greenish-yellow vaginal discharge is characteristic of which STD?
12. Which STD is characterized by remissions and exacerbations in both males and females?
13. Outline a teaching plan for a client with an STD.

See Answer Key at the end of this text for suggested responses.

BURNS

Description: Tissue injury or necrosis caused by transfer of energy from a heat source to the body

A. Categories
   1. Thermal
   2. Radiation
   3. Electrical
   4. Chemical
B. Tissue destruction results from
   1. Coagulation
   2. Protein denaturation
   3. Ionization of cellular contents
C. Critical systems affected include
   1. Respiratory
   2. Integumentary
   3. Cardiovascular
   4. Renal
   5. GI
   6. Neurologic
D. Severity is determined by burn depth (Fig. 4.10).
   1. First degree
      a. Superficial partial-thickness (e.g., sunburn)
      b. Injury to the epidermis
      c. Leaves skin pink or red, but no blisters
      d. Dry

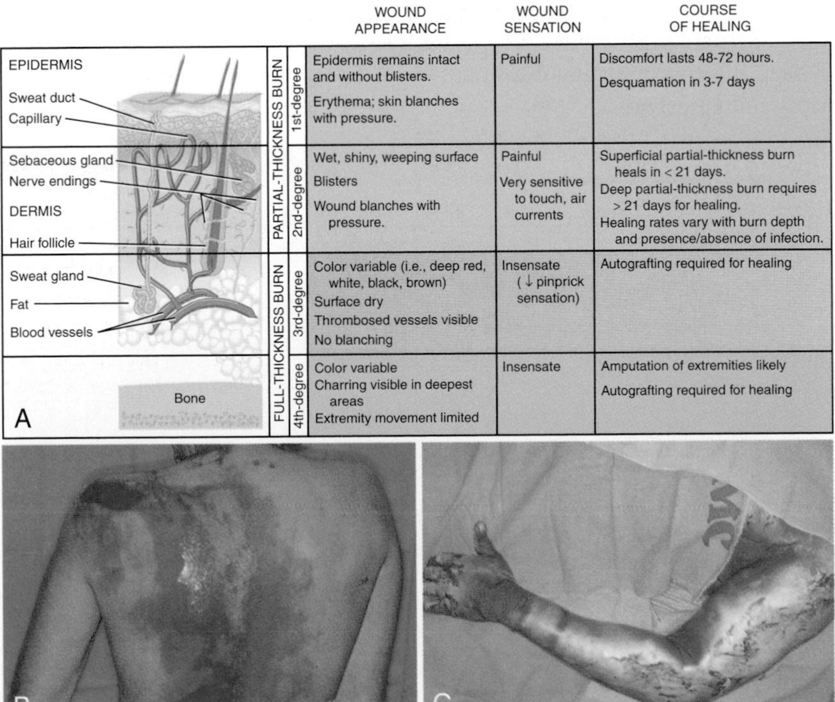

Fig. 4.10 (A) The tissues involved in burns of various depths. (B) Partial-thickness burn injury. (C) Full-thickness burn injury. (Ignatavicius, D. D., Workman, M. L., & Rebar, C. [2020]. *Medical-surgical nursing: Concepts for interprofessional collaborative care* [10th ed.]. St. Louis: Elsevier.)

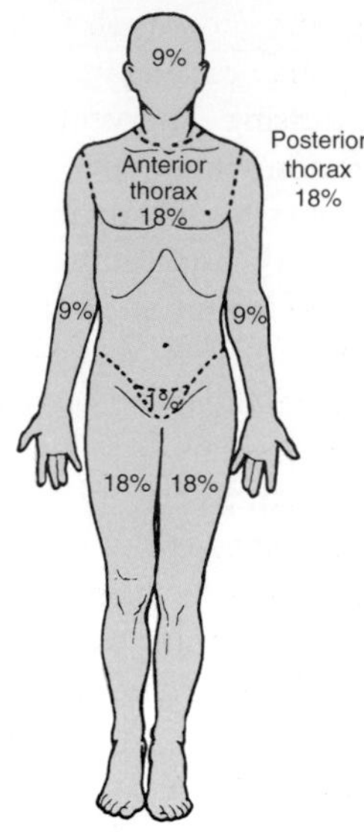

Fig. 4.11 The Rule of Nines for Estimating Burn Percentage. (Ignatavicius, D. D., Workman, M. L., & Rebar, C. [2020]. *Medical-surgical nursing: Concepts for interprofessional collaborative care* (10th ed.). St. Louis: Elsevier.)

e. Painful (relieved by cooling)
f. Slight edema
g. No scarring and skin grafts are not required

2. Second degree
   a. Deep partial-thickness destruction of epidermis and upper layers of dermis
   b. Injury to deeper portions of the dermis
   c. Painful (sensitive to touch and cold air)
   d. Appears red or white, weeps fluid, blisters present
   e. Hair follicles intact (i.e., hair does not pull out easily)
   f. Very edematous
   g. Blanching followed by capillary refill
   h. Heals without surgical intervention, usually does not scar
3. Third degree
   a. Full-thickness and deep full-thickness; involves total destruction of dermis and epidermis
   b. Skin cannot regenerate
   c. Requires skin grafting
   d. Underlying tissue (fat, fascia, tendon, bone) may be involved
   e. Wound appears dry and leathery as eschar develops
   f. Painless

E. Severity is determined by extent of surface area burned.
   1. Rule of nines: head and neck 9%, upper extremities 9% each, lower extremities 18% each, front trunk 18%, back trunk 18%, perineal area 1% for adults (Fig. 4.11)
   2. Lund and Browder method: estimates the percentage of the body surface area burned; percentages are assigned to specific body parts based on the client's age; critical body areas are face, hands, feet, and perineum (Table 4.40).

F. Three stages of burn care
   1. Stage I: resuscitative/emergent phase
      a. Begins at the time of injury and concludes with the restoration of capillary permeability, which typically reverses 48 to 72 hours after the injury.
      b. Is characterized by fluid shift from intravascular to interstitial and shock; focus of care is to preserve vital organ functioning.
      c. Expect to administer large volumes of fluid in this phase based on the client's weight and extent of injury.
      d. Fluid replacement formulas are calculated from the time of injury and not from the time of arrival at the hospital.
   2. Stage II: acute phase
      a. Occurs from beginning of diuresis (48 to 72 hours after injury) to near completion of wound closure.
      b. Is characterized by fluid shift from interstitial to intravascular.
      c. Focus is on infection control, wound care and closure, pain management, nutritional support, and physical therapy.
   3. Stage III: rehabilitation phase

TABLE 4.40 Lund and Browder Chart

Area	1 Year	1–4 Years	5–9 Years	10–14 Years	15 Years	Adult
Head	19	17	13	11	9	7
Neck	2	2	2	2	2	2
Anterior trunk	13	13	13	13	13	13
Posterior trunk	13	13	13	13	13	13
Right buttock	2½	2½	2½	2½	2½	2½
Left buttock	2½	2½	2½	2½	2½	2½
Genitalia	1	1	1	1	1	1
Right upper arm	4	4	4	4	4	4
Left upper arm	4	4	4	4	4	4
Right lower arm	3	3	3	3	3	3
Left lower arm	3	3	3	3	3	3
Right hand	2½	2½	2½	2½	2½	2½
Left hand	2½	2½	2½	2½	2½	2½
Right thigh	5½	6½	8	8½	9	9½
Left thigh	5½	6½	8	8½	9	9½
Right leg	5	5	5½	6	6½	7
Left leg	5	5	5½	6	6½	7
Right foot	½	3½	3½	3½	3½	3½
Left foot	3½	3½	3½	3½	3½	3½

a. Occurs from major wound closure to return to optimal level of physical and psychosocial adjustment (approximately 5 years)
b. Is characterized by grafting and rehabilitation specific to the client's needs

Nursing Assessment

A. Absence of bowel sounds indicating paralytic ileus
B. Radically decreased urinary output in the first 72 hours after injury, with increased specific gravity
C. Radically increased urinary output (diuresis) 72 hours to 2 weeks after initial injury
D. Signs of inadequate hydration
  1. Restlessness
  2. Disorientation
  3. Decreased urinary volume and urinary sodium and increased urine specific gravity
E. Signs of inhalation burn
  1. Red or burned face
  2. Singed facial and nasal hairs
  3. Circumoral burns
  4. Conjunctivitis
  5. Sooty nasal mucus or bloody sputum
  6. Hoarseness
  7. Asymmetry of chest movements with respirations and use of accessory muscles indicative of hypoxia
  8. Rales, wheezing, and rhonchi denoting smoke inhalation
  9. Impaired speech and drooling indicating laryngeal edema
F. Description of physiologic responses to burns (Fig. 4.12)
G. Preexisting conditions or illnesses that may influence recovery

Nursing Plans and Interventions

A. Emergent phase: Efforts are directed toward stabilization with ongoing assessment.
  1. Assist with admission care.
    a. Extinguish source of burn (burning may continue with clothing attached to skin).
      1) Thermal: Remove clothing, cool burns by immersion in tepid water, apply dry sterile dressings.
      2) Chemical: Flush with water or normal saline.
      3) Electrical: Separate client from electrical source.
        a) Provide an open airway; intubation may be necessary if laryngeal edema is a risk.
        b) Determine baseline data: vital signs, blood gases, weight.
        c) Determine depth and extent of burn.
        d) Administer tetanus toxoid.
        e) Initiate fluid and electrolyte therapy: Ringer's lactate solution with electrolytes and colloids adjusted according to laboratory results and fluid resuscitation formula used. Hemodynamic

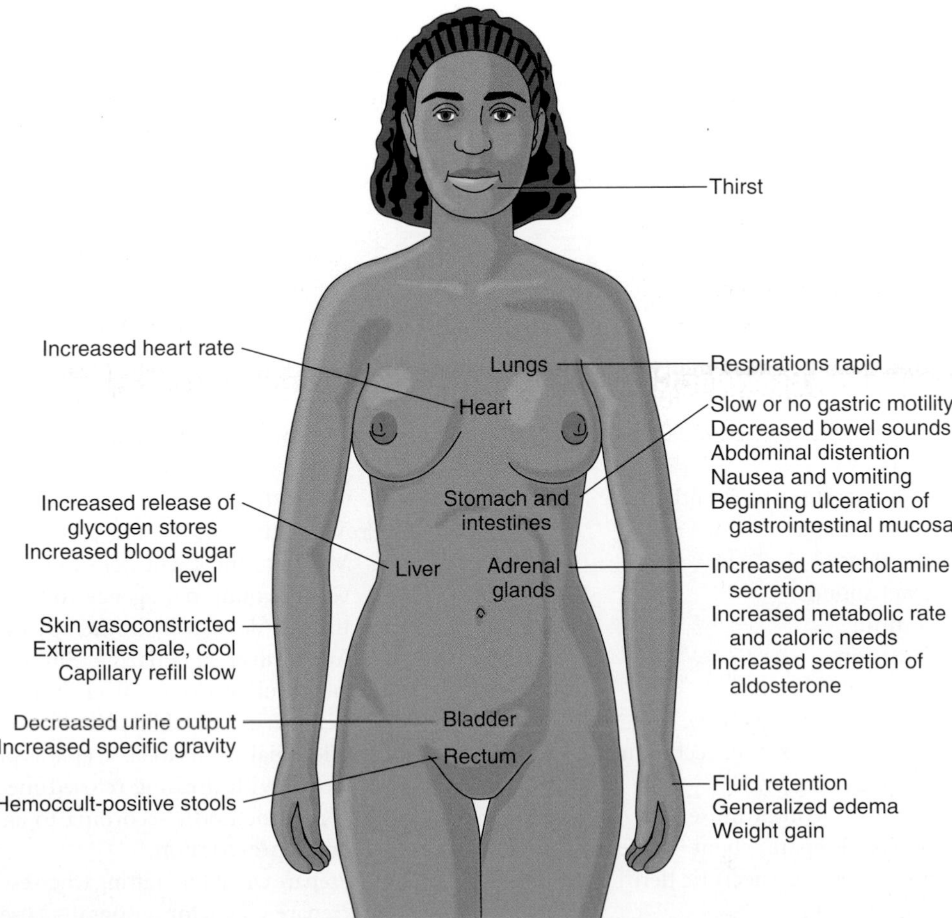

Fig. 4.12 The physiologic actions of the sympathetic nervous system's compensatory responses to burn injury (early phase). (From Ignatavicius, D. D., & Workman, M. L.: *Medical-surgical nursing: Client-centered collaborative care* [7th ed.]. St. Louis: Saunders; Ignatavicius, D. D., Workman, M. L., & Rebar, C. [2020]. *Medical-surgical nursing: Concepts for interprofessional collaborative care* [10th ed.]. St. Louis: Elsevier.)

monitoring must be closely observed to be sure the client is supported with fluids but is not overloaded.
    f) Insert NG tube to prevent vomiting, abdominal distention, and gastric aspiration.
    g) Administer IV pain medication as prescribed.
2. Monitor hydration status.
   a. Record urinary output hourly (30 to 100 mL/h is normal range).
   b. Maintain IV fluids titrated to keep urine output at 30 to 100 mL/h.
   c. Accurately record I&O.
   d. Weigh daily.
   e. Observe for signs of inadequate hydration.
      1. Restlessness
      2. Disorientation
      3. Hypothermia
      4. Decreased urine output
3. Monitor respiratory functioning.
   a. Provide care for the intubated client.
   b. Suction endotracheal or nasotracheal tube, when needed.
   c. Monitor ABGs.
   d. Observe for cyanosis, disorientation.
   e. Administer O_2.
   f. Encourage use of incentive spirometer, coughing, and deep breathing.
   g. Elevate the head of the bed to 30 degrees or more for burns of the face and head.
4. Provide wound care.
   a. Use strict aseptic technique.

HESI HINT Infection is a life-threatening risk for those with burns.

   b. Perform debridement and dressing changes according to client's condition.
   c. Change dressings in minimum time (very painful); premedicate client; maintain sterile technique.
   d. Maintain room temperature above 90°F, humidified and free of drafts.
   e. Monitor body temperature frequently; have hyperthermia blankets available.
5. Assess for paralytic ileus.
   a. Absence of bowel sounds
   b. Nausea and vomiting
   c. Abdominal distention
6. Assist with management of pain.
   a. Administer analgesics intravenously.
   b. Teach distraction and relaxation techniques.
   c. Teach use of guided imagery.
7. Assess for circulatory compromise in burns that constrict body parts. Prepare client for escharotomy (surgical incision in an eschar [necrotic dermis] to lessen constriction).
8. Provide proper nutrition.
   a. Maintain NPO status until bowel sounds are heard, and then advance to clear liquids as prescribed.
   b. Provide a diet high in protein, carbohydrates, fats, and vitamins.
   c. Monitor caloric intake.

B. Acute phase: characterized by fluid shift from interstitial to intravascular (diuresis begins); occurs from 72 hours to 2 weeks after initial injury to near completion of wound closure.
1. Provide infection control, including the following:
   a. Maintain protective isolation of entire burn unit.
   b. Cover hair at all times.
   c. Wear masks during dressing changes.
   d. Use sterile technique for hydrotherapy, dressing change, and debridement.
   e. Administer IV antibiotics if indicated.
   f. Be sure any live plants and flowers are removed from room; they are prohibited.
2. Splint and position client to prevent contractures. Avoid use of pillows in cases of neck burns.
3. Perform ROM exercises; they are painful.
   a. Administer pain medication immediately before performing ROM exercises.
   b. Perform active ROM exercises for 3 to 5 minutes frequently during day.
   c. Mobilize as soon as possible using splints designed for the client.
   d. Encourage active ROM exercises when out of bed.
4. Provide fluid therapy; may use colloids to keep fluid in vascular space.
   a. Monitor serum chemistries at all times.
   b. Keep an IV site available; a saline lock or peripherally inserted central catheter (PICC) for long-term use is helpful.
   c. Maintain strict I&O.
   d. Encourage oral intake of fluids.
5. Provide adequate nutrition.
   a. Provide high-calorie (up to 5000 calories/day), high-protein, high-carbohydrate diet.
   b. Give nutritional supplements via NG tube or enteral tube feeding at night if caloric intake is inadequate.
   c. Keep accurate calorie counts.
   d. Administer all medications with either milk or juice.
   e. May require TPN
   f. Weigh daily.
6. Provide burn and wound care.
   a. Medicate the client before the procedure.
   b. Clean wound per agency routine (daily or up to three times a day) in hydrotherapy or shower.
   c. Apply silver sulfadiazine (Silvadene) or mafenide acetate (Sulfamylon); silver impregnated dressings like Acticoat can be left in place for 3 to 14 days or other antimicrobial agents to burn area as prescribed (Table 4.41).
   d. Cover with dressing (closed method) or leave open (open method), according to agency policy or physician's prescription.
   e. Prepare client for grafting when eschar has been removed.
   f. Prepare client for autografts (use of client's own skin for grafting).
   g. Use heat lamp to donor site after graft to allow the area to reepithelialize.

TABLE 4.41 **Topical Antimicrobial Agents**

Drugs	Indications	Adverse Reactions	Nursing Implications
• Mafenide acetate	• Treatment of burns • Usually used with open method of wound care	• Painful • Causes mild acidosis	• Administer pain medication *before* dressing change. • Penetrates wound rapidly
• Silver sulfadiazine	• Treatment of burns • Usually used with open method of wound care • Used to avoid acid–base complications • Keeps eschar soft, making debridement easier	• Penetrates wound slowly	• Administer pain medication *before* dressing change.

HESI HINT Preexisting conditions that might influence burn recovery are age, chronic illness (diabetes, cardiac problems, etc.), physical disabilities, disease, medications used routinely, and drug or alcohol abuse.

C. Rehabilitation phase: characterized by the absence of infection risk
   1. Ongoing discharge planning occurs.
   2. Client may return home when the danger of infection has been eliminated.
   3. High-protein fluids with vitamin supplements are recommended.
   4. Pressure dressings or garments may be worn continuously to prevent hypertrophic scarring and contractures.

REVIEW OF BURNS

1. List four categories of burns.
2. Burn depth is a measure of severity. Describe the characteristics of superficial partial-thickness, deep partial-thickness, and full-thickness burns.
3. Describe fluid management in the emergent phase, acute phase, and rehabilitation phase of the burned client.
4. Describe pain management of the burned client.
5. Outline admission care of the burned client.
6. Nutritional status is a major concern when caring for a burned client. List three specific dietary interventions used with burned clients.
7. Describe the method of extinguishing each of the following burns: thermal, chemical, and electrical.
8. List four signs of an inhalation burn.
9. Why is the burned client allowed no "free" water?
10. Describe an autograft.

See Answer Key at the end of this text for suggested responses.

CLINICAL JUDGMENT SCENARIO 4.1

Cardiac Arrest

History & Physical (H&P)

Subjective: Chief concern (CC): Chest heaviness and difficulty breathing x 5 days

History of present illness (HPI): B. S. is a 68-year-old Caucasian female admitted to the hospital with a CC of chest heaviness and shortness of breath (SOB) over the last 5 days. Heaviness is located in the center of the chest, is intermittent, associated with movement, SOB, and nausea, alleviated by resting; pain radiates to the left jaw. SOB has worsened over the course of 5 days and is now progressed to orthopnea, is worsened by walking, and alleviated by resting.

Past medical history (PMH): Type 2 DM, hypertension, hypothyroidism, psoriasis, transitional bladder carcinoma with TURP tumor in 2001, carcinoid of the pancreas status/post Whipple procedure in 2001, lung nodules status/post lung resection in 2001 with subsequent intraprocedure cardiac arrest with normal coronary arteries, carcinoid of the small intestine with metastasis to the liver status/post right colectomy in 2010 and subsequent biliary tube insertion in 2015. Previous hospitalization for septicemia secondary to the biliary drains in 2015. No injuries or accidents. No history of childhood or infectious diseases.

Social history (SH): Lives at home with husband and dog. Quit smoking 40 years ago, used to smoke ½ pack per day (PPD) × 10 years. Doesn't drink, doesn't use other types of recreational drugs. Has health insurance and adequate access to resources to manage health care needs.

Medications

Daily

Insulin glargine 60 units daily
Novolog insulin sliding scale before meals: 6 units if 100–150 mg/dL (5.7–8.57 mmol/L); 8 units if 151–200 mg/dL (8.6–11.4 mmol/L); 10 units if 201–250 mg/dL (11.48–14.2 mmol/L); 12 units if >250 mg/dL (14.2 mmol/L)
Levothyroxine 175 mcg alternate with 150 mcg daily
Ramipril 10 mg daily
Hydrochlorothiazide 12.5 mg twice daily
Metoprolol 50 mg daily
Clobetasol 0.05% daily to foot
Calcipotriene 0.005% daily to foot

Monthly

Octreotide acetate 20 mg IM every 4 weeks
Cyanocobalamin injection 1 mL monthly

Every 3 weeks

Immunotherapy IV infusions

PRN

Albuterol inhaler 1–2 puffs twice daily
Zolpidem 10 mg at bedtime

Continued

CLINICAL JUDGMENT SCENARIO 4.1

Cardiac Arrest—cont'd

Loratadine 10 mg daily
Tramadol 50 mg every 4–6 h

Nonprescription

B Plus complex daily
Calcium 1200 mg daily
CoQmax 400 mg daily
Vitamin C 500 mg daily
Omega daily
Biotin daily
Vitamin D 5000 IU daily
Milk thistle daily
Multivitamin daily
UltraFlora (probiotics) daily

Allergies: Morphine sulfate (rash)

Review of Systems (ROS)

Subjective

General: Denies fevers. Reports recent weight gain of 11 lb in 7 days despite dieting for weight loss. Denies changes in appetite.

Integumentary: Denies skin changes, small psoriasis patch on bottom of left foot, diaphoresis.

HEENT (head, eyes, ears, nose, throat): Denies headache, head trauma. Reports recent vision changes, described as double vision for 2–3 weeks, which resolved completely 1 week ago (brain scan negative). Denies ear pain, nasal drainage, throat pain.

Breast: Denies breast changes.

Respiratory: Reports SOB over the last 5 days (see HPI). Denies cough, wheezing, sputum production.

Cardiovascular: Reports chest heaviness over the last 5 days (see HPI). Reports palpitations. Denies peripheral edema, color changes in the extremities.

Gastrointestinal: Reports bilateral biliary drain insertion, which are replaced every 4 months. Reports nausea. Denies vomiting. Reports diarrhea but states this is consistent with her typical routine secondary to abdominal surgeries. Denies abdominal distention, flatus.

Genitourinary: Denies burning on urination, vaginal discharge.

Musculoskeletal: Denies muscle/joint pain, warmth, weakness.

Neurological: Denies difficulty concentrating, gait changes, numbness, tingling.

Psychiatric: Denies mood changes, anxiety, depression.

Objective

Physical Examination

Vital signs: Temperature 36.5°C (97.7°F) oral, HR: 140 bpm (beats per minute), RR (respiratory rate): 20 bpm (breaths per minute), BP: 118/59 mmHg, Spo_2: 96%, oxygen at 3LNC (liters via nasal cannula)

General: Appears nontoxic, in no acute distress, well-nourished, well-hydrated. Answering questions appropriately.

Integumentary: Warm and dry, consistent with ethnic background.

HEENT: Head is normocephalic, atraumatic. No scleral icterus, conjunctival injection. Ear canals free of redness, swelling. Bilateral TM (tympanic membrane) pearly gray and intact. No nasal drainage, no bogginess to nasal turbinates. Oropharynx pink, moist, tonsillar pillars 2+ with no exudates, no halitosis. Neck supple, no rigidity, trachea midline.

Breast: Deferred.

Respiratory: Eupneic. Lungs clear to auscultation bilaterally (CTAB), no adventitious sounds. No use of accessory muscles.

Cardiovascular: Irregularly irregular, rate 120–140 bpm. S1S2 noted, no S3S4, no murmurs, rubs, gallops. No cyanosis, clubbing.

Gastrointestinal: Abdomen soft, nontender, nondistended. Bowel sounds (BS) + × 4 quadrants. External biliary drains × 2 noted.

Genitourinary: Deferred.

Musculoskeletal: Full active range of motion (AROM). Muscle strength intact.

Neurological: Cranial nerves II-XII grossly intact. Deep tendon reflexes (DTRs) 2+ at biceps, triceps, knee, ankle.

Psych: Appropriate, conversational.

Laboratory Results

Urinalysis (UA)

Appearance: Hazy	Color: Yellow	Urine specific gravity: 1.018
Squamous epithelial: Rare	Blood: Negative	Bacteria: Negative
Bilirubin: Negative	Leukocyte esterase: Negative	Glucose: Negative
Ketones: Negative	pH: 5	Mucous: Rare
Nitrite: Negative	WBC (white blood cells): 0–2	Protein: Negative
RBC (red blood cells): 0–2		

Glucose Point-of-Care

379 mg/dL (21.6 mmol/L)

Lipid Panel	Cardiac Markers	CXR 2 Views
Cholesterol 152 mg/dL (3.8 mmol/L) Triglycerides 60 mg/dL (1.8 mmol/L) HDL (high-density lipoprotein) 48 mg/dL (1.24 mmol/L) LDL (low-density lipoprotein) 92 mg/dL (2.38 mmol/L)	Troponin I: 4.002 ng/mL (4.002 mcg/L) Troponin I: 3.051 ng/mL (3.051 mcg/L) (6 h later) BNP (brain natriuretic peptide): 1196 ng/mL (1196 mcg/L)	Cardiac size is normal. The lungs are normally inflated and clear. There is no pleural effusion or pneumothorax. No acute findings.

ECG (Electrocardiogram)	Chemistry	Hematology
Atrial fibrillation with rapid ventricular response	Sodium: 135 mEq/L (135 mmol/L)	WBC (white blood cells): 13.7
Lateral MI, acute	Potassium 4.5 mEq/L (4.5 mmol/L)	RBC (red blood cells): 4.22
Inferior MI, acute	Chloride: 105 mEq/L (105 mmol/L)	Hgb (hemoglobin): 12 g/dL (120 mmol/L)
Intraventricular conduction delay	CO_2 content: 19 mEq/L (19 mmol/L)	Hct (hematocrit): 38.3% (0.38.3)
No ST elevation	Glucose level: 219 mg/dL (12.5 mmol/L)	MCH (mean corpuscular hemoglobin [Hgb/RBC]): 29.6 pg (29.6 pg)
	BUN (blood urea nitrogen): 40 mg/dL (14.4 mmol/L)	MCHC (mean corpuscular hemoglobin concentration [Hgb/Hct]): 32.6% (32.6 g/dL)
	Cr (creatinine): 1.17 mg/dL (131.7 mcmol/L)	MCV (mean corpuscular volume [Hct/RBC]): 90.7 mm^3 (90.7 fL)
	BUN/Cr ratio: 34.2	RDW (red cell distribution width): 16.4% (16.4%)
	Calcium: 9.1 mg/dL (2.25 mmol/L) eGFR (estimated glomerular filtration rate): 46 mL/min	

CLINICAL JUDGMENT SCENARIO 4.1

Cardiac Arrest—cont'd

Assessment

Admitting Diagnoses	Problem List/Past Medical Hx	Surgical Procedures
Atypical chest pain	Bladder cancer	Biliary drain × 2
Dyspnea on exertion	Pancreatic cancer	Colectomy
Atrial fibrillation with rapid ventricular response	Colon cancer	Lung wedge resection
Pulmonary nodule	Liver cancer	Whipple procedure
Acute MI: NSTEMI	Biliary obstruction	Liver ablation
	Hypertension	
	Diabetes	
	Hypothyroidism	

Plan

Admit to intermediate medical care unit (IMCU) for continuous cardiac monitoring. Initial plan to include
Diltiazem
Amiodarone
Low-dose carvedilol
Echocardiogram
Check TSH, serial troponins
D-dimer, computed tomography angiogram (CTA) if D-dimer is elevated
Antiemetics
GI & venous thromboembolism (VTE) prophylaxis
Accu-Check (blood glucose) checks AC & HS
Insulin sliding scale
Titrate BP to Joint National Committee (JNC) criteria
Cardiology consultation

Dictated by: Edward Ramsen, MD

Clinical Judgment Scenario Questions

Multiple Response

1. Given this client's presenting problem, admitting diagnoses, and past medical history, which problem(s) should the nurse be prepared to monitor for? **Select all that apply.**
    1. Thrombocytopenia
    2. Bronchoconstriction
    3. Fluid volume overload
    4. Diminished cardiac output
    5. Decreased renal perfusion
    6. Venous thromboembolism

Extended Drag and Drop

2. The nurse is analyzing the primary health care provider's documentation in the medical record. Match the clinical presentation findings/prescriptions with Ms. S's known or suspected diagnoses since hospital admission. ***All options (clinical presentations/prescriptions) must be used. Options may be used with more than one known or suspected diagnosis.***

Clinical Presentation/Prescription

- HR: irregularly irregular, rate 120–140 bpm
- SOB over the last 5 days
- Recent weight gain of 11 lb in 7 days despite dieting
- Chest heaviness over the last 5 days
- Reports palpitations
- Troponin I: 4.002
- BNP: 1196
- eGFR: 46
- Diltiazem for rate control
- Amiodarone
- Low-dose carvedilol
- Echocardiogram
- TSH
- Serial troponins
- D-dimer, CTA if elevated
- Cardiology consultation

Multiple Choice

3. In addition to the diagnostic tests prescribed, what additional test should the nurse anticipate will be necessary for Ms. S?
    1. Abdominal x-ray
    2. Cardiac catheterization
    3. Ultrasound of bilateral lower extremities
    4. CT of the abdomen with and without contrast

Clinical Judgment Scenario Continued

Progress Report

A cardiac catheterization was performed on Ms. S. The major coronary arteries showed no blockage. Serial troponin I levels are beginning to show a downward trend. Ms. S's TSH level is reported as 2 mLU/L (2 mcLU/mL).

Clinical Judgment Scenario Questions

Multiple Choice

4. If thyroid function is the suspected cause for Ms. S's tachydysrhythmia, what should the nurse anticipate on the results of the TSH level?
    1. Low TSH
    2. High TSH
    3. Normal TSH
    4. Critically high TSH

Cloze Item

5. The nurse is providing Ms. S with information on the therapeutic effect for home medications. How should the nurse explain the new medications to the client? **Complete the following sentences by choosing from the choice below.**
6. The apixaban is given to ____________________.
    - prevent thrombus formation
    - reduce lipid deposits and coronary calcifications
    - prevent cardiac remodeling following acute MI
7. The lisinopril is given ____________________.
    - to treat HF and promotes diuresis of excess fluid volume
    - as a supplement to prevent hypokalemia in a client taking furosemide
    - to prevent cardiac remodeling following acute MI
8. The digoxin is given ____________________.
    - to prevent thrombus formation
    - to promote cardiac inotropic activity and promote effective heart pumping
    - as a preventive measure following acute MI to reduce lipid deposits and coronary calcifications
9. The simvastatin is given ____________________.
    - to manage the atrial fibrillation
    - as a supplement to prevent hypokalemia in a client taking furosemide
    - as a preventive measure following acute MI to reduce lipid deposits and coronary calcifications
10. The potassium is given ____________________.
    - to lower the BP
    - to treat HF and promote diuresis of excess fluid volume
    - as a supplement to prevent hypokalemia in a client taking furosemide

Continued

CLINICAL JUDGMENT SCENARIO 4.1

Cardiac Arrest—cont'd

11. The amiodarone is given to_________________.
    - prevent angina
    - prevent excess fluid buildup
    - manage the atrial fibrillation
12. The furosemide is given to_________________.
    - lower the BP
    - treat HF and promote diuresis of excess fluid volume
    - prevent cardiac remodeling following an acute MI
13. The spironolactone is given _________________.
    - to prevent thrombus formation
    - as a preventive measure following acute MI to reduce lipid deposits and coronary calcifications
    - to prevent cardiac remodeling following an acute MI and can also be used to offset the potassium-wasting effects of furosemide
14. The nitroglycerin is given _________________.
    - as needed for stable angina
    - to prevent thrombus formation
    - to prevent the development of lipid plaques in the coronary vessels

Clinical Judgment Scenario Answers

1. 1. 2, 3, 4, 5, 6. As a result of the atrial fibrillation with rapid ventricular response and myocardial injury due to ischemia, the client is at risk for diminished cardiac output. Due to the injury to the heart muscle, there is the potential for diminished overall cardiac compliance. Also, as a result of diminished cardiac output, there is a risk of decreased renal perfusion. The client is at risk for VTE due to their history of cancer. In addition, the atrial fibrillation places the client at risk for the development of clots. Bronchoconstriction is another possibility in the event of a pulmonary embolism as a compensatory mechanism to injury to the respiratory tract. Although the client has a history of cancer, thrombocytopenia is not a specific concern at this time because the client is not being treated with chemotherapy.
2.

Known or Suspected Diagnosis	Known or Suspected Diagnosis	Known or Suspected Diagnosis
Atrial fibrillation with rapid ventricular response	Acute myocardial infarction	Pulmonary embolism
HR: irregularly irregular, rate 120–140 bpm	SOB over the last 5 days	SOB over the last 5 days
SOB over the last 5 days	Recent weight gain of 11 lb in 7 days despite dieting	D-dimer, CTA if elevated
Reports palpitations	Chest heaviness over the last 5 days	
Diltiazem	Reports palpitations	
Amiodarone	Troponin I: 4.002 ng/mL (4.002 mcg/L)	
TSH	BNP: 1196 ng/mL (1196 mcg/L)	
Cardiology consultation	eGFR: 46	
	Low-dose carvedilol	
	Echocardiogram	
	Serial troponins	
	Cardiology consultation	

An irregular heart rhythm with a rapid rate of 120–140 bpm is consistent with Bella's admitting diagnosis of atrial fibrillation with rapid ventricular response. Her report of SOB over the last 5 days is consistent with the atrial fibrillation as well as the acute MI and the possibility of a pulmonary embolism. Ms. S's report of recent weight gain of 11 lb in 7 days despite dieting is related to the acute MI, and there should be suspicion for a dilated cardiomyopathy with HF secondary to myocardial ischemia and HF. Chest heaviness over the last 5 days should be correlated with acute MI. The reports of palpitations are characteristic of the atrial fibrillation and may be a subsequent rhythm as a result of the acute MI. A troponin I level should be associated with the acute MI and is a cardiac enzyme that indicates myocardial ischemia. A BNP level of 1196 is related to the acute MI and may indicate subsequent HF. An eGFR of 46 mL/min is likely related to decreased renal perfusion from the acute MI. A normal eGFR for adults is greater than 90 mL/min. Diltiazem for rate control is to manage the rapid ventricular rate associated with the atrial fibrillation. Amiodarone is an antidysrhythmic used to manage the atrial fibrillation. The low-dose carvedilol is used to prevent cardiac remodeling following an acute MI. An echocardiogram is important for this client to evaluate LVEF and overall cardiac compliance following an acute MI. A TSH level is important because for a client with hypothyroidism on levothyroxine it is important to evaluate for a transient hyperthyroidism as a result of over supplementation. This can cause tachydysrhythmias such as atrial fibrillation with rapid ventricular response. Serial troponins are important to monitor for trends and are associated with the acute MI. The D-dimer is helpful in evaluating fibrin formation in the body and can be used as a screening tool to determine the need for another test such as CTA to rule out pulmonary embolism. The cardiology consultation is necessary to manage the new-onset atrial fibrillation and acute MI.

3. A cardiac catheterization is important for Ms. S to evaluate patency of the coronary arteries and the extent of cardiac damage. A cardiac catheterization can also provide information about valvular function and LVEF. Given the fact that Ms. S had an acute MI, it could be that there is a blockage in one of the main coronary arteries. Percutaneous intervention with coronary stenting may be indicated. An abdominal x-ray is useful in evaluating for any abdominal abnormalities including constipation and is not indicated at this time. An ultrasound of bilateral lower extremities would be helpful in ruling out lower extremity deep vein thromboses, and is not indicated at this time based on Ms. S's clinical presentation. A CT of the abdomen with and without contrast is useful in evaluating bowel function and for inflammatory conditions or perforation, and is not indicated for Ms. S.
4. A transient hyperthyroidism is a potential cause of tachydysrhythmias. Over supplementation on thyroid hormone can cause this problem. The nurse would find a low TSH and elevated free T_4 in a state of hyperthyroidism. The nurse may also note a borderline low TSH and a normal free T_4 if this was a problem started in previous weeks but has begun to resolve. The normal TSH level is 2–10 mLU/L (2–10 mcLU/mL). The excess thyroid hormone can cause the symptoms noted in Ms. S, but often occurs over a period of weeks until the heart is affected to the point of acute MI; this may be the reason for the borderline or normal values on presentation with cardiac issues.
5.
    a. prevent thrombus formation
    b. to prevent cardiac remodeling following acute MI
    c. to promote cardiac inotropic activity and promote effective heart pumping
    d. as a preventive measure following acute MI to reduce lipid deposits and coronary calcifications
    e. as a supplement to prevent hypokalemia in a client taking furosemide
    f. manage the atrial fibrillation
    g. treat HF and promote diuresis of excess fluid volume
    h. to prevent cardiac remodeling following an acute MI and can also be used to offset the potassium-wasting effects of furosemide
    i. as needed for stable angina

Written by: L3.101 Linda A. Silvestri PhD, RN

NEXT-GENERATION NCLEX (NGN) EXAMINATION-STYLE QUESTION: BOWTIE QUESTION

The nurse in the emergency department is caring for an 82-year-old client.

NURSE'S NOTES: 1600: Client is accompanied by spouse. Left-sided ptosis with facial drooping and slurred speech is noted. Left-sided weakness is noted in extremities. Client is alert but having difficulty answering questions. Spouse reports client had similar symptoms a few days earlier, but they went away after a few hours. These symptoms started at 0600 and not improved and believes the leg weakness is worse since the client cannot stand on the leg. Spouse also reports that the client is not eating well and has not voided in 24 hours. Lung sounds are clear. Pupils are reactive but the right is smaller. Bowel sounds are present in all quadrants, skin is warm and dry. Vital signs: & 98.4 F, P 130, RR 18, BP 190/94 pulse oximetry 92% on room air.

The nurse is reviewing the client's assessment to start a plan of care.

Instructions

Complete the diagram by selecting from the choices below to specify which potential condition the client is most likely experiencing, 2 actions to take, and 2 parameters the nurse would monitor to assess the client's progress.

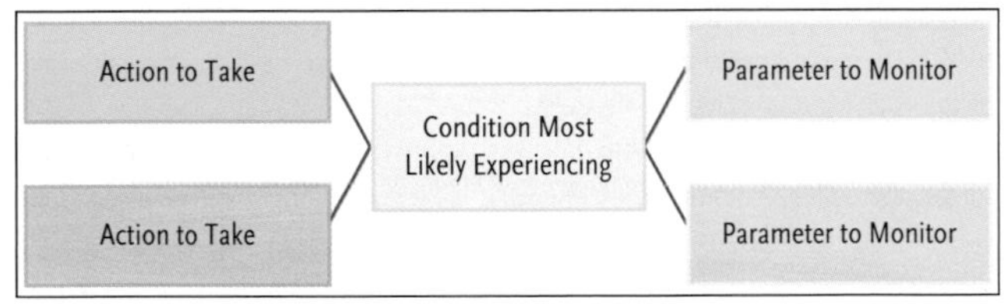

Action to take	Potential Conditions	Parameters to monitor
Obtain a blood glucose	Dehydration	Electrocardio-gram (EKG)
Obtain a urine sample for analysis	Hypoglycemia	Neurologic status
Request an order for Normal Saline to be administered intravenously	TIA/Stroke	Intake and Output
Request an order for an anti-hypertensive	Migraine	Fall precautions
Start range of motion exercises on the affected side		Serum glucose level

For more review, go to http://evolve.elsevier.com/HESI/RN for HESI's online study examinations.

Data from Burchum, J., & Rosenthal, L. (2019). *Lehne's pharmacology for nursing care* (10th 11th ed.). St. Louis: Saunders; and Ignatavicius, D. D., Workman, M. L., & Rebar, C. (2018). *Medical-surgical nursing: Concepts for interprofessional collaborative care* (10th ed.). St. Louis: Saunders, Elsevier

BIBLIOGRAPHY

ACOG Practice Guideline for Pap Smear Screening. (2021)

American College of Obstetricians and Gynecologist makes the following recommendations regarding clinical guidelines and standardization of practice to improve outcomes (2021): https://www.acog.org/clinical/clinical-guidance/committee-opinion/articles/2019/10/clinical-guidelines-and-standardization-of-practice-to-improve-outcomes

Arnold, E. (2019). Aesthetic practices of psychogeography and photography. *Geography Compass, 13*(2). https://doi.org/10.1111/gec3.12419

Arnold, E. C., & Boggs, K. U. (2019). *Interpersonal relationships: Professional communication skills for nurses* (8th ed.). Saunders.

Blazin, L. J., Sitthi-Amom, J., Hoffman, J., & Burlison, J. (2020). Improving patient handoffs and transitions through adaptation and implementation of I-pass across multiple handoff settings. *Pediatric quality and safety, 5*(4), e323. https://doi.org/10.1097/pq9.0000000000000323

Boyles, L., & Baxter, C. (2021). Premenstrual syndrome. *InnovAiT, 14*(5), 313–317. https://doi.org/10.1177/1755738021994144.

Clark, C. (2021). Aromatherapy: Essential oils and nursing: Explore this option for enhancing well-being. *American Nurse Journal, 16*(8), 34–36.

Farrar, A. J., & Farrar, F. C. (2020). Clinical aromatherapy. *Nursing Clinics of North America, 55*(4), 489–504. https://doi.org/10.1016/j.cnur.2020.06.015. Published online 2020, September 28.

Nether, K. (2018). The art of handoff communication. *The Joint Commission*. https://www.centerfortransforminghealthcare.org/why-work-with-us/blogs/patient-safety/2017/12/the-art-of-handoff-communication/?_ga=2.95413525.804021831.1636753714-89512 6800.1636753714.

Puchalsk, C. (2021). Spiritual care in health care: guideline, models, spiritual assessment and the use of the ©FICA Spiritual History Tool. *Spiritual Needs in Research and Practice*, 27–45.

Pulchaski, C. M. (2013). In J. B. Riley (Ed.), *Getting started: Communication in nursing*. (7th ed.). St. Louis, Missouri: Elsevier/Mosby.

Stussman, B. J., Nahin, R. R., Barnes, P. M., & Ward, B. W. (2020). U.S. physician recommendations to their patients about the use of complementary health approaches. *The Journal of Alternative and Complementary Medicine, 26*(1), 25–33.

World Health Organization, as adopted by the International Health conference NY 19–22 June 1946, signed on 22 July 1946 by the representatives of 61 states (official records of the EHO, no 2p100) and entered into force on 7 April 1948. The definition has not been amended since 1948.

5

Pediatric Nursing

As a nurse in a pediatric environment, the requirements include being able to connect with children in a comforting demeanor. The responsibility encompasses not only the pediatric patient but also the parent/family unit. Understanding the mindset, theoretical stages of development, and the ability to be inclusive of the child and allowing the child to make choices will facilitate a positive interaction. Being a part of the life of a child is a gratifying career choice.

The pediatric nurse encompasses a very different role and cannot be misconstrued as taking care of small adults; this is truly a psychosocial interaction with multiple implications. Conceptually, being involved with a child, infant, or adolescent means being a part of their developmental and psychosocial dynamic, which will require patience and a variety of innovative ideas to accomplish interventions. Generally, the care you provide will be all encompassing including parental education, nutrition, exercise, developmental interactions, and support of a healthy environment. Over 92% of pediatric nurses have reported that they would encourage others to have a career in pediatrics since their care can change the life of a child ("Be a Pediatric Nurse," n.d.).

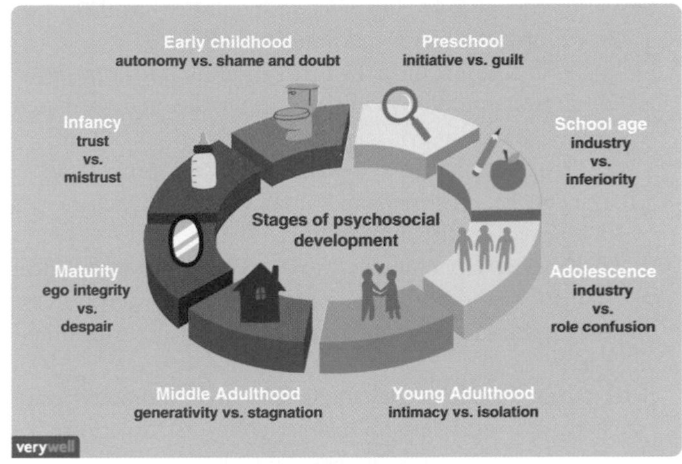

Verywell / Joshua seong

Fig. 5.1 Erikson's Stages of Psychosocial Development (Courtesy Verywell/Joshua Seong.)

Psychosocial Stages: A Summary Chart

Age	Conflict	Important Events	Outcome
Infancy (birth to 18 months)	Trust vs. Mistrust	Feeding	Hope
Early Childhood (2–3 years)	Autonomy vs. Shame and Doubt	Toilet Training	Will
Preschool (3–5 years)	Initiative vs. Guilt	Exploration	Purpose
School Age (6–11 years)	Industry vs. Inferiority	School	Confidence
Adolescence (12–18 years)	Identity vs. Role Confusion	Social Relationships	Fidelity
Young Adulthood (19 to 40 years)	Intimacy vs. Isolation	Relationships	Love
Middle Adulthood (40–65 years)	Generativity vs. Stagnation	Work and Parenthood	Care
Maturity (65 to death)	Ego Integrity vs. Despair	Reflection on Life	Wisdom

GROWTH AND DEVELOPMENT

A. Nurses need to understand the normal growth and development baselines to be able to assess developmental milestones in all pediatric individuals.
B. Knowledge of psychosocial, cognitive, and moral developmental abilities allows a nurse to adapt teaching to the level of the child.
C. Knowledge of appropriate interests of children at different ages enables the nurse to use innovative interactions to facilitate the child's development and to minimize problems caused by the exposure to a hospitalization and illness.

Theories of Development

A. Erik Erikson was a psychologist who developed one of the most popular and influential theories of development. Figure 5.1 demonstrates psychosocial & developmental milestones.
   1. Stages of Psychosocial Development
      a. Trust vs. Mistrust
      b. Autonomy vs. Shame
      c. Initiative vs. Guilt

d. Industry vs. Inferiority
e. Identity vs. Role Confusion
f. Intimacy vs. Isolation
g. Generativity vs. Stagnation
h. Integrity vs. Despair

B. Piaget. Jean Piaget was a Swiss developmental psychologist who studied children in the early 20th century. His theory of intellectual or cognitive development was published in 1936.
   1. Stages of Cognitive Development
      a. Sensorimotor, Birth 18 to 24 months: Motor activity without use of symbols. All things learned are based on experiences, or trial and error.
      b. Preoperational, 2 to 7 years old: Development of language, memory, and imagination. Intelligence is both egocentric and intuitive.
      c. Concrete Operational, 7 to 11 years old: More logical and methodical manipulation of symbols. Less egocentric, and more aware of the outside world and events.
      d. Formal Operational, adolescence to adulthood: Use of symbols to relate to abstract concepts. Able to make hypotheses and grasp abstract concepts and relationships.

C. Kohlberg. Lawrence Kohlberg was a developmental theorist of the mid-twentieth century who is best known for his specific and detailed theory of children's moral development.
   1. Moral Development
      a. Naivete and Egocentrism
      b. Punishment-Obedience Orientation
      c. Instrumental Hedonism and Concrete Reciprocity
      d. Good Boy or Good Girl Orientation
      e. Law and Order Orientation
      f. Social Contract Orientation
      g. Personal Principle Orientation
      h. Universal Principle Orientation

Clinical Implications: Birth to 1 Year

A. Developmental milestones
   1. Birth weight doubles by 6 months, triples by 12 months.
   2. Birth length increases by 50% at 12 months.
   3. The infant explores the environment by motor and oral means (Fig. 5.2).

B. Erickson's stage of development
   1. Trust vs. Mistrust

C. Clinical implications
   1. During hospitalization, the infant's emerging skills may disappear.
   2. Infant may be inconsolable due to separation anxiety.
   3. The nurse should plan and encourage the parents to be a part of the infant's care.
   4. Encourage the parents to implement a consistent routine when possible.
   5. Preparation and teaching should be directed to the family.
   6. Always speak to the infant and console the infant, use distraction while performing painful or stressful procedures.
   7. Toys for hospitalized infants include mobiles, rattles, squeaking toys, picture books, balls, colored blocks, and activity boxes.

> **HESI HINT** Understanding the milestones accomplished by the infant during each month of growth will enhance the ability of the nurse to acknowledge if the infant is at the anticipated baseline for psychosocial, cognitive, and moral development.

Toddler (1 to 3 Years)

A. Developmental milestones
   1. Birth weight quadruples by 30 months.
   2. Toddler achieves 50% of adult height by 2 years.
   3. Growth velocity slows (Fig. 5.3)

Developmental and Genetic

B. Erickson's stage of development
   1. Autonomy vs. Shame

C. Clinical implications
   1. Give simple, brief explanations immediately before procedures, keeping in mind that a 1-year-old does not benefit from the same explanation as that given to a 3-year-old.
   2. During hospitalization, enforced separation from the parents is the greatest threat to the toddler's psychological and emotional integrity.
   3. Security objects or favorite toys from home should be provided for a toddler.
   4. Teach parents to explain their plans to the child (e.g., "I will be back after your nap.").
   5. Respect the child's routine and implement whenever possible.
   6. Expect regression (e.g., bedwetting).
   7. Toys for the hospitalized toddler include a board and mallet, push-pull toys, toy telephones, stuffed animals, and storybooks with pictures. Toddlers benefit from being taken to the hospital playroom because mobility is very important to their development.
   8. Toddlers are learning to name body parts and are concerned about their bodies.
   9. Very basic explanations should be given to toddlers about procedures.
   10. Autonomy should be supported by providing guided choices when appropriate.

Preschool Child (3 to 6 Years)

A. Developmental milestones
   1. Each year, a child gains about 5 pounds and grows 2.5 to 3 inches.

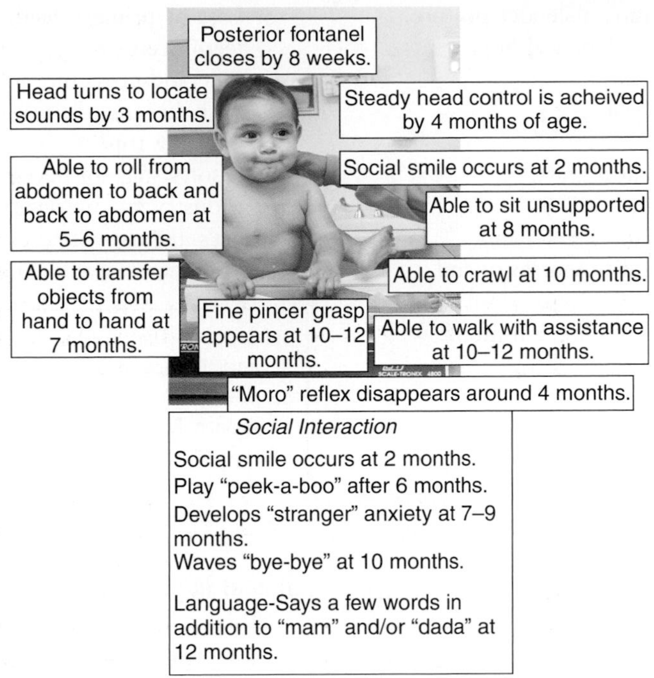

Fig. 5.2 Infant Milestones. (Modified from Hockenberry, M. J., & Wilson, D. [2011]. *Wong's nursing care of infants and children* [9th ed.]. St. Louis: Elsevier/Mosby.)

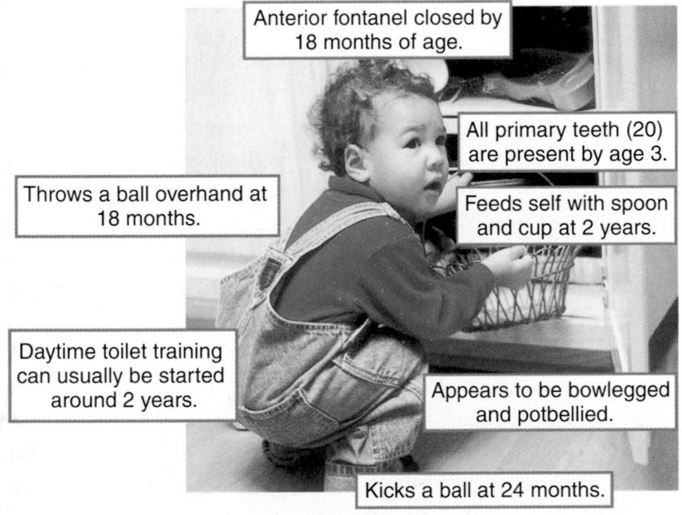

Social Interaction:

Two- to three-word sentences are spoken by 2 years.

Three- to four-word sentences are spoken by 3 years.

Own first and last name can be stated by 2½ to 3 years.

Temper tantrums are common.

Safety Issues: Curious about the world around them and like to explore. Poisonous solutions and products need to be kept out of reach from them by being stored away up high and behind locked doors.

Fig. 5.3 Toddler Milestones. (Modified from McKinney, E. S., James, S. R., Murray, S. S., Nelson, K. A., & Ashwill, J. W. [2013]. *Maternal-child nursing* [4th ed.]. St. Louis: Saunders.)

2. The child stands erect, exhibiting a slender posture.
3. The child learns to run, jump, skip, and hop.
4. Handedness is established.
5. The 3-year-old can ride a tricycle.
6. Scissors are used at 4 years.
7. Tying shoelaces is established at 5 years.
8. Colors and shapes are learned.
9. Visual acuity approaches 20/20.
   a. The child learns sexual identity (curiosity and masturbation are common).
   b. Imaginary playmates and fears are common.
   c. Aggressiveness at 4 years is replaced by more independence at 5 years.

B. Erickson's stage of development
   1. Initiative vs. Guilt

C. Piaget's theory: Preoperational thought, intuitive phase = representing things with words and images

D. Clinical implications
   1. Nursing care for hospitalized preschoolers should emphasize an understanding of the child's egocentricity. Explain that he or she did not cause the illness and that painful procedures are not a punishment for misdeeds.
   2. The child's questions should be answered at the child's developmental and learning level. Use simple words that will be understood by the child.
   3. Encourage therapeutic play or medical play that allow the child to act out his or her experiences.
   4. Fear of mutilation caused by procedures is common. A small bandage may be quite helpful in restoring body integrity.
   5. Toys and play for the hospitalized preschooler include coloring books, puzzles, cutting and pasting, dolls, building blocks, clay, and toys that allow the preschooler to work out hospitalization experiences.
   6. The preschooler requires preparation for procedures. He or she should understand what is and what is not going to be "fixed." Simple explanations and basic pictures are helpful. Let the child handle equipment or models of the equipment.

> **HESI HINT** Understanding the developmental stages at the individual ages in planning-teaching interventions. Therefore, a 5-year-old child with diabetes could choose the injection sites and provide the child some sense of control.

School-Age Child (6 to 12 Years)

A. Developmental milestones
   1. Each year, a child gains 4 to 6 pounds and about 2 inches in height.
   2. Girls may experience menarche.
   3. Loss of primary teeth and eruption of most permanent teeth occurs.
   4. Fine and gross motor skills mature.
   5. Activities include painting, drawing, riding a bicycle, and jumping rope.

B. Erickson's stage of development
   1. Industry vs. Inferiority

C. Piaget's theory: Concrete operations = thinking logically about concrete events and grasping concrete analogies

> **HESI HINT** The NGN-NCLEX-RN will test your clinical judgment to differentiate between normal and pathologic based upon the anticipated stages of development and the expectation of the child at the age of intervention. For example, what would be important to children who are school age?

Clinical Implications

1. The hospitalized school-age child may need more support from parents than the child wishes to admit.
2. Maintaining contact with peers and school activities is important during hospitalization.
3. Providing an explanation of all procedures is important. The child can learn from verbal explanations, pictures, and books, as well as by handling equipment.
4. Privacy and modesty are important and should be respected during hospitalization (e.g., close curtains during procedures, allow privacy during baths).
5. Participation in care and planning with staff fosters a sense of involvement and accomplishment.
6. Toys for the school-age child include board games, card games, and hobbies, such as stamp collecting, puzzles, and video games.

> **HESI HINT**
> **Tanner Stages of Pubertal Development (Table 5.1)**
> Girls: Breast changes, rapid increase in height and weight, growth of pubic hair, appearance of axillary hair, menstruation, abrupt deceleration of linear growth.
> Boys: Enlargement of testicles; growth of pubic hair, axillary hair, facial hair, and body hair; rapid increase in height; changes in larynx and voice; nocturnal emissions; abrupt deceleration of linear growth.

Adolescent (12 to 18 Years)

A. Developmental milestones (see Table 5.1)
   1. Girls' growth spurts during adolescence begin earlier than boys' (may begin as early as 10 years for girls).
   2. Boys catch up at around 14 years of age and continue to grow.

TABLE 5.1 Tanner Stages

Male	Stage	Female
Prepuberty	1	Prepuberty
Enlargement of scrotum and testes and darkening of scrotal sac, scarce light-pigmented pubic hair	2	Breast budding, little amount of breast tissue, enlargement of areola, scarce light pigmented pubic hair
Significant enlargement of penis, further enlargement of testes and darkening of scrotum; increase of pigmentation and amount of pubic hair	3	Further enlargement of breasts, onset of menarche 2% of females; increase of pigmentation and amount of pubic hair
Enlargement of penis, in particular the diameter, development of glands, and further enlargement of testes and darkening of scrotum; pubic hair darkens like an adult, but not as distributed; development of facial hair	4	Breast tissue and areola increase in size and nipple slightly projected; onset of menarche occurs in most females; pubic hair darkens like an adult, but not as distributed; female adult height reached approximately 2 years after onset of menarche
Penis and testes and scrotal sac adult size, continuation of growth of body hair and increase in size of muscles, 20% of males have reached final adult height		Breast tissue adult size and contour, onset of menarche 10% of females; pubic hair pigmented and distributed as an adult

Data from Marshall, W. A., & Tanner, J. M. (1969). Variations in pattern of pubertal changes in girls. *Archives of Disease in Childhood, 44*(235), 291–303; Marshall, W. A., & Tanner, J. M. (1969). Variations in pattern of pubertal changes in boys. *Archives of Disease in Childhood, 45*(239): 13–23; and Sexual Maturity Rating (Tanner Staging) in Adolescents, Copyright © 2010, World Health Organization.

3. Girls finish growth at around age 15, and boys at around age 17.
4. Secondary sex characteristics develop.
5. Adult-like thinking begins around age 15. They can problem-solve and use abstract thinking.
6. Family conflicts develop.

B. Erikson's stage of development
   1. Identity vs. Role Confusion

C. Piaget's theory: Formal operations = thinking about hypothetical scenarios and processing abstract thoughts

D. Immunizations: HPV, Meningococcal

E. Clinical implications
   1. Hospitalization of adolescents disrupts school and peer activities; it is important that teens maintain contact with both.
   2. They should share a room with other adolescents.
   3. Illnesses, treatments, and procedures that alter the adolescent's body image can be viewed by the adolescent as devastating.
   4. Teaching about procedures should include time without the parents being present, so that the teen can ask questions that they may not be comfortable asking in front of their parents. It is important to direct questions to the adolescent when the parents are present in order for all involved to hear the same information.
   5. The age of assent for making medical decisions in children and adolescents ranges from 7 to 14 years. Parental consent is also needed for treatment.
   6. For prolonged hospitalizations, adolescents need to maintain identity (e.g., have their own clothing, posters, and visitors). A teen room or teen night is very helpful. The adolescent should be part of the decision regarding a parent's rooming-in.
   7. When teaching adolescents, the focus should be on the here and now.
      a. "How will this affect me today?"

HESI HINT Clinical judgments are critical during these age categories. Understanding the different concepts of what stage of development changes will occur to know the baseline will be part of the NCLEX exam. Knowing what interventions are necessary if not meeting the baseline will be part of answering the questions for NCLEX.

PAIN ASSESSMENT AND MANAGEMENT IN THE PEDIATRIC CLIENT

A. Pediatric pain management may be undertreated, unrecognized, or undertreated. Untreated pain may lead to complications, such as delayed recovery, change in sleep patterns, and alterations in nutrition.

B. Barriers include unrecognized pain due to different manifestations of pain in the infant and/or toddler who is unable to verbalize the experience of pain and may display pain through actions and mannerisms.

C. Different tools have been developed to help health care providers recognize and identify if the infant or toddler is experiencing pain.

D. Pain assessment encompasses the pain experiences including nature, impact, and context.

E. The multidimensional pain assessment incorporates a clinical assessment on general comfort, treatment effectiveness, pain intensity, activity level, and sleep quality.

F. The tool chosen must be individualized, incorporated child and parental input, developmentally appropriate, valid, and reliable.

Clinical Assessment

A. Obtain a verbal report by the child. Children as young as 3 years of age are able to report the location and degree of pain they are experiencing.

B. Observe for nonverbal signs of pain, such as grimacing, irritability, restlessness, and difficulty in sleeping or feeding. (This is especially important in nonverbal infants and children.)

C. Include the child's parents in the assessment.
D. Observe for physiologic responses to pain, such as increased heart rate, increased respiratory rate, diaphoresis, and decreased oxygen levels.
E. Physiologic responses to pain are most often seen in response to acute pain rather than in response to chronic pain.

Clinical Judgment

A. Use a pain rating scale appropriate for the child's age and developmental level.
B. Neonates and infants
   1. Premature infants, starting around 20 weeks gestation, can perceive and respond to pain. To conserve energy, they frequently show a less-robust physical response compared to full-term infants (for example, they are more likely to close their eyes instead of grimacing and often have lower oxygen saturation levels). This unique response requires a scale specific to premature infants.
   2. The premature infant pain profile (PIPP), valid only in premature infants ≤37 weeks gestation, is well equipped to measure pain in this patient population. The Neonatal Pain, Agitation and Sedation Scale (N-PASS) includes a sedation assessment so that only one scale is needed for infants 23 weeks gestation through 100 days of life. The N-PASS scores pain/agitation from 0 to 10 and sedation from −10 to 0.
   3. Scales appropriate for full-term and older infants include the Neonatal Infant Pain Scale; the FLACC (Face, Legs, Activity, Cry, Consolability) scale; Child Facial Coding System; CRIES (Crying, Requires increased oxygen administration, Increased vital signs, Expression, Sleeplessness) score; Children's Hospital of Eastern Ontario Pain Scale; Riley Infant Pain Scale; and Children and Infants Postoperative Pain Scale.
C. Self-report measures are used to determine the behaviors of a child; respondents are asked to report directly on the child's behavior, attitudes or intentions. The scales can be used with 5 year olds or with parents to determine a child' behaviors.
   1. Faces Pain Scale-Revised (FPS-R) and Wong–Baker FACES pain rating scale. Use the same scale with a child rather than alternating between scales.
D. School age and adolescents
   1. Many older children (8 years and older) can self-report pain by using a 0 to 10 scale. Numeric rating scales are easy to use and may be verbal (Verbal Numerical Rating Scale) or written (Visual Analogue Scale) (Fig. 5.4).
E. Children with cognitive developmental delays
   1. These children are at increased risk for poor pain assessment and management. Several scales exist, each with varying levels of reliability and validity.
   2. The revised FLACC (r-FLACC) has been validated in children from age 4 to 19 years. Using the original FLACC scale as a base, additional indicators (such as head banging and breath holding) were added, along with space for parents to document any features unique to their child. The scale measures Facial expression, Leg movements, Activity, Cry, and Consolability.

0
No hurt

1 or 2
Hurts
little bit

2 or 4
Hurts
little more

3 or 6
Hurts
even more

4 or 8
Hurts
whole lot

5 or 10
Hurts
worst

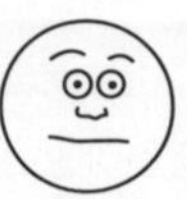

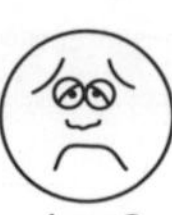

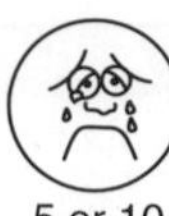

Fig. 5.4 Wong–Baker FACES Pain Rating Scale. (From Wong–Baker FACES Foundation. [2016]. *Wong-Baker FACES® Pain Rating Scale.* Retrieved June 3, 2016, with permission from http://www.WongBakerFACES.org)

   3. Another helpful tool is the Individualized Numeric Rating Scale. Caregivers are asked to assign a number to typical pain behavior seen in their child. The scale must be periodically updated because pain signs may change as the child ages.
F. Intubated and mechanically ventilated children
   1. The COMFORT scale (Van Dijk et al.) uses six behavioral and two physiological metrics for a total score from 8 to 40.

> **HESI HINT** An American Society of Pain Management Nursing position statement recommends using self-report if possible, evaluating potential sources of pain, assessing patient behaviors, incorporating physiologic measures (keeping in mind that they may not be specific to pain), soliciting input from parents, and assuming pain is present if the child is undergoing a painful procedure or has known reasons for pain (Wrona & Czarnecki, 2021).

2. Nonpharmacologic interventions
   a. Should be used according to the child's age and developmental level
   b. Infants may respond best to pacifiers, holding, and rocking.
   c. Toddlers and preschoolers may respond best to distraction. Distraction may be provided through books, music, television, and bubble blowing.
   d. School-aged children and adolescents may use guided imagery.
   e. Other interventions may include massage, application of heat or cold, and deep-breathing exercises.
3. Pharmacologic interventions
   a. Before administering a pain medication to a pediatric client, verify that the prescribed dose is safe for the child on the basis of the child's weight (mg/kg).
   b. Monitor the child's vital signs after administration of opioid medications.
   c. Children as young as 5 years of age may be taught to use a patient-controlled analgesia (PCA) pump.
4. Children may deny pain if they fear receiving an intramuscular (IM) injection.

> **HESI HINT**
> **Child Health Promotion**
> Description: Immunization of children against communicable diseases is one of the greatest accomplishments of modern medicine. Childhood mortality and

morbidity rates have greatly decreased. Protection against disease should begin in infancy according to the recommendations of the American Academy of Pediatrics and the U.S. Public Health Service.

Recommendations can be found at http://www.cdc.gov/vaccines/schedules/hcp/child-adolescent.html

A. The nursing care of children with communicable diseases is virtually the same for all, regardless of the disease (Table 5.2).

HESI HINT Protection against communicable disease should begin in infancy according to the recommendations of the American Academy of Pediatrics and the U.S. Public Health Service. Recommendations can be found at http://www.cdc.gov/vaccines/schedules/hcp/child-adolescent.html

Clinical Care for Children With Communicable Disease

A. Isolate child during period of communicability.
B. Treat fever with *nonaspirin* product.
C. Report occurrence to the health department.
D. Prevent child from scratching skin (e.g., cut nails, apply mittens, and provide soothing baths).
E. Administer diphenhydramine hydrochloride (HCl; i.e., Benadryl) as prescribed for itching.
F. Wash hands after caring for child and handling secretions or child's articles.
G. Administer vaccinations using the recommended CDC schedule Table 5.3.

HESI HINT Children with communicable disease pose a serious threat to their unborn siblings. The nurse should counsel all expectant mothers, especially those with young children, to be aware of the serious consequences of exposure to communicable diseases during pregnancy.

Pediatric Nutritional Assessment

Description: Profile of the child's and family's eating habits

A. Iron deficiency occurs most commonly in children 12 to 36 months old, in adolescent females, and in females during their childbearing years.
   1. The recommended daily amount of vitamin D is 400 international units (IU) for children up to age 12 months, 600 IU for people ages 1 to 70 years, and 800 IU for people over 70 years (Mayo Clinic, 2021e, *Vitamin D*).
   2. If a mother is not taking enough vitamin D, it is recommended that the infant receive an oral dose of 400 IU/daily.

TABLE 5.2 Communicable Disease in Children

Name of Communicable Disease	Definition	Clinical Transmission	Clinical Symptoms	Clinical Treatment
Rubeola (measles)	A highly contagious viral disease that can lead to neurologic problems or death	Transmitted by direct contact with droplets from infected persons Contagious mainly during the prodromal period	Fever and upper respiratory symptoms including the following: Classic Photophobia Koplik spots	Bed rest Fluids Isolation
Paramyxovirus (mumps)	A viral infection that affects the salivary glands below and in front of the ears. The disease spreads through infected saliva.	Incubation period: 14–21 days	Fever, headache, malaise, parotid gland swelling and tenderness; manifestations include submaxillary and sublingual infection, orchitis, and meningoencephalitis	Analgesics are used for pain and antiseptics for fever. Bed rest is maintained until swelling subsides.
Rubella (German measles)	Common viral disease that has teratogenic effects on fetus during the first trimester of pregnancy	Transmitted by droplet and direct contact with infected person	Discrete red maculopapular rash that starts on face and rapidly spreads to entire body Rash disappears within 3 days Fever, headache	Prevention: vaccination
Varicella (chickenpox)	Viral disease characterized by skin lesions.	Transmitted by direct contact, droplet spread, or freshly contaminated objects Communicable prodromal period to the time all lesions have crusted	Lesions that begin on the trunk and spread to the face and proximal extremities Progresses through macular, papular, vesicular, and pustular stages	CDC recommends two doses of varicella vaccine for everyone Children should receive their first dose of varicella vaccine between 12 and 15 months of age and their second dose at 4 to 6 years of age.

CDC, Centers for Disease Control and Prevention

TABLE 5.3 Vaccines

Type of Vaccine	Description
MMR Vaccine • Measles, mumps, rubella (MMR) • Offers protection against these three diseases	• It is generally administered at 12–15 months of age and repeated at 4–6 years or by 11–12 years. • In times of measles epidemics, it is possible to give measles protection at 6 months and repeat the MMR at 15 months. • Measles vaccine is contraindicated for persons with history of anaphylactic reaction to neomycin or eggs, those with known altered immunodeficiency, and pregnant women. It may be given to those with human immunodeficiency virus (HIV) and to breastfeeding women. • Administer subcutaneously at separate sites. • Child may have a light, transient rash 2 weeks after administration of vaccine.

DTaP Vaccine
• Diphtheria, pertussis, tetanus
• Offers protection against these diseases
	• Beginning at age 2 months, administer three doses at 2-month intervals.
	• Booster doses given at 15–18 months and at 4–6 years.
	• Administer IM (separate site from other vaccine).
	• Not given to children past the seventh birthday; they receive Td, which contains full-strength protection against tetanus and lesser-strength diphtheria protection.
	• When pertussis vaccine is contraindicated, give Delirium tremens (DT), full-strength diphtheria, and tetanus without pertussis vaccine, until seventh birthday.
	• Contraindications to pertussis vaccine include:
	  • Encephalopathy within 7 days of previous dose of DTaP
	  • History of seizures
	  • Neurologic symptoms after receiving the vaccine
	  • Systemic allergic reactions to the vaccine
	• Parents should be instructed to begin acetaminophen (Tylenol) administration after the immunization (normal dosage is 10–15 mg/kg).
	Instruct parents to report immediately any side effects of the immunization to the primary caregiver.

Polio Vaccine • Inactive polio vaccine (IPV)	• Recommended for all persons under 18 years. • Administer at 2 months of age and again at 4 months of age. Boosters are given at 6 –18 months and at 4–6 years. • Administer IPV subcutaneously or IM at separate site. • IPV is contraindicated for those with history of anaphylactic reaction to neomycin or streptomycin. • May give with all other vaccines.
Hib (*Haemophilus influenzae* Type B) Vaccine • Offers protection against bacteria that cause serious illness (epiglottitis, bacterial meningitis, septic arthritis) in small children and those with chronic illnesses such as sickle cell disease	• Three conjugate vaccines have been recommended for administration to infants: PRP-OPMs can be given beginning as early as 2 months of age; DTaP/Hib combinations should not be used as primary immunizations at ages 2, 4, or 6 months. • Vaccines have different series administration schedules; the schedules cover children through 5 years of age. • Children at high risk who were not immunized previously should be immunized after the age of 5. • Administer IM. • There are no contraindications.
Hepatitis B • Offers protection against hepatitis B • May be given to newborns before hospital discharge • All children up to 18 years of age should be vaccinated.	• Is contraindicated for persons with anaphylactic reaction to common baker's yeast.
Varicella • Offers protection against chickenpox • Is a school entry requirement in almost all states • Is safe for children with asymptomatic HIV infection	• Administer at 12–18 months of age (must be at least 12 months). • Give MMR and varicella on same day or > 30 days apart (separate site).

Continued

Tuberculosis (TB) Skin Testing • Offers screening for exposure to TB	• Screening is usually done using one of the following: • Mantoux test with purified protein derivative (PPD) (tuberculin purified protein derivative) injected intradermally on the forearm; standard method for identifying infection with Mycobacterium tubrculosis • Tine test (OT, old tuberculin), which consists of four prongs pressed into the forearm. These multiple puncture tests are unreliable and should not be used to determine the presence of a TB infection • A positive reaction represents exposure to M. tuberculosis. • Screening can be initiated at 12 months.

IM, Intramuscular; *IV*, intravenous

B. The vitamins most often consumed in less-than-appropriate amounts by preschool and school-age children are
   1. Vitamin A
   2. Vitamin C
   3. Vitamin B_6
   4. Vitamin B_{12}

Clinical Interventions

A. Determine dietary history.
   1. The 24-hour recall: Ask the family to recall all food and liquid intake during the past 24 hours.
   2. Food diary: Ask the family to keep a 3-day record (2 weekdays and 1 weekend day) of all food and liquid intake and the amount of each.
   3. Food frequency record: Provide a questionnaire and ask family to record information regarding the number of times per day, week, or month a child consumes items from the four food groups.
B. Perform a clinical assessment/clinical judgment examination
   1. Assess skin, hair, teeth, lips, tongue, and eyes.
   2. Use anthropometry: Measurement of height, weight, body mass index (BMI), head circumference in young children, proportion, skinfold thickness, and arm circumference.
      a. Height and head circumference reflect past nutrition.
      b. Weight, skinfold thickness, and arm circumference reflect present nutritional status (especially protein and fat reserves).
      c. Skinfold thickness provides a measurement of the body's fat content (half of the body's total fat stores are directly beneath the skin).
C. Obtain biochemical analysis.
   a. Plasma, blood cells, urine, or tissues from liver, bone, hair, or fingernails can be used to determine nutritional status.
   b. Laboratory testing of hemoglobin (Hgb), hematocrit (Hct), albumin, creatinine, and nitrogen are commonly used to determine nutritional status.
D. Implement appropriate nursing judgment, including client and family teaching, to correct identified nutritional deficits (Table 5.4).

Diarrhea

Description: Increased number or decreased consistency of stools

A. Diarrhea can be a serious or fatal symptom, especially in infancy.
B. Causes include but are not limited to
   1. Infections: Bacterial, viral, parasitic
   2. Malabsorption problems
   3. Inflammatory diseases
   4. Dietary factors
C. Conditions associated with diarrhea are
   1. Dehydration
   2. Metabolic acidosis
   3. Shock

Clinical Assessment

A. Usually occurs in infants
B. History of exposure to pathogens, contaminated food, dietary changes
C. Signs of dehydration
   1. Poor skin turgor/tenting of skin
   2. Absence of tears
   3. Dry and sticky mucous membranes
   4. Weight loss (5% to 15%)
   5. Depressed fontanel
   6. Decreased urinary output, increased specific gravity
   7. Acidotic state
D. Laboratory signs of acidosis
   1. Loss of bicarbonate (serum pH < 7.35)
   2. Loss of sodium and potassium through stools
   3. Elevated Hct
   4. Elevated blood urea nitrogen (BUN)
E. Signs of shock (late signs)
   1. Decreased blood pressure
   2. Rapid, weak pulse
   3. Skin: Mottled to gray color; cool and clammy to touch
   4. Delayed capillary refill greater than (+) 4 seconds
   5. Changes in mental status

HESI HINT Capillary refill is best evaluated on the infant's sternum. To obtain capillary refill in newborn infants, capillary refill time can be measured by **pressing on the sternum for 5 s with a finger or thumb**, and noting the time needed for the color to return once the pressure is released. The upper normal limit for capillary refill in newborns is 3 s.

TABLE 5.4 Nutritional Assessment

Nutrient	Signs of Deficiency	Food Sources
• Iron	• Anemia • Pale conjunctiva • Pale skin color • Atrophy of papillae on tongue • Brittle, ridged, spoon-shaped nails • Thyroid edema	• Iron-fortified formula • Infant high-protein cereal • Infant rice cereal • Liver • Beef • Pork • Eggs
• Vitamin B_2 (riboflavin)	• Redness and fissuring of eyelid corners; burning, itching, tearing eyes; photophobia • Magenta-colored tongue, glossitis • Seborrheic dermatitis, delayed wound healing	• Prepared infant formula • Liver • Cow's milk • Cheddar cheese • Some green leafy vegetables (broccoli, green beans, spinach) • Enriched cereals
• Vitamin A (retinol)	• Dry, rough skin • Dull cornea; soft cornea; Bitot spots • Night blindness • Defective tooth enamel • Retarded growth; impaired bone formation • Decreased thyroxine formation	• Liver • Sweet potatoes • Carrots • Spinach • Peaches • Apricots
• Vitamin C (ascorbic acid)	• Scurvy • Receding gums that are spongy and prone to bleeding • Dry, rough skin; petechiae • Decreased wound healing • Increased susceptibility to infection • Irritability, anorexia, apprehension	• Strawberries • Oranges and orange juice • Tomatoes • Broccoli • Cabbage • Cauliflower • Spinach
• Vitamin B_6 (pyridoxine)	• Scaly dermatitis • Weight loss • Anemia • Irritability • Convulsions • Peripheral neuritis	• Meats, especially liver • Cereals (wheat and corn) • Yeast • Soybeans • Peanuts • Tuna • Chicken • Bananas

Clinical Judgment

A. Assess hydration status and vital signs frequently.
B. Monitor intake and output.
C. Do not take temperature rectally.
D. Rehydrate as prescribed with fluids and electrolytes.
E. Calculate intravenous (IV) hydration to include maintenance and replacement fluids.
F. Add potassium to IV fluids only when the client has an adequate urine output. Standard IV fluids used to treat pediatric dehydration are isotonic (e.g., Ringer's lactate [LR]) or normal saline (NS). The amount is a fluid bolus of 20 mL/kg.
G. Collect specimens to aid in diagnosis of cause.
H. Check stools for pH, glucose, and blood.
I. Administer antibiotics as prescribed.
J. Check urine for specific gravity.
K. Institute careful isolation precautions; wash hands with soap and water.
L. Teach home care of child with diarrhea.
   1. Provide child with oral rehydration solution such as Pedialyte or Lytren.
   2. Child may temporarily need lactose-free diet.
   3. Children should not receive antidiarrheals (e.g., Imodium A-D).
   4. Do not give child grape juice, orange juice, apple juice, cola, or ginger ale. These solutions have high osmolality.

HESI HINT Antibiotics are not recommended for diarrhea. They are only prescribed if the child has diarrhea caused by a bacterial, fungal, or parasitic infection.

Burns

Description: Tissue injuries caused by heat, electricity, chemicals, or radiation

A. Burns are a major cause of accidental death in children younger than 15 (after automobile accidents).

B. Nearly 75% of all scalding burns in children are preventable. Toddlers and children are more often burned by a scalding or flames. Most children ages 4 and under who are hospitalized for burn-related injuries suffer from scald burn (65%) or contact burns (20%) (*Burns in Children,* Johns Hopkins Medicine, 2021).

C. Scald burns
   1. Children younger than 5 are one of the two highest risk groups.
   2. Ranked the top cause of burns (accidentally or purposeful) to children younger than 4 years old.
   3. Hot water heater temperature greater than 140 degrees can cause a third-degree burn on a child in 15 seconds and is responsible for 20% of childhood admissions for scald burns.

D. Children younger than age 2 have a higher mortality rate due to
   1. Greater central body surface area. In a child younger than 2, a greater part of the body surface area is concentrated in the head and trunk compared with an older child or an adult; therefore; the younger child is more likely to have serious effects from burns to the trunk and head (Fig. 5.5). Update to latest edition
   2. Greater fluid volume (proportionate to body size)
   3. Less effective cardiovascular responses to fluid volume shifts

E. In childhood, a partial-thickness burn is considered a major burn if it involves more than 25% of body surface.

F. A full-thickness burn is considered major if it involves more than 10% of body surface.

G. Because of the changing proportions of the child, especially the infant, the rule of nines cannot be used to assess the percentage of burn (see Fig. 5.5).

H. An assessment tool such as the Lund–Browder chart, which takes into account the changing proportions of the child, should be used.

I. Fluid needs should be calculated from the time of the burn.

J. The Parkland formula is a commonly used guideline for calculating fluid replacement and maintenance, which is based on the child's body surface area and should include volume for burn losses and maintenance.

K. Adequacy of fluid replacement is determined by evaluating urinary output.

> **HESI HINT** Urinary output for infants and children should be 1–2 mL/kg/h.

L. Specific gravity should be less than 1.025.

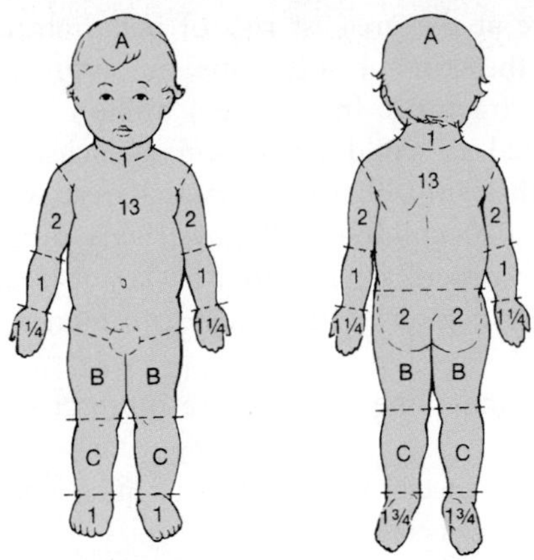

RELATIVE PERCENTAGES OF AREAS AFFECTED BY GROWTH

A

AREA	BIRTH	AGE 1 YR	AGE 5 YR
A = ½ of head	9½	8½	6½
B = ½ of one thigh	2¾	3¼	4
C = ½ of one leg	2½	2½	2¾

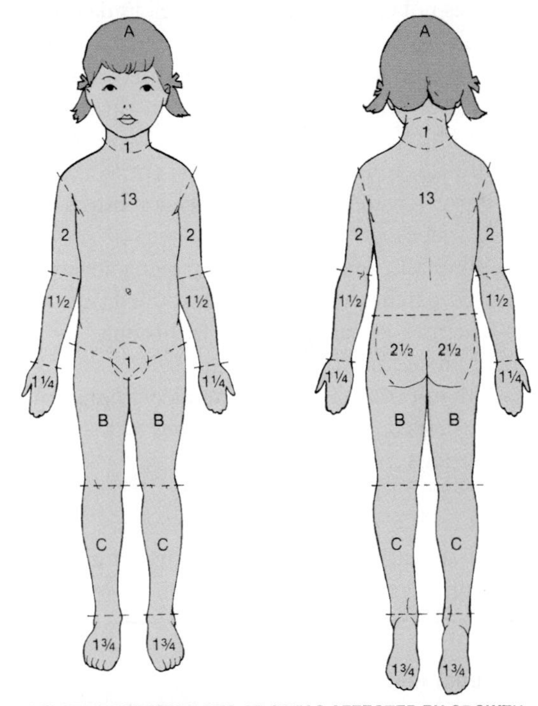

RELATIVE PERCENTAGES OF AREAS AFFECTED BY GROWTH

B

AREA	AGE 10 YR	AGE 15 YR	ADULT
A = ½ of head	5½	4½	3½
B = ½ of one thigh	4½	4½	4¾
C = ½ of one leg	3	3¼	3½

Fig. 5.5 Estimated Distribution of Burns in Children. (A) Children from birth to age 5 years. (B) Older children. (From Hockenberry, M. J., & Wilson, D. [2020]. *Wong's nursing care of infants and children* [8th ed.]. St. Louis: Elsevier, Mosby.)

Non-accidental Trauma (NAT)

Description: NAT is an injury that is purposefully inflicted upon a child—in other words, child abuse, intentional or nonintentional physical and mental injury, sexual abuse, and emotional and physical neglect of a child. Children under the age of 1 are at the greatest risk of being abused. Often the injury is to the skin and soft tissue, but approximately a third of NATs are fractures. In 2011, 3.4 million instances of NAT were reported to child protection agencies in the United States. Death from inflicted injury that year was estimated at 2.1 per 100,000 children. All physicians, nurses, and other health care workers are required by law to report suspected abuse. Child neglect is the most common form of abuse (80%).

A. Children under the age of 4 are more at risk for being a victim.
B. Children of special needs are at an increased risk of being abused or neglected.
C. Abused individuals are at an increased risk of becoming a perpetrator of abuse (Weber, 2015).

Clinical Assessment

A. Most important indicators of NAT
  1. Injuries not congruent with the child's developmental age or skills
  2. Injuries not correlated with the stated cause of injury
    a. Bruises in unusual places and in various stages of healing
    b. Bruises, welts caused by belts, cords, etc.
    c. Burns (cigarette, iron); immersion burns (symmetrical in shape)
    d. Whiplash injuries caused by being shaken
    e. Bald patches where hair was pulled out
    f. Fractures in various stages of healing
  3. Delay in seeking medical care
  4. Failure to thrive (FTT), unattended-to physical problems
  5. Torn, stained, bloody underclothes
  6. Lacerations of external genitalia
  7. Older child bedwetting or soiling
  8. Child with sexually transmitted diseases
  9. Child appearing frightened and withdrawn in the presence of parent or other adult

Clinical Judgment

A. Nurses are legally required to report all cases of suspected NAT to the appropriate local or state agency.
B. Take color photographs of injuries, upload in Electronic medical records (EMRs).
C. Document factual, objective statements about child's physical condition, child–family interactions, and interviews with family.
D. Establish trust, and care for the child's physical problems; these are the primary and immediate needs of these children.
E. Recognize own feelings of anger toward the parents.
F. Utilize principles of crisis intervention.
G. Assist child and family to develop self-esteem.
H. Teach basic child development and parenting skills to family.
I. Support the need for family therapy.

HESI HINT When NAT is suspected, look for patterns of injury. If getting the patient's history raises concerns, primary care providers should evaluate the patient for cutaneous, cranial, ocular, visceral, and orthopedic injuries.

Poisonings

Every day, over 300 children in the United States ages 0 to 19 are treated in an emergency department, and two children die, as a result of being poisoned. It is not just chemicals in your home marked with clear warning labels that can be dangerous to children (Centers for Disease Control and Prevention [CDC], *Poisoning Prevention,* 2019, February 6).

Description: Ingesting, inhaling, or absorbing a toxic substance

A. Poisoning, particularly by ingestion, is a common cause of childhood injury and illness.
B. While young children (younger than 6 years) comprise a disproportionate percentage of the cases, poisoning affects ALL age groups, from infants to seniors. Peak poisoning frequency occurs in 1- and 2-year-olds, but poisonings in teens and adults are more serious (Poison Statistics, 2019 Poison Control).

More than 90% of the time, poisonings happen in people's homes. The majority of these poisonings occur in the kitchen, bathroom, and bedroom (Health Resources & Service Administration [HRSA], 2021, *Poison Help and Prevention Tips*).

Clinical Assessment

A. Child found near source of poison
B. Gastrointestinal (GI) disturbance: Nausea, abdominal pain, diarrhea, vomiting
C. Burns of mouth, pharynx
D. Respiratory distress
E. Seizures, changes in level of consciousness (LOC)
F. Cyanosis
G. Shock

Clinical Judgment

A. Identify the poisonous agent as soon as suspected
B. Assess the child's respiratory, cardiac, and neurologic status.
C. Instruct parent to bring any emesis, stool, etc., to the emergency department.
D. Determine the child's age and weight.

HESI HINT Put the nationwide poison control center phone number, 1-800-222-1222, on or near every telephone in your home and program it into your cell phone. Call the poison control center if you think a child has been poisoned but they are awake and alert. Call 911 if you have a poison emergency and your child has collapsed or is not breathing.

A. Poison removal and care may require gastric lavage, activated charcoal, *N*-acetylcysteine, or naloxone HCl.
B. Teach home safety.

1. Poison-proof and child-proof the home.
   a. Identify location of poisons: Under the sink (cleaning supplies, drain cleaners, bug poisons); medicine cabinets; storage rooms (paints, varnishes); garages (antifreeze, gasoline); poisonous plants (philodendron, dieffenbachia).
   b Put locks on cabinets.
   c. Use safety containers: Do not place poisonous materials in non–child-proof containers.
   d. Discard unused medications.
2. Make sure child is always under adult supervision.
3. Put the nationwide poison control center phone number, 1-800-222-1222, near all phones.
4. Examine the environment from the child's viewpoint (the height to which a 2- to 5-year-old can reach).
5. Be aware of changes in the child's environment because of house guests or visiting a relative or friends.

C. Contact community health nurse or child welfare agency if necessary.

> **HESI HINT** Common household products that are poisonous to children if ingested: Perfume and aftershave, sunburn relief products, alcohol, cigarettes or any type of tobacco products, and mouthwash.

Lead Poisoning

Description: CDC now uses a blood lead reference value of 5 micrograms per deciliter (μg/dL) to identify children with blood lead levels (BLLs) that are much higher than most children's levels. This new level is based on the U.S. population of children ages 1 to 5 years who are in the highest 2.5% of children when tested for lead in their blood. There is no established "safe" level of lead for children. Every system in the human body can be affected by lead exposure. Lead exposure and elevated levels have been linked to decreased IQs (Center for Disease Control and Prevention, 2021, *Childhood Lead Poisoning Prevention*).

Children 6 years of age and younger are most vulnerable to the effects of lead because children tend to put things in their mouths.

A. Though lead can be found in many places in a child's environment, lead exposure is preventable. The key is stopping children from coming into contact with lead. Parents can take simple steps to make their homes more lead-safe. The major cause of lead poisoning is deteriorating lead-based paint.

B. Lead enters the body through ingestion, inhalation, or, in the case of an unborn child, placental transfer when the mother is exposed. The most common route is ingestion either from hand-to-mouth behavior via contaminated hands, fingers, toys, or pacifiers or, less often, from eating sweet-tasting loose paint chips found in a home built before the 1950s or in a play area.

C. The renal, neurologic, and hematologic systems are the most seriously affected by lead.

D. The BLL test is currently used for screening and diagnosis. BLL testing is currently required at 12 and 24 months for all Medicaid-enrolled children, unless the state has a Centers for Disease Control and Prevention and the Centers for Medicare and Medicaid Services (CDC/CMS) waiver indicating that children enrolled in Medicaid are not at higher risk for high BLLs than other children.

Clinical Assessment

A. Screen for lead poisoning using CDC guidelines of blood lead surveillance and other risk factor data collected over time to establish the status and risk of children throughout the state.

B. In areas without available data, universal screening is recommended.
1. All children should have a BLL test at the ages of 1 and 2 years.
   a. Collect blood in a capillary tube and send to the laboratory.
   b. During collection, avoid contamination of blood specimen and lead on the skin.
2. Any child between 3 and 6 years of age who has not been screened should also be tested.

C. Obtain a history of possible sources of lead in the child's environment.

D. Physical assessment
1. General signs/symptoms
   a. Anemia
   b. GI
      1) Acute cramping; abdominal pain
      2) Vomiting
      3) Constipation
      4) Anorexia
   c. Neurologic
      1) Headache
      2) Lethargy
   d. Impaired growth
2. Central nervous system (CNS) signs (early)
   a. Hyperactivity
   b. Aggression
   c. Impulsiveness
   d. Decreased interest in play
   e. Irritability
   f. Short attention span
3. CNS signs (late)
   a. Mental retardation
   b. Paralysis
   c. Blindness
   d. Convulsions
   e. Coma
   f. Death

Clinical Judgment

A. Identify sources of lead in the environment to prevent further exposure.

B. Administer prescribed chelating agents to reduce high BLL levels.

C. Dimercaprol (chelating agent) is contraindicated in patients with a peanut allergy or hepatic insufficiency.

D. IM and IV administration

1. Calcium disodium ethylenediaminetetraacetic acid (EDTA) is generally administered IM.
2. Dimercaprol (also called BAL) is given in conjunction with calcium disodium EDTA (may contain peanut oil) to help in efficacy of treatment.
3. Considerations for administration.
   a. Rotate injection sites if chelating agent is given IM.
   b. Reassure child that injections are a treatment, not a punishment.
   c. Administer the local anesthetic procaine with IM injection of calcium disodium EDTA to reduce discomfort.
   d. Apply EMLA cream over puncture site 2½ hours before the injection to reduce discomfort.

> **HESI HINT** Monitor client's renal functioning and complete blood count (CBC) while client is receiving chelating agents.

E. Avoid giving iron during chelation because of possible interactive effects.
F. If home oral chelation therapy is used, teach family proper administration of medication.
G. Administer prescribed cleansing enemas or cathartic for acute lead ingestion.
H. Assist family to obtain sources of help for removing lead from the environment.
   1. Do not vacuum hard-surfaced floors or windowsills or window wells in homes built before 1960 because this spreads dust.
   2. Wash and dry child's hands and face frequently, especially before the child eats.
   3. Wash toys and pacifiers frequently.
   4. Make sure that home exposure is not occurring from parental occupations or hobbies.

REVIEW OF CHILD HEALTH PROMOTION

1. List two contraindications to live virus immunization.
2. List different techniques to assess pain in children.
3. Discuss the signs and symptoms of NAT.
4. List the signs and symptoms of iron deficiency.
5. What measurements reflect present nutritional status?
6. List the signs and symptoms of dehydration in an infant.
7. List the laboratory findings that can be expected in a dehydrated child.
8. How should burns in children be assessed?
9. How can the nurse best evaluate the adequacy of fluid replacement in children?
10. How should a parent be instructed to childproof a house?
11. What interventions should the nurse perform first in caring for a child who has ingested a poison?
12. What early signs should the nurse assess for if lead poisoning is suspected?

See Answer Key at the end of this text for suggested responses.

RESPIRATORY DISORDERS

Clinical Assessment in Children

A. Normal pulse and respiratory rates (Table 5.5)
B. Signs of respiratory distress in children
   1. Tachypnea. An increase in the number of breaths per minute
   2. Tachycardia. An increased heart rate. Low oxygen levels may cause an increase in heart rate.
   3. Color changes. Circumoral cyanosis: A bluish color seen around the mouth, on the inside of the lips, or on the fingernails; color of the skin may also appear pale or gray.
   4. Grunting. This grunting is the body's way of trying to keep air in the lungs
   5. Nose flaring. The openings of the nose spreading open while breathing may indicate that a person is having to work harder to breathe.
   6. Retractions. The chest appears to sink in just below the neck and/or under the breastbone with each breath—one way of trying to bring more air into the lungs.
   7. Sweating. There may be increased sweat on the head, but the skin does not feel warm to the touch. More often, the skin may feel cool or clammy.

TABLE 5.5 Normal Pulse and Respiratory Rates for Children

Age	Pulse	Respirations	Nursing Implications
Newborn	100–160	30–60	These ranges are averages only and vary with the sex, age, and condition of the child. Always note whether the child is crying, febrile, or in some distress.
1–11 months	100–150	25–35	
1–3 years (toddler)	80–130	20–30	
3–5 years (preschooler)	80–120	20–25	
6–10 years (school age)	70–110	18–22	
10–16 years (adolescent)	60–90	16–20	

8. Wheezing. A tight, whistling or musical sound heard with each breath can indicate that the air passages may be smaller, making it more difficult to breathe.
9. Stridor. An inspiratory sound heard in the upper airway.
10. Accessory muscle use. The muscles of the neck appear to be moving and can also be seen under the rib cage or even the muscles between the ribs.
11. Head bobbing in alertness. Low oxygen levels may cause your child to act very tired and may indicate respiratory fatigue.
12. Body positions. Low oxygen and difficulty breathing may force your child to thrust his or head.
13. Alterations in blood gases: Decreased partial pressure of oxygen (Po_2), elevated partial pressure of carbon dioxide (Pco_2)

The signs of respiratory distress may resemble other problems or medical conditions (Stanford Children's' Health, 2021, *Signs of Respiratory Distress in Children.*).

SYMPTOMS OF HYPOXIA
Early: Restlessness, anxiety, tachycardia/tachypnea
Late: Bradycardia, extreme restlessness, severe dyspnea
Pediatrics: Difficulty feeding, inspiratory stridor, nares flaring, grunting with expirations, sternal retractions

C. Clinical Judgment
  1. Child often goes into respiratory failure before cardiac failure.
  2. Identify signs of respiratory distress.

Asthma

Description: Inflammatory reactive airway disease that is commonly chronic

A. The airways become edematous.
B. The airways become congested with mucus.
C. The smooth muscles of the bronchi and bronchioles constrict.
D. Air trapping occurs in the alveoli.
E. Differences with the anatomy in children:
  1. Infants have smaller nares, and are obligate nose breathers (until about 1 to 2 months of age).
  2. Children eight and younger have immature cartilage, and the epiglottis is more flaccid, making it difficult to completely close.
  3. The trachea has a narrower diameter than in adults.
  4. Lung tissue develops and grows from birth to about the age of 12.
  5. The alveoli multiply over 10 times the amount an infant is born with.
  6. Children younger than six breathe with their abdominal muscles, as there is weak musculature with thoracic muscles.

Clinical Assessment

A. History of asthma in the family
B. History of allergies and/or eczema
C. Home environment containing pets or other allergens
D. Tight cough (nonproductive cough) usually occurs and/or worsens at nighttime
E. Breath sounds: Coarse expiratory wheezing, rales, crackles
F. Chest diameter enlarges (late sign and symptom)
G. Increased number of school days missed during past 6 months
H. Signs of respiratory distress (Table 5.6)

Clinical Judgment

A. Monitor carefully for increasing respiratory distress.
B. Administer rapid-acting bronchodilators and steroids for acute attacks.
C. Maintain hydration (oral fluids or IV).
D. Monitor blood gas values for signs of respiratory acidosis.
E. Administer oxygen or nebulizer therapy as prescribed.
F. Monitor pulse oximetry as prescribed (usually >95% is normal).
G. Monitor beta-adrenergic agonists, as well as anti-inflammatory corticosteroids, which are commonly used medications (Table 5.7).
H. Teach home care program, including:
  1. Identifying precipitating factors
  2. Eliminating triggers
  3. Reducing allergens in the home
  4. Using metered-dose inhaler/nebulizer
  5. Monitoring peak expiratory flow rate at home
  6. Doing breathing exercises
  7. Monitoring drug actions, dosages, and side effects
  8. Managing acute episode and when to seek emergency care
I. Refer child and family for emotional and psychological counseling.

Cystic Fibrosis

A. Description: An autosomal-recessive disease caused by a defective gene that inhibits the transport of water and sodium in and out of cells. As a result, secretions become tenacious, which causes dysfunction of the exocrine glands. This disease can affect any race, but Caucasians are mostly affected.
  1. Lung insufficiency (most critical problem)
  2. Pancreatic insufficiency
  3. Increased loss of sodium and chloride in sweat

Clinical Assessment

A. Meconium ileus at birth (10% to 20% of cases)
B. Recurrent respiratory infection
C. Pulmonary congestion
D. Steatorrhea (excessive fat, greasy stools)
E. Foul-smelling bulky stools
F. Delayed growth and poor weight gain
G. Skin that tastes salty when kissed (caused by excessive secretions from sweat glands)
H. End stages: Cyanosis, nail-bed clubbing, congestive heart failure (CHF)

Clinical Judgment

A. Monitor respiratory status.

TABLE 5.6 Clinical Judgment Measures: Pediatric Respiratory System

Clinical Judgment Measure	Assessment Characteristics
Recognize cues	Note any tachypnea Observe for increased heart rate (low oxygen levels may cause an increase in heart rate). Color changes: a bluish color seen around the mouth, on the inside of the lips, or on the fingernails, color of the skin may also appear pale or gray. Grunting Nose flaring Retractions Sweating Wheezing Stridor Accessory muscle use
Analyze cues	Breathing patterns are consistent with age of patient (without Shortness of breath (SOB), confusion, orthopnea). Respiratory rate is consistent with age and diagnosis of patient. Nares clear without mucus. Productive/non-productive cough. Either use or no use of accessory muscles.
Prioritize cues	Keep in mind any emergent issue related to airway, breathing, or circulation (A, B, C). Observe for any change in the child's ability to respond to you, needs to be based on the child's age and developmental age. Note alertness (mentation is what is expected for age and diagnosis) Change in skin color (pale, cyanosis)
Solutions	Provide interventions at the level of need Remember that hypoxia can manifest differently from infancy to young adult Provide oxygen consistent with underlying disease pathology Teach family breathing techniques to ensure relaxation and to facilitate respirations. Encourage routine vaccinations that are required for age.
Actions	Perform resuscitation as indicated Check vital signs for normalcy of age and development Note that respiratory rate is within normal limits Auscultate lungs for consolidation. Teach family members to provide rest and exercise consistent with the patient's underlying diagnosis.
Evaluate outcomes	Respiratory status has improved (respiratory rate normal, color good, use of oxygen properly if ordered for age and patient's diagnosis). Response to questions noted by observation if infant, by response if older: Mentation within normal limits (recites date, time, mini-mental exam as an adolescent) Respiratory rate consistent with activity (walking, ADL).

TABLE 5.7 Adrenergics

Drugs/Route	Indications	Adverse Reactions	Nursing Implications
• Epinephrine Hydrochloric acid (HCl) isonicotinic acid hydrazide (INH), subcutaneous, IM, IV	• Rapid-acting bronchodilator • Drug of choice for acute asthma attack	• Tachycardia • Hypertension • Tremors • Nausea	• Give subcutaneously, IV, via nebulizer • May be repeated in 20 min

IM, Intramuscular; *IV*, intravenous

B. Assess for signs of respiratory infection.
C. Administer IV antibiotics as prescribed; manage vascular access.
D. Administer pancreatic enzymes (Cotazym-S, Pancrease: For infants, with applesauce, rice, or cereal; for an older child, with food).
E. Administer fat-soluble vitamins (A, D, E, K) in water-soluble form.
F. Administer oxygen (Box 5.1) and nebulizer treatments (recombinant human deoxyribonuclease or dornase alfa as prescribed).
G. Evaluate effectiveness of respiratory treatments.
H. Teach family percussion and postural-drainage techniques.
I. Teach dietary recommendations: High in calories, high in protein, moderate to high in fat (more calories per volume), and moderate to low in carbohydrates (to avoid an increase in carbon dioxide [CO_2] drive).

BOX 5.1 Respiratory Client

Administration of Oxygen

- Oxygen hood: used for infants.
- Nasal prongs: provide low to moderate concentrations of oxygen (up to 4 to 6 L).
- Tents: provide mist and oxygen. Monitor child's temperature. Keep edges tucked in. Keep child dry.

Measurement of Oxygenation

- Pulse oximetry measures oxygen saturation (Sa_{O_2}) of arterial Hgb non-invasively via a sensor that is usually attached to the finger or toe, or, in an infant, to sole of foot.
- Nurse should be aware of the alarm parameters signaling decreased Sa_{O_2} (usually <95%).
- Blood gas evaluation is usually monitored in respiratory clients through arterial sampling.
- Norms: P_{O_2}: 80–100 mm Hg; P_{CO_2}: 35–45 mm Hg for children (not infants and newborns)

J. Provide age-appropriate activities.
K. Refer family for genetic counseling.

HESI HINT Cystic fibrosis is now screened with newborn screening (NBS) tests performed after birth. The newborn screening test can provide a diagnosis in the child's first month of life before signs and symptoms occur.

Epiglottitis

Description: Severe life-threatening infection of the epiglottis is a medical emergency

A. Epiglottitis progresses rapidly, causing acute airway obstruction.
B. The organism usually responsible for epiglottitis is *Haemophilus influenzae* (primarily type B).

Clinical Assessment

A. Sudden onset
B. Restlessness
C. High fever
D. Sore throat, dysphagia
E. Drooling
F. Muffled voice
G. Child assuming upright sitting position with chin out and tongue protruding ("tripod position")

Clinical Judgment

A. Encourage prevention with *H. influenzae* type B (Hib) vaccine.
B. Maintain child in upright sitting position.
C. Prepare for intubation or tracheostomy.
D. Administer IV antibiotics as prescribed.
E. Prepare for hospitalization in intensive care unit (ICU).
F. Restrain as needed to prevent extubation.
G. Employ measures to decrease agitation and crying.

Bronchiolitis

Description: Viral infection of the bronchioles that is characterized by thick secretions

A. Bronchiolitis is usually caused by respiratory syncytial virus (RSV) and is found to be readily transmitted by close contact with hospital personnel, families, and other children.
B. Bronchiolitis occurs primarily in young infants.

Clinical Assessment

A. History of upper respiratory symptoms
B. Irritable, distressed infant
C. Paroxysmal coughing
D. Poor eating
E. Nasal congestion
F. Nasal flaring
G. Prolonged expiratory phase of respiration
H. Wheezing, rales can be auscultated
I. Deteriorating condition that is often indicated by shallow, rapid respirations

Clinical Judgment

A. Isolate child (isolation of choice for RSV is contact isolation).
B. Monitor respiratory status; observe for hypoxia.
C. Clear airway of secretions using a bulb syringe for suctioning.
D. Provide care in mist tent; administer oxygen as prescribed.
E. Maintain hydration (oral and IV fluids).
F. Evaluate response to respiratory therapy treatments.
G. Administer palivizumab to provide passive immunity against RSV in high-risk children (younger than 2 years of age with a history of prematurity, lung disease, or congenital heart disease [CHD]).

HESI HINT Only severe RSV lower respiratory tract infection should be treated with VIRAZOLE (ribavirin). The vast majority of infants and children with RSV infection have disease that is mild, self-limited, and does not require hospitalization or antiviral treatment. Ribavirin is a Pregnancy: Category X medication; pregnant mothers of children who are receiving ribavirin inhalation therapy and nurses who may be pregnant should not be exposed to the ribavirin aerosol.

Otitis Media

Description: Inflammatory disorder of the middle ear

A. Otitis media may be suppurative or serous.
B. Anatomic structure of the ear predisposes young child to ear infections.
C. The major cause of conductive hearing loss in children is otitis media with effusion.

Clinical Assessment

A. Fever, pain; infant may pull at ear

B. Enlarged lymph nodes
C. Discharge from ear (if drum is ruptured)
D. Upper respiratory symptoms
E. Vomiting, diarrhea

Clinical Judgment

A. Treatment of AOM includes administration of antipyretics and analgesics.
B. Antimicrobial therapy in only select patients.
C. Position child on affected side with head of bed elevated.
D. Provide comfort measure: Warm compress on affected ear.
E. Teach home care.
   1. Follow-up visit.
   2. Monitor for hearing loss.
F. Teach preventive care: Wash hands and toys frequently to reduce your chances of getting a cold or other respiratory infection.
G. Avoid cigarette smoke.
H. Get seasonal flu shots and pneumococcal vaccines.
I. Breastfeed infants instead of bottle feeding them if possible.
J. If the child has a eustachian tube malfunction leading to chronic infections, then the MD may perform a procedure called a myringotomy with placement of tympanostomy tubes that equalize pressure in the eustachian tubes.

> **HESI HINT** Respiratory disorders are the primary reason most children and their families seek medical care. Therefore, these disorders are frequently tested on the NGN-NCLEX-RN. Knowing the normal parameters of respiratory rates and the key signs of respiratory distress in children is essential!

> **HESI HINT** Watchful waiting can be applied in selected children with nonsevere acute otitis media by withholding antibiotics and observing the child for clinical improvement. Antibiotics should be promptly provided if the child's infection worsens or fails to improve within 24–48 h.

Tonsillitis

Description: Inflammation of the tonsils

Pharyngeal tonsils (adenoids) are two glands of tissue visible in the back of the throat. The tonsils function as a part of the immune system protecting the body from infections.

A. Tonsillitis may be viral or bacterial.
B. Tonsillitis may be related to infection by a Streptococcus species.
C. A complication of tonsillitis is a peritonsillar abscess, which happens when the infection spreads behind the tonsils. Early treatment is indicated as it may cause airway obstruction.

If tonsillitis is related to strep, treatment is very important because of the risk for developing post-streptococcal glomerulonephritis (PSGN), a rare kidney disease that can develop after group A strep infections. The main way to prevent PSGN is to prevent group A strep infections.

Clinical Assessment

A. Sore throat and may have difficulty swallowing that lasts longer than 48 hours
B. Fever
C. Enlarged tonsils (may have purulent discharge on tonsils)
D. Breathing may be obstructed (tonsils touching)
E. Throat culture to determine viral or bacterial cause (see Table 5.6)

Clinical Judgment

A. Collect throat culture if prescribed.
B. Instruct parents in home care.
   1. Encourage warm saline gargles.
   2. Administer antibiotics if prescribed.
   3. Manage fever with acetaminophen.
C. If a tonsillectomy is indicated:
   1. Provide preoperative teaching and assessment.
   2. Monitor for signs of postoperative bleeding.
      a. Frequent swallowing
      b. Vomiting fresh blood
      c. Clearing throat
   3. Encourage soft foods and oral fluids (avoid red fluids, which mimic signs of bleeding); do not use straws.
   4. Provide comfort measures: Ice collar helps with pain and with vasoconstriction.
   5. Provide education. Post-tonsillectomy hemorrhage is considered a surgical emergency. Hemorrhage after tonsillectomy can be classified as primary or secondary. If bleeding occurs within the first 24 hours after surgery, it is referred to as a primary hemorrhage. Secondary hemorrhage risk occurs after 24 hours. The risk of primary hemorrhage is 0.2% to 2.2%, and secondary hemorrhage is 0.1% to 4.8%, with an increase in the risk of post-tonsillectomy hemorrhage, including age above 5, chronic tonsillitis
   6. In children with hemophilia or Von Willebrand disease, rates of hemorrhage immediately after tonsillectomy are similar but are substantially higher with delayed hemorrhage.

> **HESI HINT** Teach parents why it is important to administer pain medication as prescribed. (Pain medication for this procedure generally has a cough suppressant property to suppress coughing.)

Coughing may loosen sutures, or clots, at the surgical site, causing active bleeding.

REVIEW OF RESPIRATORY DISORDERS

1. Describe the purpose of bronchodilators.
2. What are the physical assessment findings for a child with asthma?
3. What nutritional support should be provided for a child with cystic fibrosis?
4. Why is genetic counseling important for the family of a child with cystic fibrosis?
5. List signs of respiratory distress in a pediatric client.
6. What position does a child with epiglottitis assume?
7. Why are IV fluids important for a child with an increased respiratory rate?
8. Children with chronic otitis media are at risk for developing what problem?
9. What is the most common postoperative complication after a tonsillectomy? Describe the signs and symptoms of this complication.

See Answer Key at the end of this text for suggested responses.

CARDIOVASCULAR DISORDERS

Congenital Heart Disorders

Description: Heart anomalies that develop in utero and manifest at birth or shortly thereafter (Table 5.8)

A. Congenital heart disorders (CHDs) are the most common birth defects. CHDs occur in almost 1% of births. Congenital heart occurs in 4 to 10 children per live birth.
B. We can classify the different types of CHD into several categories in order to better understand the problems your baby may experience, include: *problems that cause too much blood to pass through the lungs. These defects allow oxygen-rich blood that should be traveling to the body to recirculate through the lungs, causing increased pressure and stress in the lungs. They include:*
   1. Acyanotic
      a. Left-to-right shunts or increased pulmonary blood flow
      b. Obstructive defects
      c. Cyanotic: Right to left shunts to left shunts or decreased blood flow; mixed blood flow

Acyanotic Heart Defects

Ventricular Septal Defect (Increased Pulmonary Blood Flow)

A. In this condition, a hole in the ventricular septum (a dividing wall between the two lower chambers of the heart—the right and left ventricles) occurs. Because of this opening, blood from the left ventricle flows back into the right ventricle, due to higher pressure in the left ventricle. This causes an extra volume of blood to be pumped into the lungs by the right ventricle, often creating congestion in the lungs.
B. Oxygenated blood from left ventricle is shunted to right ventricle and recirculated to the lungs.
C. Small defects may close spontaneously.
D. Large defects cause Eisenmenger syndrome or CHD and require surgical closures (Fig. 5.6).

Atrial Septal Defect (Increased Pulmonary Blood Flow)

A. In this condition, there is an abnormal opening between the two upper chambers of the heart—the right and left atria—causing an abnormal blood flow through the heart.
B. Oxygenated blood from the left atrium is shunted to the right atrium and lungs.
C. Most defects do not compromise children seriously.
D. Surgical closure is recommended before school age. It can lead to significant problems, such as CHF or atrial dysrhythmias later in life, if not corrected (Fig. 5.7).

Patent Ductus Arteriosus (Increased Pulmonary Blood Flow)

A. Patent ductus arteriosus (PDA): There is an abnormal opening between the aorta and the pulmonary artery. This defect short circuits the normal pulmonary vascular system and allows blood to mix between the pulmonary artery and the aorta. Prior to birth, there is an open passageway between the two blood vessels. This opening closes soon after birth. When it does not close, some blood

TABLE 5.8 Congenital Heart Disorders

Congenital Heart Defects	Conditions	Hemodynamics	Classical Symptoms
ACYANOTIC L → R shunt	ASD VSD PDA	Increased pulmonary blood flow	Increase fatigue Murmur Increase risk of endocarditis
	Coarctation/stenosis of aorta	Obstructive pulmonary blood flow	CHF Growth retardation
CYANOTIC R → L shunt	Tetralogy of Fallot	Decreased pulmonary blood flow	Squatting
	Transposition of the great vessels (TGV) TA	Mixed pulmonary blood flow	Cyanosis Clubbing Syncope

ASD, Atrial septal defect; *CHF,* congestive heart failure, *PDA,* patent ductus arteriosus; *TA,* truncus arteriosus; *VSD,* ventricular septal defect
Created by Katherine, T. Ralph MSN, RN, Curriculum Manager, Elsevier-NHE.

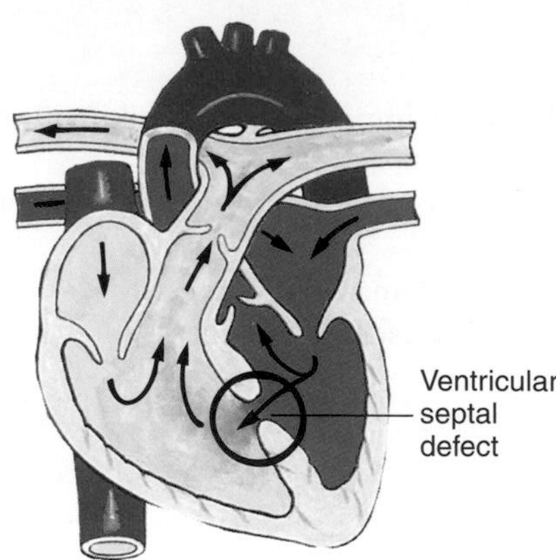

Fig. 5.6 Ventricular Septal Defect. (From Hockenberry, M. J., & Wilson, D. [2011]. *Wong's nursing care of infants and children* [9th ed.]. St. Louis: Mosby.)

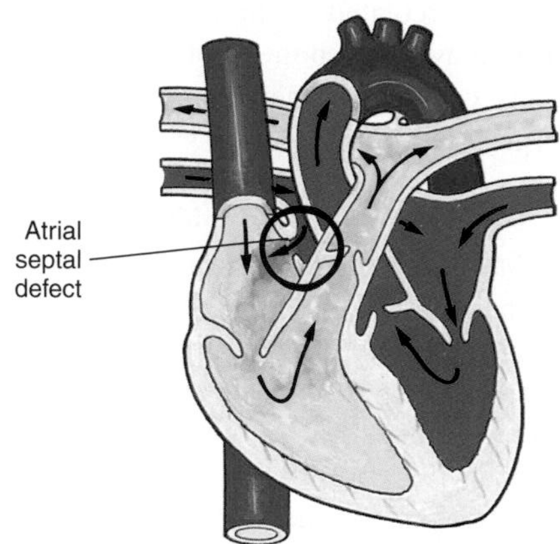

Fig. 5.7 Atrial Septal Defect. (From Hockenberry, M. J., & Wilson, D. [2011]. *Wong's nursing care of infants and children* [9th ed.]. St. Louis: Mosby.)

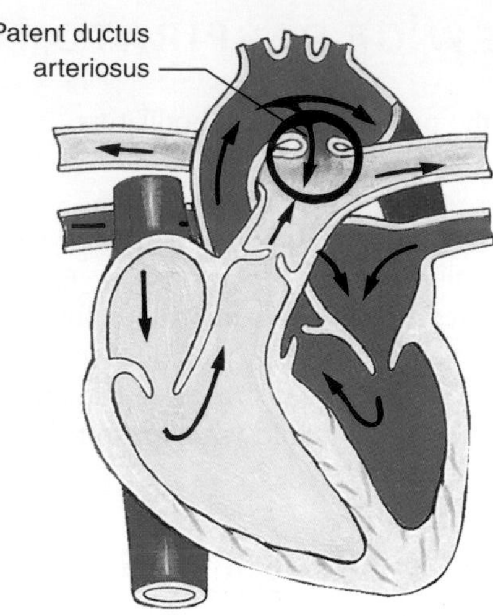

Fig. 5.8 Patent Ductus Arteriosus. (From Hockenberry, M. J., & Wilson, D. [2011]. *Wong's nursing care of infants and children* [9th ed.]. St. Louis: Mosby.)

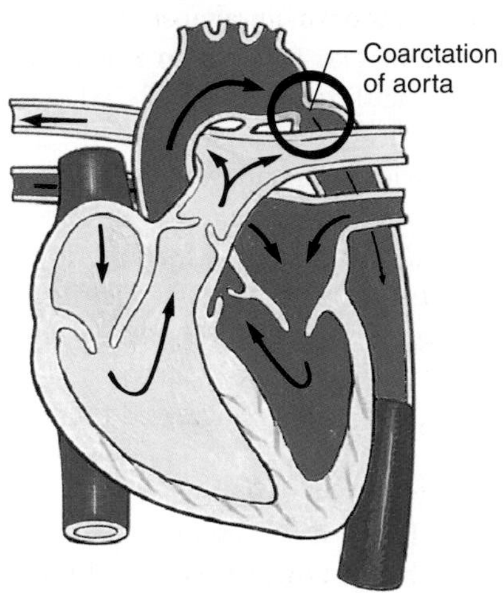

Fig. 5.9 Coarctation of the Aorta. (From Hockenberry, M. J., & Wilson, D. [2011]. *Wong's nursing care of infants and children* [9th ed.]. St. Louis: Mosby.)

returns to the lungs. PDA is often seen in premature infants.

B. Usually closes within 72 hours after birth.
C. Remains patent; oxygenated blood from the aorta returns to the pulmonary artery.
D. Increased blood flow to the lungs causes pulmonary hypertension.
E. May require medical intervention with indomethacin (Indocin), Ibuprofen or Tylenol/Ofirmev administration, or surgical closure (Fig. 5.8).
F. Characteristic machine-like murmur

Atrioventricular canal (AVC or AV canal): AVC is a complex heart problem that involves several abnormalities of structures inside the heart, including atrial septal defect (ASD), ventricular septal defect (VSD), and improperly formed mitral and/or tricuspid valves.

Problems That Cause Too Little Blood to Travel to the Body

These defects are a result of underdeveloped chambers of the heart or blockages in blood vessels that prevent the proper amount of blood from traveling to the body to meet its needs. They include:

Coarctation of the Aorta
Plaque build up
Blood clots
Narrowed blood vessels

Coarctation of the Aorta (Obstruction of Blood Flow From Ventricles)

A. In this condition, the aorta is narrowed or constricted, obstructing blood flow to the lower part of the body and increasing blood pressure above the constriction.
B. The most common sites are the aortic valve and the aorta near the ductus arteriosus.
C. A common finding is hypertension in the upper extremities and decreased or absent pulses in the lower extremities.
D. Defect may require surgical correction (Fig. 5.9).

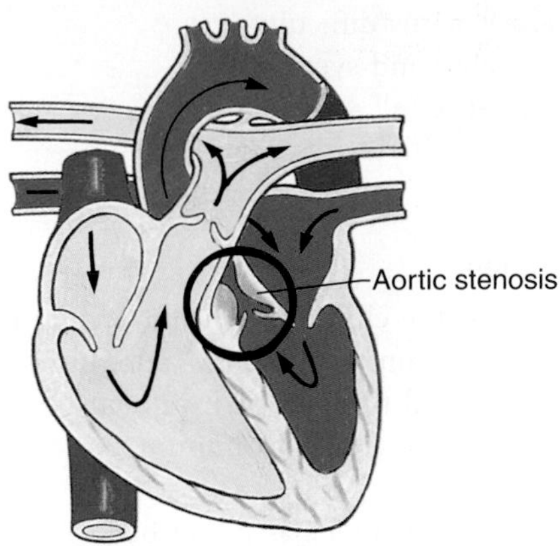

Fig. 5.10 Aortic Stenosis. (From Hockenberry, M. J., & Wilson, D. [2011]. *Wong's nursing care of infants and children* [9th ed.]. St. Louis: Mosby.)

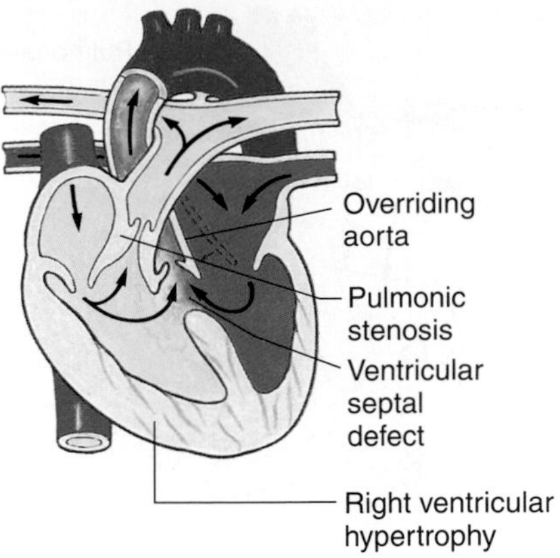

Fig. 5.11 Tetralogy of Fallot. (From Hockenberry, M. J., & Wilson, D. [2011]. *Wong's nursing care of infants and children* [9th ed.]. St. Louis: Mosby.)

Aortic Stenosis (Obstruction of Blood Flow From Ventricles)

A. In this condition, the aortic valve between the left ventricle and the aorta did not form properly and is narrowed, making it difficult for the heart to pump blood to the body.
B. Oxygenated blood flow from the left ventricle into systemic circulation is diminished.
C. Symptoms are caused by low cardiac output.
D. May require surgical correction (Fig. 5.10).

Hypoplastic left heart syndrome (HLHS): A combination of several abnormalities of the heart and the great blood vessels.

Problems That Cause Too Little Blood to Pass Through the Lungs

These conditions allow blood that has not been to the lungs to pick up oxygen to travel to the body. The body does not receive enough oxygen with these heart problems. Babies with these forms of CHD may be cyanotic. These conditions include:

2. Cyanotic
   a. Right-to-left shunts or decreased blood flow
   b. Mixed blood flow

Tetralogy of Fallot (Decreased Pulmonary Blood Flow)

A. Tetralogy of Fallot (TOF): This condition is characterized by four defects, including an abnormal opening, or VSD; a narrowing (stenosis) at or just beneath the pulmonary valve that partially blocks the flow of blood from the right side of the heart to the lungs; a right ventricle that is more muscular than normal and often enlarged; and an aorta that lies directly over the VSD.

TOF requires staged surgery for correction (Fig. 5.11).

> **HESI HINT** HLHS: A combination of several abnormalities of the heart and the great blood vessels.

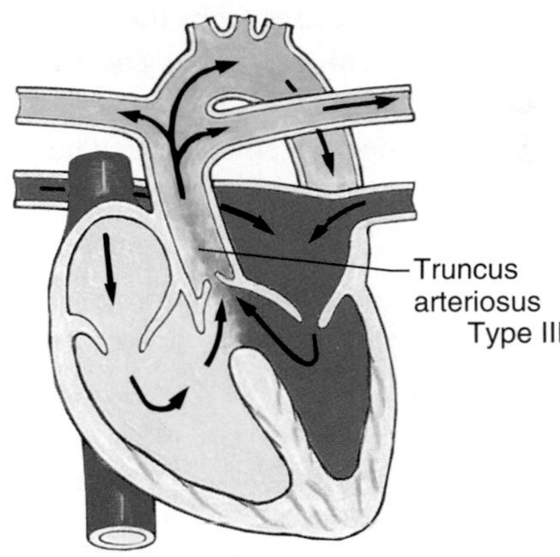

Fig. 5.12 Truncus Arteriosus. (From Hockenberry, M. J., & Wilson, D. [2011]. *Wong's nursing care of infants and children* [9th ed.]. St. Louis: Mosby.)

Truncus Arteriosus (Mixed Blood Flow)

A. In this condition, the aorta and pulmonary artery start as a single blood vessel, which eventually divides and becomes two separate arteries. Truncus arteriosus (TA) occurs when the single great vessel fails to separate completely, leaving a connection between the aorta and pulmonary artery.
B. One main vessel receives blood from the left and right ventricles together.
C. Blood mixes in right and left ventricles through a large VSD, resulting in cyanosis.
D. Increased pulmonary resistance results in increased cyanosis.
E. This congenital defect requires surgical correction; only the presence of the large VSD allows for survival at birth (Fig. 5.12).

Transposition of the Great Vessels (Mixed Blood Flow)

A. Transposition of the great vessels (TGA): With this condition, the positions of the pulmonary artery and the aorta are reversed.
B. The great vessels are reversed; the pulmonary artery leaves the left ventricle, and the aorta exits from the right ventricle.

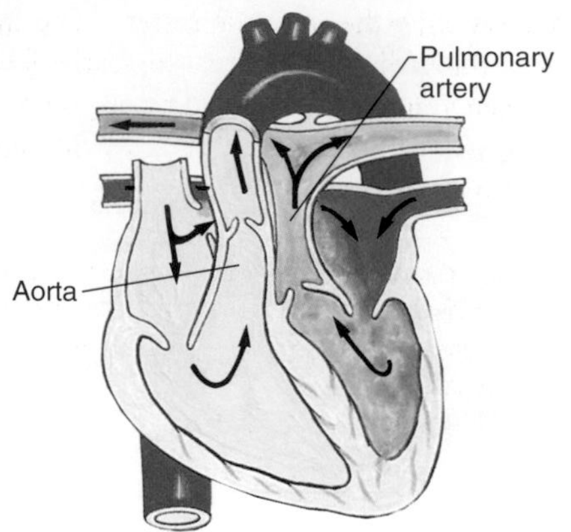

Fig. 5.13 Transposition of the Great Vessels. (From Hockenberry, M. J., & Wilson D. [2011]. *Wong's nursing care of infants and children* [9th ed.]. St. Louis: Mosby.)

C. The pulmonary circulation arises from the left ventricle, and the systemic circulation arises from the right ventricle.
D. This is incompatible with life unless coexisting VSD, ASD, and/or PDA is present.
E. The diagnosis is a medical emergency. The child is given prostaglandin E (PGE) to keep the ductus open (Fig. 5.13).

BOX 5.2 Congenital Heart Disease Conditions.

Double outlet right ventricle (DORV): In this condition, both the aorta and the pulmonary artery are connected to the right ventricle.
Tricuspid atresia: In this condition, there is no tricuspid valve, which means no blood flows from the right atrium to the right ventricle.
Pulmonary atresia: This is a complicated CHD in which there is abnormal development of the pulmonary valve.

F. Hemodynamic classification may be used.
   1. Increased pulmonary blood flow defects (ASD, VSD, PDA)
   2. Obstructive defects (coarctation of aorta, aortic stenosis [AS])
   3. Decreased pulmonary blood flow defects (TOF)
   4. Mixed defects (TGA, TA)

Care of Children With Congenital Heart Disease

Clinical Assessment

A. Manifestations of CHD
   1. Murmur (present or absent; thrill or rub)
   2. Cyanosis, clubbing of digits
   3. Poor feeding, poor weight gain, FTT
   4. Frequent regurgitation
   5. Frequent respiratory infections
   6. Activity intolerance, fatigue
B. The following are assessed:
   1. Heart rate and rhythm and heart sounds
   2. Respiratory status/difficulty
   3. Pulses (quality and symmetry)
   4. Blood pressure (all 4 extremities)
   5. Feeding difficulties; tires easily

Clinical Judgment

A. Provide care for the child with cardiovascular dysfunction.
   1. Monitor hydration; defects may cause heart failure (HF).
   2. Maintain neutral thermal environment.
   3. Organize activities to help minimize the child's energy expenditure.
   4. Administer medications as prescribed.
   5. Monitor laboratory data closely.
   6. Monitor for signs of deteriorating condition or HF.
   7. Teach family how to monitor for HF.
B. Assist with diagnostic tests and support family during diagnosis.
   1. Electrocardiogram (ECG)
   2. Echocardiography

HESI HINT Congenital heart problems range from simple to complex. Some heart problems can be monitored and medically managed while others will require heart surgery or cardiac catheterization often in the first few hours after birth (Stanford Children's' Health, 2021 *Congenital Heart Disease*).

Prepare family and child for cardiac catheterization (conducted when surgery is probable or as an intervention for certain procedures).

1. Risks of catheterization are similar to those for a child undergoing cardiac surgery:
   a. Arrhythmias
   b. Bleeding
   c. Perforation
   d. Phlebitis
   e. Arterial obstruction at the entry site
2. Child requires reassurance and close monitoring after catheterization:
   a. Vital signs
   b. Pulses
   c. Incision site
   d. Cardiac rhythm
3. Prepare family and child (as able) for surgical intervention if necessary.

Prepare child as appropriate for age.

1. Show ICU.
2. Explain chest tubes, IV lines, monitors, dressings, and ventilator.
3. Show family and child waiting area for families.
4. Use a doll or a drawing for explanations.
5. Provide emotional support.
6. Include and incorporate family as much as possible in client teachings.

HESI HINT Basic differences between cyanotic and acyanotic defects:
- Acyanotic: Has abnormal circulation; however, all blood entering the systemic circulation is oxygenated.
- Cyanotic: Has abnormal circulation with unoxygenated blood entering the systemic circulation.

Heart Failure

CHF is more often associated with acyanotic defects.

Description: Condition in which the heart is unable to effectively pump the volume of blood that is presented to it (see Table 5.8).

HESI HINT CHF is a common complication of CHD. HF reflects the increased workload of the heart caused by shunts or obstructions. The two objectives in treating CHF are to reduce the workload of the heart and increase cardiac output.

Clinical Assessment

A. Edema (face, eyes of infants), weight gain

Clinical Assessment

A. Monitor vital signs frequently and report signs of increasing distress.
B. Maintain neutral thermal environment.
C. Monitor for signs of deteriorating condition or HF.
D. Assess respiratory functioning frequently.
E. Elevate head of bed or use infant seat.
F. Administer oxygen therapy if prescribed.
G. Administer medications as prescribed.
H. Monitor hydration, maintain strict input and output (I&O); defects may cause HF (weigh infant and report unusual weight gains).
I. Monitor laboratory data closely.
J. Gavage-feed infants if unable to get adequate nutrition by mouth.
K. Teach family how to monitor for HF. Organize activities to help minimize the child's energy expenditure.

HESI HINT When frequent weights are required, weigh child on the same scale at the same time of day so that accurate comparisons can be made.

Rheumatic Fever

Description: Rheumatic fever is the most common cause of acquired health disease in children. It affects the aortic and mitral valves of the heart and is associated with an antecedent beta-hemolytic streptococcal infection. Most importantly it is a collagen disease that injures the heart, blood vessels, joints, and subcutaneous tissue. Group A Streptococcus (GAS) causes strep throat and scarlet fever. It usually takes about 1 to 5 weeks after strep throat or scarlet fever for rheumatic fever to develop. Rheumatic fever is thought to be caused by a response of the body's defense system—the immune system. The immune system responds to the earlier strep throat or scarlet fever infection and causes a generalized inflammatory response. Rheumatic fever can be treated with appropriate antibiotics such as penicillin or erythromycin.

HESI HINT People cannot catch rheumatic fever from someone else because it is an immune response and not an infection. However, people with strep throat or scarlet fever can spread group A strep to others, primarily through respiratory droplets.

Inform dentist and other health care providers of diagnosis so they can evaluate the necessity for prophylactic antibiotics.

Rheumatic fever with carditis and clinically significant residual heart disease requires antibiotic treatment for a minimum of 10 years after the latest episode; prophylaxis is required until the patient is aged at least 40 to 45 years and is sometimes continued for life.

Rheumatic fever with carditis and no residual heart disease aside from mild mitral regurgitation requires antibiotic treatment for 10 years or until age 25 years (whichever is longer).

Rheumatic fever without carditis requires antibiotic treatment for 5 years or until the patient is aged 18 to 21 years (whichever is longer).

HESI HINT Early diagnosis of these infections and treatment with antibiotics are key to preventing rheumatic fever.

Pediatric Patients With Congenital Heart Disease (CHD)

Children born with a birth defect such as CHD may need prophylactic antibiotics because they may be susceptible to infection. However, if a child is put on antibiotics, it should be because of cyanotic heart disease (birth defects with oxygen levels lower than normal) that has not been fully repaired or children who may have surgical shunts. Other CHD defects that may need prophylaxis treatment would be defects repaired with prosthetic material or a first device that was implanted within 6 months. Those with CHD have residual defects such as abnormal flow or persistent leaks ("Infective Endocarditis," n.d.).

Clinical Assessment

A. Chest pain, shortness of breath (pericarditis), heart murmur, cardiomegaly
B. Tachycardia, even during sleep
C. Migratory large-joint pain, painful, tender joints (arthritis), most commonly in the knees, ankles, elbows, and wrists; with nodules under skin near joints
D. Fatigue
E. Chorea (irregular involuntary movements)
F. Rash (erythema marginatum)
G. Fever

H. Laboratory findings
  1. Elevated erythrocyte sedimentation rate (ESR)
  2. C reactive protein
  3. Elevated antistreptolysin O (ASO) titer

ASO is an antibody targeted against streptolysin O, a toxic enzyme produced by group A Streptococcus bacteria.

Elevated ESR
  4. EKG
  5. Echocardiogram

Clinical Interventions

A. Monitor vital signs.
B. Assess for increasing signs of cardiac distress.
C. Encourage bed rest (as needed for fatigue).
D. Assist with ambulation.
E. Reassure child and family that chorea is temporary.
F. Administer prescribed medications.
  1. Penicillin or erythromycin
  2. Aspirin for antiinflammatory and anticoagulant actions
G. Teach home care program

Explain the necessity for prophylactics.

  1. Antibiotics taken either orally or IM
  2. Children given penicillin G benzathine at a dose of 1.2 million U IM q4w
  3. IM penicillin G each month (Table 5.10)
    a. Long-term administration of oral penicillin may be used in lieu of the IM route. Erythromycin or sulfadiazine may be used in patients who are allergic to penicillin.

Kawasaki Disease (Mucocutaneous Lymph Node Syndrome)

Description: Kawasaki disease causes swelling (inflammation) in the walls of medium-sized arteries throughout the body. It primarily affects children. The inflammation tends to affect the coronary arteries, which supply blood to the heart muscle.

Kawasaki disease is sometimes called mucocutaneous lymph node syndrome because it also affects glands that swell during an infection (lymph nodes), skin, and the mucous membranes inside the mouth, nose, and throat.

Signs of Kawasaki disease, such as a high fever and peeling skin, can be frightening. The good news is that Kawasaki disease is usually treatable, and most children recover from Kawasaki disease without serious problems.

Risk Factors

Three things are known to increase your child's risk of developing Kawasaki disease.

- Age. Children under 5 years old are most at risk of Kawasaki disease.
- Sex. Boys are slightly more likely than girls to develop Kawasaki disease.

Ethnicity. Children of Asian or Pacific Island descent, such as Japanese or Korean, have higher rates of Kawasaki disease.

Complications

Kawasaki disease is a leading cause of acquired heart disease in children. However, with effective treatment, only a few children have lasting damage.

Heart complications include:

Inflammation of blood vessels, usually the coronary arteries, that supply blood to the heart

Inflammation of the heart muscle

Heart valve problems

Any of these complications can damage your child's heart. Inflammation of the coronary arteries can lead to weakening and bulging of the artery wall (aneurysm). Aneurysms increase

TABLE 5.9 Congestive Heart Failure Signs and Symptom

CONGESTIVE HEART FAILURE			
Cardiac	**Pulmonary**	**Gastrointestinal**	**Integumentary**
1. Tachycardia 2. Poor circulation 3. Weight gain (excessive fluid)	1. Tachypnea 2. Shortness of breath 3. Cyanosis 4. Grunting 5. Wheezing 6. Pulmonary congestion	1. Difficulty feeding 2. Hepatomegaly	Diaphoresis (especially head) Edema (face, eyes in infants)

TABLE 5.10 Anti-Infective

Drug/Route	Indications	Adverse Reactions	Nursing Implications
• Penicillin G IM	• Prophylaxis for recurrence of rheumatic fever	• Allergic reactions ranging from rashes to anaphylactic shock and death	• Penicillin G is released very slowly over several weeks, giving sustained levels of concentration. • Have emergency equipment available wherever medication is administered. • Always determine existence of allergies to penicillin and cephalosporins; check chart and record and inquire of client and family.

the risk of blood clots, which could lead to a heart attack or cause life-threatening internal bleeding.

For a very small percentage of children who develop coronary artery problems, Kawasaki disease can cause death, even with treatment (Mayo Clinic, 2021a, *Kawasaki Disease*).

Clinical Assessment

Kawasaki disease signs and symptoms usually appear in three phases.

Phase 1

Signs and symptoms of the first phase may include:

- A fever that often is higher than 102.2°F (39°C) and lasts more than 3 days
- Extremely red eyes without a thick discharge
- A rash on the main part of the body and in the genital area
- Red, dry, cracked lips and an extremely red, swollen tongue
- Swollen, red skin on the palms of the hands and the soles of the feet
- Swollen lymph nodes in the neck and perhaps elsewhere
- Irritability

Phase 2

In the second phase of the disease, your child may develop:

- Peeling of the skin on the hands and feet, especially the tips of the fingers and toes, often in large sheets
- Joint pain
- Diarrhea
- Vomiting
- Abdominal pain

Phase 3

In the third phase of the disease, signs and symptoms slowly go away unless complications develop. It may be as long as 8 weeks before energy levels seem normal again.

Clinical Judgment

A. Initial treatment for KD patients includes IV immune globulin (IVIG; 2 g/kg) administered as a single infusion over 8 to 12 hours
B. Aspirin (30 to 50 mg/kg daily during IV infusion)
C. Administer acetaminophen for fever as prescribed.
D. Cardiac status needs to be monitored.
  1. Monitor I&O
  2. Obtain daily weights
E. Minimize skin discomfort with lotions and cool compresses.
F. Initiate meticulous mouth care.
G. Monitor intake of clear liquids and soft foods.
H. Support family as they comfort child during periods of irritability.
I. Provide discharge teaching and home referral (Table 5.11).

REVIEW OF CARDIOVASCULAR DISORDERS

1. Differentiate between: Problems that cause too much blood to pass through the lungs. Problems that cause too little blood to pass through the lungs. Problems that cause too little blood to travel to the body.
2. List the four defects associated with TOF.
3. List the common signs of cardiac problems in an infant.
4. What are the two objectives in treating CHF?
5. Describe nursing judgment to reduce the workload of the heart.
6. What cardiac complications are associated with rheumatic fever?
7. What medications are used to treat rheumatic fever?

See Answer Key at the end of this text for suggested responses.

NEUROMUSCULAR DISORDERS

Down Syndrome

Description: Most common chromosomal abnormality in children

A. Down syndrome is evidenced by various physical characteristics and by cognitive impairment (Fig. 5.14).
B. Down syndrome occurs when cell division is abnormal; as a result, there is extra genetic material from chromosome 21 and, in less than 5% of cases, a translocation of chromosome 21.
C. Common associated problems
  1. Cardiac defects
  2. Respiratory infections
  3. Feeding difficulties
  4. Delayed developmental skills
  5. Low IQ range of 20 to 70
  6. Skeletal defects
  7. Altered immune function
  8. Endocrine dysfunctions; hypothyroidism

Clinical Interventions

A. Assist and support parents during the diagnostic process and management of child's associated problems.
B. Assess and monitor growth and development.
C. Teach use of bulb syringe for suctioning nares.
D. Teach signs of respiratory infection.
E. Assist family with feeding problems.
F. Feed to back and side of mouth.

TABLE 5.11 Clinical Judgment Measures: Pediatric Cardiovascular

Clinical Judgment Measure	Assessment Characteristics
Recognize cues	Abnormal heart rate for age/abnormal rhythm if on monitor or during pulse evaluation Note paleness/abnormal color/duskiness Note tachypnea Fatigue or fatigue with exertion, even just nibbling or eating Syncope Not on growth curve Squatting or leaning forward to breath Diaphoresis Edema Audible wheezing Shortness of breath
Analyze cues	Pulse evaluation abnormal, analyze on monitor Saturation monitor Tachypnea related to abnormal heart capabilities such as pulmonary edema and congestive heart failure Tachypnea, shortness of breath, or audible wheezing, respiratory or cardiac in origin Diaphoresis cardiac versus inability to manage heat Below growth curve due to fatigue or inability to sustain weight due to work of breathing/cardiac failure
Prioritize cues	Remember Circulation-Airway-Breathing (CAB) in resuscitation with cardiac failure. Analyze rhythm on a monitor for fibrillation; only cure is defibrillation (automated external defibrillator (AED) may be only cure) For younger children oxygen may be the initial cure if respiratory system is functional. Tachypnea relieve work of breathing/oxygen/diuretic may be needed
Solutions	Interventions may vary based on age and underlying conditions. Cardiac congenital lesions, cyanotic repaired/single ventricle/pulmonary overload versus need for oxygen Pulmonary hypertension requiring need for afterload reduction, evaluating symptoms to clinically intervene
Actions	Evaluate vital signs and intervene as indicated Resuscitation based on underlying known cardiac anomaly Saturation monitor Monitor and/or baseline ECG/AED if indicated. Auscultate for murmur. Provide preload support or afterload reduction as indicated. Teach family home interventions to sustain child.
Evaluate outcomes	Able to sustain vital signs with normal rhythm and saturations. Able to sustain caloric intake and maintain and gain weight based on growth curve. Respiratory rate is normalized for age. Diaphoresis is resolved. Edema is treated. Color has normalized.

G. Monitor for signs of cardiac difficulty or respiratory infection.
H. Refer family to early intervention program.
I. Refer to other specialists as indicated: Nutritionist, speech therapist, physical therapist, and occupational therapist.

> **HESI HINT** The nursing goal in caring for a child with Down syndrome is to help the child reach his or her optimal level of functioning.

Cerebral Palsy

Description: Cerebral palsy (CP) is a group of disorders that affect a person's ability to move and maintain balance and posture. CP is the most common motor disability in childhood. CP is caused by abnormal brain development or damage to the developing brain that affects a person's ability to control his or her muscles.

Nonprogressive injury to the motor centers of the brain causing neuromuscular problems of spasticity or dyskinesia (involuntary movements). This injury can occur to a healthy infant during uterine development, the birthing process, exposure to an infection such as meningitis during the early years of development; it is irreversible. The extent of the damage is dependent on the location of trauma to the brain; the symptoms either worsen or improve over time.

A. Associated problems may include cognitive impairment and seizures.
B. Causes include
   1. Anoxic injury before, during, or after birth
   2. Maternal infections
   3. Kernicterus
   4. Low birth weight (major risk factor)

HEAD to TOE

A. Common physical characteristics
1. Small head
2. Flat, wide nasal bridge
3. Inner epicanthal eye fold
4. Upward, outward slant of eyes
5. Brushfield spots on the iris (white spots)
6. Small, irregularly shaped ears; low-set
7. Small mouth and protruding tongue
8. Short neck
9. Short, stubby hands with a single crease in palm (Simian crease)
10. Short arms and legs in comparison to their body
11. Short in stature
12. Hypotonic flexibility
13. Atlantoaxial instability
14. Short, stubby toes with an enlarged space between the big toe and other toes.
15. Hyperextensible and lax joint (hypotonia)

Fig. 5.14 Head-to-Toe Common Characteristics of Down Syndrome. (Created by: Katherine T. Ralph MSN, RN, Curriculum Manager, Elsevier-NHE.)

Clinical Assessment

Cerebral palsy (CP) according to the main type of movement disorder involved. Depending on which areas of the brain are affected, one or more of the following movement disorders can occur:
Stiff muscles (spasticity)
Uncontrollable movements (dyskinesia)
Poor balance and coordination (ataxia)

A. Spastic diplegia/diparesis—In this type of CP, muscle stiffness is mainly in the legs, with the arms less affected or not affected at all. People with spastic diplegia might have difficulty walking because tight hip and leg muscles cause their legs to pull together, turn inward, and cross at the knees (also known as scissoring).
B. Spastic hemiplegia/hemiparesis—This type of CP affects only one side of a person's body; usually the arm is more affected than the leg.
C. Spastic quadriplegia/quadriparesis—Spastic quadriplegia is the most severe form of spastic CP and affects all four limbs, the trunk, and the face. People with spastic quadriparesis usually cannot walk and often have other developmental disabilities such as intellectual disability; seizures; or problems with vision, hearing, or speech.

Dyskinetic Cerebral Palsy (also includes athetoid, choreoathetoid, and dystonic cerebral palsies). People with dyskinetic CP have problems controlling the movement of their hands, arms, feet, and legs, making it difficult to sit and walk. The movements are uncontrollable and can be slow and writhing or rapid and jerky. Sometimes the face and tongue are affected and the person has a hard time sucking, swallowing, and talking. A person with dyskinetic CP has muscle tone that can change (varying from too tight to too loose) not only from day to day, but even during a single day.

Ataxic Cerebral Palsy. People with ataxic CP have problems with balance and coordination. They might be unsteady when they walk. They might have a hard time with quick movements or movements that need a lot of control, like writing. They might have a hard time controlling their hands or arms when they reach for something.

Mixed Cerebral Palsy. Some people have symptoms of more than one type of CP. The most common type of mixed CP is spastic-dyskinetic CP.

Clinical Interventions

A. Identify CP through follow-up of high-risk infants such as premature infants, breech births, cardiac and/or respiratory distress during birth, low Apgar scores, a product of multiple pregnancies, and/or severe jaundiced.
B. Refer to community-based agencies.
C. Coordinate with physical therapist, occupational therapist, speech therapist, nutritionist, orthopedic surgeon, and neurologist (Centers for Disease Control and Prevention, 2021e, December 2, *Cerebral Palsy*).

> **HESI HINT** Feed an infant or child with CP using nursing judgment aimed at preventing aspiration. Position child upright and support the lower jaw.

I. Support family through grief process at diagnosis and throughout the child's life. Caring for severely affected children is very challenging.
II. Administer anticonvulsant medications such as phenytoin (Dilantin) if prescribed (see Table 5.12).
III. Administer diazepam (Valium) for muscle spasms if prescribed (see Table 7.4).

TABLE 5.12 **Anticonvulsants**

Drugs/Routes	Indications	Adverse Reactions	Nursing Implications
• Phenobarbital the medication is taken by mouth (PO), IM, IV	• Tonic-clonic and partial seizures • Is the longest acting of common barbiturates • Usually combined with other drugs	• Drowsiness • Nystagmus • Ataxia • Paradoxic excitement	• Therapeutic levels: 15.40 mcg/mL • Avoid rapid IV infusion. • Monitor blood pressure during IV infusion.
• Phenytoin PO, IV	• Tonic-clonic and partial seizures	• Gingival hyperplasia • Dermatitis • Ataxia • Nausea, anorexia • Bone marrow depression • Nystagmus	• Therapeutic levels: 10–20 mcg/mL • Monitor any drug interactions. • Do not administer with milk. • Ensure meticulous oral hygiene. • Monitor CBC. • Report to physician if any rash develops. • For IV administration, flush IV line before and after with normal saline only.
• Fosphenytoin sodium IM, IV	• Generalized convulsive status epilepticus • Prevention and treatment of seizures during neurosurgery • Short-term parenteral replacement for phenytoin oral (Dilantin)	• Rapid IV infusion can cause hypotension. • Severe: ataxia, CNS toxicity, confusion, gingival hyperplasia, irritability, lupus erythematosus, nervousness, nystagmus, paradoxic excitement, Stevens–Johnson syndrome, toxic epidural necrosis	• Use for short-term parenteral use (IV infusion or IM injection) only. • Should always be prescribed and dispensed in phenytoin sodium equivalents (PEs) • Before IV infusion, dilute in D_5W or NS to administer. • Infuse at IV rate of no more than 150 mg PE/min.
• Valproic acid PO	• Absence seizures • Myoclonic seizures	• Hepatotoxicity, especially in children less than 2 years • Prolonged bleeding times • GI disturbances	• Monitor liver function. • Potentiates phenobarbital and Dilantin, altering blood levels • Therapeutic levels: 50–100 mEq/mL
• Carbamazepine PO	• Tonic-clonic, mixed seizures • Drowsiness • Ataxia	• Hepatitis • Agranulocytosis	• Monitor liver function while on therapy. • Therapeutic levels: 6–12 mcg/mL
• Lamotrigine PO	• Partial seizures • Tonic-clonic seizures • Absence seizures	• Dizziness • Headache • Nausea • Rash	• Withhold drug if rash develops. • Do not discontinue abruptly.
• Clonazepam PO	• Absence seizures • Myoclonic seizures	• Drowsiness • Hyperactivity • Agitation • Increased salivation	• Therapeutic levels: 20–80 mcg/mL • Do not abruptly discontinue drug. • Monitor liver function, CBC, and renal function periodically.

CBC, Complete blood count; *CNS,* central nervous system; *IM,* intramuscular; *IV,* intravenous

Attention-Deficit/Hyperactivity Disorder

Description: Attention-deficit/hyperactivity disorder (ADHD) is one of the most common neurodevelopmental disorders of childhood. It is usually first diagnosed in childhood and often lasts into adulthood. Children with ADHD may have trouble paying attention, controlling impulsive behaviors, or be overly active.

There are three different types of ADHD, depending on which types of symptoms are strongest in the individual:

Predominantly Inattentive Presentation: It is hard for the individual to organize or finish a task, to pay attention to details, or to follow instructions or conversations. The person is easily distracted or forgets details of daily routines.

Predominantly Hyperactive-Impulsive Presentation: The person fidgets and talks a lot. It is hard to sit still for long (e.g., for a meal or while doing homework). Smaller children may run, jump, or climb constantly. The individual feels restless and has trouble with impulsivity. Someone who is impulsive may interrupt others a lot, grab things from people, or speak at inappropriate times. It is hard for the person to wait their turn or listen to directions. A person with impulsiveness may have more accidents and injuries than others.

Combined Presentation: Symptoms of the above two types are equally present in the person.

Symptoms can change over time; the presentation may change over time as well. In most cases, several treatment options may be used. These include a combination of medications, behavior therapy, dietary changes, or specific treatment plans specific for one's age (Centers for Disease Control and Prevention, 2021, September 23, *Attention Deficit Hyperactivity Disorder*, Centers for Disease Control and Prevention).

Spina Bifida

Description: Malformation of the vertebrae and spinal cord, which can happen anywhere along the spine if the neural tube does not close all the way, which causes damage to the spinal cord and nerves, resulting in varying degrees of disability and deformity depending on the location of the malformation (Fig. 5.15).

Spina bifida might cause physical and intellectual disabilities that range from mild to severe. The severity depends on:

- The size and location of the opening in the spine.
- Whether part of the spinal cord and nerves are affected.

Types of spina bifida

1. Spina bifida occulta. There is a small gap in the spine, but no opening or sac on the back. The spinal cord and the nerves usually are normal and may not be discovered until late childhood or adulthood. This type of spina bifida usually does not cause any disabilities.
2. Meningocele. There is a sac of fluid that comes through an opening along the back, contains only meninges and spinal fluid, but the spinal cord is not in this sac. There is usually little or no nerve damage, and this type of spina bifida can cause minor disabilities.
3. Myelomeningocele is the most serious type of spina bifida. There is a sac of fluid that comes through an opening in the back. Part of the spinal cord and nerves are in this sac and are damaged. This type of spina bifida causes moderate to severe disabilities, causing incontinence, parathesis, and paralysis.

A. Prevention
   1. Women in childbearing years before and during pregnancy should consume a minimum of 400 mcg of folic acid daily.

B. Avoid latex in children with spina bifida.

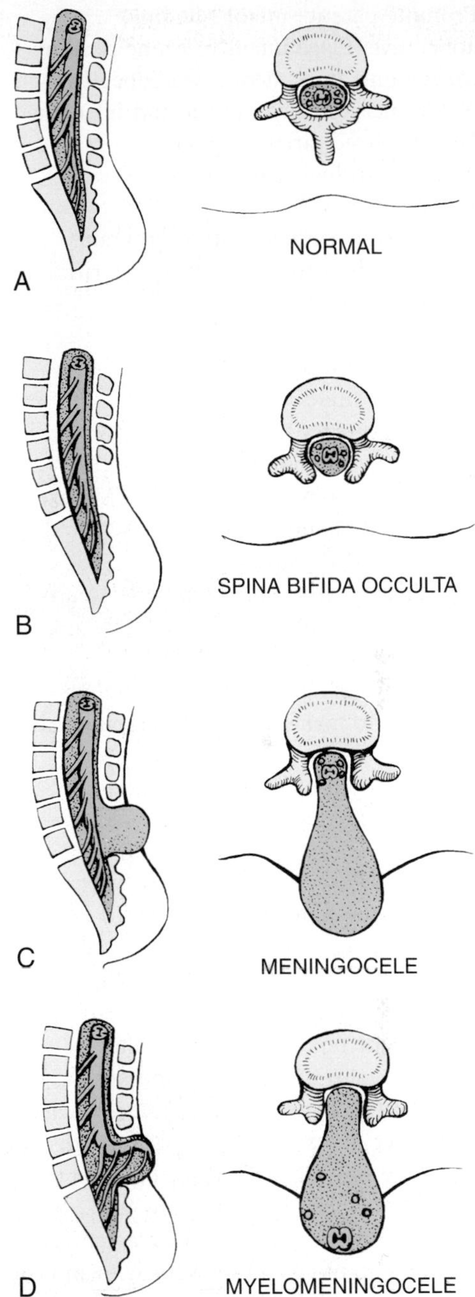

Fig. 5.15 Midline Defects of Osseous Spine With Varying Degrees of Neural Herniations. (A) Normal. (B) Spina bifida occulta. (C) Meningocele. (D) Myelomeningocele. (From Hockenberry, M. J., & Wilson, D. [2013]. *Wong's essentials of pediatric nursing* [9th ed.]. St. Louis: Mosby.)

Clinical Assessment

A. Spina bifida occulta: Dimple with or without hair tuft at base of spine
B. Presence of sac in myelomeningocele
C. Paralysis and parathesis below the defect
D. Head circumference at variance with norms on growth grids
E. Associated problems
   1. Hydrocephalus (90% with myelomeningocele)
   2. Neurogenic bladder, poor anal sphincter tone
   3. Congenital dislocated hips
   4. Club feet
   5. Skin problems associated with parathesis below the defect
   6. Scoliosis

Clinical Judgment

A. Preoperative: Place infant in prone position.
   1. Keep sac free of stool and urine.
   2. Cover sac with moist sterile dressing.
   3. Position child on abdomen, legs in natural position.
   4. Measure head circumference at least every 8 hours or every shift; check fontanel.
   5. Assess neurologic function.
   6. Monitor for signs of infection.
   7. Catheterize routinely (usually every 6 hours).

8. Promote parent–infant bonding.

B. Postoperative: Place infant in prone position.
   1. Make same assessments as preoperatively.
   2. Assess incision for drainage and infection.
   3. Monitor head circumference.
   4. Assess neurologic function.

C. Long-term care.
   1. Teach family catheterization program.
   2. Older children to learn self-catheterization.
   3. Develop bowel program.
      a. High-fiber diet
      b. Increased fluids
      c. Regular fluids
      d. Suppositories as needed
   4. Assess skin condition frequently.
   5. Assist with range-of-motion (ROM) exercises, ambulation, and bracing as indicated by physical therapy and occupational therapy.
   6. Coordinate with team members: Neurologist, orthopedist, urologist, physical therapist, occupational therapist, and nutritionist.

D. Support independent functioning of child.

E. Assist family to make realistic developmental expectations of child.

(Centers for Disease Control and Prevention, 2020, September 3, *What Is Spina Bifida?*)

Hydrocephalus

Description: Condition characterized by an abnormal accumulation of cerebrospinal fluid (CSF) within the ventricles of the brain that does not drain properly from the cranium.

The two major types of hydrocephalus are called communicating hydrocephalus and non-communicating hydrocephalus.

Communicating hydrocephalus occurs when the flow of CSF is blocked after it exits the ventricles. This form is called communicating since the CSF flows between the ventricles; the passages remain open. Reduced flow and absorption of CSF into specialized blood vessels called arachnoid villi can also result in a buildup of CSF in the ventricles and communicating hydrocephalus.

Non-communicating hydrocephalus: The flow of CSF is blocked along one or more of the narrow passages connecting the ventricles (U.S. Department of Health and Human Services, 2020, May 13, *Hydrocephalus fact sheet*).

A. Caused by an obstruction in the flow of CSF between the ventricles.

B. Results in enlargement of the ventricles, which causes pressure on the brain tissue.

C. Hydrocephalus is most often associated with spina bifida; it can be a complication of meningitis.

> **HESI HINT** Infants with hydrocephalus have enlarged head circumference as a result of widening fontanels that compensate for accumulating cerebral spinal fluid and relieve pressure of the developing brain.

Clinical Assessment

A. Toddlers and older children show classic signs of intracranial pressure (ICP).
   1. Change in LOC
   2. Irritability
   3. Vomiting
   4. Headache on awakening
   5. Motor dysfunction
   6. Unequal pupil response
   7. Seizures
   8. Decline in academics
   9. Change in personality

B. Signs of increased ICP in infants
   1. Irritability, lethargy
   2. Increasing head circumference
   3. Bulging fontanels
   4. Widening suture lines
   5. "Sunset" eyes
   6. High-pitched cry
   7. Feeding difficulties
   8. Decreased muscle tone and strength

Clinical Judgments

A. Prepare infant and family for diagnostic procedures.

B. Monitor for signs of increased ICP.

C. Maintain seizure precautions.

D. Elevate head of bed.

E. Prepare parents for surgical procedure (e.g., ventricular shunt placement).

F. Purpose of the shunt is to drain the excess fluid off the brain.

G. Postoperative care
   1. Assess for signs of shunt malfunction.
      a. Infant
         1) Change in size, signs of bulging, tenseness in fontanels, and separation of suture lines
         2) Irritability, lethargy, or seizure activity
         3) Altered vital signs and feeding behavior
      b. Older child: Increase in ICP
         1) Change in LOC
         2) Complaint of headache
         3) Changes in customary behavior (sleep patterns, developmental capabilities)
   2. Assess for signs of infection (meningitis).
      a. Increase fever greater than 38.6°C (100.5°F).
      b. Shunt tract may appear erythemic, tender, and swollen; drainage may be present.
      c. Decrease feeding/increase vomiting
      d. Stiff neck and headache
   3. Monitor I&O closely.
   4. Assess surgical sites (head and abdomen).

H. Teach home care program.
   1. Teach to watch for signs of increased ICP or infection.
   2. Follow up appointments for shunt function and potential need for shunt revision.
   3. Provide anticipatory guidance for potential problems with growth and development.

Seizures

Description: Uncontrolled electrical discharges of neurons in the brain which may be caused by:

An imbalance of nerve-signaling brain chemicals (neurotransmitters)

Genetics

Brain tumor

Stroke

Brain damage from illness or injury, including those at birth

Medicines or illegal drugs

Immaturity of the CNS, fever, infection, neoplasms, cerebral anoxia, and metabolic disorders.

In most cases, the cause of a seizure can't be found.

A. Seizures are categorized as generalized or partial/focal.

A generalized seizure occurs in both sides of the brain causing lost consciousness and a postictal state. Types of generalized seizures include:

1. Absence seizure. This is also called petit mal seizure. This seizure causes a brief changed state of consciousness, staring and posturing with twitching and possibly rapid blinking. The seizure usually lasts no longer than 30 seconds. There is usually no recall of what just occurred and the child may go on with activities as though nothing happened. These seizures may occur several times a day. Absence seizures almost always start between ages 4 and 12.
2. Atonic seizure. A sudden loss of muscle tone, and may fall from a standing position or suddenly drop his or her head. During the seizure, child will be limp and unresponsive.
3. Generalized tonic-clonic seizure (GTC)/grand mal seizure which has five distinct phases: a. body, arms, and legs will flex (contract), b. extend (straighten out), and tremor (shake), c. followed by contraction and relaxation of the muscles (clonic period), d. postictal period/ sleepy and possible problems with vision or speech, and e. subsequent bad headache, fatigue, or body aches (not all of these phases occur in everyone).
4. Myoclonic seizure. Quick movements or sudden jerking of a group of muscles. These seizures tend to occur in clusters. This means that they may occur several times a day, or for several days in a row.

Focal seizures take place when abnormal electrical brain function occurs in one or more areas of one side of the brain. Before a focal seizure, some may experience an aura, or signs that a seizure is about to occur, which is more common with a complex focal seizure. The most common aura involves feelings, such as déjà vu, impending doom, fear, or euphoria. There may also be visual changes, hearing abnormalities, or changes in sense of smell.

The two types of focal seizures are:

1. Simple focal seizure. The symptoms depend on which area of the brain is affected. If the abnormal electrical brain function occurs in the occipital lobe, which involves vision, then sight may be altered. More often, muscles are affected, and the seizure activity is limited to an isolated muscle group such as fingers, or larger muscles in the arms and legs. There may be sweating, nausea, or paleness, but no loss of consciousness.
2. Complex focal seizure. This type of seizure often occurs in the temporal lobe, which controls emotion and memory function causing altered consciousness or loss of consciousness or just a loss of awareness of surroundings while still looking awake, but have a variety of unusual behaviors including but not limited to gagging, lip smacking, running, screaming, crying, or laughing and then become postictal.

Clinical Assessment

A. Generalized
   1. Aura (a warning sign of impending seizure)
   2. LOC
   3. Generalized stiffness of entire body
   4. Apnea, cyanosis
   5. Spasms followed by relaxation
   6. Pupils dilated and nonreactive to light
   7. Incontinence
   8. Post ictal disoriented, sleepy

B. Absence seizures (petit mal)
   1. Onset between 4 and 12 years of age
   2. Lasts 5 to 10 seconds
   3. Child appears to be inattentive, daydreaming
   4. Poor performance in school

> **HESI HINT** Medication noncompliance is the most common cause of increased seizure activity.

Nursing Judgment

A. Maintain airway during seizure: Turn client on side to aid ventilation.

B. Do not restrain client.

C. Protect client from injury during seizure and support head (avoid neck flexion).

D. Document seizure, noting all data in assessment.

E. Maintain seizure precautions.
   1. Reduce environmental stimuli as much as possible.
   2. Pad side rails or crib rails.
   3. Have suction equipment and oxygen quickly accessible; set up at the bedside/crib side. Tape oral airway to the head of the bed.

> **HESI HINT** Do not use tongue blade, padded or not, during a seizure as this may cause traumatic damage to the oral cavity.

A. Support during diagnostic tests: Electroencephalogram (EEG), computed tomography (CT) scan

B. Support during workup for infections such as meningitis

C. Administer anticonvulsant medications as prescribed (see Table 5.12).
   1. For tonic-clonic seizures: Carbamazepine, Phenytoin, Valproic acid, Oxcarbazepine, Lamotrigine Gabapentin, Topiramate, Phenobarbital

2. For focal seizures: Carbamazepine, Oxcarbazepine, Lacosamide
3. For absence seizures: Ethosuximide or valproate

D. Monitor therapeutic drug levels.
E. Teach family about drug administration: Dosage, action, and side effects.
F. Consider Ketogenic diet
G. Vagus nerve stimulator
H. Possible surgical interventions (Stanford Children's Health, 2021, *Epilepsy and Seizures in Children*)

Bacterial Meningitis

Bacterial meningitis is very serious and death can occur in a few hours. Most will recover, but may have permanent disabilities (such as brain damage, hearing loss, and learning disabilities).

Description: Bacterial inflammatory disorder of the meninges that cover the brain and spinal cord

Meningitis is usually caused by:

Streptococcus pneumoniae
Group B Streptococcus
Neisseria meningitidis
H.influenzae
Listeria monocytogenes

These bacteria can also be associated with another serious illness, sepsis, which is extreme response to infection. Without timely treatment, sepsis can quickly lead to tissue damage, organ failure, and death.

Causes

Usual Source: Bacterial invasion from the middle ear, nasopharynx, and wounds including fractures of the skull, lumbar punctures, and shunts.

A. Exudate covers brain and cerebral edema occurs.
B. Lumbar puncture shows
   1. Increased white blood cells (WBCs)
   2. Decreased glucose
   3. Elevated protein
   4. Increased ICP
   5. Positive culture for meningitis

Clinical Assessment

A. Older children
   1. Classic signs of increased ICP (see the section "Hydrocephalus" earlier)
   2. Fever, chills
   3. Neck stiffness, opisthotonos
   4. Photophobia
   5. Positive Kernig sign (inability to extend leg when thigh is flexed anteriorly at hip)
   6. Positive Brudzinski sign (neck flexion causing adduction and flexion movements of lower extremities)
B. Infants and young children (3 months to 2 years old)
   1. Absence of classic signs demonstrating generalized symptoms
   2. Poor feeding with vomiting, irritability
   3. Bulging fontanel (an important sign)
   4. Seizures
C. Neonates (birth to 2 months)
   1. Very difficult to diagnose
   2. Temperature nonspecific: May be normal, hypothermia, or hyperthermia
   3. Symptoms can appear a few days after birth.
   4. Infant has difficulty eating and refuses to eat when prompted.
   5. Weak cry
   6. Vomiting and diarrhea may be present.
   7. Movement decreases, along with tone
   8. Restless, sleep pattern changes
   9. Late sign: Bulging and tense fontanel

Clinical Interventions

A. Administer antibiotics (may be ampicillin, and appropriate cephalosporin) and antipyretics as prescribed.
B. Isolate for at least 24 hours.
C. Monitor vital signs and neurologic signs.
D. Keep environment quiet and darkened to prevent overstimulation.
E. Implement seizure precautions.
F. Position for comfort: Head of the bed slightly elevated, with client on side if prescribed.
G. Measure head circumference daily in infants.
H. Monitor I&O closely.

> **HESI HINT** With meningitis, there may be inappropriate antidiuretic hormone (ADH) secretions causing fluid retention (cerebral edema) and dilutional hyponatremia.

I. Administer Hib vaccine to protect against *H. influenzae* infection.

Reye Syndrome

First recognized about 19 years ago, Reye syndrome is a rare, acute, life-threatening condition characterized by vomiting and lethargy that may progress to delirium and coma. Most commonly it occurs in children who are recovering from viral infections, particularly influenza and chickenpox (Box 5.2).

Brain Tumors

Description: Brain cancers account for about 15% of pediatric cancers and are the second most common type of cancer in children. Since the brain controls learning, memory, senses (hearing, visual, smell, taste, touch), emotions, muscles, organs, and blood vessels, the presentation of symptoms varies accordingly.

Third most common cancer in children after leukemia and lymphomas

A. Most pediatric brain tumors are infratentorial, making them difficult to excise surgically.
B. Tumors usually occur close to vital structures.
C. Medulloblastomas account for the largest percentage of pediatric brain cancers, are more common in boys than girls, usually occur between the ages of 2 and 6, and frequently

BOX 5.3 Use of Reye Syndrome & Use of Aspirin

Because the use of salicylates such as aspirin for children with influenza and chickenpox has been associated with Reye syndrome, the Surgeon General advises against use of salicylate and salicylate-containing medications for children with these diseases. The association of salicylates with Reye syndrome is based upon evidence from epidemiologic studies that are sufficiently strong to justify this warning to parents and health care personnel.

From Center for Disease Control and Prevention. (1982). National surveillance of Reye syndrome (1982).

spreads (American Childhood Cancer Organization [ACCO], 2021, *Brain Cancer*).

Clinical Assessment

A. Headache
B. Vomiting (usually in the morning), often without nausea
B. Loss of concentration
C. Change in behavior or personality
D. Balance issues
E. Vision hearing and speech changes, tilting of the head
F. Seizures
G. In infants: Widening sutures, increasing frontal occipital circumference, tense fontanel

HESI HINT Many children with a brain tumor experience headaches before their diagnosis

Clinical Interventions

A. Identify baseline neurologic functioning.
B. Support child and family during diagnostic workup and treatment.
C. If surgery is treatment of choice, provide preoperative teaching.
   1. Explain changes including head will be shaved and describe ICU, dressings, IV lines, etc.
   2. Identify child's developmental level and plan teaching accordingly.
   3. Radiation to the tumor site is sometimes performed before surgical excision of the tumor, in attempt to shrink the size of the tumor and to save as much brain tissue as possible.
D. Assess family's response to the diagnosis and treat family appropriately.
E. After surgery, position client as prescribed by the health care provider.
F. Postoperatively, after the operation to remove the tumor, the child may have a drain coming out of the incision that allows excess CSF to drain from the skull. Other tubes may be placed to allow blood that builds up after surgery to drain from under the scalp.

HESI HINT Most postoperative clients with infratentorial tumors are prescribed to lie flat or turn to either side. A large tumor may require that the child not be turned to the operative side.

A. Monitor IV fluids and output carefully. Overhydration can cause cerebral edema and increased ICP.
B. Steroids and osmotic diuretics may be prescribed
C. Brain tumors are treated with surgery, radiation, and chemotherapy. The specific treatment and prognosis depend on the type, grade, and location of the tumor. Depending on the type of tumor and the promptness of diagnosis, the 5-year survival rate is 40% to 80%. Long-term management of brain cancer survivors is complex and requires a multidisciplinary approach.
D. Support child and family to promote optimum functioning postoperatively.

Muscular Dystrophy

Muscular dystrophies are a group of genetic disorders that result in muscle weakness over time. Each type of muscular dystrophy is different and has no cure, but acting early may help an individual with muscular dystrophy get the services and treatments he or she needs to lead a full life.

Description: Inherited disease of the muscles, causing muscle atrophy and weakness

A. Duchenne muscular dystrophy (DMD) and Becker muscular dystrophy (BMD) can have the same symptoms and are caused by mutations in the same gene. BMD symptoms can begin later in life and be less severe than DMD. However, because these two kinds are very similar, they are often studied and referred to together (DBMD).
B. DMD is a rare muscle disorder but it is one of the most frequent genetic conditions affecting approximately 1 in 3500 male births worldwide, which is usually recognized between 3 and 6 years of age. DMD is characterized by weakness and atrophy of the muscles of the pelvic area followed by the involvement of the shoulder muscles. As the disease progresses, muscle weakness and atrophy spread to affect the trunk and forearms and gradually progress to involve additional muscles of the body. The disease is progressive and most affected individuals require a wheelchair by the teenage years. Serious life-threatening complications may ultimately develop including cardiomyopathy and respiratory difficulties.
C. DMD is caused by mutations of the DMD gene on the X chromosome. The gene regulates the production of a protein called dystrophin that is found in association with the inner side of the membrane of skeletal and cardiac muscle cells. Dystrophin is thought to play an important role in maintaining the membrane (sarcolemma) of muscle cells.

From Muscular Dystrophy. CDC. Retrieved from: https://www.cdc.gov/ncbddd/musculardystrophy/index.html and Acsadi, G. Rare Disease Database. Duchenne Muscular Dystrophy. National Organization of Rare Diseases (NORD) Duchenne. Retrieved October 8, 2021 from https://rarediseases.org/rare-diseases/duchenne-muscular-dystrophy/

Clinical Assessment

A. Waddling gait, lordosis
B. Increasing clumsiness, muscle weakness

C. Gowers sign: Difficulty rising from a squatting position; has to use arms and hands to "walk" up legs to stand erect
D. Pseudohypertrophy of muscles (especially noted in calves) due to fat deposits
E. Muscle degeneration, especially the thighs, and fatty infiltrates (detected by muscle biopsy); cardiac muscle also involved
F. Delayed cognitive development, severity of the cognitive impairment varies
G. Later in disease: Scoliosis, respiratory difficulty, and cardiac difficulties
H. Eventual wheelchair dependency, confinement to bed (Table 5.13)

Clinical Interventions

A. Provide supportive care.
B. Provide exercises (active and passive).
C. Prevent exposure to respiratory infection.
D. Encourage a balanced diet to avoid obesity.
E. Support family's grieving process.
F. Support participation in the Muscular Dystrophy Association: https://www.mda.org/.
G. Coordinate with health care team: physical therapist, occupational therapist, nutritionist, neurologist, orthopedist, and geneticist.

> **HESI HINT** Encourage the parents of children who are diagnosed with any type of neuromuscular disease to allow the child to do as much as possible as an effort to try to maintain muscle function and independence.

REVIEW OF NEUROMUSCULAR DISORDERS

1. What are the physical features of a child with Down syndrome?
2. Describe scissoring.
3. What are two priorities for a newborn with myelomeningocele?
4. List the signs and symptoms of increased ICP in older children.
5. What teaching should parents of a newly shunted child receive?
6. State the three main goals in providing care for a child experiencing a seizure.
7. What are the side effects of Dilantin?
8. Describe the signs and symptoms of a child with meningitis.
9. What antibiotics are usually prescribed for bacterial meningitis? Review
10. How is a child usually positioned after brain tumor surgery?
11. Describe the function of an osmotic diuretic.
12. What increases ICP?
13. Describe the mechanism of inheritance of DMD.
14. What is the Gowers sign?

See Answer Key at the end of this text for suggested responses.

RENAL DISORDERS

Post-streptococcal Glomerulonephritis

Description: Post-streptococcal glomerulonephritis (PSGN) is an immunologically mediated sequela of pharyngitis or skin infections caused by nephritogenic strains of *Streptococcus pyogenes. S. pyogenes* are also called group A Streptococcus or group A strep. PSGN is usually an immunologically mediated, nonsuppurative, delayed sequela of pharyngitis or skin infections caused by a nephritogenic strain of *S. pyogenes*. Antigen—antibody complexes become trapped in the membrane of the glomeruli, causing inflammation and decreased glomerular filtration. Reported outbreaks of PSGN caused by group C streptococci are rare.

Clinical Assessment

A. The clinical features of acute glomerulonephritis include:
   1. Recent streptococcal infection (e.g., strep throat)
   2. Edema (often pronounced facial and orbital edema, especially on arising in the morning)
   3. Hypertension
   4. Proteinuria
   5. Macroscopic hematuria, with urine appearing dark, reddish-brown
   6. Complaints of lethargy, generalized weakness, or anorexia
A. Laboratory examination usually reveals:
   1. Mild normocytic normochromic anemia
   2. Slight hypoproteinemia
   3. Elevated blood urea nitrogen and creatinine
   4. Elevated ESR
   5. Low total hemolytic complement and C3 complement
B. Patients usually have decreased urine output. Urine examination often reveals protein (usually <3 g/day) and hemoglobin with red blood cell (RBC) casts.

Additionally, some evidence from epidemic situations indicates that subclinical cases of PSGN may occur. Thus, some individuals may have symptoms that are mild enough to not come to medical attention.

> **OCCURRENCE OF POST-STREPTOCOCCAL GLOMERULONEPHRITIS** PSGN occurs after a latent period of approximately 10 days following group A strep pharyngitis. Generally, PSGN occurs up to 3 weeks following group A strep skin infections (Centers for Disease Control and Prevention, 2021, *Group A Streptococcal [GAS] Disease*).

Clinical Interventions

A. Provide supportive care.

TABLE 5.13 Clinical Judgment Measures: Pediatric Neuromuscular

Clinical Judgment Measure	Assessment Characteristics
Recognize cues	Lethargy Hyperactivity Aggression Impulsiveness Decreased interest in play Irritability Short attention span Stiff muscles (spasticity) Uncontrollable movements (dyskinesia) Poor balance and coordination (ataxia)
Analyze cues	Headache Hydrocephalus, measure head circumference Neurogenic bladder, Catheterize routinely Full fontanel check fontanel Evaluate neurologic function Monitor for signs of infection Brain tumor Stroke Brain damage from illness or injury, including those at birth Medicines or illegal drugs Immaturity of the CNS
Prioritize cues	Keep in mind any emergent issue related to: airway, breathing, or circulation (A, B, C). Observe for any change in the child's ability to respond to you, needs to be based on the child's age and developmental age. (Tanner Stages) Note alertness (mentation is what is expected for age and diagnosis) Change in skin color (pale, cyanosis)
Solutions	Normalize vital signs Position for comfort: head of the bed slightly elevated Manage pain Control fever Control seizures Promote parent—infant bonding.
Actions	Treat fever. Evaluate for infection, neoplasms, cerebral anoxia, and metabolic disorders. Identify baseline neurologic functioning. Monitor vital signs and neurologic signs. Keep environment quiet and darkened to prevent overstimulation. Implement seizure precautions. Measure head circumference daily in infants. Monitor I&O closely.
Evaluate outcomes	Coordinate with team members: neurologist, orthopedist, urologist, physical therapist, occupational therapist, and nutritionist. Coordinate with genetics if indicated. Refer to community-based agencies.

CNS, Central nervous system

B. Monitor vital signs including blood pressure frequently.
C. Monitor I&O closely.
D. Weigh daily.
E. Provide low-sodium diet with no added salt; low potassium, if oliguric.
F. Encourage bed rest during acute phase (usually 4 to 10 days).
G. Administer antihypertensives if prescribed.
H. Monitor for seizures (hypertensive encephalopathy).
I. Monitor for signs of CHF.
J. Monitor for signs of renal failure (uncommon).

HESI HINT Decreased urinary output is the first sign of renal failure.

Nephrotic Syndrome

Description: Childhood nephrotic syndrome is not a disease in itself; rather, it is a group of symptoms that indicate kidney damage—particularly damage to the glomeruli resulting in the release of too much protein from the body into the urine causing protein albumin, normally found in the blood, to leak into the urine.

A. The two types of childhood nephrotic syndrome are
   1. Primary—the most common type of childhood nephrotic syndrome, which is idiopathic, or unknown, begins in the kidneys and affects only the kidneys.
   2. Secondary—the syndrome is caused by other diseases.

   Refer to Table 5.14.

Clinical Assessment

A. Edema that begins insidiously becomes severe and generalized.
B. Lethargy
C. Anorexia
D. Pallor
E. Urine
   1. Frothy-appearing urine
   2. Massive proteinuria
F. Laboratory findings
   1. Hypoproteinemia
   2. Hypercholesterolemia

Clinical Judgment

Congenital Nephrotic Syndrome: Researchers have found that medications are not effective in treating congenital nephrotic syndrome, and that most children will need a kidney transplant by the time they are 2 or 3 years old.

In order to attempt to sustain a child until transplant:

- albumin injections to make up for the albumin lost in urine
- diuretics
- antibiotics to treat the first signs of infection
- growth hormones to promote growth and help bones mature
- removal of one or both kidneys to decrease the loss of albumin in the urine
- dialysis to artificially filter wastes from the blood if the kidneys fail

A. Provide supportive care.
B. Monitor temperature; assess for signs of infection.
C. Protect from persons with infections.
D. Provide skin care to specifically vulnerable edematous areas.
E. Maintain bed rest during edematous phase.
F Administer medications as ordered.
G. Monitor I&O.
H. Teach dietary changes.
   1. limiting the amount of sodium, often from salt, they take in each day
   2. reducing the amount of liquids they drink each day
   3. eating a diet low in saturated fat and cholesterol to help control elevated cholesterol levels
I. Teach home care.
   1. Instruct to weigh child daily.
   2. Train to prevent infection.

Secondary childhood nephrotic syndrome. Treat the underlying cause of the primary illness

J. Prescribing antibiotics for an infection
K. Adjusting medications to treat lupus, HIV, or diabetes
L. Changing or stopping medications that are known to cause secondary childhood nephrotic syndrome

Urinary Tract Infection (UTI)

Description: Bacterial infection; most common is *Escherichia coli* (*E. coli*) bacteria. A UTI is not common in children younger than age 5. A UTI is much more common in girls, due to a shorter urethra. A UTI can occur in boys if part of the urinary tract is blocked. Uncircumcised boys are more at risk for a UTI than circumcised boys. A child with a part or full blockage in the urinary tract is more likely to develop a UTI.

Clinical Assessment

A. In infants
   1. Vague symptoms
   2. Fever
   3. Irritability
   4. Poor food intake
   5. Diarrhea, vomiting, jaundice
   6. Foul smelling urine
   7. Signs of sepsis
B. In older children
   1. Urinary frequency
   2. Hematuria
   3. Enuresis
   4. Dysuria
   5. Fever
   6. 1Signs of sepsis, fever chills

Clinical Interventions

A. Suspect and assess for UTI in infants who are ill.

TABLE 5.14 Comparison of Acute Glomerulonephritis and Nephrotic Syndrome

Variable	Acute Glomerulonephritis	Nephrotic Syndrome
Causes	Follows streptococcal infection	Usually idiopathic
Edema	Mild, usually around eyes	Severe, generalized
Blood pressure	Elevated	Normal
Urine	Dark, tea-colored (hematuria)	Dark, frothy yellow
	Slight or moderate proteinuria	Massive proteinuria
Blood	Normal serum protein	Decreased serum protein
	Positive ASO titer	Negative ASO titer

ASO, Antistreptolysin O.

B. Assess for recurrent UTI. In infants and young boys, UTI may indicate structural abnormalities of the urinary system.
C. Collect clean voided or catheterized specimen, as prescribed (Table 5.15).
D. Administer antibiotics as prescribed.
E. Teach home program.
   1. Finish all prescribed medication.
   2. Follow-up specimens may be indicated.
   3. Increase oral fluids.
   4. Instruct to void frequently and fully empty bladder.
   5. Teach females to clean genital area from front to back.
   6. Note symptoms of recurrence (John Hopkins Medicine, 2021, *Urinary Tract Infections*).

Vesicoureteral Reflex

Description: Result of valvular malfunction and backflow of urine into the ureters (and higher) from the bladder (severe cases are associated with hydronephrosis)

Clinical Assessment

A. Recurrent UTI
B. Reflux (common with neurogenic bladder)
C. Reflux noted on voiding cystourethrogram (VCUG)

Clinical Interventions

A. Teach home program for prevention of UTI.
B. Teach family the importance of medication compliance, which usually leads to resolution of mild cases.
C. Provide support for children and families requiring surgery.
D. Surgery to remove a blockage
E. Antibiotics to prevent or treat UTIs
F. Surgery to correct an abnormal bladder or ureter
G. Intermittent urinary catheterization
H. Monitor postoperative urinary drainage.
   1. Measure output.
   2. Assess dressing and incision for drainage.
I. Maintain hydration with IV or oral fluids.
J. Manage pain relief postoperatively.
   1. Surgical pain
   2. Bladder spasms (National Institute of Diabetes and Digestive and Kidney Diseases, 2018, *Vesicoureteral Reflux*).

Wilms Tumor (Nephroblastoma)

Description: Malignant renal tumor. Wilms tumor is the most frequent tumor of the kidney in infants and children. Wilms tumor typically develops in otherwise healthy children without any predisposition to developing cancer; however, approximately 10% of children with Wilms tumor have been reported to have a congenital anomaly. Children with Wilms tumor may have associated hemihyperplasia and urinary tract anomalies, including cryptorchidism and hypospadias. Children may have recognizable phenotypic syndromes such as overgrowth, aniridia, genetic malformations, and others. These syndromes have provided clues to the genetic basis of the disease.

A. Wilms tumor is embryonic in origin.
B. The tumor tends to be encapsulated and vascularized.
C. Occurs most often in children 3 to 4 years of age and is much less common after age 5.
D. Can affect one or both kidneys.
E. It is important to recognize that the absolute risk of Wilms tumor varies with the underlying condition or anomaly.
   Caregiver-Education/Fact-Sheets/Hydrocephalus-Fact-Sheet

Clinical Assessment

A. A lump, swelling, or pain in the abdomen. Most children present with an asymptomatic mass that is noted when they are bathed or dressed. Abdominal pain is present in 40% of children.
B. Blood in the urine. Gross hematuria occurs in about 18% of children with Wilms tumor at presentation, and microscopic hematuria is seen in 24% of patients.
C. Hypertension. About 25% of children have hypertension at presentation, which is attributed to activation of the renin-angiotensin system.
D. Hypercalcemia. Symptomatic hypercalcemia can sometimes be seen at presentation of rhabdoid tumors.
E. Constitutional symptoms such as fever, anorexia, and weight loss occur in 10% of cases (National Cancer Institute, 2021, *Wilms Tumor and Other Childhood Kidney Tumors Treatment*).

Clinical Interventions

A. Support family during diagnostic period.
B. Protect child from injury; place a sign on bed stating, "no abdominal palpation" (to prevent accidental fragmentation and dislodging of tumor pieces into the abdominal cavity).
C. Prepare family and child for possible surgery.

TABLE 5.15 Collection of Urine Specimens

Method	Description for Children and Infants
Clean catch	• Best obtained by using a urine bag to catch the specimen. • Apply from side to side or back to front. Diaper should be applied over the bag. • Check child frequently to note urination.
Catheterization	• Sterile feeding tube is often used to catheterize small children and infants.
Sterile specimen	• In small infants, it is best collected by the physician performing a bladder tap. Urine is aspirated through a needle inserted directly into the bladder. The nurse is responsible for making sure infant is appropriately hydrated and restrained during the procedure.

D. Provide postoperative care.
   1. Monitor for increased blood pressure.
   2. Monitor kidney function: I&O, urine specific gravity.
   3. Plan care for abdominal surgery.
      a. Maintain nasogastric tube.
      b. Check for bowel sounds.
   4. Support child and family during interventions.

Hypospadias

Description: Congenital defect of urethral meatus in males; urethra opens on ventral side of penis behind the glans.

Clinical Assessment

A. Abnormal placement of meatus
B. Altered voiding stream
C. Presence of chordee
D. Undescended testes and inguinal hernia (may occur concurrently)

Clinical Judgments

A. Prepare child and family for surgery (no circumcision before surgery).
B. Assess circulation to tip of penis postoperatively.
C. Monitor urinary drainage after urethroplasty.
   1. Plan for possible tubes and drains post-op.
D. Maintain hydration (IV and oral fluids).
E. Teach home care.
   1. Teach care of drains and tubes.
   2. Instruct to increase oral fluids.
   3. Describe signs of infection.

REVIEW OF RENAL DISORDERS

1. Compare the signs and symptoms of PSGN with those of nephrosis.
2. What antecedent event occurs with PSGN?
3. Compare the dietary interventions for PSGN and nephrosis.
4. What is the physiologic reason for the laboratory finding of hypoproteinemia in nephrosis?
5. What interventions can be taught to prevent UTIs in children?
6. Describe the pathophysiology of vesicoureteral reflux.
7. What are the priorities for children with a Wilms tumor?
8. Explain why hypospadias correction is performed before the child reaches preschool age.
9. See Answer Key at the end of this text for suggested responses.

GASTROINTESTINAL DISORDERS

Cleft Lip or Palate

Description: Malformations of the face and oral cavity that seem to be multifactorial in hereditary origin (Fig. 5.16)
A. Cleft lip is readily apparent.
B. Cleft palate may not be identified until the infant has difficulty with feeding.
C. Initial surgical closure of cleft lip is performed ~3 months of age.
D. Surgical closure of palate defect is usually performed at ~10 to 12 months of age.

Clinical Assessment

A. Failure of fusion of the lip, palate, or both
B. Difficulty sucking and swallowing
C. Parent reaction to facial defect

Clinical Judgment Measures

A. Promote family bonding.
B. Discuss surgical options.
C. In newborn period, assist with feeding.
   1. Feed in upright position.
   2. Feed slowly, with frequent burping.
   3. Use appropriate nipples and speech therapy.
   4. Support mother's breastfeeding if possible.
D. Provide postoperative care.
   1. Maintain patent airway and proper positioning.
   2. Sutures are self-dissolving.
   3. Provide soft foods.
   4. Use special sleeves ("no-nos") that prevent the elbows from bending.
   5. Remove oral secretions carefully.
   6. Protect surgical site.
   7. HESI Hint: The surgical closure for repair of the cleft lip will occur at ~3 months for cleft lip and ~10 to 12 months for palate.
   8. Provide age-appropriate stimulation.
   9. Feeding as prescribed. Cleanse suture site with sterile water after feeding.
   10. Teach family care and feeding.

Usually for cleft palate: Coordinate long-term care with other team members: Plastic surgeon, ear/nose/throat (ENT) specialist, nutritionist, speech therapist, orthodontist, pediatrician, nurse (Nemours Kids Health, 2021, *Cleft Palate With Cleft Lip*).

> **HESI HINT** Typical parent and family reactions to a child with an obvious malformation such as cleft lip or palate are guilt, disappointment, grief, sense of loss, and anger. Therefore, it is helpful for the families to be provided pictures of before and after surgical repair of children with cleft lip or cleft palate.

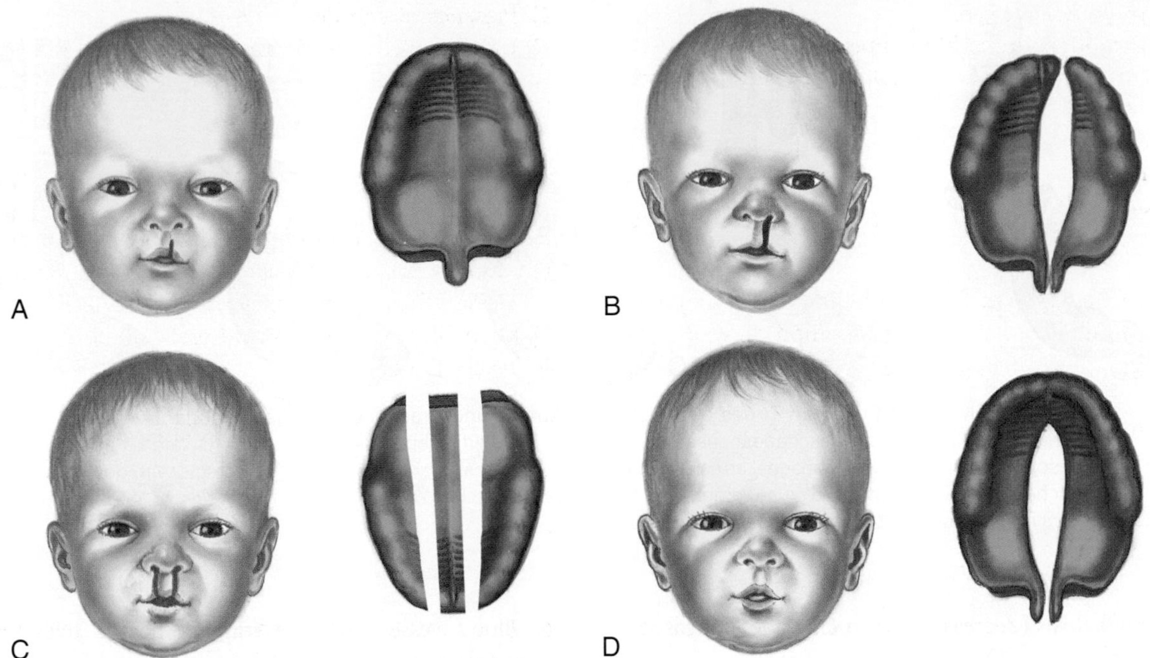

Fig. 5.16 **Variations in Clefts of Lip and Palate at Birth.** (A) Notch in vermilion border. (B) Unilateral cleft lip and cleft palate. (C) Bilateral cleft lip and cleft palate. (D) Cleft palate. (From Hockenberry, M. J., & Wilson, D. [2011]. *Wong's nursing care of infants and children* [9th ed.]. St. Louis: Mosby.)

Esophageal Atresia With Tracheoesophageal Fistula (TEF)

Description: Congenital anomaly in which the esophagus does not fully develop (Fig. 5.17)

A. Most common: Upper esophagus ends in a blind pouch, and the lower part of the esophagus is connected to the trachea.
B. This condition is a clinical and surgical emergency.

Clinical Assessment

A. Three Cs of TEF in the newborn
   1. Choking
   2. Coughing
   3. Cyanosis
      a. Excess salivation
      b. Respiratory distress
      c. Aspiration pneumonia

Clinical Judgment Measures

A. Provide preoperative care.
   1. Monitor respiratory status.
   2. Remove excess secretions (suction is usually continuous due to the blind pouch).
   3. Provide oxygen if needed.
   4. Maintain NPO.
   5. Administer IV fluids as prescribed.
B. Provide postoperative care.
   1. Maintain NPO.
   2. Administer IV fluids.
   3. Monitor I&O.
   4. Provide tube feedings as prescribed.
   5. Provide pacifier to meet developmental needs.
   6. Monitor child for postoperative stricture of the esophagus.
      a. Poor feeding
      b. Dysphagia
      c. Drooling
      d. Regurgitating undigested food
C. Promote parent—infant bonding for high-risk infant.

Pyloric Stenosis

Description: Pyloric stenosis: the pylorus muscles thicken and become abnormally large, blocking food from reaching the small intestine, which is an uncommon condition in infants.

Pyloric stenosis can lead to forceful vomiting, dehydration, and weight loss. Babies with pyloric stenosis may seem to be hungry all the time.

Surgery Cures Pyloric Stenosis

Clinical Assessment

A. Vomiting after feeding (projectile vomiting). Vomiting might be mild at first and gradually become more severe as the pylorus opening narrows.
B. Persistent hunger
C. Stomach contractions (peristalsis) that ripple across upper abdomen
D. Dehydration, subsequent lethargy
E. Changes in bowel movements/constipation
F. Weight loss
G. Usually occurs in first-born males
H. Hungry

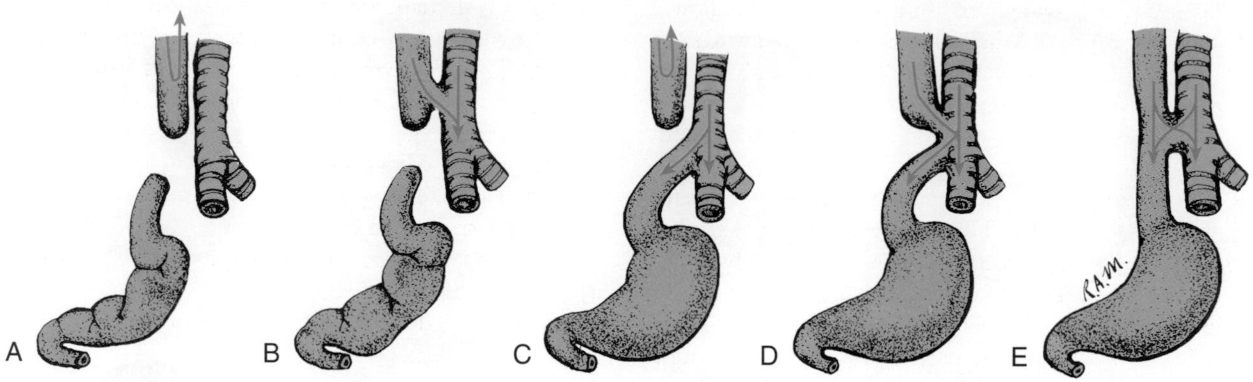

Fig. 5.17 Five Most Common Types of Esophageal Atresia and Tracheoesophageal Fistula. (A) esophageal atresia with distal tracheoesophageal fistula, (B) Isolated esophageal atresia, (C) Isolated tracheoesophageal fistula, (D) esophageal atresia with tracheoesophageal fistula, (E) esophageal atresia with double tracheoesophageal fistu. (From Hockenberry, M. J., & Wilson, D. [2013]. *Wong's essentials of pediatric nursing* [9th ed.]. St. Louis: Mosby.)

I. Metabolic alkalosis (decreased serum chloride, increased pH and bicarbonate or CO_2 content)
J. Palpable olive-shaped mass in upper-right quadrant of the abdomen

Clinical Judgment Measures

A. Preoperative care
  1. Assess for dehydration.
  2. Administer IV fluids and electrolytes as prescribed.
  3. Weigh daily; monitor I&O.
B. Prepare family for surgery by teaching that
  1. The hypertrophied wall is surgically corrected to allow proper drainage from the stomach into the small intestines.
C. Postoperative care
  1. Continue IV fluids as prescribed.
  2. Provide small oral feedings with electrolyte solutions or glucose as ordered.
  3. Position on right side in semi-Fowler position after feeding.
  4. Burp frequently to avoid stomach becoming distended and putting pressure on surgical site.
  5. Weigh daily; monitor I&O (Mayo Clinic, 2021b, *Pyloric Stenosis*).

Intussusception

Description: Telescoping of one part of the intestine into another part of the intestine, usually the ileum into the colon (called ileocolic). Most common cause for bowel obstruction in children under 3 years old. Intussusception more often affects boys.

- Abnormal intestinal formation at birth. Intestinal malrotation: The intestine does not develop or rotate correctly, which increases the risk of intussusception.
- Certain conditions—cystic fibrosis, Henoch-Schonlein purpura (also known as IgA vasculitis), Crohn disease, and celiac disease—can increase the risk of intussusception

A. Partial to complete bowel obstruction occurs.
B. Blood vessels become trapped in the telescoping bowel, causing necrosis.

Clinical Assessment

A. Acute, intermittent abdominal pain
B. Screaming, with legs drawn up to abdomen
C. Vomiting
D. "Currant jelly" stools (mixed with blood and mucus)/ diarrhea
E. Sausage-shaped mass in upper right quadrant and lower-right quadrant is empty

Clinical Judgment

A. Monitor carefully for shock and bowel perforation.
B. Administer IV fluids as prescribed.
C. Monitor I&O.
D. Prepare family for emergency intervention.
E. Prepare child for barium enema (which provides hydrostatic reduction). Two of three cases respond to this treatment; if not, surgery is necessary.
F. Provide postoperative care for clients who require abdominal surgery.

HESI HINT Nutritional needs and fluid and electrolyte balance are key problems for children with GI disorders. The younger the child, the more vulnerable to fluid and electrolyte imbalances; increases the need for the caloric intake required for growth.

Certain conditions—cystic fibrosis, Henoch-Schonlein purpura (also known as IgA vasculitis), Crohn disease, and celiac disease—can increase the risk of intussusception.

Congenital Aganglionic Megacolon (Hirschsprung Disease)

Description: Congenital absence of autonomic parasympathetic ganglion (HSCR). This disorder is characterized by the absence of particular nerve cells (ganglions) in a segment of the bowel in an infant. The absence of ganglion cells causes the muscles in the bowels to lose their ability to move stool through the intestine (peristalsis). Symptoms in the newborn period, including failure to pass a meconium for 24 to 48 hours, are suggestive of HSCR.

HSCR can sometimes lead to a condition called enterocolitis, which is inflammation of the small intestines and colon. This is often referred to as Hirschsprung-associated enterocolitis. Hirschsprung-associated enterocolitis is the most frequent complication of HSCR, occurring in 30% to 40% of individuals with HSCR.

Untreated Hirschsprung-associated enterocolitis may develop sepsis, which also can lead to toxic megacolon.

Approximately 90% of initial HSCR diagnoses in the United States are made within the first year of life. Most of the remaining 10% are made in early childhood.

A. There is a lack of peristalsis in the area of the colon where the ganglion cells are absent.
B. Fecal contents accumulate above the aganglionic area of the bowel.
C. Correction may involve several surgical procedures.
   1. A temporary colostomy with reanastomosis and closure of the colostomy

Clinical Assessment

A. Suspicion in newborn who fails to pass meconium within 24 hours
B. Distended abdomen, chronic constipation alternating with diarrhea
C. Nutritionally deficient child
D. Enterocolitis that occurs as an emergency event
E. Ribbonlike stools in the older child

Clinical Judgment

A. Provide preoperative care.
   1. Begin preparation for abdominal surgery.
   2. Provide bowel-cleansing program as prescribed.
   3. Observe for symptoms of bowel perforation.
      a. Abdominal distention (measure abdominal girth)
      b. Vomiting
      c. Increased abdominal tenderness
      d. Irritability
      e. Dyspnea and cyanosis
   4. Initiate preoperative teaching regarding colostomy.
B. Provide postoperative care.
   1. Check vital signs, axillary temperature.

HESI HINT Symptoms in the newborn period, including failure to pass a meconium for 24–48 h, are suggestive of HSCR.

HSCR can sometimes lead to a condition called enterocolitis, which is inflammation of the small intestines and colon.

NORD, 2017, https://rarediseases.org/rare-diseases/hirschsprungs-disease/

   2. Administer IV fluids as prescribed.
   3. Monitor I&O.
   4. Care for nasogastric tube with connection to intermittent suction.
   5. Check abdominal and perineal dressings.
   6. Assess bowel sounds and bowel function.

Prepare family for home care.

1. Teach care of temporary colostomy.
2. Teach skin care.
3. Refer family to enterostomal therapist, GI specialist, nutritionist, OT/PT and speech therapy, and social services.

Prepare child and family for closure of temporary colostomy.

After closure, encourage family to be patient with child when toileting.

Teach family to begin toilet training after age 2.

REVIEW OF GASTROINTESTINAL (GI) DISORDERS

1. Describe feeding techniques for a child with cleft lip or palate.
2. List the signs and symptoms of esophageal atresia with TEF.
3. What actions are initiated for the newborn with suspected esophageal atresia with TEF?
4. Describe the postoperative care for an infant with pyloric stenosis.
5. Describe the preoperative care for a child with Hirschsprung disease.
6. What care is needed for a child with a temporary colostomy?
7. What are the signs of anorectal malformation?
8. What are the priorities for a child undergoing abdominal surgery?
9. See Answer Key at the end of this text for suggested responses.

HEMATOLOGIC DISORDERS

Iron Deficiency Anemia

Description: Hgb levels below normal range because of the body's inadequate supply, intake, or absorption of iron

A. Iron deficiency anemia is the leading hematologic disorder in children.
B. The need for iron is greater in children than in adults because of accelerated growth.
C. Anemia may be caused by the following:
   1. Inadequate stores during fetal development
   2. Deficient dietary intake
   3. Chronic blood loss
   4. Poor utilization of iron by the body

Clinical Assessment

A. Pallor, paleness of mucous membranes
B. Tiredness, fatigue
C. Usually seen in infants 6 to 24 months old (times of growth spurt); toddlers and female adolescents most affected
D. Dietary intake low in iron
E. Pica habit (eating nonfood substances)
F. Laboratory values
  1. Decreased Hgb
  2. Low serum iron level
  3. Elevated total iron binding capacity (TIBC)

> **HESI HINT** Remember the Hgb norms:
> - Newborn: 14 to 24 g/dL
> - Infant: 9.5 to 14 g/dL
> - Child: 10.5 to 15 g/dL

Clinical Judgment Measures

A. Support child's need to limit activities.
B. Provide rest periods.
C. Administer oral iron (ferrous sulfate) as prescribed.

> **HESI HINT** Teach the family about administration of oral iron:
> Give on empty stomach (as tolerated, for better absorption).
> Give with citrus juices (vitamin C) for increased absorption.
> Use dropper or straw to avoid discoloring teeth.
> Teach that stools will become tarry.
> Teach that iron can be fatal in severe overdose; keep away from other children.
> Do not give with any dairy products.

A. Teach family nutritional facts concerning iron deficiency.
  1. Teach about dietary sources of iron.
    a. Meat
    b. Green, leafy vegetables
    c. Fish
    d. Liver
    e. Whole grains
    f. Legumes
    g. For infants: Iron-fortified cereals and formula
  2. Teach about appropriate nutrition for child's age.
B. Be aware of family's income and cultural food preferences.
C. Refer family to nutritionist.
D. Refer to Women, Infants, and Children's (WIC) nutrition program, if available to family.

Hemophilia

Description: Inherited bleeding disorder
A. Known as factor VIII (8), which is a genetic disorder caused by a clotting protein that is transmitted by an X-linked recessive chromosome (mother to her sons).
B. Hemophilia A is the same as factor VIII that is passed down from parents to children; however, 1/3 of the cases have no previous family history (CDC, 2021).

Clinical Assessment

A. Male child: First red flag may be prolonged bleeding at the umbilical cord or injection site (vitamin K)
B. Prolonged bleeding with minor trauma
C. Hemarthrosis (most frequent site of bleeding)
D. Spontaneous bleeding into muscles and tissues (less severe cases have fewer bleeds)
E. Loss of motion in joints
F. Pain
G. Laboratory values
  1. Partial thromboplastin time (PTT) is prolonged.
  2. Factor assays less than 25%

Clinical Judgment Measures

A. Administer fresh-frozen plasma
B. Administer pain medication as prescribed (analgesics containing no aspirin).
C. Follow blood precautions: Risk for hepatitis.
D. Teach child and family home care.
  1. Teach to recognize early signs of bleeding into joints.
  2. Teach local treatment for minor bleeds (pressure, splinting, ice).
  3. Teach administration of factor replacement (if receiving routine treatments of the clotting factors may have an indwelling catheter).
  4. Discuss dental hygiene: Use soft toothbrushes.
  5. Provide protective care: Give child soft toys; use padded bed rails.
  6. Have child wear medical alert identification.
E. Refer family for genetic counseling.
F. Support child and family during periods of growth and development when increased risk for bleeding occurs (e.g., learning to walk, tooth loss).

> **HESI HINT** Inherited bleeding disorders (hemophilia and sickle cell disease [SCD]) are often used to test knowledge of genetic transmission patterns. Remember this:
> - Autosomal recessive: Both parents must be heterozygous, or carriers of the recessive trait, for the disease to be expressed in their offspring. With each pregnancy, there is a one in four chance that the infant will have the disease. However, all children of such parents can get the disease—not just 25% of them. This is the transmission pattern of SCD, cystic fibrosis, and phenylketonuria (PKU).
> - X-linked recessive trait: The trait is carried on the X chromosome; therefore, it usually affects male offspring, as in hemophilia. With each pregnancy of a woman who is a carrier, there is a 25% chance of having a child with hemophilia. If the child is male, he has a 50% chance of having hemophilia. If the child is female, she has a 50% chance of being a carrier.

Sickle Cell Disease

Description: Sickle cell anemia is one of a group of disorders known as SCD. Sickle cell anemia is an inherited RBC disorder without enough healthy RBCs to carry oxygen throughout the body. Flexible, round RBCs move easily through blood vessels. In sickle cell anemia, the red blood are shaped like sickles or crescent moons. These rigid, sticky cells can get stuck in small blood vessels, which can slow or block blood flow and oxygen to parts of the body.

Genetics: Both parents must carry a sickle cell gene. In the United States, sickle cell anemia most commonly affects black people. There is no cure for sickle cell anemia, usually diagnosed after 6 months of age.

A. Hemoglobin S (HgbS) replaces all or part of the normal Hgb, which causes the RBCs to sickle when oxygen is released into the tissues.
   1. Sickled cells cannot flow through capillary beds (Fig. 5.18).
   2. Dehydration promotes sickling.
   3. Increased sickling episodes occur with cold because cold causes constriction of the vessels (Mayo Clinic, 2021c, *Sickle Cell Anemia*).

HESI HINT Hydration is very important in the treatment of SCD because it promotes hemodilution and circulation of red cells through the blood vessels.

Tissue ischemia causes widespread pathologic changes in spleen, liver, kidney, bones, and the CNS.

HESI HINT Important terms

Heterozygous gene (HgbAS)—sickle cell trait

Homozygous gene (HbSS)— SCD

Abnormal hemoglobin (HgbS)—disease and trait

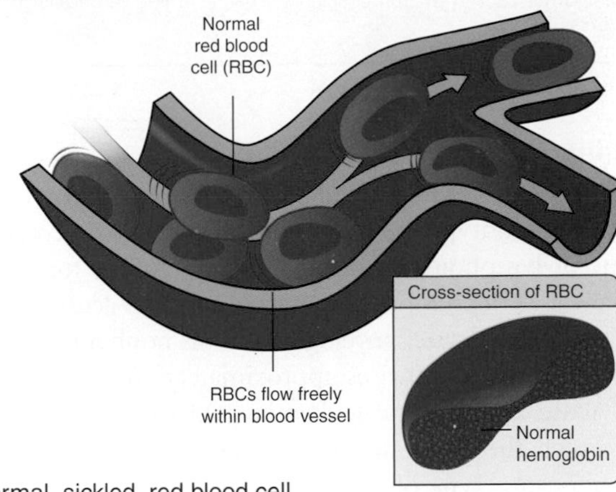

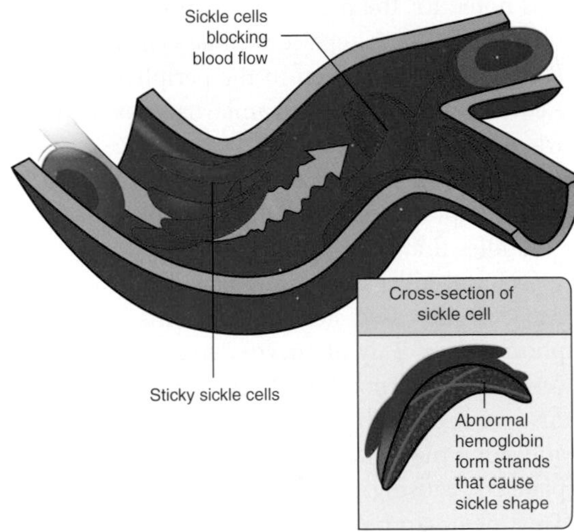

Fig. 5.18 Normal Red Cells and Sickle Red Cells. (A) Normal red blood cells flowing freely in a blood vessel. The inset image shows a cross-section of a normal red blood cell with normal Hgb. (B) Abnormal, sickled red blood cells blocking blood flow in a blood vessel. The inset image shows a cross-section of a sickle cell with abnormal (sickle) Hgb forming abnormal stiff rods. (From NIH: National Heart, Lung, and Blood Institute. Retrieved from http://www.nhlbi.nih.gov/health/health-topics/topics/sca)

Clinical Assessment

A. Children of African descent, usually over 6 months of age
B. Parents with sickle cell trait or SCD
C. Laboratory diagnosis: Hgb electrophoresis (differentiates trait from disease)
D. Frequent infections (nonfunctional spleen)
E. Fatigue
F. Chronic hemolytic anemia
G. Delayed physical growth
H. Vasoocclusive crisis; the classic signs include the following:
   1. Fever
   2. Severe abdominal pain
   3. Hand–foot syndrome (infants); painful edematous hands and feet
   4. Arthralgia
I. Leg ulcers (adolescents)
J. Cerebrovascular accidents (increased risk with dehydration)

Clinical Judgment Measures

A. Teach family that to prevent crisis (hypoxia), they should
   1. Keep child from exercising strenuously.
   2. Keep child away from high altitudes.
   3. Avoid letting child become infected and seek care at first sign of infection.
   4. Keep child well hydrated.
   5. Do not withhold fluids at night because enuresis is a complication of both the disease and the treatment.
B. For a child hospitalized with a vaso-occlusive crisis
   1. Administer IV fluids and electrolytes, as prescribed, to increase hydration and treat acidosis.
   2. Monitor I&O.
   3. Administer blood products as prescribed.
   4. Administer analgesics, including parenteral morphine for severe pain, as prescribed.
   5. Use warm compresses (not ice).
   6. Administer prescribed antibiotics to treat infection.
C. Administer pneumococcal vaccine, meningococcal vaccine, and Hib vaccine as prescribed.
D. Administer hepatitis B vaccine as prescribed.
E. Refer family for genetic counseling.
F. Support child and family experiencing chronic disease.

HESI HINT Supplemental iron is not given to clients with SCD. The anemia is not caused by iron deficiency. Folic acid is given orally to stimulate RBC synthesis.

Acute Lymphocytic Leukemia (ALL)

Description: Cancer of the blood and bone marrow. The most common subtype, acute lymphoblastic (also termed lymphocytic or lymphoid) leukemia (ALL), accounts for 75% to 80% of all cases of childhood leukemia, whereas acute myeloid (also termed myelocytic, myelogenous, or nonlymphoblastic) leukemia (AML) comprises approximately 20%.

A. Acute lymphocytic leukemia (ALL) is a type of cancer in which the bone marrow makes too many immature lymphocytes (type of WBC).
B. Leukemia may affect RBCs, WBCs, and platelets.
C. It is noted for the presence of lymphoblasts (immature lymphocytes), which replace normal cells in the bone marrow.
D. Blast cells are also seen in the peripheral blood.
E. Acute lymphocytic leukemia is classified according to whether it involves
   1. B lymphocytes that make antibodies to help fight infection
   2. T lymphocytes that help B lymphocytes make the antibodies that help fight infection
   3. Natural killer cells that attack cancer cells and viruses
F. ALL has increased stem cells become lymphoblasts, B lymphocytes, or T lymphocytes/leukemia cells, which do not function as normal lymphocytes and do not fight infection. Also, as the number of leukemia cells increases in the blood and bone marrow, there are less healthy WBCs, RBCs, and platelets, causing infection, anemia, and easy bleeding.
G. Treatment can be divided into four phases.
   1. First phase—induction chemotherapy
   2. Second phase—consolidation chemotherapy
   3. Third phase—maintenance chemotherapy
   4. Fourth phase—CNS prophylaxis

Clinical Assessment

A. Pallor, tiredness, weakness, lethargy
B. Petechia, bleeding, bruising
C. Infection
D. Bone joint pain
E. Enlarged lymph nodes; hepatosplenomegaly
F. Headache and vomiting (signs of CNS involvement)
G. Anorexia, weight loss
H. Laboratory data: A diagnosis of ALL generally requires that at least 20% of the cells in the bone marrow are blasts.
I. A bone marrow aspiration and biopsy is the only definitive way to diagnose leukemia.

Clinical Judgment Measures

A. Isolation if prescribed.
B. Provide child with age-appropriate explanations for diagnostic tests, treatments, and care.
C. Examine child for infection of skin, needle-stick sites, and dental problems.
D. Administer blood products as prescribed.
E. Administer antineoplastic chemotherapy.
F. Monitor for side effects of chemotherapeutic agents.
G. Provide care directed toward managing side effects and toxic effects of antineoplastic agents.

HESI HINT Corticosteroids are often given with chemotherapy to help destroy leukemia cells or to reduce allergic reactions to some chemotherapy drugs. The most commonly used steroids for ALL include prednisolone and dexamethasone.

1. Administer antiemetics as prescribed.
2. Monitor fluid balance.
3. Monitor for signs of infection.
4. Monitor for signs of bleeding.
5. Monitor for cumulative toxic effects of drugs: Hepatic toxicity, cardiac toxicity, renal toxicity, and neurotoxicity.
6. Provide oral hygiene.
7. Provide small, appealing meals; increase calories and protein; refer to nutritionist.
8. Promote self-esteem and positive body image if child has alopecia, severe weight loss, or other disturbance in body image.
9. Provide care to prevent infection.
10. Provide emotional support for family in crisis.
11. Encourage family's and child's input and control in determining plans and treatment.

REVIEW OF HEMATOLOGIC DISORDERS

1. Describe the information families should be given when a child is receiving oral iron preparations.
2. List dietary sources of iron.
3. What is the genetic transmission pattern of hemophilia?
4. Describe the sequence of events in a vaso-occlusive crisis in SCD.
5. Explain why hydration is a priority in treating SCD.
6. What should families and children do to avoid triggering sickling episodes?
7. Interventions and treatments for a child with leukemia are based on what three physiologic problems?
8. Interventions and treatments for a child with retinoblastoma are based on what type of treatment?
9. See Answer Key at the end of this text for suggested responses.

METABOLIC AND ENDOCRINE DISORDERS

Congenital Hypothyroidism

Description: Congenital condition resulting from inadequate thyroid tissue development in utero. Cognitive impairment and growth failure occur if it is not detected and treated in early infancy.

Clinical Assessment

A. NBS reveals low thyroxine (T_4) and high thyroid-stimulating hormone (TSH).
B. Symptoms in the newborn
   1. Long gestation (>42 weeks)
   2. Large hypoactive infant
   3. Delayed meconium passage
   4. Feeding problems (poor suck)
   5. Prolonged physiologic jaundice
   6. Hypothermia
C. Symptoms in early infancy if untreated with T_4
   1. Large, protruding tongue
   2. Coarse hair/hairline will appear low.
   3. Lethargy, sleepiness
   4. Flat expression
   5. Constipation
   6. Hypotonia
   7. Large soft spots of the skull
   8. Hoarse cry
   9. Distended stomach with outpouching of the belly button (umbilical hernia)
   10. Feeding problems, including needing to be awakened for feedings and difficulty swallowing
   11. "Floppy" (poor muscle tone, also called hypotonia)
   12. Delay of serum phenylalanine testing will lead to CNS damage, delays in learning.
D. Prognosis is good if the condition is recognized and treated. The infant's development is usually not affected if treatment is initiated within the first month of life.

> **HESI HINT** Congenital hypothyroidism is a condition resulting from inadequate thyroid tissue development in utero. Cognitive impairment and growth failure occur if it is not detected and treated in early infancy. Testing includes a newborn screen based on state requirements, which will reveal low thyroxine (T_4) and high TSH.

Clinical Judgment Measures

A. Perform NBS programs per state regulations.
B. Assess newborn for signs of congenital hypothyroidism.

Once identified, teach family about replacement therapy with thyroid hormone.

C. Treatment involves monitoring of blood thyroid hormone levels (TSH and free T4) to make sure that the amount of medication is adjusted to keep up with how fast the baby is growing. Generally, blood tests are checked every 1 to 2 months up to 6 months of age and then every 2 to 3 months thereafter.
D. Family Teaching
   1. Explain that child will have a lifelong need for the therapy.
   2. Tell parents to give child a single dose in the morning.
   3. Signs of overdose include rapid pulse, irritability, fever, weight loss, and diarrhea.
   4. Signs of underdose include lethargy, fatigue, constipation, and poor feeding.
   5. Periodic thyroid testing is necessary (American Thyroid Association (ATA), 2021, *Congenital Hypothyroidism*).

Phenylketonuria

Description: Rare autosomal-recessive disorder in which the body cannot metabolize the essential amino acid phenylalanine, which accumulates in the blood after the infant begins consuming breast milk or formula and is in all foods containing protein. PKU can cause intellectual and developmental disabilities (IDDs) if not treated. High phenylalanine will damage the brain. Children and adults who are treated early and consistently develop normally.

All children born in U.S. hospitals are tested routinely for PKU soon after birth, making it easier to diagnose and treat affected children early.

Clinical Assessment (If Undetected and/or Untreated)

A. NBS using the Guthrie test; positive result; serum phenylalanine level of 4 mg/dL
B. Frequent vomiting, failure to gain weight
C. Irritability
D. Musty odor of urine
   1. Delayed growth and development
   2. Signs of FTT
   3. Unpleasant peculiar body odor and urine
   4. In the United States, PKU is most common in people of European or Native American ancestry. It is much less common among people of African, Hispanic, or Asian ancestry.
   5. May have microcephaly
E. Mothers diagnosed with PKU disease who do not maintain a low-phenylalanine diet during pregnancy can cause problems for their children who do inherit PKU. Those infants are at risk for:
   1. Cognitive impairment
   2. Microcephaly
   3. Birth weight below 2500 grams
   4. Disrupted growth and development
   5. Congenital heart anomalies

> **HESI HINT** Early detection of hypothyroidism and PKU is essential for preventing cognitive impairment in infants. Knowledge of normal growth and developmental patterns is important because a lack of attainment can be used to detect the presence of a disease and to evaluate the treatment's effects.

Clinical Interventions

A. Perform NBS based on state requirements. Obtain a subsequent sample as notified by NBS. Screen infants born at home who have no hospital contact, as well as infants adopted internationally.
B. Once identified, teach family dietary management.
   1. Stress the importance of strict adherence to prescribed low-phenylalanine diet.
   2. Instruct family to provide special formulas for infant.
   3. Teach family to avoid foods high in phenylalanine; that is, high-protein foods and encourage family to work with nutritionist.
   4. Refer for genetic counseling (National Institute of Health, 2021, *Phenylketonuria (PKU) Condition Information*).

> **HESI HINT** Ensure family is educated regarding a low-phenylalanine diet.
>
> **Insulin-Dependent Diabetes Mellitus (IDDM), or Type 1 Diabetes**
>
> Description: Metabolic disorder in which the insulin-producing cells of the pancreas are nonfunctioning as a result of some insult. The child's body no longer produces the hormone (insulin).
>
> A. The exact cause of type 1 diabetes is unknown. The body's immune system destroys insulin-producing (islet) cells in the pancreas, stopping the production of insulin. Genetics and environmental factors have a role in this process.
>
> B. Diabetes causes altered metabolism of carbohydrates, proteins, and fats. Insulin replacement and dietary management are the recommended treatments. The missing insulin needs to be replaced with injections or with an insulin pump.

Clinical Assessment

A. Classic three Ps:
   1. Polydipsia
   2. Polyphagia
   3. Polyuria, enuresis (bedwetting) in previously continent child
B. Unintentional weight loss
C. Fatigue
D. Irritability or behavior changes
E. Fruity-smelling breath
F. Abdominal complaints, nausea, and vomiting
G. Usually occurs in school-age children but can occur even in infancy
H. See Table 4.27.

Complications can include:

Heart and blood vessel disease. Diabetes increases risk of developing conditions such as narrowed blood vessels, high blood pressure, heart disease, and stroke later in life.

Nerve damage. Excess sugar can injure the walls of the tiny blood vessels causing tingling, numbness, burning, or pain. Nerve damage usually happens gradually over a long period of time.

Kidney damage. Diabetes can damage the numerous tiny blood vessel clusters that filter waste.

Eye damage. Diabetes can damage the blood vessels of the retina, which may lead to vision problems.

Osteoporosis. Diabetes may lead to lower-than-normal bone mineral density, increasing your child's risk of osteoporosis as an adult.

> **HESI HINT** DM in children was typically diagnosed as insulin-dependent diabetes (type 1) until recently. Adolescence frequently causes difficulty in management because growth is rapid, and the need to be like peers makes compliance difficult. Remember to consider the child's age, cognitive level of development, and psychosocial development when answering NCLEX-RN questions.

Clinical Judgment Measures

A. Assist with diagnosis (fasting blood sugar >120 mg/dL glucose).
B. If child is in ketoacidosis, provide care for seriously ill child (may be unconscious).
   1. Monitor vital signs and neurologic status.
   2. Monitor blood glucose, pH, and serum electrolytes.
   3. Administer IV fluids, insulin, and electrolytes as prescribed.

> **HESI HINT** When a child is in ketoacidosis, administer regular insulin IV in NS as prescribed.

   4. Assess hydration status.
   5. Maintain strict I&O.

Initiate home teaching program as soon as possible; involve child and family.

1. Teach insulin administration.
   a. Child usually receives multiple doses daily.
   b. May be administered subcutaneously or via insulin pump.
2. Teach dietary management (carbohydrate counting preferred).
   a. Meals and snacks
   b. Growth and exercise needs
   c. Four basic food groups, no concentrated sweets
   d. Advice from nutritionist
3. Teach about exercise.
   a. Regular, planned activities
   b. Diet modification; snacks before or during exercise
4. Teach about home glucose monitoring and urine testing.
5. Teach the signs and symptoms of hyperglycemia and hypoglycemia.
6. Ensure that the parents involve the school nurse and/or day-care in daily management.

Initiate program for school-age child, as appropriate.

1. Identify issues specific to school.
   a. Physical education class and exercise
   b. Scheduled times for meals and snacks
   c. Need to be like peers
2. Teach that a school-age child should be responsible for most management.
3. Advise regarding a medical alert ID (Mayo Clinic, 2021d, *Type 1 Diabetes in Children*).

REVIEW OF METABOLIC AND ENDOCRINE DISORDERS

1. How is congenital hypothyroidism diagnosed?
2. What are the symptoms of congenital hypothyroidism in early infancy?
3. What are the outcomes of untreated congenital hypothyroidism?
4. What are the metabolic effects of PKU?
5. List foods type high in phenylalanine.
6. What are the three classic signs of diabetes?
7. Differentiate the signs of hypoglycemia and hyperglycemia.
8. Describe the care of a child with ketoacidosis.
9. Describe developmental factors that would affect the school-age child with diabetes.
10. What is the relationship between hypoglycemia and exercise?
11. See Answer Key at the end of this text for suggested responses.

SKELETAL DISORDERS

Fractures

Description: Traumatic injury to bone. Younger children diagnosed with fractures may be at risk for child abuse. 4.4 million child maltreatment referral reports received. Child abuse reports involved 7.9 million children. 45.4% of children who die from child abuse are under 1 year. Boys had a higher child fatality rate than girls. The history of the incident matches the physical injury and sounds feasible (American Society for Preventive Care of Children, 2021, *Children maltreatment*).

Fractures are classified according to type.

Open and closed fractures. Open fracture (compound fracture): The bone pokes through the skin and can be seen. Or a deep wound exposes the bone through the skin. Closed fracture (simple fracture): The bone is broken, but the skin is intact.

1. Complete fractures: Bone fragments are completely separate.
2. Incomplete fractures: Bone fragments remain attached (e.g., greenstick, bowing, buckles).
3. Comminuted fractures: Bone fragments from the fractured shaft break free and lie in the surrounding tissue usually associated with high impact and trauma.
4. Spiral fractures: Fracture line results from twisting force; forms a spiral encircling the bone. *Pediatric fractures*, see https://www.amboss.com/us/knowledge/Pediatric_fractures

> **HESI HINT** Fractures in older children are common because they fall during play and are involved in motor vehicle accidents.
> - Spiral fractures (caused by twisting) and fractures in infants may be related to child abuse.
> - Fractures involving the epiphyseal plate (growth plate) can have serious consequences in terms of the growth of the affected limb.

Clinical Assessment

A. General condition
   1. Visible bone fragments
   2. Misalignment of the limb
   3. Pain
   4. Swelling
   5. Contusions
   6. Child guarding or protecting the extremity
   7. Limited range of motion

B. The five Ps are a late indication of compartment syndrome:
   1. Pain
   2. Pallor
   3. Pulselessness
   4. Paresthesia
   5. Paralysis

Clinical Interventions

A. Obtain baseline data and frequently perform neurovascular assessments.
   1. Pulses: Check pulses distal to the injury to assess circulation.
   2. Color: Check injured extremity for pink, brisk, capillary refill.
   3. Movement and sensation: Check injured extremity for nerve impairment; compare for symmetry with uninjured extremity (child may guard injury).
   4. Temperature: Check extremity for warmth.
   5. Swelling: Check for an increase in swelling. Elevate extremity to prevent swelling.
   6. Pain: Monitor for severe pain that is not relieved by analgesics (Table 5.16).
   7. Newly fractured sites are generally splinted and braced until swelling goes down. Once the swelling has subsided, a cast is applied to the affected extremity.

B. Report abnormal neurovascular assessments promptly!

> **HESI HINT** Compartment syndrome is a progressive decrease of tissue perfusion occurring as a result of increased pressure from edema or swelling that presses on the tissues and vessels. Compromised circulation with abnormal neurovascular checks is the result of compartment syndrome. If compartment syndrome occurs and is not treated immediately with a fasciotomy, it can result in permanent nerve and vasculature damage, possibly leading to amputation of the limb.

C. Maintain traction if prescribed. Note bed position, type of traction, weights, pulleys, pins, pin sites, adhesive strips, Ace wraps, splints, and casts.
   1. Skin traction: Force is applied to skin.

> **HESI HINT** Skin traction for fracture reduction should not be removed unless the health care provider prescribes its removal.

TABLE 5.16 Medications Used in Skeletal Disorders

Drugs/Route	Indications	Adverse Reactions	Nursing Implications
• Infliximab IV • Methocarbamol PO, IM, IV • Cyclobenzaprine PO	• Nonnarcotics to treat pain, stiffness, and discomfort	• Nausea • Vomiting • Fever • Chills • Dizziness • Drowsiness • Chest pain • Allergic response: rash, difficulty breathing, etc.	• Review history: heart disease (all); thyroid disorders, and use of Monoamine oxidase inhibitors (MAOIs) • Remicade use can worsen TB.

IM, Intramuscular; *IV*, intravenous; *TB*, tuberculosis.

a. Buck extension traction: Lower extremity, legs extended, no hip flexion
b. Dunlop traction: Two lines of pull on the arm
c. Russell traction: Two lines of pull on the lower extremity, one perpendicular, one longitudinal
d. Bryant traction: Both lower extremities flexed 90 degrees at hips (rarely used because extreme elevation of lower extremities causes decreased peripheral circulation)

Skeletal traction: Pin or wire applies pull directly to the distal bone fragment.

e. Ninety-degree traction: 90-degree flexion of hip and knee; lower extremity is in a boot cast; can also be used on upper extremities.
f. Dunlop traction: May be used as skeletal traction.

HESI HINT Pin sites can be a source of infection. Monitor for signs of infection. Cleanse and dress pin sites as prescribed.

HESI HINT When moving the client in bed, with either skin or skeletal traction, it is necessary for someone to hold and move the weights of the traction as the client changes position to avoid additional tension on the traction and fracture sites.

A. Maintain child in proper body alignment; restrain if necessary.
B. Monitor for problems of immobility.
C. Provide age-appropriate play and toys.
D. Prepare child for cast application; use age-appropriate terms when explaining procedures.
E. Provide routine cast care after application; petal cast edges.
F. Teach home cast care to family, including
   1. Neurovascular assessment of casted extremity
   2. Not to get cast wet
   3. Teach that, in the presence of a hip spica, family may use a Bradford frame under a small child to help with toileting; they must not use an abduction bar to turn child.
   4. Teach to seek follow-up care with health care provider.

HESI HINT Skeletal disorders affect the infant's or child's physical mobility, and typical NCLEX-RN questions focus on appropriate toys and activities for the child who is confined to bed rest and who is immobilized.

Developmental Dysplasia of Hip (DDH)

Description: Abnormal development of the femoral head in the acetabulum, usually diagnosed at birth. Although developmental dysplasia of hip (DDH) is most often present at birth, it may also develop during a child's first year of life. Recent research shows that babies whose legs are swaddled tightly with the hips and knees straight are at a notably higher risk for developing DDH after birth. As swaddling becomes increasingly popular, it is important for parents to learn how to swaddle their infants safely, and to understand that when done improperly, swaddling may lead to problems like DDH.

In all cases of DDH, the socket (acetabulum) is shallow, meaning that the ball of the thighbone (femur) cannot firmly fit into the socket. Sometimes, the ligaments that help to hold the joint in place are stretched. The degree of hip looseness, or instability, varies among children with DDH.

Dislocated. In the most severe cases of DDH, the head of the femur is completely out of the socket.

Dislocatable. In these cases, the head of the femur lies within the acetabulum, but can easily be pushed out of the socket during a physical examination.

Subluxatable. In mild cases of DDH, the head of the femur is simply loose in the socket. During a physical examination, the bone can be moved within the socket, but it will not be dislocated.

Contributing factors: DDH tends to run in families and can be present in either hip and in any individual. It usually affects the left hip and is predominant in:

1. Girls
2. Firstborn children
3. Babies born in the breech position (especially with feet up by the shoulders). The American Academy of Pediatrics now recommends ultrasound DDH screening of all female breech babies.
4. Family history of DDH (parents or siblings)
5. Oligohydramnios

A. Treatment
   1. When DDH is detected at birth, it can usually be corrected with the use of a harness or brace. If the hip is not dislocated at birth, the condition may not be noticed until the child begins walking. At this time, treatment is more complicated, with less predictable results.
   2. Newborns. The baby is placed in a soft positioning device, called a Pavlik harness, for 1 to 2 months to keep the thighbone in the socket. This special brace is designed

to hold the hip in the proper position while allowing free movement of the legs and easy diaper care. The Pavlik harness helps tighten the ligaments around the hip joint and promotes normal hip socket formation.

3. 1 month to 6 months. Similar to newborn treatment, a baby's thighbone is repositioned in the socket using a harness or similar device. This method is usually successful, even with hips that are initially dislocated.
4. 6 months to 2 years. Older babies are also treated with closed reduction and spica casting. In most cases, skin traction may be used for a few weeks prior to repositioning the thighbone. Skin traction prepares the soft tissues around the hip for the change in bone positioning. It may be done at home or in the hospital.

Clinical Assessment

A. Infant
   1. Positive Ortolani sign ("clicking" with abduction; the sound heard when the health care provider maneuvers the femoral head and it slips back into the acetabulum)
   2. Positive Barlow maneuver ("feel" the dislocation as the femur leaves the acetabulum when the health care provider adducts and extends the hips while stabilizing the pelvis; Fig. 5.19)

B. Older child
   1. Limp on affected side
   2. Trendelenburg sign

HESI HINT A positive Trendelenburg sign usually indicates weakness in the hip abductor muscles gluteus medius and gluteus minimus.

Clinical Judgment Measures

A. Perform newborn assessment at birth.

B. Apply abduction device or splint (Pavlik harness) as prescribed. Therapy involves positioning legs in flexed abducted position.

C. Teach parents home care.
   1. Teach application and removal of device (worn 24 hours a day).
   2. Teach skin care and bathing (physician may allow parents to remove device for bathing).
   3. Teach that follow-up care involves frequent adjustments because of growth.

D. Teach how to provide care for an infant if splinting is ineffective.
   1. Instruct to monitor circulation to feet.
   2. Instruct to meet developmental needs of an immobilized infant.
   3. Incorporate family in care.
   4. Prepare family for spica cast application.

E. Provide care for a child requiring surgical correction.
   1. Perform preoperative teaching of child and family, including cast application.
   2. Perform postoperative care.
      a. Assess vital signs.
      b. Check cast for drainage and bleeding.
      c. Perform neurovascular assessment of extremities.
      d. Promote respiratory hygiene.
      e. Administer narcotic analgesics or morphine either IV (preferred) or IM.
      f. Teach family cast care when child gets home, including checking the cast for "hot spots" (possibly indicative of infection).

Scoliosis (Idiopathic, Congenital, and Neuromuscular)

Description: Lateral curvature of the spine that generally occurs during rapid growth spurts in adolescents. Hereditary conditions, neuromuscular diseases, congenital spinal defects, and trauma or infections to the spine may factor in the development of scoliosis. Treatment depends on the curvature of the spine.

- Idiopathic scoliosis, which means the exact cause is not known, is a condition that causes the spine to curve sideways. Idiopathic scoliosis curves vary in size, and mild curves are more common than larger curves. If a child is still growing, a scoliosis curve can worsen rapidly during a growth spurt. Although it can develop in toddlers and young children, idiopathic scoliosis most often begins during puberty. Both boys and girls can be affected; however, girls are more likely to develop larger curves that require medical care.
- Congenital scoliosis. Problems in the spine sometimes develop before a baby is born. Babies with congenital scoliosis may have spinal bones that are not fully formed or are fused together.
- Neuromuscular scoliosis. Medical conditions that affect the nerves and muscles, such as muscular dystrophy or CP, can lead to scoliosis. These types of neuromuscular conditions can cause imbalance and weakness in the muscles that support the spine.

From OrthoInfo. Idiopathic Scoliosis in Children and Adolescents. Retrieved from: https://orthoinfo.aaos.org/en/diseases–conditions/idiopathic-scoliosis-in-children-and-adolescents/ Reproduced with permission as adapted from OrthoInfo. © American Academy of Orthopaedic Surgeons. https://orthoinfo.org/

Clinical Assessment

A. Occurs most commonly in adolescent females (10 until fully grown)
   1. Elevated shoulder or hip
   2. Head and hips not aligned
   3. While child is bending forward, a rib hump is apparent. (Ask child to bend forward from the hips with arms hanging free, and examine child for a curve of the spine, rib hump, and hip asymmetry.)

Clinical Judgment Measures

A. Screen all adolescent children, especially females, during growth spurt.

B. Prepare child and family for conservative treatment, such as the use of a brace.

C. Observation. If spinal curve is less than 25 degree or if almost full-grown, monitor the curve to make sure it does not get worse, including a recheck about every 6 to 12 months and schedule follow-up x-rays until child is fully grown.

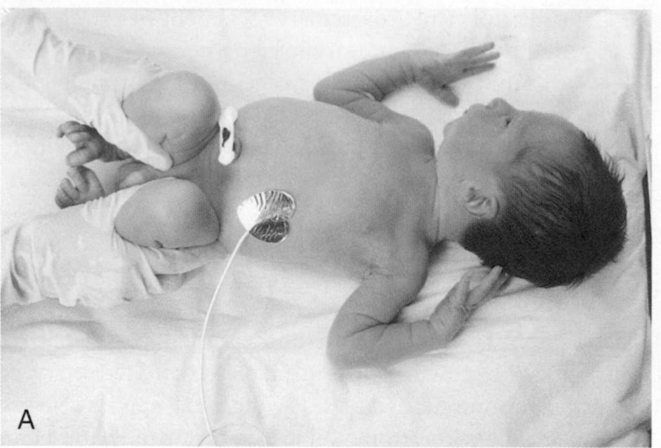

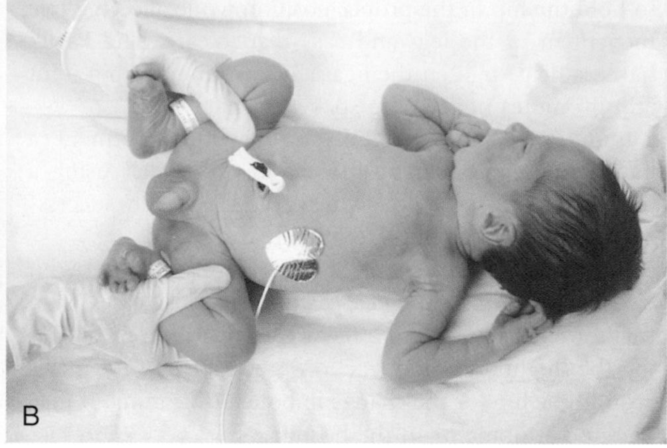

Fig. 5.19 Hip examination: (A) Barlow test and (B) Ortolani test. (From McKinney, E. S., James, S. R., Murray, S. S., Nelson, K. A., & Ashwill, J. W. [2013]. *Maternal-child nursing* [4th ed.]. St. Louis: Saunders.)

D. Bracing. If the spinal curve is between 25 degrees and 45 degrees and is still growing, bracing may be recommended. Although bracing will not straighten an existing curve, it often prevents it from getting worse to the point of requiring surgery. Braces are underarm braces that are custom-made to fit the child's body comfortably.

E. Spinal Fusion. For a curve that is greater than 45 degrees to 50 degrees or if bracing did not stop the curve from reaching this point. Severe curves that are not treated could eventually worsen to the point where they affect lung function. This will straighten the curve and then fuse the vertebrae together so that they heal into a single, solid bone. This will stop growth completely in the part of the spine affected by scoliosis. Metal rods are typically used to hold the bones in place until the fusion happens. The rods are attached to the spine by hooks, screws, and/or wires.
   1. Suggest clothing modifications to camouflage brace.
   2. Reinforce prescribed exercise regimen for back and abdominal muscles.
   3. Plan ways of improving self-concept with the adolescent.
   4. Teach family that severe, untreated scoliosis can cause respiratory difficulty.
   5. A brace does not correct the spine's curve in a child with scoliosis; it only stops or slows the progression.

F. Prepare child and family for surgical correction if required.
   1. Teach child and family log-rolling technique.
   2. Teach how to practice respiratory hygiene.
   3. Orient child to ICU.
   4. Discuss possible postoperative tubes.
   5. Describe postoperative pain management; PCA may be used.
   6. Obtain a baseline neurologic assessment.

G. Provide postoperative care.
   1. Perform frequent neurologic assessments.
   2. Log-roll for 5 days.
   3. Administer IV fluids and analgesics as prescribed.
   4. Perform oral hygiene.
   5. Assist with ambulation.
   6. Encourage child's participation in care to promote self-esteem.

Juvenile Arthritis (JA) or Juvenile Idiopathic Arthritis (JIA)

Description: Juvenile arthritis affects nearly 300,000 kids and teens in the United States.

Juvenile arthritis (JA), also known as pediatric rheumatic disease, and is an umbrella term to describe the inflammatory and rheumatic diseases that develop in children under the age of 16.

Most kinds of JA are autoimmune or autoinflammatory diseases. The immune system is confused and releases inflammatory chemicals that attack healthy cells and tissue. In most JA cases this causes joint inflammation, swelling, pain, and tenderness, but some types of JA have few or no joint symptoms or only affect the skin and internal organs.

Causes

The exact causes of JA are unknown, but researchers believe that certain genes may cause JA when activated by a virus, bacteria, or other external factors. There is no evidence that foods, toxins, allergies, or lack of vitamins cause the disease.

Treatment

There is no cure for JA, but with early diagnosis and aggressive treatment, remission is possible.

Chronic inflammatory disorder of the joint synovium is considered one of the most common rheumatoid conditions occurring in children under the age of 17. JIA is diagnosed when the client presents with the following symptoms for a minimum of 6 weeks:

A. Continuous arthritic pain in single or multiple joints
B. Repetitive fevers up to 39.44°C (103°F)
C. Systematic indications appearing as pinkish/reddish rash on the legs, arms, and trunk
D. The exact cause is unknown; the child's immune system attacks the synovial lining of the joints

Clinical Assessment

A. Joint swelling and stiffness (usually large joints)
B. Painful joints

C. Generalized symptoms: Fever, malaise, and rash
D. Periods of exacerbations and remissions
E. Varying severity: Mild and self-limited or severe and disabling

Clinical Judgment Measures

A. A well-rounded plan includes medication, physical activity, complementary therapies (acupuncture, massage, mind-body therapies), and healthy eating habits.
B. Medications: Drugs that control disease activity include corticosteroids and disease-modifying antirheumatic drugs (DMARDs).
C. Support the maintaining of school schedule and activities appropriate for age.

> **HESI HINT** A well-rounded plan includes medication, physical activity, complementary therapies (acupuncture, massage, mind-body therapies), and healthy eating habits.

REVIEW OF SKELETAL DISORDERS

1. List normal findings in a neurovascular assessment.
2. What is compartment syndrome?
3. What are the signs and symptoms of compartment syndrome?
4. Why are fractures of the epiphyseal plate a special concern?
7. What discharge instructions should be included concerning a child with a spica cast?
7. What are the signs and symptoms of congenital dislocated hip in infants?
8. How would the nurse conduct a scoliosis screening?
10. What care is indicated for a child with juvenile rheumatoid arthritis?

See Answer Key at the end of this text for suggested responses.

For more review, go to http://evolve.elsevier.com/HESI/RN for HESI's online study examinations.

NEXT-GENERATION NCLEX (NGN) EXAMINATION-STYLE QUESTION: BOWTIE QUESTION

Medical Record

Jamie Smith, a 15-year-old adolescent woman, is admitted to the emergency room with joint pain, nausea, and vomiting. Jamie loves track and was at track practice when she had excruciating pain in her joints and fell on the track. She had difficulty getting up from the track and trying to walk. She was brought to the emergency room with shortness of breath, pain, and a possible sprained ankle. Jamie told the doctor that she was diagnosed with Sickle Cell Anemia since she was five years old. She is very aware of her symptoms and tries to avoid being hospitalized. Unfortunately, today she was running, fell on the track, and was extremely fatigued.

Orders

02 oxygen at 2L, Toradol 40 mg q.3–4 h.; IV 1000 NS @ 100 cc/h. routine laboratory, daily I & O, ambulate, safety parameters.

Instructions

Complete the diagram by selecting from the choices below to specify which potential condition the client is most likely experiencing, 2 actions to take, and 2 parameters the nurse would monitor to assess the client's progress.

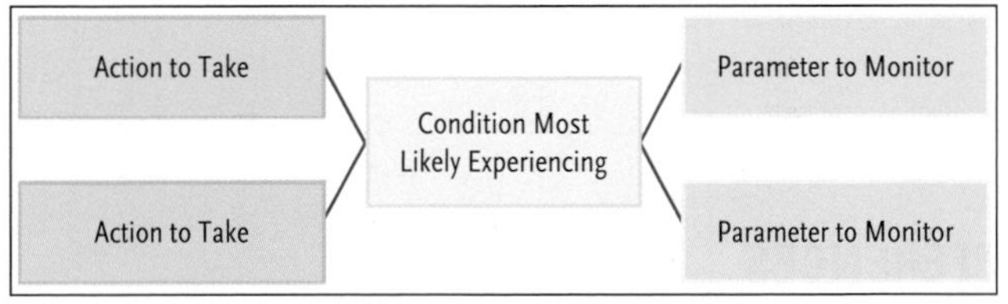

Actions to Take	Potential Conditions	Parameters to Monitor
Administer oxygen 2 L/min NC	Fracture to right ankle	Pulse oximetry
Administer pain medication	Exacerbated flu syndrome	>1000 cc fluid intake per day
Initiate fall precautions	Sickle cell crisis	Oriented to time, person, and place
Monitor I&O	Acute appendicitis	Check bowel sounds
Obtain daily weights		Monitor for skin breakdown

Answers are highlighted in the Answer Key

Medical Record

Baby Carlos Mejaho is a 6-month-old infant who is admitted to the pediatric medical floor with difficulty eating, coughing and vomiting, mild nasal flaring, retractions, and grunting. Carlos is usually happy and breast feeds regularly. He is having trouble with sucking and swallowing and trying to latch due to difficulty with breathing. His mother brought him to the hospital due to dry diapers and increasing lethargy. He is being admitted with viral syndrome, and his past medical history has no known allergies or birth history of concern. Her concern was worsened today due to his dry diapers and his lack of interest in eating including his increasing inability to suck, swallow, and breathe while seemingly fatigued.

- Weight (17 lb 8 oz (7.9 kg))
- Vaccines (CDC, https://www.cdc.gov/vaccines/parents/by-age/months-6.html)
- Diphtheria, tetanus, and whooping cough (pertussis) (DTaP) (3rd dose)
- *H. influenzae* type b disease (Hib) (3rd dose)
- Polio (IPV) (3rd dose)
- Pneumococcal disease (PCV13) (3rd dose)
- Rotavirus (RV) (3rd dose)

Orders

02 oxygen 2 to 6 L high flow, Tylenol 15 mL/kg/dose every 6 hours prn for comfort, report all temperatures; IV D5 0.45 NS with 10 meq/L at 150 mL/kg/day. Routine laboratory, Hourly I&O, safety parameters.

Instructions

Complete the diagram by selecting from the choices below to specify which potential condition the client is most likely experiencing, 2 actions to take, and 2 parameters the nurse would monitor to assess the client's progress.

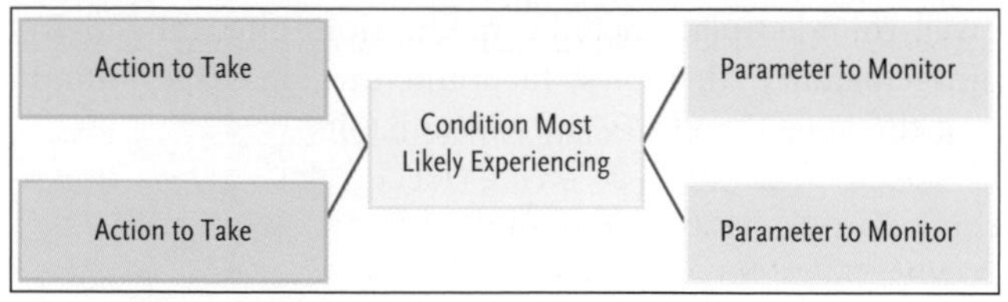

Actions to Take	Potential Conditions	Parameters to Monitor
Administer oxygen 2–6 L/min NC		Pulse oximetry
Administer pain medication	Viral syndrome	Pain level
	Vaccine hesitancy	Need of catch-up vaccines
Obtain MRI	<50% percentile	Percentile in growth chart
Initiate safety precautions	Falls	Fatigue and lethargy
Monitor strict I&O		

Answers are highlighted in the Answer Key

REFERENCES

American Childhood Cancer Organization (ACCO). (2021). *Brain cancer*. Retrieved October 21, 2021, from https://www.acco.org/brain-cancers/

American Society for Preventive Care of Children. (2021). *Children maltreatment*. Retrieved December 4, 2021, from https://americanspcc.org/child-abuse-statistics/

American Thyroid Association (ATA). (2021). *Congenital hypothyroidism*. Retrieved October 21, 2021, from https://www.thyroid.org/congenital-hypothyroidism/

Ballantyne, M., Stevens, B., McAllister, M., Dionne, K., & Jack, A. (1999). Validation of the premature infant pain profile in the clinical setting. *The Clinical Journal of Pain, 15*(4), 297–303. https://doi.org/10.1097/00002508-199912000-00006. PMID: 10617258.

Be a Pediatric Nurse. (n.d.). Retrieved from https://www.herzing.edu/become/pediatric-nurse

Boerlage, A., Ista, E., Duivenvoorden, H., de Wildt, S., Tibboel, D., & van Dijk, M. (2015). The COMFORT behaviour scale detects clinically meaningful effects of analgesic and sedative treatment. *European Journal of Pain, 19*(4), 473–479. https://doi.org/10.1002/ejp.569 Epub 2014 Jul 29. PMID: 25070754.

Center for Disease Control and Prevention. (1982). National surveillance of Reye syndrome 1982: Update, Reye syndrome and salicylate usage: Surgeon General's Advisory on the Use of Salicylates and Reye Syndrome. MMWR. *Morbidity and Mortality Weekly Report, 31*(22), 289–290. Retrieved from: https://www.cdc.gov/mmwr/preview/mmwrhtml/00001108.htm#:~:text=First%20recognized%20about%2019%20years,infections%2C%20particularly%20influenza%20and%20chickenpox.

Centers for Disease Control and Prevention. (2019). *Poisoning prevention*. Centers for Disease Control and Prevention. Retrieved October 8, 2021, from https://www.cdc.gov/safechild/poisoning/index.html

Center for Disease Control and Prevention. (2021c). *Childhood lead poisoning prevention*. Retrieved from https://www.cdc.gov/nceh/lead/data/blood-lead-reference-value.htm

Center for Disease Control and Prevention. (2021d). *Group A streptococcal (GAS) disease*. Retrieved from https://www.cdc.gov/groupastrep/diseases-public/rheumatic-fever.html#diagnosis

Center for Disease Control and Prevention. (2021e). *Cerebral palsy*. Retrieved from https://www.cdc.gov/ncbddd/cp/facts.html#:~:text=Cerebral%20palsy%20(CP)%20is%20a,problems%20with%20using%20the%20muscles

Cherry, K. (2021, July 18). *Understanding Erikson's stages of psychosocial development*. Verywell mind. Retrieved October 7, 2021, from https://www.verywellmind.com/erik-eriksons-stages-of-psychosocial-development-2795740

Child Maltreatment & Neglect Statistics. American SPCC. (2021, September 28). Retrieved October 8, 2021, from https://americanspcc.org/child-abuse-statistics/

Congenital Heart Disease. (2021). *Children's Hospital of Philadelphia.* Retrieved October 30, 2021, from https://www.chop.edu/conditions-diseases/congenital-heart-disease

Congenital Heart Disease Facts and Statistics. (2021). Retrieved October 29, 2021, from https://mendedhearts.org/story/chd-facts-and-statistics/

Health Resources & Service Administration (HRSA). (2021). *Poison help and prevention tips.* Retrieved October 10, 2021, from https://poisonhelp.hrsa.gov/what-you-can-do/prevention-tips

Hirschsprung disease. (2017, February 1). *NORD (National Organization for Rare Disorders).* Retrieved October 8, 2021, from https://rarediseases.org/rare-diseases/hirschsprungs-disease/

Infective Endocarditis. (n.d.). Retrieved from https://rarediseases.info.nih.gov/diseases/6337/infective-endocarditis/cases/29688

Johns Hopkins Medicine. (2021a). *Burns in children.* Retrieved October 8, 2021, from https://www.hopkinsmedicine.org/health/conditions-and-diseases/burns/burns-in children#:~:text=Nearly%2075%25%20of%20all%20scalding,or%20contact%20burns%20(20%25)

John Hopkins Medicine. (2021b). *Urinary tract infections.* Retrieved December 8, 2021, from https://www.hopkinsmedicine.org/health/conditions-and-diseases/urinary-tract-infections/urinary-tract-infections-uti-in-children.

Kim, A. H., & Erby, M. (2020). *Physical abuse (non-accidental trauma).* PM&R KnowledgeNow. Retrieved October 8, 2021, from https://now.aapmr.org/physical-abuse-nonaccidental-trauma/

Mayo Clinic. (2021a). *Kawasaki disease.* Retrieved December 1, 2021, from https://www.mayoclinic.org/diseases-conditions/kawasaki-disease/symptoms-causes/syc-20354598

Mayo Clinic. (2021b). *Pyloric stenosis.* Retrieved December 1, 2021, from https://www.mayoclinic.org/diseases-conditions/pyloric-stenosis/symptoms-causes/syc-20351416

Mayo Clinic. (2021c). *Sickle cell anemia.* Retrieved December 3, 2021, from https://www.mayoclinic.org/diseases-conditions/sickle-cell-anemia/symptoms-causes/syc-20355876

Mayo Clinic. (2021d). *Type 1 diabetes in children.* Retrieved December 3, 2021, from https://www.mayoclinic.org/diseases-conditions/type-1-diabetes-in-children/symptoms-causes/syc-20355306

Mayo Clinic. (2021e). *Vitamin D.* Retrieved December 28, 2021, from https://www.mayoclinic.org/drugs-supplements-vitamin-d/art-20363792

Mayo Foundation for Medical Education and Research. (2020a). *Type 1 diabetes in children.* Mayo Clinic. Retrieved October 8, 2021, from https://www.mayoclinic.org/diseases-conditions/type-1-diabetes-in-children/symptoms-causes/syc-20355306

National Cancer Institute. (2021). *Wilms Tumor and Other Childhood Kidney Tumors Treatment (PDQ®)—Health.* Retrieved October 30, 2021, from https://www.cancer.gov/types/kidney/hp/wilms-treatment-pdq

National Institute of Diabetes and Digestive and Kidney Diseases. (2018). *Vesicoureteral reflux.* Retrieved October 10, 2021, from https://www.niddk.nih.gov/health-information/urologic-diseases/hydronephrosis-newborns/vesicoureteral-reflux

National Institute of Health. (2021). *Phenylketonuria (PKU) condition information.* Retrieved September 8, 2021, from https://www.nichd.nih.gov/health/topics/pku/conditioninfo/default

Nemours Kids Health. (2021). *Cleft palate with cleft lip.* Retrieved November 10, 2021, from https://kidshealth.org/en/parents/cleft-palate-cleft-lip.html

Pediatric fractures—knowledge @ amboss. ambossIcon. (2021, October 13). Retrieved October 8, 2021, from https://www.amboss.com/us/knowledge/Pediatric_fractures

Potter, P., Perry, A.Q., Stockert, P. Hall, A. (2021). Fundamentals of Nursing (10th ed) Elsevier, St. Louis Missouri.

Poison Control. (2019). *Poison control.* Retrieved November 1, 2021, from https://www.poison.org/poison-statistics-national

Stanford Childrens' Health. (2021a). *Congenital heart disease.* Retrieved November 8, 2021, from https://www.stanfordchildrens.org/en/topic/default?id=signs-of-respiratory-distress-in-children-90-P02960

Stanford Childrens' Health. (2021b). *Epilepsy and seizures in children.* Retrieved November 20, 2021, from https://www.stanfordchildrens.org/en/topic/default?id=seizures-and-epilepsy-in-children-90-P02621

Stanford Childrens' Health. (2021c). *Signs of respiratory distress in children.* Retrieved November 8, 2021, from https://www.stanfordchildrens.org/en/topic/default?id=congenital-heart-disease-90-P02346

Vogel-Scibilia, S., McNulty, K., Baxter, B., Miller, S., Dine, M., & Frese, F. (2009). The recovery process utilizing Erikson's stages of human development. *Community Mental Health Journal, 45*(6), 405–414. https://doi.org/10.1007/s10597-009-9189-4

Weber, L. (2015). *Guidelines for non-accidental trauma pediatric perspectives.* Retrieved October 8, 2021, from https://www.gillettechildrens.org/assets/uploads/for-medical-professionals/Guidelines_for_Non-Accidental_Trauma_Pediatric_Perspectives_Vol._24_No.2.pdf.

Wrona, S., & Czarnecki, M. L. (2021). Pediatric pain management. *American Nurse Journal, 16*(3), 6–12.

6

Maternity Nursing

THE MENSTRUAL CYCLE

Menarche

Description: Menarche is defined as the onset of menstruation. Menarche usually occurs between 11 to 13 years with a median age of 12.8 years, or 2 to 3 years after breast budding (thelarche). The first menstrual cycles are typically anovulatory, often irregularly spaced, and can produce heavy bleeding. Regularity and predictability of cycles generally occur within three years of menarche. While ovulation can occur at the time of menarche, it most often takes several months to establish regular ovulatory patterns. However, while most women will have ovulatory cycles within 2 years of menarche, young women should be aware that pregnancy can occur after the onset of menarche.

Menarche is viewed very differently among different cultures; some celebrate the event and others treat it as taboo. Providing education about menarche can increase the comfort of young women. It signifies an important transition into adulthood for young women.

The complete menstrual cycle is under physiological control of the hypothalamic-pituitary ovarian (H-P-O) axis. The HPO axis releases hormones in a pulsatile fashion and triggers changes on both the uterine endometrium (endometrial cycle) and the ovaries (ovarian cycle); whatever happens in the endometrium during the menstrual cycle matches with ovarian activities.

The hypothalamus initially releases gonadotropin-releasing hormone (GnRH). GnRH then stimulates the pituitary gland to produce luteinizing hormone (LH) and follicle-stimulating hormone (FSH), along with several other thyroid, adrenal, and pancreatic hormones. LH and FSH in turn stimulate ovarian production of estrogen and progesterone. LH and FSH regulate the activities of the menstrual cycle through a complex system of negative and positive feedback loops. These feedback loops work synergistically to control functional changes to the endometrial lining and ovulation from the ovaries.

The normal menstrual cycle length is approximately 21 to 35 days. The menstrual cycle can be further defined through ovarian activities and endometrial changes.

Ovarian Cycle

There are three phases in the ovarian cycle.

A. **Follicular phase:** Begins the first day of menstruation (day 1) through day 14 of a typical 28-day cycle. In this preovulatory phase, FSH is secreted by the anterior pituitary and rises triggering one dominant follicle to emerge. As the dominant follicle further develops it moves toward the surface of the ovary in anticipation of the LH surge.

B. **Ovulatory phase:** Ovulation is the process that releases the mature ovum from the dominant follicle. About 34 to 36 hours prior to ovulation, there is a marked rise in LH that prompts the final maturation of the ovum and its release. The ovum is picked up by the fimbriated end of the fallopian tube and transported to the uterus.

   1. Indications of ovulation. A slight drop in temperature occurs 1 day before ovulation (basal body temperature may be less than 37°; a rise of 0.5 degree to 1 degree in temperature occurs at ovulation). Temperature remains elevated for approximately 10 to 12 days. Preovulatory and postovulatory mucus is thick, but at ovulation, cervical mucus is abundant, watery, thin, and clear (it resembles egg white, called spinnbarkeit). The cervical os dilates slightly, softens, and rises in the vagina. Some women have localized abdominal pain (mittelschmerz) that coincides with ovulation. Ferning can be seen microscopically.

C. **Luteal phase:** Begins immediately after ovulation and ends with initiation of menstruation. This phase is relatively constant at 14 days. The influence of LH helps form the corpus luteum. The corpus luteum secretes progesterone and some estrogen to start the negative feedback loop to the HPO axis and prevents further ovulation in the current cycle. Corpus luteum reaches its peak of functional activity 8 days after ovulation. If conception occurs, the fertilized ovum is implanted in the prepared endometrium. In the absence of implantation, the corpus luteum regresses, estrogen and progesterone levels decrease, and the endometrium is shed via menstruation.

Endometrial Cycle

There are four phases of the endometrial cycle (Fig. 6.1).

A. **Menstrual phase:** Begins with initiation of menses. Periodic vasoconstriction in the upper layers of the endometrium initiates shedding of functional 2/3 of the endometrium. Menses, or menstrual flow, typically lasts three to five days but normal variations are noted with as little as 2 days up to 7 days of flow. The average amount of flow ranges from 35 to 80 mL with an average of 50 ml.

B. **Proliferative phase**: Primarily influenced by estrogen. Typically begins on day 4 to 5 and replenishes the endometrium after menses. This phase lasts about 10 days.

C. **Secretory phase**: Primarily influenced by progesterone. Begins at ovulation, usually day 15, and lasts through day 28.

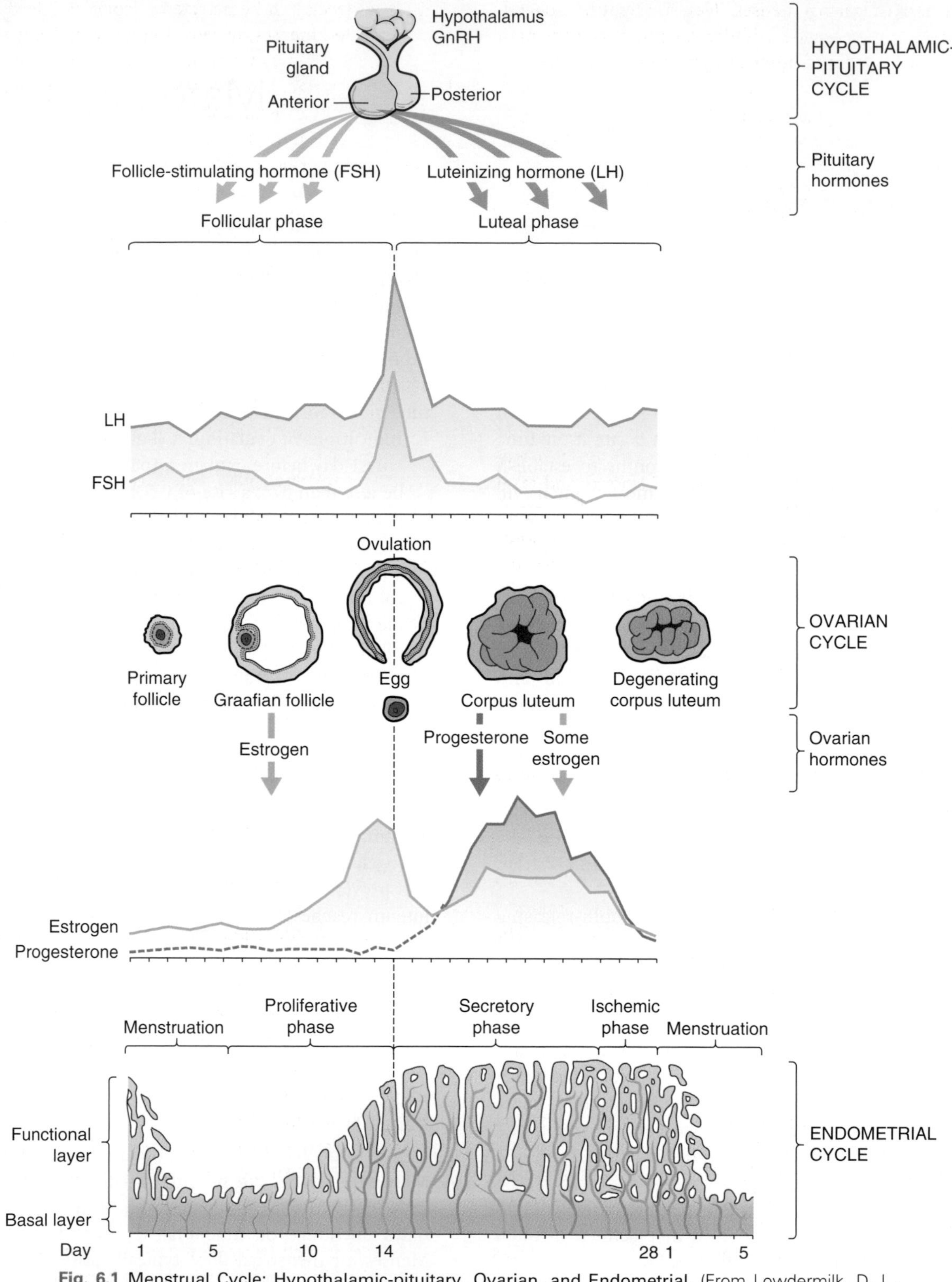

Fig. 6.1 Menstrual Cycle: Hypothalamic-pituitary, Ovarian, and Endometrial. (From Lowdermilk, D. L., Perry, S. E., Cashion, K., Alden, K., & Olshansky, E. [2020]. *Maternity and women's health care* [12th ed., p. 54]. St. Louis: Elsevier.)

During this phase, the endometrium becomes thick and nutritive as it prepares for implantation of a fertilized ovum. Implantation of a fertilized ovum usually occurs about 7 to 10 days after ovulation. If fertilization and implantation do not occur, the corpus luteum regresses and a rapid decrease in progesterone and estrogen occurs.

D. **Ischemic phase:** Blood supply to the superficial endometrial layers decreases to the superficial endometrial layers causing ischemia and triggering menses. Newer literature suggests that estrogen-progesterone withdrawal prompts enzymatic autodigestion of the endometrium and initiates menses.

> **HESI HINT** To avoid pregnancy, a woman should abstain from unprotected sexual intercourse during her fertile days. The fertile period begins 4 to 5 days prior to ovulation and ends 24 to 48 h after ovulation. A couple should not engage in unprotected intercourse before an anticipated ovulation and for approximately 3 days after ovulation to prevent a mistimed pregnancy.

Conception

The union of a single egg and sperm.

Fertilization

Description: The process of fusing the sperm and the ovum (23 chromosomes each) to create a diploid cell with 46 chromosomes. Fertilization usually occurs in 18 to 24 hours and takes place in ampulla (outer third) of the fallopian tube. The zygote is formed. Mitotic cellular replication begins within 30 hours after fertilization. Three to four days later, the zygote has traveled into the uterus and gone through rapid cell division to create additional cells becoming a morula (12 to 16 cells) and then a blastocyst. Implantation then occurs approximately 7 to 10 days post-conception. Some women may experience slight bleeding at the time of implantation.

Embryo and Fetal Development

A. **Embryo.** The embryonic period lasts between 2 and 8 weeks following fertilization. At the end of this stage, the embryo is approximately 3 cm.
   1. During this period of organogenesis, the embryo is most vulnerable to teratogens (viruses, drugs, radiation, or infections), which can cause major congenital anomalies.

B. **Fetus.** The fetal period lasts from 9 weeks until birth. The age of the fetus is measured in gestational weeks and refers to the number of weeks after fertilization (Fig. 6.2).

Maternal Physiologic Changes During Pregnancy

Signs of Pregnancy

A. **Presumptive (subjective):** fatigue, amenorrhea, nausea and vomiting, urinary frequency, breast changes, quickening

B. **Probable (objective):** Hegar sign (softening of the isthmus of cervix), Goodell sign (softening of cervix at approximately 4 weeks gestation), Chadwick's sign (bluish-violet color of cervix and vagina at approximately 6 to 8 weeks gestation), positive pregnancy test.

C. **Positive (Objective):** fetal heart tones, visualization of fetus on ultrasound

Pregnancy Testing

A. **Blood or urine testing**: Recognizes or measures human chorionic gonadotropin (hCG) or a beta subunit of hCG (B-hCG).
   1. hCG levels can be detected as soon as 7 to 8 days before expected menses, usually double every 2 days for the first 4 weeks of pregnancy and peak at about 60 to 70 days.

B. **Gestational age.** Most women do not know the exact date of fertilization, so historically the estimated due date is calculated as 280 days (40 weeks) from the first day of her last menstrual period (LMP). This is approximately 266 days (38 weeks) from ovulation.
   1. Naegele's rule estimates the due date. To calculate, 7 days are added to the LMP and then 3 months are subtracted. This is based on a 28-day cycle.

C. The prenatal period is divided into three trimesters each lasting about 12 to 13 weeks
   1. First trimester: From the first day of LMP through 12 weeks
   2. Second trimester: 13 weeks through 27 weeks
   3. Third trimester: 28 weeks to 40 weeks

Maternal Physiological Adaptations to Pregnancy and Nurse's Clinical Response

First trimester.

A. Maternal Adaptations
   1. Uterus begins to change from pear shape to globular (ball) shape. Size remains below symphysis pubis.
   2. There is often no noticeable weight gain.
   3. Vaginal discharge may start to increase (Leukorrhea)
   4. Breast tenderness is often present
   5. Urinary frequency is noticeable
   6. Weight gain is 2 to 4 lb during the first trimester

B. Clinical Judgment Measures
   1. Common discomforts of pregnancy
      a. Nausea may be relieved by eating small, frequent meals, avoiding fried fatty foods with strong odors, avoiding skipping meals. Antiemetic medications may be prescribed by obstetric provider.
      b. Breast tenderness may be lessened by wearing a supportive bra.
      c. Constipation may occur secondary to effects of first trimester progesterone changes. Increase fluids, drink warm liquids, eat foods with natural fiber, and avoid castor oil.
      d. Fatigue may improve with regular, approved exercise and increased rest.
      e. Urinary frequency is common in first trimester but monitor for signs of a urinary tract infection.
   2. Safety
      a. Avoid hot tubs, saunas, and steam rooms throughout pregnancy (may increase risk for neural tube defects [NTDs] in first trimester; hypotension may cause fainting).
      b. Avoid known teratogens like alcohol, tobacco/nicotine, and substances of abuse.
      c. Report any unusual pain or vaginal bleeding throughout pregnancy.
      d. Report persistent nausea and vomiting or inability to keep any food and fluids down.

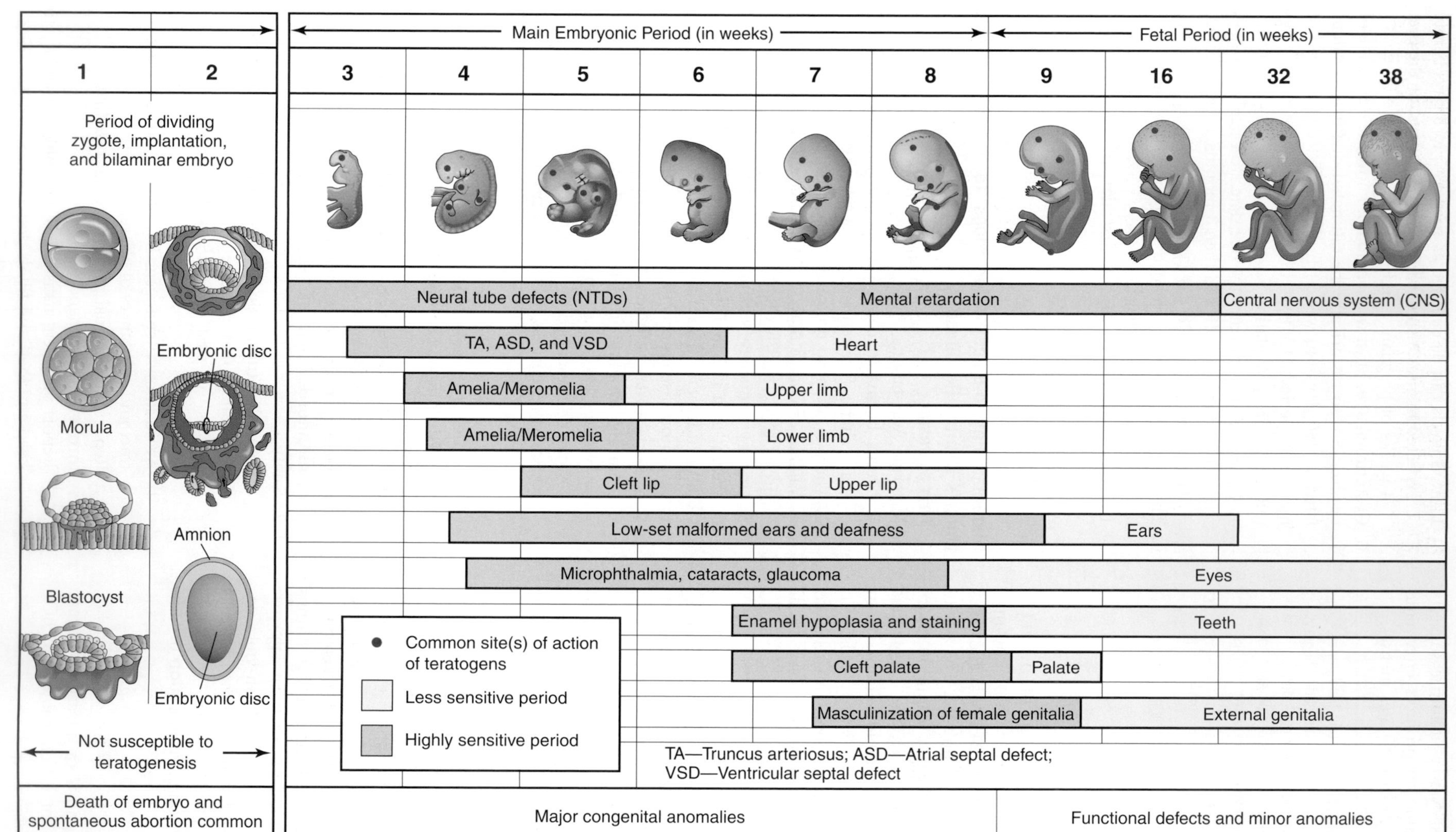

Fig. 6.2 Critical Periods in Human Prenatal Development. Purple denotes highly sensitive periods; green indicates stages that are less sensitive to teratogens. (From Moore, K. L., Persaud, T. V. N., & Torchia, M. G. [2016]. *Before we were born: Essentials of embryology and birth defects* [9th ed.]. Philadelphia: Elsevier.)

e. Report urinary tract infection (UTI) symptoms throughout pregnancy.
f. Screen for intimate partner violence.
g. Educate about perinatal mental health (especially depression and anxiety).
3. Preparation for pregnancy
a. Orient to schedule of prenatal care visits and cost of prenatal care and birth.
b. Discuss choice of obstetric provider.
c. Discuss early pregnancy classes that focus on what to expect during pregnancy.
d. Provide information about childbirth preparation classes.
e. Include partner and family in preparation for childbirth (Table 6.1).

HESI HINT For many women, intimate partner violence or perinatal intimate partner violence (emotional and/or physical abuse) begins during pregnancy. Women should be assessed for abuse in private, away from the partner, by a nurse who is familiar with local resources and can offer information about available services.

TABLE 6.1 Clinical Judgment Measures: First Trimester Common Discomforts

Clinical Judgment Measure	Assessment Characteristics
Recognize Cues	Nausea Breast tenderness Vaginal spotting Fatigue Mild cramping
Analyze Cues	Determine frequency of nausea, ability to hold down food, fluids Determine when breast tenderness began, unilateral or bilateral Determine characteristics of vaginal bleeding: amount, color, time of occurrence, associated pain Discuss fatigue noting onset, alleviating factors Verify constitution of cramping (location, frequency, degree of intensity)
Prioritize Cues	Determine LMP, possible date of conception, date of first positive pregnancy test, gestational age Verify obstetric history and determine risk factors for ectopic pregnancy and spontaneous abortion Determine ability to hold down food and fluids
Solutions	Discuss possible reasons for vaginal spotting in first trimester Discuss potential lab work, US to further evaluate vaginal spotting Provide information about small frequent meals to treat nausea, when to contact provider for additional evaluation of nausea Teach to wear a supportive bra to help alleviate breast tenderness Encourage frequent rest periods (urinary tract infection) ***For more information on potential first trimester concerns, see "Antepartum Complications"**

LMP, Last menstrual period

Second trimester.

A. Maternal Adaptations
1. Uterus rises above pelvic brim. Fundus reaches level of umbilicus by approximately 20 weeks. Two to four fingerbreadths above the umbilicus by 24 weeks, and is halfway between umbilicus and xiphoid process by the end of 27 weeks.
2. Areolas darken and superficial veins noted.
3. Colostrum may be present from the nipples by 16 weeks.
4. Striae gravidarum (stretch marks) may become more noticeable.
5. Quickening, the mother's first perception of fetal movement, may be noted between 16 and 20 weeks.
6. Varicose veins may begin to develop.
7. Glomerular filtration rate increases by 50% over prepregnant levels and peaks at 12 weeks.
8. Placenta is fully functioning and producing hormones.
9. Amniotic sac holds approximately 400 mL of fluid. (Average amount is 700 to 800 mL at term.)
10. Postural hypotension may occur. Blood pressure decreases gradually from pre-pregnancy values reaching its nadir in the second trimester then gradually increases at 24 to 32 weeks and returns to pre-pregnancy levels by term.
11. Serum cholesterol increases from 16 to 32 weeks of pregnancy and remains at this level until after birth.
12. Insulin resistance begins as early as 14 to 16 weeks of gestation and continues to rise until it stabilizes during the last few weeks of pregnancy.
13. Approximate weight gain of 1 lb per week beginning in the second trimester and continuing until delivery.

B. Clinical Judgment Measures
1. Common discomforts of pregnancy
a. Flatulence and gas may be improved with approved exercise.
b. Nasal congestion may be relieved with humidifier. Best to avoid nasal sprays with epinephrine.
c. Round ligaments increase in length and stretch as uterus rises in abdomen and may cause pain. May change position to lessen tension on round ligament or wear maternity abdominal supports as directed by provider.
d. Remaining active may help with constipation, fatigue.
e. Lower extremity edema. Elevate feet when possible. Avoid prolonged sitting and crossing legs. Teach about use of support stockings if directed.
f. Suggest that cool-air vaporizer or saline nasal spray may help with nasal stuffiness.
g. Lower back pain may start to increase. Encourage proper body mechanics.

h. Dyspareunia may be present. Positional changes to accommodate enlarging uterus may help. Report any unusual vaginal discharge or odor.
i. Mild dyspnea may be noticeable by end of second trimester and continue to increase. Educate about expected physiologic changes and warning signs.

2. Safety
   a. Review diet and exercise.
   b. Teach prevention of UTIs.
   c. Remind of importance of dental care throughout pregnancy as needed.
   d. Report leg cramps.
   e. Report heart palpitations.
   f. Report any unresolved nausea or vomiting.
   g. Report any vaginal bleeding or cramping, unusual back pain, or discomfort.
   h. Be aware of signs of intimate partner violence.
   i. Review body mechanics to avoid increased back discomfort.
3. Preparation for pregnancy
   a. Discuss nutrition and regular exercise.
   b. Discuss possible effects of pregnancy on sexual relationship. Recognize partner's role as partner learns to incorporate the parental role into self-identity.
   c. Discuss screening and diagnostic rests for fetal aneuploidy or carrier testing for cystic fibrosis, hemoglobinopathies, spinal muscular atrophy. Typically performed in first or second trimester. May include ultrasound and blood tests, chorionic villus sampling (CVS), testing for nuchal translucency/thickness (NT) or open neural tube defects (ONTDs). Maternal serum markers or noninvasive prenatal testing may be options.
      1) Maternal serum alpha-fetoprotein (AFP) screens for NTD
         a) Performed between 15 and 20 weeks of gestation, 16 to 18 weeks ideal
         b) Elevated levels associated with open NTD
         c) Low levels associated with Down syndrome
         d) Abnormal levels are confirmed with additional testing.
      2) Multiple-marker screens for fetal chromosomal abnormalities, particularly trisomy 21 (Down syndrome) and NTDs. Can be performed in place of maternal serum alpha-fetoprotein (MSAFP). Includes serum levels of hCG, AFP, estriol, inhibin A
         a) May be performed in first trimester with serum testing and ultrasound or performed in second trimester as "quad screen" at 16 to 18 weeks
         b) Elevated levels of AFP associated with risk for NTD
         c) Low levels of AFP associated with Down syndrome and other chromosomal abnormalities
         d) Elevated levels of hCG and inhibin A associated with risk for Down syndrome
         e) Low levels of estriol associated with risk for Down syndrome
      3) Explain screening for gestational diabetes that is usually done between 24 and 28 weeks' gestation.
      4) Sign up for prepared childbirth classes if desired.
      5) A doula is a trained labor support person who may be contracted by the mother to provide emotional and physical support during labor and postpartum.
      6) Discuss desire to breastfeed or bottle feed and provide education accordingly.

Third trimester.

A. Maternal Adaptations
   1. Fundus is halfway between umbilicus and xiphoid process at 28 weeks, is about 3 to 4 fingerbreadths below xiphoid process at 32 weeks, and 1 fingerbreadth below xiphoid process at 36 to 38 weeks. If lightening occurs, may be 2 to 3 fingerbreadths below xiphoid process
   2. Thoracic breathing replaces abdominal breathing.
   3. Cardiac output increases by 30% to 50% and peaks at about 30 weeks. Blood volume increases by 40% to 50% over the pregnancy, reaching a maximum at about 32 weeks.
   4. Heartburn may begin.
   5. Hemorrhoids may develop.
   6. Urinary frequency may increase and nocturia become more prevalent throughout remainder of pregnancy.
   7. Breasts are full and tender. Colostrum may be present.
   8. Swollen ankles may occur.
   9. Sleeping problems may develop.
   10. Dyspnea may be more noticeable and persist until delivery.
   11. Lightening may occur. Around 36 weeks and on.
   12. Backaches may increase.
   13. Braxton Hicks contractions may be more noticeable.

B. Clinical Judgment Measures
   1. Common discomforts of pregnancy
      a. Discuss eating small, frequent meals, avoiding fatty foods, avoiding laying down after meals to help with heartburn. Review medications and over-the-counter treatments as prescribed.
      b. Educate about any prescribed interventions for hemorrhoids like stool softeners or topical agents.
      c. Encourage to wear a well-fitting bra.
      d. Teach measures to decrease lower leg edema and encourage leg elevation one or two times per day. Report of any varicosities.
      e. Encourage sleeping on side for comfort during rest and to help prevent symptoms of supine hypotensive syndrome.
      f. Encourage proper posture and review correct body mechanics.
   2. Safety
      a. Encourage to report any vaginal bleeding, loss of fluid, unusual back pain

b. Discuss third trimester warning signs of pre-eclampsia:
   1) Visual disturbances
   2) Swelling of face, fingers, or sacrum
   3) Severe, continuous headache
   4) Persistent vomiting
   5) Epigastric pain
c. Discuss signs of Infection
   1) Chills
   2) Temperature over 38°C
   3) Dysuria. Pain in abdomen.
d. Report any change in fetal movement. Review fetal movement kick counting.
e. Review signs of labor. Report any preterm labor symptoms. Discuss when to notify obstetric provider about onset of labor symptoms.

HESI HINT Daily fetal movement counting (kick counting) is done by the mother at home. The presence of fetal movements is a generally reassuring sign of fetal health.

3. Preparation for labor, delivery, and parenthood.
   a. Discuss mother's and support person's expectations of labor and delivery. Assess partner's role during childbirth.
   b. Encourage woman to start childbirth-preparation classes.
   c. Discuss location of delivery, i.e., birth center, hospital, homebirth plans; and tour of area.
   d. Encourage review of any birth plans with obstetric provider.
   e. Encourage to pack supplies for hospital or birth center.
   f. Answer questions regarding breastfeeding.
   g. Discuss postpartum choices and decisions: circumcision, rooming-in, initiation of breastfeeding or bottle feeding, support partner's role, cultural beliefs and practices, plans for discharge. If adoption is anticipated, discuss postpartum plans.
   h. Review signs of postpartum blues/postpartum depression.
   i. Review expected postpartum changes and discomforts like vaginal bleeding, any incisional or episiotomy pain, care for vaginal health, voiding, and changes to bowel movements.
   j. Review postpartum warning signs for UTIs, pre-eclampsia, unusual vaginal bleeding, development of blood clots (deep vein thrombosis, pulmonary embolis (DVT, PE)).
   k. Confirm choice and provide education for any desired contraception (Table 6.2).

TABLE 6.2 Clinical Judgment Measures: Third Trimester Common Discomforts

Clinical Judgment Measure	Assessment Characteristics
Recognize Cues	Low back pain Mild abdominal cramping History of preterm labor Frequent voiding
Analyze Cues	Determine where pain is located Verify constitution of pain (constant, intermittent, only with voiding, increasing in intensity) Ascertain ability to stop pain with activity (change of position alleviates discomfort or worsens it) Determine frequency of voiding and characteristics Clarify gestational age
Prioritize Cues	Determine risk factors for preterm labor Verify normalcy of voiding patterns in pregnancy Clarify any loss of fluids Establish fetal well-being (FHR, movement)
Solutions	Teach about preterm labor symptoms, Braxton Hicks contractions, and differences between true labor and false labor Provide guidelines for when to contact obstetric provider with concerns Prevent UTIs with adequate hydration, frequent voiding, and fully emptying of bladder Teach clients about proper body mechanics, appropriate exercises and activity, and adequate rest after activity Teach clients to assess for fetal well-being through fetal kick counting

FHR, Fetal heart rate

PSYCHOSOCIAL RESPONSES TO PREGNANCY

Description: Adaptation to pregnancy is a complex process for the mother, the father or the non-pregnant partner, and the entire family. It is influenced by culture, societal trends, family beliefs, and available supports. Adaptation will vary with each pregnancy and with every person involved. There is no one perfect pathway, but there are similar steps in the process as each person accepts the pregnancy, identifies with their emerging roles, adapts to changing personal relationships (including a relationship with the fetus), and prepares for the birth.

Examples of Psychosocial Responses

A. First trimester
   1. Ambivalence: Whether pregnancy is planned or mistimed, ambivalence is normal and discussions may include attitudes toward pregnancy and desire to continue pregnancy.
   2. Financial worries about increased responsibility and care of an infant are often experienced.
   3. Career concerns may arise.
B. Second trimester
   1. Quickening occurs and fetal movement is experienced by the mother and her partner. Pregnancy may feel more "real" and prompt acceptance of pregnancy.
   2. There may still be some ambivalence toward the pregnancy and the mother and partner may still be considering parenting or other options like adoption.

C. Third trimester
   1. The pregnant person may appear more introverted or self-absorbed as she contemplates delivery, parenting.
   2. Pregnant woman and partner may feel strain in the relationship or experience differing views on delivery, postpartum recovery, and changing roles as each plan for transition into parenthood individually and as a couple.

Antepartum Nursing Care

Description: The antepartum period (pregnancy) is a time of physical and psychological preparation for the birth. The routine prenatal visit schedule typically includes a first visit within the first trimester of pregnancy, monthly visits during weeks 16 to 28, visits every 2 weeks from weeks 29 to 36, and weekly visits until birth.

The First Prenatal Visit

A. Obtain history
   1. Medical history
      a. Family history
      b. Social history
      c. Mental health screening (i.e., history of mood and anxiety disorders)
      d. Substance use screening
      e. Sexual health screening: STDs, TORCH infections (see Chapter 4)
      f. IPV screening
   2. Obstetrical history. Pregnancy count can be determined by two common methods.
      a. Two digits: G/P only records the gravida and para of a client.
         1) Gravida refers to the number of times a woman has been pregnant (regardless of the duration or outcome). The count includes the current pregnancy.
         2) Para refers to the number of times a woman has given birth to a fetus of at least 20 weeks or greater gestation (viable or nonviable). Multiple births count as one birth.
      b. Five digits nomenclature, (gravity-parity, number of pregnancies (GTPAL)) provides more detailed information about the client's obstetrical history.
         1) Gravida—total number of pregnancies, including current pregnancy
         2) Term—total number of pregnancies that reached 37 0/7 weeks gestation or greater
         3) Preterm—total number of pregnancies that reached 20 0/7 weeks gestation to 36 6/7 weeks gestation regardless of fetal outcome or number of fetuses
         4) Abortions—total number of spontaneous and induced abortions prior to 20 0/7 weeks
         5) Living Children—total number of living children. This usually equals the total of term and preterm numbers but may be greater if woman has had multiples or less if any children have died.
      c. History and status of current pregnancy. Including presumptive, probable, and positive signs of pregnancy.

HESI HINT Practice determining gravidity and parity. A woman who is 6 weeks pregnant has the following maternal history:
- She has healthy 2-year-old male fraternal twins.
- She had a miscarriage at 22 weeks.
- She had an induced abortion at 6 weeks, 5 years earlier.
- G/P: Gravida 4, Para 2.
- GTPAL: 4 1-1-1-21 (G-4 pregnancies [twins, miscarriage, induced abortion, current pregnancy]): T-1 (twins count as one birth); P-1 (22-week miscarriage); A-1 (induced abortion at 6 weeks); L-2 (twins).

HESI HINT Practice calculating estimated date of birth using Naegele's rule. The first day of a woman's last normal menstrual period was December 9. What is her EDB?
Answer: September 16. Count back 3 months and add 7 days (always give February 28 days).

B. Assist with physical examination
   1. Vital signs (T, P, R, BP), height and weight
      a. Blood pressure (BP): systolic: slight or no decrease from pre-pregnancy level. Diastolic: slight decrease to mid-pregnancy (24 to 32 weeks) and gradual return to pre-pregnancy levels by end of pregnancy
      b. Heart rate: increases 15 to 20 beats/min
   2. Abdominal exam (including auscultation of fetal heart tones and fundal height measurement as applicable)
   3. Pelvic exam (may include pelvimetry, pap testing, sexually transmitted infection (STI) testing, vaginal discharge screening)

HESI HINT Some women may decline a pelvic exam for cultural, religious, or personal reasons. Pelvic and/or breast exams may trigger adverse emotions if the woman has experienced sexual abuse or is currently experiencing abuse.

C. Routine laboratory data (see Appendixxxxxxx)
   1. Complete blood count
      a. Hemoglobin (Hgb): values during pregnancy greater than 1 at least 11 g/dL first trimester and 10.5 g/dL second trimester
      b. Hematocrit (Hct): values during pregnancy greater than 33% first and third trimesters and at least 32% in second trimester
      c. Mean corpuscular volume or size of red blood cell (MCV)
      d. Platelets
   2. Human immunodeficiency virus (HIV)
   3. Hepatitis B (HBsAg)
   4. Hepatitis C (if high risk)
   4. Rubella titer (>1:10 = immunity)
   5. Syphilis (rapid plasma regain [RPR], Venereal Disease Research Laboratory [VDRL])
   6. Blood type, RH, antibody screen
   7. Varicella immunity (if applicable)
   8. Hgb electrophoresis (sickle cell) (if applicable)
   9. Pap smear (if applicable)

10. Additional STI screening
    a. Gonorrhea
    b. Chlamydia
11. Tuberculin skin testing (if applicable)
12. Urinalysis and culture
13. Genetic Testing, Carrier Screening, Fetal Aneuploidy Screening as applicable and desired

Subsequent Antepartum Visits

A. Vital Signs
B. Check urine
   1. Albumin: No more than a trace is a normal finding (related to preeclampsia)
   2. Glucose: No more than 1+ is a normal finding (related to gestational diabetes)
   3. Protein: A trace amount of protein may be present in the urine; a higher presence may indicate contamination by vaginal secretions, kidney disease, or preeclampsia.
C. Graph weight gain.
   1. 2 to 4 lb weight gain in the first trimester is recommended
   2. 1 lb per week weight gain thereafter is recommended
   3. Total weight gain during the pregnancy for a woman with a pre-pregnancy normal body mass index (BMI), should be approximately 25 to 35 lb
D. Check fundal height
E. Check fetal heart rate (FHR)
   1. 10 to 12 weeks: detectable by using Doppler
   2. 15 to 20 weeks: detectable by using fetoscope
   3. 110 to 160 beats/min: normal FHR range

HESI HINT The normal baseline FHR is 110 to 160 beats/min. Changes in FHR are often the first and most important indicators of compromised blood flow to the fetus.

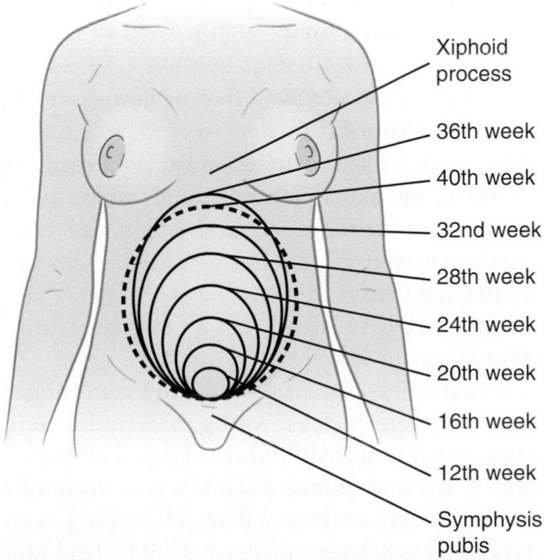

Fig. 6.3 Fundal Height Assessment. (from Murray SS, McKinny ES. Foundations of Maternal Newborn and Women's Health Nursing, 5th ed. Philadelphia: Saunders; 2010)

F. Screen for and address psychosocial concerns: i.e., depression, IPV, substance use

PRENATAL NUTRITION

A. Diet
   1. Use a questionnaire to determine routine dietary habits, individual deficiencies, vegetarian needs, current food aversions, and any subsequent nausea and/or vomiting
   2. Determine food insecurity.
   3. Any symptoms of pica (this should be an ongoing assessment)
   4. Review foods that are less safe during pregnancy and should be avoided.
      a. Unpasteurized cheeses
      b. Raw eggs, meat, fish
      c. Fish containing high levels of mercury
   5. Determine BMI.
      a. Weight (those who weigh <100 lb or >200 lb may be at higher risk)
   6. Note symptoms of malnutrition.
      a. Glossitis
      b. Cracked lips
      c. Dry, brittle hair
B. Determine history of dental care, dental caries, periodontitis.
C. Educate about increased nutritional needs in pregnancy.
   1. Increase intake by about 340 to 450 calories per day (starting in the second trimester) for women carrying one fetus.
   2. Have a minimum of 60 g of protein a day.
   3. Review Daily Recommended Amounts of key nutrients as directed by obstetric provider. Typically:
      a. Iron—27 mg (Box 6.1)
      b. Calcium—1000 mg
      c. Vitamin A—770 μg
      d. Folic acid—600 μg. This amount may be increased by the obstetric provider if the pregnant woman has a history of having a child with an NTD.
      e. Review use of prenatal vitamins. A balanced diet typically provides all the nutrients needed for a healthy pregnancy; however, many women in the United States consume an inadequate diet that does not provide the vitamins and micronutrients needed in pregnancy.
      f. Explain that poor nutrition can lead to anemia, preterm labor, obesity, and intrauterine growth restriction (IUGR).
      g. Drink 8 to 10 glasses of water per day.
      h. Provide a copy of daily food guide for quick reference. Consider cultural food patterns in choices given. Include the following:
         1) 3 servings from dairy group (milk, cheese)
         2) 3 servings of protein (meats, eggs, legumes)
         3) 4 to 5 servings of vegetables (green and deep yellow vegetables are good sources of vitamin C)
         4) 9 to 11 servings of breads or cereals
         5) 3 to 4 servings of fruit

BOX 6.1 Iron Supplementation

- Iron supplements should be taken upon the recommendation of the health care provider.
- A diet rich in vitamin C (in citrus fruits, tomatoes, melons, and strawberries) and heme iron (in meats) increases the absorption of the iron supplement; therefore, include these in the diet often.
- Bran, tea, coffee, milk, oxalates (in spinach and Swiss chard), and egg yolk decrease iron absorption. Avoid consuming them at the same time as the supplement.
- Iron is absorbed best if it is taken when the stomach is empty; that is, take it between meals with a beverage other than tea, coffee, or milk.
- Iron can be taken at bedtime if abdominal discomfort occurs when it is taken between meals.
- If an iron dose is missed, take it as soon as it is remembered if that is within 13 h of the scheduled dose. Do not double up on the dose.
- Keep the supplement in a childproof container and out of the reach of any children in the household.
- The iron may cause stools to be black or dark green.
- Constipation is common with iron supplementation. A diet high in fiber with adequate fluid intake is recommended.

From Lowdermilk, D. L., Perry, S. E., Cashion, K., Alden, K., & Olshansky, E. (2020). *Maternity and women's health care* (12th ed.). St. Louis, MO: Elsevier.

REVIEW OF ANATOMY AND PHYSIOLOGY OF REPRODUCTION AND ANTEPARTUM NURSING CARE

1. State the objective signs that signify ovulation.
2. Ovulation occurs how many days before the next menstrual period?
3. State three ways to identify the chronological age of a pregnancy (gestation).
4. Name the major discomforts of the first trimester and one suggestion for amelioration of each.
5. At 20 weeks' gestation, the fundal height would be _____.
6. State three principles relative to the pattern of weight gain in pregnancy.
7. FHR can be auscultated by Doppler at _____ weeks' gestation.
8. Describe the schedule of prenatal visits for a low-risk pregnant woman.

See Answer Key at the end of this text for suggested responses.

ANTEPARTUM FETAL AND MATERNAL ASSESSMENTS

Description: Assessments to obtain data regarding fetal and maternal physiologic status.

A. Assess maternal risk factors which include but are not limited to
   1. Age under 17 or over 34 years
   2. High parity (>5)
   3. Recent pregnancy history including recent pregnancy loss (3 months or less since last delivery)
   4. Hypertension, preeclampsia in current pregnancy
   5. Anemia, history of hemorrhage, or current hemorrhage
   6. Multiple gestations
   7. Rh incompatibility
   8. History of dystocia or previous operative delivery
   9. A height of 60 inches (5 feet) or less
   10. Malnutrition (15% under ideal weight) or extreme obesity (20% over ideal weight)
   11. Medical disease during pregnancy (diabetes, hyperthyroidism, hyperemesis, clotting disorders)
   12. Infection in pregnancy: **T**oxoplasmosis, **O**ther agents, **R**ubella, **C**ytomegalovirus, **H**erpes simplex (**TORCH** diseases); influenza; HIV; STIs *(chlamydia or gonorrhea)*; human papillomavirus (HPV)
   13. History of family violence, lack of social support
   14. History of assisted reproductive technology

B. Various examinations used to determine fetal and maternal well-being.

Ultrasonography

Description: High-frequency sound waves are used to produce an image of the fetus and surrounding structures to record the fetus's location, size, biophysical status. Used in first trimester to determine number of fetuses, presence of fetal cardiac movement and rhythm, uterine abnormalities, gestational age. Used in second and third trimesters to determine fetal viability and gestational age, size–date discrepancies, amniotic fluid volume (AFV), placental location and maturity, uterine anomalies and abnormalities, cervical length and status, and during amniocentesis.

A. Ultrasound Findings
   1. Fetal heart activity is apparent as early as 6 to 7 weeks' gestation.
   2. Serial evaluation of biparietal diameter and limb length can differentiate between wrong dates and true IUGR.
   3. A biophysical profile (BPP) is made to ascertain fetal well-being. It uses both ultrasound and a non-stress test (NST).
      a. Five variables are assessed: fetal breathing movements (FBM), gross body movements (FM), fetal tone (FT), reactivity of FHR (FHR typically assessed over 20 minutes), and AFV and index.

b. A score of 2 or 0 can be obtained for each variable. An overall score of 8 to 10 designates that the fetus appears well on the day of the examination.

B. Clinical Judgment Measures
1. Explain procedure.
2. Instruct the woman to drink 3 to 4 glasses of water before coming for examination and not to urinate. In the first and second trimesters the client's bladder must be full during the examination in order for the uterus to be supported for imaging. (A full bladder is not needed if ultrasound is done transvaginally instead of abdominally.)
3. Position the woman with pillows under neck and knees to keep pressure off bladder; late in the third trimester, place wedge under right hip to displace uterus to the left.
4. Position display so woman can watch if she wishes.
5. Have bedpan or bathroom immediately available.

C. Complications
1. There are no known complications or risks to mother or fetus.
2. There is controversy regarding routine use of ultrasound in pregnancy.

CHORIONIC VILLI SAMPLING

Description: Chorionic villi sampling (CVS) is the collection of placental tissue between 10 and 12 weeks' gestation. It is collected transcervically or transabdominally under ultrasound guidance.

A. Findings
1. The test determines genetic karyotyping for detection of aneuploidy during the first trimester.

B. Clinical Judgment Measures
1. Have informed consent signed before any procedure.
2. Assist with confirmation of gestational age prior to procedure. (Documented risk of limb reduction birth defects if performed at an earlier age.)
3. Collect appropriate medical history, including blood type and Rh.
4. Warn of slight sharp pain upon catheter insertion.

C. Complications
1. Slightly higher risk of spontaneous abortion over average risk
2. Risk of infection, cramping, bleeding, leaking of amniotic fluid
3. Risk for fetal limb loss
4. Risk for Rh sensitization

AMNIOCENTESIS

Description: Removal of amniotic fluid sample from the uterus for testing or treatment. Typically performed between 15 and 20 weeks. Procedure is used to determine fetal genetic and chromosomal testing, assess for NTD (usually in the second trimester), fetal lung maturity (last trimester), fetal well-being, uterine infection, Rh disease, may be used for follow-up after abnormal maternal serum screening tests.

A. Findings
1. Genetic disorders
   a. Karyotype: Determines Down syndrome (trisomy 21), other trisomies, and sex-linked disorders
   b. Biochemical analysis: Determines more than 60 types of metabolic disorders (Tay-Sachs)
   c. AFP: Elevations may be associated with neutral tube defects; low levels may indicate trisomy 21.
2. Fetal lung maturity
   a. L/S ratio: 2:1 ratio indicates fetal lung maturity unless mother is diabetic or has Rh disease or fetus is septic.
   b. Presence of blood or meconium in the sample can alter the result.
   c. L/S ratio and presence of phosphatidylglycerol (PG): Most accurate determination of fetal maturity. PG is present after 35 weeks' gestation.
   d. Lung maturity is the best predictor of extrauterine survival.
3. Fetal well-being
   a. Analysis of amniotic fluid for bilirubin (usually collected after 28 weeks' gestation) is helpful to evaluate severity of hemolytic disease of a newborn.
   b. Meconium in amniotic fluid may indicate fetal distress.

B. Clinical Judgment Measures
1. Obtain and document baseline vital signs and FHR before procedure.
2. Collect appropriate medical history, including blood type and Rh.
3. Explain procedure and obtain informed consent.
4. Have client empty bladder.
5. Place client in supine position.
6. Provide emotional support and stay with the client. Monitor vital signs, FHR, contractions throughout procedure.
7. After specimen is drawn, wash abdomen; assist woman to empty bladder. A full bladder can irritate the uterus and cause contractions.
8. Monitor vital signs, FHR, contractions for 30 minutes to 1 hour after procedure.
9. Administer Rho(D) immune globin to mother if Rh-negative.
10. Instruct woman to report any contractions, change in fetal movement, or fluid leaking from vagina, vaginal bleeding for symptoms of infection (chills, fever).

C. Complications
1. Risk of spontaneous abortion (1%)
2. Fetal injury
3. Infection
4. Bleeding or leaking of amniotic fluid from puncture site or vagina
5. Preterm labor

Nonstress Test

Description: Noninvasive test to determine fetal well-being. The FHR is recorded for 20 minutes but may be extended to 40 minutes if needed.

A. Findings
   1. A healthy fetus will usually respond to its own movement by means of an FHR acceleration of 15 beats/min, lasting for at least 15 seconds after the movement, twice in a 20-minute period.
   2. The fetus that responds with the 15/15 acceleration within a 20-minute tracing is considered "reactive" and healthy.

B. Clinical Judgment Measures
   1. Apply fetal monitor, ultrasound, and tocodynamometer to maternal abdomen.
   2. Mother placed in semi-recumbent or side-lying position.
   3. Give mother handheld event marker and instruct her to push the button whenever fetal movement is felt. Monitor client for 20 minutes, observing for reactivity.
   4. Vibroacoustic stimulation (VAS) may be used to elicit an acceleration, increase FHR variability, or change the fetal wake/sleep cycle during an NST. After obtaining a 5-minute baseline, the artificial larynx is placed near fetal head.
   5. Stimulus applied for 1 to 3 seconds and fetal response is observed.
      a. Do not use VAS during episodes of bradycardia or during a deceleration

Contraction Stress Test or Oxytocin Challenge Test

Description: The purpose of test is to detect late decelerations with uterine contractions which are due to uteroplacental insufficiency (UPI). Contractions can be induced by nipple stimulation or by infusing a dilute solution of oxytocin.

A. Findings
   1. The contraction stress test (CST) is positive if fetus has late decelerations with at least 50% of contractions in 10 minutes. A negative test suggests fetal well-being (i.e., no occurrence of late decelerations).

B. Clinical Judgment Measures
   1. Assess for contraindications: prematurity, preterm labor, placenta previa, multiple gestation, previous uterine classical scar, previous uterine rupture, preterm rupture of membranes (ROM).
   2. Explain procedure. Place mother in semi-Fowler's position. Place external monitors on abdomen (FHR ultrasound monitor and tocodynamometer).
   3. Record a 20-minute baseline strip to determine fetal well-being (reactivity) and presence or absence of contractions.
   4. To assess for fetal well-being, a recording of at least three contractions in 10 minutes must be obtained.
   5. If no spontaneous contractions are noted, nipple stimulation is attempted. Patient may brush, massage, or roll one nipple for 10 minutes. A warm, wet washcloth may be applied to nipples prior to massaging. If contractions do not begin in 10 minutes, may proceed with oxytocin infusion to stimulate uterine contractions.

> **HESI HINT** With nipple stimulation, there is no control of the "dose" of oxytocin delivered by the posterior pituitary. The chance of hyperstimulation or tachysystole (5 contractions within 10 min or contractions lasting longer than 90 s) may be increased. The test should be discontinued if this occurs.

Biophysical Profile

Description: Combines real-time ultrasonography with an NST to evaluate fetal health by assessing FBM, gross body movement, FT, AFV, and FHR reactivity. Each variable receives 2 points for a normal response or 0 points for an abnormal or absent response.

A. Findings
   1. A score of 8 to 10 indicates fetal well-being.

B. Clinical Judgment Measures
   1. Prepare client for procedure.
   2. Inform client of purpose of examination.
   3. Provide psychological support, especially if testing will continue throughout the pregnancy.
   4. Advise client that a low score indicates fetal compromise that would warrant more detailed investigation.
   5. A score of 8 to 10 indicates fetal well-being.

> **HESI HINT** Percutaneous umbilical blood sampling (PUBS) is the removal of fetal blood from the umbilical cord. It can be done during pregnancy (usually second trimester) under ultrasound for prenatal diagnosis and therapy. Hemoglobinopathies, infections, fetal karyotyping, metabolic disorders can be done using this method.

REVIEW OF FETAL AND MATERNAL ASSESSMENT TECHNIQUES

1. Name five maternal variables associated with diagnosis of a high-risk pregnancy.
2. What does the BPP determine?
3. List necessary nursing actions before an ultrasound examination for a woman in the first trimester of pregnancy.
4. State the advantage of CVS over amniocentesis.
5. Why are serum or amniotic AFP levels done prenatally?
6. What is an important determinant of fetal maturity for extrauterine survival?
7. What is a reactive nonstress test?
8. What are the dangers of the nipple-stimulation stress test?

See Answer Key at the end of this text for suggested responses.

ANTEPARTUM COMPLICATIONS

Spontaneous Abortion

Description: A pregnancy that ends through natural causes before 20 weeks of gestation and a fetal weight less than 500 g. It is also referred to as a miscarriage. About 80% of spontaneous abortions occur before 12 weeks gestation and are not clinically recognized. Ten percent to 15% of clinically recognized pregnancies will end in spontaneous abortion. Possible causes include chromosomal abnormalities, various medical disorders (especially if poorly controlled), substance use, environmental toxins, or trauma.

Types of Spontaneous Abortions

1. Threatened: painless vaginal bleeding without cervical changes; uterine size is equal to dates
2. Inevitable: moderate vaginal bleeding, uterine cramping, and cervical dilation and/or ROM; uterine size is equal to dates
3. Incomplete: moderate to heavy vaginal bleeding, uterine cramping with passage of some fetal or placental tissue through the dilated cervix
4. Complete: spontaneous expulsion of all fetal and placental tissue from uterine cavity; uterus is pre-pregnancy size, cervix may be closed or dilated.
5. Missed: nonviable products of conception are retained; vaginal bleeding may be present or has occurred, then stopped and reoccurred. Possible history of uterine cramping.
6. Recurrent: three or more spontaneous abortions occurring consecutively

A. Common symptoms
   1. Uterine cramping
   2. Backache
   3. Pelvic pressure
   4. Abnormal uterine bleeding
      a. May be bright-red, dark maroon, scant or heavy, intermittent, or continuous
B. Clinical Judgment Measures
   1. Care of the woman will vary by type of spontaneous abortion. Provider may advise expectant management at home (threatened) or follow-up treatment if symptoms worsen and progress. Fifty percent to 85% of spontaneous abortions will complete with expectant management. Medical or surgical management may also be ordered (incomplete or missed abortion). The nurse must assess client's and family's emotional status, needs, and support systems regardless of type of abortion.
C. Labs
   1. Pregnancy test (usually serum, quantitative hCG)
   2. WBC
   3. Hgb/Hct
   4. Confirmation of maternal blood type and Rh factor (Rh_0(D) immune globin may be ordered for women who are Rh-negative).
D. Diagnostic assessment

   Provider may order US and see the client for a physical exam with cervical assessment.
E. Expectant Management
   1. Teach client to notify provider of:
      a. Temperature above 38°C
      b. Foul-smelling vaginal discharge
      c. Bright-red bleeding accompanied by any tissue larger than a dime; client should also monitor amount and color of bleeding
      d. Worsening cramping or unmanaged pain
   2. Acetaminophen-based analgesics may be ordered.
   3. Avoid sexual intercourse, inserting anything into vagina, or tub baths.
   4. Discuss follow-up with provider as directed. Follow-up hCG tests or US may be ordered.
F. Medical or surgical management (D&C) if pregnancy loss confirmed (incomplete, missed)
   1. Nurse should follow admission protocols and assessments, monitor vital signs, ensure intravenous (IV) access, educate woman, and support persons about treatment.
   2. Post-medical or post-surgical care will include monitoring vital signs, administering medications if ordered (oxytocin, antibiotics, Rh (D) immune globin), providing compassionate psychosocial care that addresses perinatal loss. Families are often provided with an opportunity to see the fetus or products of conception.
   3. Educate on follow-up care.

HYPEREMESIS GRAVIDARUM

Description: The inability to control nausea and vomiting during pregnancy. Hyperemesis gravidarum is characterized by excessive vomiting that causes weight loss, electrolyte imbalance, nutritional deficiencies, and ketonuria. It occurs in up to 3% of pregnancies. Pregnancy and nonpregnancy risk factors include first pregnancy, younger maternal age, multifetal gestation, gestational trophoblastic disease (GTD), chronic medical conditions (asthma, DM, hyperthyroid disorders), and history of this condition.

A. Symptoms
   1. Excessive vomiting
   2. Weight loss
   3. Dehydration
   4. Dry mucous membranes, poor skin turgor
   5. Low BP, increased pulse
B. Clinical Judgment Measures
   1. Assess frequency, severity, duration of vomiting
   2. Monitor I&O
   3. Monitor vital signs
   4. Establish and maintain IV access, IV fluids as ordered
   5. Administer antiemetics, antihistamines as ordered
      a. Provide emotional support
C. Labs
   1. Chemistry panel
   2. Urinalysis
   3. Mean corpuscular volume (size of red blood cells) (CBC)

D. Discharge
   1. Discuss advancement of diet once vomiting has stopped
   2. Review medications as prescribed
   3. Review follow up care and importance of regular prenatal assessment of maternal weight gain, fetal growth, and well-being

MOLAR PREGNANCY (HYDATIDIFORM MOLE)

Description: Proliferative growth of placental trophoblast where chorionic villi develop into edematous, cystic, transparent vesicle; appear as a grapelike cluster. Embryo is not viable. The molar pregnancy is a form of GTD that can be associated with pregnancy-related cancers. Cause is unknown but risk is higher for those who have had a previous molar pregnancy and those at extreme ages for reproduction; occurs in 1 in 1000 pregnancies. May be complete (absence of fetal tissue) or partial (nonviable fetal tissue).

A. Symptoms
   1. Vaginal bleeding; dark red or brown, may be intermittent
   2. Abdominal tenderness
   3. Severe nausea and vomiting persisting beyond 12 weeks
   4. Uterus may be larger than expected by dates
   5. Fatigue
   6. Woman may pass vesicles
   7. Early symptoms of preeclampsia may present
B. Clinical Judgment Measures
   1. Assess vital signs, vaginal discharge, uterine cramping.
C. Labs
   1. Serum B-hCG levels are ordered (typically high or rising)
D. Diagnostics
   1. US ordered
E. Surgical intervention (D&C) likely
   1. Provide preoperative and postoperative education and care.
F. Provide discharge instructions.
   1. Follow-up care includes frequent physical exams.
   2. Teach to report signs of complications to obstetric provider immediately.
      a. Bright-red, frank vaginal bleeding
      b. Temperature spike over 100.4°F
      c. Foul-smelling vaginal discharge
   3. Weekly, then monthly serum B-hCG levels are usually monitored for 6 to 12 months to ensure B-hCG levels return to normal. Rising B-hCG levels and an enlarging uterus may indicate malignancy.
G. Refer to community resources for grief and loss.

Ectopic Pregnancy

Description: Fertilized ovum is implanted outside the uterine cavity, about 90% are located in a fallopian tube. Occurs in about 2% of pregnancies and carries increased risk for pregnancy loss, tubal rupture, excessive blood loss, and possible future infertility. Potential risk factors include previous history of ectopic pregnancy, previous tubal surgeries, pelvic infections, use of intrauterine contraceptive devices. It is considered a medical emergency.

A. Symptoms
   1. The three most classic symptoms include abdominal pain (dull to colicky and progresses to constant and severe), delayed menses or may report a very light or irregular menses, abnormal vaginal bleeding (dark brown or red or intermittent spotting).
   2. May report full feeling in lower abdomen, lower quadrant tenderness.
   3. Referred shoulder pain
B. Clinical Judgment Measures
   1. Provide admission care including education, psychological support, preparation for surgery.
   2. Assess vital signs every 15 minutes and as needed.
   3. Start IV to administer fluids.
   4. Assess for active bleeding (associated with tubal rupture). A vaginal exam or abdominal palpation should only be done with caution.
C. Labs
   1. Serum pregnancy test (quantitative B-hCG). When B-hCG levels are greater than 1500 to 2000 milli International Units/mL, a normal intrauterine pregnancy should be visible on transvaginal US.
   2. Progesterone
   3. CBC
   4. Blood type and Rh
D. Diagnostics
   1. Transvaginal US
E. Medical or surgical intervention likely
   1. Those with early diagnosis of ectopic pregnancy may be treated with methotrexate.
   2. Surgical management depends on location of ectopic pregnancy, extent of tissue involved, woman's desires for future pregnancies. Salpingectomy or salpingostomy are options.
F. Post-treatment care
   1. May include serial B-hCG levels (after methotrexate) and physical exam.
   2. Education should include discussion of contraceptive options as pregnancy should be delayed for at least 3 months. Future fertility should be discussed.

> **HESI HINT** Suspect ectopic pregnancy in any woman of childbearing age who presents at an emergency department, clinic, or office with unilateral or bilateral abdominal pain.

ABRUPTIO PLACENTAE AND PLACENTA PREVIA

Description: Two of the major causes of bleeding in late pregnancy are abruptio placentae and placenta previa. It is important to rapidly assess and intervene with these two

TABLE 6.3 Major Causes of Late Pregnancy Bleeding: Abruptio Placentae versus Placenta Previa

Abruptio Placentae	Placenta Previa
A. Partial or complete premature detachment of the placenta from its site of implantation in the uterus, a medical emergency	A. Abnormal implantation of placenta in lower uterine segment near or over the cervical os
B. Occurs in 1 of 80 to 250 pregnancies	B. Occurs in 1 of 200 pregnancies
C. Usually occurs in third trimester or in labor	C. Bleeding usually occurs in the second or third trimester
D. Classification of abruption	D. Classification of previas
1. Retroplacental: blood collection between placenta and uterine wall	1. Incomplete (Partial): Placenta lies over part of cervical os.
2. Subchorionic: bleeding between placenta and membranes	2. Complete: Placenta lies over entire cervical os.
3. Preplacental: blood collection between placenta and amniotic fluid (within the amnion and chorion)	3. Marginal: Edge of placenta 2.5 cm or closer to the cervical os.
E. Associated with	4. Low lying: Placenta implants in lower uterine segment with a placental edge lying near the cervical os, extent not determined.
1. Hypertensive disorders	E. Associated with
2. High gravidity	1. Previous uterine scars
3. Blunt, external abdominal trauma (Motor Vehicular Accident (MVA) or intimate partner violence [IPV])	2. Surgery, cesarean birth
4. Short umbilical cord	3. Smoking
5. Substance use (i.e., cocaine)	4. History of previa

conditions to prevent both maternal and fetal morbidity and mortality (Tables 6.3–6.5).

HESI HINT A client who is at 32 weeks' gestation calls the health care provider because she is experiencing dark-red vaginal bleeding. She is admitted to the emergency department, where the nurse determines the FHR to be 100 beats/min. The client's abdomen is rigid and boardlike, and she is complaining of severe pain. Which actions should the nurse take?

1. Differentiate between abruptio placentae (this client) and placenta previa (painless bright-red bleeding occurring in the third trimester).
2. Notify the health care provider.
3. Do not perform any abdominal or vaginal manipulation or examinations.
4. Administer O_2 by facemask.
5. Monitor for bleeding at IV sites and gums because of the increased risk for DIC.
6. Prepare for emergency cesarean section because uteroplacental perfusion to the fetus is being compromised by early separation of the placenta from the uterus.

HESI HINT DIC is a syndrome of abnormal clotting that is systematic and pathologic. Large amounts of clotting factors, especially fibrinogen, are depleted, causing widespread external and internal bleeding. DIC is related to fetal demise, infection and sepsis, gestational hypertension, preeclampsia, and abruptio placentae. (DIC is discussed in greater detail in Chapter 3: Advanced Clinical Concepts.)

HYPERTENSIVE DISORDERS OF PREGNANCY

Classification

A. **Gestational Hypertension:** Onset of hypertension without proteinuria or other systemic findings after 20 weeks' gestation in a previously normotensive woman; resolves after birth.
B. **Preeclampsia:** Pregnancy-specific condition; hypertension and proteinuria developed after 20 weeks' gestation in a previously normotensive woman. In the absence of proteinuria, preeclampsia may be diagnosed when hypertension is accompanied by multisystem changes as noted below. Can also develop in early postpartum period.
   1. Occurs in 2% to 8% of all pregnancies.
   2. There is no known cause of preeclampsia. Pathophysiology is characterized by
      a. Generalized vasospasm and vasoconstriction leading to vascular damage, poor tissue perfusion to major organs, intravascular protein and fluid loss, and less plasma volume
   3. Preeclampsia is characterized by:
      a. BP of ≥140/90 mm Hg on two occasions at least 4 hours apart after 20 weeks of gestation in a woman with a previously normal blood pressure OR
      b. Systolic blood pressure of ≥160 mmHg or diastolic blood pressure of 110 mm Hg, AND

TABLE 6.4 Symptoms of Abruptio Placentae and Placenta Previa

Abruptio Placentae	Placenta Previa
A. Symptoms vary with degree of separation	A. Painless, bright-red vaginal bleeding in second or third trimester
B. Vaginal bleeding, dark red	B. Uterus soft, nontender
C. Uterine tenderness, often a sudden onset	C. Vital signs usually normal, unless significant blood loss
D. Persistent abdominal pain	D. Placenta in lower uterine segment (indicated by ultrasound)
E. Contractions; may have a rigid, boardlike abdomen (hypertonicity)	E. FHR is usually reassuring
F. FHR abnormalities	

FHR, Fetal heart rate

TABLE 6.5 Clinical Judgment Measures for Abruptio Placentae Versus Placenta Previa

Abruptio Placentae	Placenta Previa
A. Institute bed rest with *no* vaginal or rectal examinations, no internal monitoring, and notify obstetric provider immediately. B. Monitor vital signs frequently. C. Apply continuous, external uterine and fetal monitoring. D. Assess ongoing vaginal bleeding. Serial fundal height measurements may be ordered (increasing fundal height indicates concealed bleeding). E. Start and maintain large bore IV access; administer IV fluids, medications, blood products as ordered. F. Labs: Complete blood count (CBC), coagulation studies, blood type and screen; Kleihauer-Betke test may be ordered. G. US and BPP may be ordered. H. Watch for signs of Disseminated intravascular coagulation (DIC) (can be associated with moderate to severe abruption). 1. Bleeding from three unrelated sites; spontaneous nosebleed 2. Petechiae 3. Ecchymosis 4. Hypotension 5. Tachycardia 6. Abnormal coagulation tests I. Prepare for immediate birth (vaginal or cesarean). J. Expectant management is usually only implemented if both woman and fetus are stable and fetus is between 20 and 34 weeks. K. Provide emotional support; teach regarding usual management and expected outcomes of abruption.	A. Do not perform vaginal examination, rectal examination, or internal monitoring, notify obstetric provider. B. Expectant management: Initial hospitalization with bed rest to extend the period of gestation, continuous external fetal and uterine monitoring. Home care may be a later option if stable. C. If previa determined during labor, institute bed rest immediately and notify obstetric provider. D. Monitor vital signs frequently. E. Start and maintain large bore IV access F. Labs: blood type and screen, CBC, coagulation studies. G. If less than 34 weeks, corticosteroids may be ordered H. Continuous assessment of blood loss I. Prepare client and family for probable cesarean birth emergently if indicated or at 36 weeks or beyond 36 weeks if stabilized. J. Provide emotional support and appropriate teaching regarding usual management and outcomes of placenta previa.

BPP, Biophysical profile; *IV*, intravenous

c. Concomitant evidence of proteinuria.
d. OR, in the absence of proteinuria, hypertension with any of the following is diagnostic:
1) Thrombocytopenia
2) Renal insufficiency
3) Pulmonary edema
4) Impaired liver function

4. Woman may present with visual changes, right upper quadrant (RUQ) pain or epigastric pain, nausea, central nervous system (CNS) symptoms (headache, irritability), edema (especially around eyes, face, and fingers), reflexes may be normal or 2+, weight gain.
5. Risk factors include nulliparity, maternal age ≥35years, previous hypertension or previous pregnancy with preeclampsia, diabetes, thrombophilia, multifetal gestation, autoimmune disorders, family history of preeclampsia.

C. Clinical Judgment Measures

Nursing care will vary based on time of diagnosis during the antepartum, intrapartum, or postpartum period.

A. Antepartum
1. Expectant management: If symptoms are mild in women less than 34 weeks, home management may be an option and guidelines will be established by obstetric provider. If symptoms progress, hospitalization may be necessary and nursing actions will be implemented.
2. Upon hospital admission:
a. Monitor level of consciousness.
b. Frequent vital signs (correct BP monitoring is critical)
c. Assess deep tendon reflexes (DTRs) frequently for evidence of clonus
d. Oxygen status
e. Measure input and output, daily weights.
f. Assess for vaginal bleeding and abdominal pain.
g. Maintain large bore IV access.
h. Typically bedrest with left side-lying position
i. Administer antihypertensive medications if ordered.
j. Nifedipine, hydralazine, methyldopa, or labetalol are common choices (Table 6.6).
k. Administer magnesium sulfate if ordered.
1) Magnesium sulfate (IV) is the medication of choice for preventing and treating seizure activity.
2) Must be aware of risk of magnesium toxicity (absent DTRs, decreased respiratory rate, decreased level of consciousness); if suspected, infusing should be discontinued immediately. Calcium gluconate is the antidote.
3) Never abbreviate magnesium sulfate as $MgSO_4$ in documentation as it is a high alert medication.
3. Obtain fetal assessment continuously; apply external fetal monitor.
4. Assess lab findings daily (Table 6.7).
5. Prepare client for delivery if symptoms worsen, mother or fetus are showing evidence of complications, labor begins.
a. Imminent or actual eclampsia
b. Uncontrolled hypertension

TABLE 6.6 Pharmacologic Control of Hypertension in Pregnancy

Action	Target Tissue	Maternal Effects	Fetal Effects	Nursing Actions
Hydralazine (Apresoline, Neopresol)				
Arteriolar vasodilator	Peripheral arterioles: to decrease muscle tone, decrease peripheral resistance; hypothalamus and medullary vasomotor center for minor decrease in sympathetic tone	Headache, flushing, palpitations, tachycardia, some decrease in uteroplacental blood flow, increase in heart rate and cardiac output, increase in oxygen consumption, nausea and vomiting	Tachycardia; late decelerations and bradycardia if maternal diastolic pressure <90 mm Hg	Assess for effects of medication; alert woman (family) to expected effects of medication; assess blood pressure frequently because precipitous drop can lead to shock and perhaps placental abruption; if giving multiple doses, wait at least 20 min after the first dose is given to administer an additional dose to allow time to assess the effects of the initial dose; assess urinary output; maintain bed rest in lateral position with side rails up; use with caution in presence of maternal tachycardia.
Labetalol Hydrochloride (Normodyne, Trandate)				
Combined alpha- and beta-blocking agent causing vasodilation without significant change in cardiac output	Peripheral arterioles (see Hydralazine)	Lethargy, fatigue, sleep disturbances; Minimal: flushing, tremulousness, orthostatic hypotension; minimal change in pulse rate	Minimal, if any May be associated with small-for-gestational-age infant	See hydralazine; less likely to cause excessive hypotension and tachycardia; less rebound hypertension than hydralazine. Do not use in women with asthma, heart disease, or congestive heart failure. Do not exceed 80 mg in a single dose. Do not give more than 300 mg total in a 24-h period.
Methyldopa (Aldomet)				
Maintenance therapy if needed: 250–500 mg orally every 8 h (α_2-receptor agonist)	Postganglionic nerve endings: interferes with chemical neurotransmission to reduce peripheral vascular resistance; causes CNS sedation	Sleepiness, postural hypotension, constipation, hepatic dysfunction and necrosis, hemolytic anemia; rare: drug-induced fever in 1% of women and positive Coombs test result in 20% of women	After 4 months of maternal therapy, positive Coombs test result in infant	See Hydralazine.
Nifedipine (Adalat, Procardia)				
Calcium channel blocker	Arterioles: to reduce systemic vascular resistance by relaxation of arterial smooth muscle	Headache, flushing, tachycardia; may interfere with labor	Minimal	See Hydralazine. Avoid concurrent use with magnesium sulfate because skeletal muscle blockade can result. Avoid immediate release or sublingual form due to increased risk for profound maternal hypotension

CNS, Central nervous system.

From Lowdermilk, D. L., Perry, S. E., Cashion, K., Alden, K., & Olshansky, E. (2020). *Maternity and women's health care* (12th ed.). St. Louis: Elsevier. Data from Harvey, C., & Sibai, B. (2013). Hypertension in pregnancy. In N. Troiano, C. Harvey, & B. Chez (Eds.), *AWHONN's high risk and critical care obstetrics* (3rd ed.). Philadelphia: Wolters Kluwer/Lippincott Williams & Wilkins; Poole, J. H. (2014). Hypertensive disorders of pregnancy. In K. R. Simpson & P. Creehan (Eds.), *AWHONN's perinatal nursing* (4th ed.). Philadelphia: Lippincott Williams & Wilkins; Sibai, B. (2017). Preeclampsia and hypertensive disorders. In S. G. Gabbe, J. R. Niebyl, & J. L. Simpson, et al. (Eds.), *Obstetrics: Normal and problem pregnancies* (7th ed.). Philadelphia: Elsevier; Witcher, P. M. (2017). Caring for the laboring woman with hypertensive disorders complicating pregnancy. In B. B. Kennedy & S. M. Baird (Eds.), *Intrapartum management modules: A perinatal education program* (5th ed.). Philadelphia: Wolters Kluwer.

TABLE 6.7 Common Laboratory Changes in Preeclampsia

	Normal Nonpregnant	Preeclampsia	HELLP
Hemoglobin, hematocrit	12–16 g/dL, 37%–47%	May ↑	↓
Platelets (cells/mm^3)	150,000–400,000/mm^3	<100,000/mm^3	<100,000/mm^3
Prothrombin time (PT), partial thromboplastin time (PTT)	12–14 s, 60–70 s	Unchanged	Unchanged
Fibrinogen	200–400 mg/dL	300–600 mg/dL	↓
Fibrin split products (FSPs)	Absent	Absent or present	Present
Blood urea nitrogen (BUN)	10–20 mg/dL	↑	↑
Creatinine	0.5–1.1 mg/dL	>1.1 mg/dL	↑
Lactate dehydrogenase (LDH)[a]	45–90 units/L	↑	↑ (>600 units/L)
Aspartate aminotransferase (AST)	4–20 units/L	↑	↑ (>70 units/L)
Alanine aminotransferase (ALT)	3–21 units/L	↑	↑
Creatinine clearance	80–125 mL/min	130–180 mL/min	↓
Burr cells or schistocytes	Absent	Absent	Present
Uric acid	2–6.6 mg/dL	>5.9 mg/dL	>10 mg/dL
Bilirubin (total)	0.1–1 mg/dL	Unchanged or ↑	↑ (>1.2 mg/dL)

[a]LDH values differ according to the test or assays being performed.

From Lowdermilk, D. L., Perry, S. E., Cashion, K., Alden, K., & Olshansky, E. (2020). *Maternity and women's health care* (12th ed.). St. Louis: Elsevier. Data from American College of Obstetricians and Gynecologists (ACOG). (2002). *Practice Bulletin No. 33: Diagnosis and management of preeclampsia and eclampsia.* Washington, DC: ACOG; American College of Obstetricians and Gynecologists. (2013). Executive summary: Hypertension in pregnancy. *Obstetrics & Gynecology, 122*(5), 1122–1131; Dildy, G. (2004). Complications of preeclampsia. In G. Dildy, M. Belfort, G. Saade, et al. (Eds.), *Critical care obstetrics* (4th ed.). Malden, MA: Blackwell Science; Witcher, P. M., & Shah, S. S. (2019). Hypertension in pregnancy. In N. H. Troiano, P. M. Witcher, & S. M. Baird (Eds.), *AWHONN's high risk and critical care obstetrics* (4th ed.). Philadelphia: Wolters Kluwer.

c. Placental abruption
d. DIC
e. Non-reassuring fetal status

B. Intrapartum
1. Continue same, frequent assessments as noted in antepartum care.
2. Have emergency medications, oxygen, and suction equipment available.
3. Control the amount of stimulation in the labor room.
   a. Keep nurse-to-client ratio at 1:1.
   b. If possible, put client in darkened, quiet private room.
   c. Keep client on absolute bed rest, side-lying, and with side rails up.
   d. Disturb client as little as possible with nursing interventions.
   e. Have client choose support person to stay with her and limit other visitors.
4. Continuously explain rationale for procedures and care.
5. Ongoing assessment of labor status and progress
   a. Promptly identify FHR abnormalities.
   b. Ongoing assessment of maternal central nervous, cardiovascular, pulmonary, hepatic, and renal systems
5. If seizures occur
   a. Stay with client, summon help, and contact obstetric team immediately.
   b. Turn client onto side to prevent aspiration.
   c. Do *not* attempt to force objects inside mouth or put fingers into woman's mouth.
   d. Administer oxygen and have suction available.

C. Immediate Postpartum

Nurse should continue to monitor for signs and symptoms of preeclampsia. Preeclampsia usually resolves within 48 hours after birth.

1. Ongoing, frequent assessment of vital signs, I & O, DTRs and level of consciousness
2. Magnesium sulfate infusion is typically continued for first 24 hours postpartum.
   a. Continue to monitor for side effects and toxicity.
3. Carefully assess uterine tone and fundal height for uterine atony.
4. Monitor for blood loss.
5. Instruct client to report headache, visual disturbances, or epigastric pain.
6. Check with the health care provider before administration of *any* ergot derivatives.
7. Upon discharge, client and support persons should be educated about symptoms of preeclampsia in the postpartum recovery period and be advised to report any new or ongoing symptoms to obstetric provider immediately or return to the hospital. Home BP monitoring may be ordered and antihypertensive medications may be restarted or ordered and directions should be followed as ordered.

D. **Eclampsia:** Onset of seizures or coma in a woman with preeclampsia who has no history of preexisting seizure pathology; life-threatening complication of preeclampsia.

E. **HELLP syndrome:** Severe form of preeclampsia associated with increased maternal morbidity and mortality. HELLP stands for hemolysis (H), elevated liver enzymes (EL), and low platelets (LP).

Gestational Diabetes Mellitus

Description: Impaired glucose tolerance that occurs during pregnancy. Occurs in about 10% of pregnancies. Risk factors include family history, personal history of gestational diabetes mellitus (GDM) in previous pregnancy, previous pregnancy that ended in stillbirth, previous delivery of a macrosomic infant, obesity, hypertension (HTN). Associated with increased incidence of macrosomia, birth trauma, neonatal hypoglycemia, and hydramnios.

Women with GDM typically fall into one of two classes:

1. Class A1: Two or more abnormal values on oral glucose tolerance test (OGTT) but fasting and postprandial glucose values are diet controlled
2. Class A2: Not known to have diabetes prior to pregnancy but requires either insulin or oral hypoglycemic mediation for blood glucose control (see Diabetes Mellitus in Chapter 4)

A. Symptoms
   1. May be asymptomatic or describe similar symptoms to diabetes mellitus
      a. The three Ps: **p**olyphagia, **p**olydipsia, and **p**olyuria
      b. Assessment of maternal central nervous, cardiovascular, pulmonary

B. Clinical Judgment Measures
   1. Educate about physiological changes of blood glucose and insulin needs during pregnancy and pathology of GDM.
      a. Hypoglycemia risk in first trimester
      b. Hyperglycemia risk in second and third trimesters: maternal nutrient ingestion contributes to greater and sustained level of blood glucose; maternal insulin resistance increases. If woman unable to compensate for insulin resistance, GDM can result.
   2. Educate about risks and adverse outcomes associated with GDM.
   3. Explain screening for GDM and lab testing procedures.

C. Labs
   1. Early prenatal screening may be done for women considered high risk.
   2. Routine screening typically done between 24 and 28 weeks gestation
      a. Two step screening: (non-fasting) 50-g oral glucose load followed by plasma glucose measurement 1 hour later
      b. Value of 130 to 140 mg/dL or higher considered positive screen; follow-up step of a fasting 3-hour OGTT: fasting glucose level obtained, followed by a 100-g oral glucose load, and then plasma glucose levels obtained at 1-, 2-, and 3-hour intervals

D. Education
   1. If woman determined to have GDM, educate on prescribed medications, diet, exercise.
      a. Refer client to dietitian for individualized diet management.
   2. Explain self-monitoring of blood glucose levels.
   3. Educate on increased fetal surveillance like NSTs, BPPs, amniocentesis.
   4. Teach fetal kick counting.
   5. Teach client signs and symptoms of ketoacidosis and to seek immediate assistance should it occur.
   6. Discuss possibility of scheduled induction between 38 and 40 weeks' gestation, dependent on maternal-fetal well-being.

E. Intrapartum Care for Client with GDM
   1. Establish IV access. Client may need IV insulin and maintenance fluids (once in active labor), or if glucose levels fall below 70 mg/dL, client may need fluids containing 5% dextrose.
   2. Monitor glucose levels per orders.
   3. Check urine for ketones.
   4. Monitor fetus continuously (FHR).
   5. Prepare for complications at birth like dystocia, macrosomic infant, or need for cesarean birth.

F. Postpartum Care for Client with GDM
   1. Insulin administration and maintenance fluids may be continued until stable. Monitor glucose levels per orders and observe for symptoms of hypoglycemia or hyperglycemia.
   2. Check for urine ketones.
   3. Monitor for complications.
      a. Preeclampsia
      b. Postpartum hemorrhage (PPH; postpartum uterine atony associated with uterine overdistention)
      c. Infection
   4. Encourage breastfeeding.
   5. Postpartum education should include guidelines for glucose monitoring, continuation of any insulin or oral hypoglycemic medications, and follow-up care.

> **HESI HINT** Insulin requirements decrease during the first 24 hours after delivery and can drop precipitously; therefore, clients should be monitored closely.

Anemia

Description: A decrease in the O_2-carrying capacity of blood. Occurs in 20% to 50% of pregnant women; often related to iron deficiency. Risk factors include diet low in iron, shortened interval between pregnancies. Associated with increased incidence of preterm birth and low-birth-weight infants. Sickle cell anemia can be reviewed in Chapter 5.

A. Symptoms
   1. Fatigue
   2. Pallor
   3. Weakness
   4. Pica

B. Clinical Judgment Measures
   1. Dietary history
   2. Educate about maternal and fetal concerns associated with iron deficiency anemia.
   3. Discuss labs

TABLE 6.8 Iron

Drug	Indications	Adverse Reactions	Nursing Implications
Ferrous sulfate	Iron deficiency anemia	• Constipation • Diarrhea • Gastric irritation Nausea or vomiting	• Iron is best absorbed on an empty stomach. • To be taken with vitamin C source such as orange juice to increase absorption. • Should not be taken with cereal, eggs, or milk, which decrease absorption. • Should be taken in the evening if problem exists with morning sickness. • Stools will turn dark green to black. • Laboratory values should be checked for increased reticulocytes and rising Hgb and Hct.

C. Labs
  1. Hgb and Hct.
    a. Hgb <11 g/dL, Hct <37% in first, third trimesters
    b. Hgb <10.5 g/dL, Hct <35% in second trimester
    c. Hct <33%
D. Medical treatment
  1. Oral iron supplementation is often ordered (Table 6.8).

Infections

Description: Maternal infection during pregnancy can cause significant concerns for both the woman and the fetus. The woman is typically screened for STDs at her first antepartum appointment and as needed during the remainder of the pregnancy (see Chapter 4 for review of STIs and HIV/AIDS).

A. Symptoms
  Description: Maternal and fetal symptoms will vary with each disease process.

Sexually Transmitted Infections (STIs)

STIs can cause significant maternal and fetal morbidity. Many can be vertically transmitted to the fetus during pregnancy or through the birth canal in labor (Table 6.9).

TORCH Infections

Description: TORCH is a collective acronym for toxoplasmosis, other infections (hepatitis), rubella, cytomegalovirus (CMV), and herpes simplex. These infections can cause significant maternal and fetal morbidity (Table 6.10).

TABLE 6.9 Maternal and Fetal Effects of Common Sexually Transmitted Infections

Infection	Maternal Effects	Fetal Effects
Chlamydia	Prelabor rupture of membranes Preterm labor Postpartum endometritis	Low birth weight
Gonorrhea	Miscarriage Preterm labor Prelabor rupture of membranes Chorioamnionitis Postpartum endometritis Postpartum sepsis	Preterm birth IUGR
Group B streptococcus	Urinary tract infection Chorioamnionitis Postpartum endometritis Sepsis Meningitis (rare)	Preterm birth
Herpes simplex virus	Intrauterine infection (rare)	Congenital infection (rare)
Human papillomavirus	Dystocia from large lesions Excessive bleeding from lesions after birth trauma	None known
Syphilis	Miscarriage Preterm labor	IUGR Preterm birth Stillbirth Congenital infection
Trichomoniasis	Yellow-green vaginal discharge; may be frothy and mucopurulent. Often copious amounts. Cervix and vaginal walls may have tiny petechiae (strawberry spots).	Preterm labor and birth Premature ROM

IUGR, Intrauterine growth restriction; *ROM,* rupture of membranes
Adapted from Lowdermilk, D. L., Perry, S. E., Cashion, K., Alden, K., & Olshansky, E. (2020). *Maternity and women's health care* (12th ed.). St. Louis: Elsevier. Data from Gilbert, E. (2011). *Manual of high risk pregnancy & delivery* (5th ed.). St. Louis: Mosby; Duff, P., Sweet, R., & Edwards, R. (2013). Maternal and fetal infections. In R. K. Creasy, R. Resnik, J. D. Iams, C. J. Lockwood, T. R. Moore, & M. F. Greene (Eds.), *Creasy and Resnik's maternal-fetal medicine: Principles and practice* (7th ed.). Philadelphia: Saunders.

TABLE 6.10 **TORCH Infections: Maternal and Fetal**

Infection	Maternal Effects	Fetal Effects	Counseling: Prevention, Identification, and Management
Toxoplasmosis (protozoa)	Most infections asymptomatic Acute infection similar to mononucleosis Woman immune after first episode (except in immunocompromised clients)	Congenital infection is most likely to occur when maternal infection develops during the third trimester. The risk of fetal injury, however, is greatest when maternal infection occurs during the first trimester.	Good handwashing technique should be used. Eating raw or rare meat and exposure to litter used by infected cats should be avoided; *Toxoplasma* titer should be checked if there are cats in the house. If titer is rising during early pregnancy, therapeutic abortion may be considered an option.
Other Infections			
Hepatitis A (infectious hepatitis) (virus)	Liver failure (extremely rare) Low-grade fever, malaise, poor appetite, right upper quadrant pain and tenderness, jaundice, and light-colored stools	Perinatal transmission virtually never occurs.	Spread by fecal-oral contact especially by culinary workers; gamma globulin can be given as prophylaxis for hepatitis A. Hepatitis A vaccine is available.
Hepatitis B (serum hepatitis) (virus)	May be transmitted sexually Approximately 10% of clients become chronic carriers. Some people with chronic hepatitis B eventually develop severe chronic liver disease, such as cirrhosis or hepatocellular carcinoma.	Infection occurs during birth. Maternal vaccination during pregnancy should present no risk for fetus; however, data are not available.	Generally passed by contaminated needles, syringes, or blood transfusions; also can be transmitted PO or by coitus (but incubation period is longer); hepatitis B immune globulin can be given prophylactically after exposure. Hepatitis B vaccine recommended for populations at risk
Rubella (3-day or German measles) (virus)	Rash, fever, mild symptoms such as headache, malaise, myalgias, and arthralgias; postauricular lymph nodes may be swollen; mild conjunctivitis	Approximately 50%–80% of fetuses exposed to the virus within 12 weeks after conception will show signs of congenital infection. Very few fetuses are affected if infection occurs after 18 weeks of gestation. The most common fetal anomalies associated with congenital rubella syndrome are deafness, eye defects (e.g., cataracts or retinopathy), central nervous system defects, and cardiac defects.	Vaccination of pregnant women is contraindicated; non-immune women should be vaccinated in the early postpartum period; pregnancy should be prevented for 1 month after vaccination. Women may breastfeed after vaccination and the vaccine can be administered along with immunoglobulin preparations such as Rh immune globulin.
Cytomegalovirus (CMV) (a herpesvirus)	Most adults are asymptomatic or have only mild influenza-like symptoms. The presence of CMV antibodies does not totally prevent reinfection.	The fetus can be infected transplacentally. Infection is much more likely with a primary maternal infection. The most common indications of congenital infection include hepatosplenomegaly, intracranial calcifications, jaundice, growth restriction, microcephaly, chorioretinitis, hearing loss, thrombocytopenia, hyperbilirubinemia, and hepatitis.	The virus is transmitted by transplantation of an infected organ, transfusion of infected blood, sexual contact, or contact with contaminated saliva or urine. Virus may be reactivated and cause disease in utero or during birth in subsequent pregnancies; fetal infection may occur during passage through infected birth canal. Prevention includes use of CMV-negative blood products if transfusion of pregnant women is necessary and teaching all women to wash hands carefully after handling infant diapers and toys.

Continued

TABLE 6.10 TORCH Infections: Maternal and Fetal—cont'd

Infection	Maternal Effects	Fetal Effects	Counseling: Prevention, Identification, and Management
Herpes Genitalis (herpes simplex virus, type 1 or type 2 [HSV-1 or HSV-2])	Primary infection with painful blisters, tender inguinal lymph nodes, fever, viral meningitis (rare) Recurrent infections are much milder and shorter.	Transplacental infection resulting in congenital infection is rare and usually occurs with primary maternal infection. The risk mainly exists with infection late in pregnancy.	As many as two-thirds of women with HSV-2 antibodies acquired the infection asymptomatically; however, asymptomatic women can give birth to seriously infected neonates. Risk of transmission is greatest during vaginal birth if woman has active lesions; thus cesarean birth is recommended. Acyclovir can be used to treat recurrent outbreaks during pregnancy or as suppressive therapy late in pregnancy to prevent an outbreak during labor and birth.

TORCH, Toxoplasmosis, other infections, rubella, cytomegalovirus, herpes genitalis.
From Lowdermilk, D. L., Perry, S. E., Cashion, K., Alden, K., & Olshansky, E. (2020). *Maternity and women's health care* (12th ed.). St. Louis: Elsevier. Data from Duff, P., Sweet, R., & Edwards, R. (2013). *Maternal and fetal infections.* In R. K. Creasy, R. Resnik, J. D. Iams, C. J. Lockwood, T. R. Moore, & M. F. Greene (Eds.), *Creasy and Resnik's maternal-fetal medicine: Principles and practice* (7th ed.). Philadelphia: Saunders.

Group B Streptococcus

Description: Group B streptococcus (GBS) can be found in normal vaginal flora and will be present in about 25% of pregnant women. While many women with GBS will be asymptomatic or experience mild symptoms, this infection can cause significant neonatal morbidity and mortality.

Pregnant women with GBS may experience UTIs, develop uterine infections like chorioamnionitis or postpartum endometritis, sepsis, or experience a stillbirth. GBS can cause preterm labor and birth, preterm ROM, or cause intrapartum maternal fever. At birth, GBS infection can cause the neonate to have a fever, difficulty feeding, be irritable or lethargic, or have difficulty breathing.

HIV/AIDS

Description: Women should be universally screened for HIV early in pregnancy, and again in the third trimester for those who are considered to be high risk, so that treatment can be started expeditiously, and the likelihood of perinatal transmission can be reduced. Women with HIV may be asymptomatic, or laboratory studies may reveal leukopenia, thrombocytopenia, anemia, or an elevated erythrocyte sedimentation rate (see Chapter 4). Decisions to proceed with a vaginal birth or a cesarean birth will depend on the degree of the maternal viral load. In the United States, women with HIV are advised not to breastfeed their infants.

Other Vaginal Infections

Bacterial Vaginosis

Description: The most common vaginal infection in women of childbearing age. Bacterial vaginosis (BV) can be sexually associated but it is not an STI. It occurs secondary to a reduction in the normal lactobacilli found in vaginal flora. Characteristically, women will complain of vaginal discharge that is milky, white, or grayish and is accompanied by a fishy odor. BV can cause preterm labor and birth.

Candidiasis

Description: This is sometimes known as a "yeast infection" or vulvovaginal candidiasis and is the second most common type of vaginal infection in the United States. Predisposing factors include antibiotic therapy, diabetes, obesity, and immunosuppressed states. Vaginal discharge is often thick, white, clumpy, or cottage cheese–like and accompanied by vaginal and vulvar itching. It may be connected to oral thrush in the neonate.

A. Clinical Judgment Measures
   1. All pregnant clients should be screened for risk factors for infections.
   2. All prenatal clients should be screened for symptoms of infections.
   3. A thorough sexual history should include asking about Partners, Practices, Protection from STDs, Past history of STDs, Prevention of pregnancy (prior to conception and postpartum plans).
   4. Educate the mother about infections, possible maternal and fetal effects, and treatment options.
   5. Administer medications as prescribed.

B. Labs
   1. May include serology (HIV, syphilis, TORCH), endocervical swabs (chlamydia, gonorrhea), vaginal and rectal swabs (GBS), urine, vaginal, or anal cultures, pap testing, antibody titers.
   2. Labs are typically completed at the first prenatal appointment, repeated as applicable, and third trimester

screening is recommended for women who continue to be at high risk.

C. Diagnostics
   1. May include additional fetal surveillance, i.e., US, if mother is positive for infection and fetal growth appears to be impacted or there is concern of congenital anomalies or infection.

Substance Use Disorders (See Chapter 7)

All women should be universally screened for substance use and substance use disorders (SUDs) during pregnancy and in the postpartum period. SUDs can contribute to significant maternal morbidity and mortality as well as obstetric complications. They can impact fetal growth and development. Treatment options that are safe for both the mother and infant are available during the perinatal period.

Review of Antepartum Complications

1. What instructions should the nurse give the woman with a threatened abortion?
2. Identify the nursing plans and interventions for a woman hospitalized with hyperemesis gravidarum.
3. Describe discharge counseling for a woman after hydatidiform mole evacuation by D&C.
4. What condition should the nurse suspect if a woman of childbearing age presents to an emergency department with bilateral or unilateral abdominal pain, with or without bleeding?
5. List three symptoms of abruptio placentae and three symptoms of placenta previa.
6. All pregnant women should be taught preterm labor recognition. Describe the warning symptoms of preterm labor.
7. List the factors predisposing a woman to preterm labor.
8. Magnesium sulfate is used to treat preeclampsia.
   a. What is the purpose of magnesium sulfate?
   b. What is the main action of magnesium sulfate?
   c. What is the antidote for magnesium sulfate?
   d. List the three main assessment findings indicating toxic effects of magnesium sulfate.
9. What are the major symptoms of preeclampsia?
10. A woman on the oral hypoglycemic tolbutamide asks the nurse if she can continue this medication during pregnancy. How should the nurse respond?
11. Name three maternal and three fetal complications of gestational diabetes.
12. State three priority nursing actions in the postdelivery period for the client with preeclampsia.
13. What are the two most difficult times for control in the pregnant diabetic?
14. Why is regular insulin used in labor?
15. List three conditions clients with diabetes mellitus are more prone to developing.

See Answer Key at the end of this text for suggested responses.

Intrapartum Nursing Care

Description: The process of labor and birth.

Five key factors affect the process of labor and birth. They are noted as the 5 P's:

1. Passengers (fetus and placenta)
2. Passageway (birth canal)
3. Powers (contractions)
4. Position of the mother
5. Psychologic response

Stages of Labor

A First stage of labor: from the beginning of regular contractions to 10 cm dilatation and 100% effacement (Table 6.11)
   a. Latent phase: 0 to 3 cm
   b. Active phase: 4 to 7 cm
   c. Transition phase: 8 to 10 cm

A. Second stage of labor: 10 cm to delivery of the fetus

B. Third stage of labor: From delivery of the fetus to delivery of the placenta. Typically the shortest phase of labor.

C. Fourth stage of labor: About 1 to 2 hours after delivery of the placenta (immediate recovery)

True or False Labor

A. True labor
   1. Pain accompanied by rhythmic contractions that become stronger, longer, and more regular

TABLE 6.11 First Stage of Labor

Phase	Description	Psychological and Physical Responses
Latent	From beginning of true labor until 3–4 cm cervical dilatation	• Mildly anxious, conversant • Able to continue usual activities • Contractions mild, initially 10–20 min apart, 15–20 s duration; later 5–7 min apart, 30–40 s duration
Active	From 4 to 7 cm cervical dilatation	• Increased anxiety • Increased discomfort • May not want to be left alone • Contractions moderate to severe, 2–3 min apart, 30–60 s duration

Transition	From 8 to 10 cm cervical dilatation	• Changed behavior:
		  • Sudden nausea, hiccups
		  • Increased irritability, may not want to be touched, although desirous of companionship and support
		  • Contractions severe, 1 ½ min apart, 60–90 s duration

2. Contractions that intensify with ambulation or activity change
3. Progressive cervical softening, dilatation, and effacement

B. False labor
1. Discomfort may be localized in abdomen
2. Contractions decrease in intensity or frequency with ambulation or changing position
3. No cervical change in dilation or effacement

C. Impending labor signs may include the following:
1. Lightening (fetal presenting part drops into true pelvis)
2. Braxton Hicks contractions (irregular contractions)
3. Lower back pain
4. Increase in vaginal discharge, bloody show, or expulsion of mucous
5. Burst of energy, "nesting instinct"

Initial Nursing Assessment of Client Presenting in Labor

Interview to determine reason client is presenting for care
1. Triage for obstetrical emergencies, (i.e., vaginal bleeding, no fetal movement, ROM, trauma, abnormal vital signs) (Fig. 6.4)
2. Client report of status of membranes
3. Pain assessment
4. Review of prenatal records, obstetric problems (i.e., diabetes mellitus, gestational hypertension), pertinent laboratory and diagnostic test results
   a. Gravidity and parity
   b. Gestational age
5. Psychosocial assessment
   a. General appearance and behavior
   b. Presence of support person
6. Physical examination
   a. General systems assessment with vital signs
   1. Laboratory and diagnostic tests as ordered, i.e., urinalysis, blood tests (hematocrit, CBC, ABO typing and Rh-factor), group B streptococcus status if not known
   b. Fetal assessment

Leopold's maneuvers: abdominal palpation to determine which fetal part is in the fundus, where the fetal back is located, and what is the presenting part. Leopold's may help determine the number of fetuses (Box 6.2, Fig. 6.5).

Fetal lie: The relationship of the long axis (spine) of the fetus to the long axis (spine) of the mother. It can be longitudinal (up and down), transverse (perpendicular), or oblique (slanted; see Fig. 6.6).

Fetal presentation: The part of the fetus that presents to the inlet (see Fig. 6.6)
a. Cephalic (Vertex, face brow)
b. Shoulder (acromion)
c. Breech (buttocks)

Fetal position: Determine location of fetal back. The location of the back in the anterior, lateral, or posterior portion of the abdomen also helps determine the variety (position). Fetal small parts (hands, feet, knees) should be opposite the fetal back. The relationship of the point of reference (occiput, sacrum, acromion) on the fetal presenting part (cephalic, breech, shoulder) to the mother's pelvis. Most common is left occiput anterior (LOA). The point of reference on the vertex (occiput) is pointed up toward the symphysis and directed toward the left side of the maternal pelvis (Fig. 6.7).

Fetal station: Relationship of presenting part to an imaginary line drawn between the maternal ischial spines. Measures degree of descent of presenting fetal part through birth canal. Expressed as cm above or below the ischial spines. Best assessed as part of the vaginal exam and should be determined when labor begins so that rate of fetal descent can be assessed regularly and accurately (Fig. 6.8).
a. Station 0 is engaged.
b. Negative stations are above the ischial spines.
c. Positive stations are below the ischial spines.

Fetal attitude:

A. Relationship of the fetal parts to one another
B. Flexion or extension
C. Flexion is desirable so that the smallest diameters of the presenting part move through the pelvis.
D. FHR and pattern assessment
   1. FHR best heard over fetal back (see Fig. 6.5 and Box 6.2)
E. Assessment of uterine contractions
   1. Frequency. Time contractions from beginning of one contraction to the beginning of the next (measured in minutes apart).
   2. Duration. Time the length of the entire contraction (from beginning to end).
   3. Strength. Assess the intensity of strongest part (peak) of contraction. It is measured by clinical estimation of the indentability of the fundus through palpation (use gentle pressure of fingertips to determine it).
      a. Very indentable (mild)
      b. Moderately indentable (moderate)
      c. Unindentable (firm)

HESI HINT Internal electric monitoring with an intrauterine pressure catheter is the most accurate way to assess uterine contraction intensity and uterus resting tone.

F. Sterile vaginal examination (performed only when indicated by the status of the client and the fetus). Nurse should obtain permission to touch the woman prior to the exam.
   1. Sterile gloves are worn.
   2. Examinations are not done routinely. They are sharply curtailed after membranes rupture to prevent infection.
   3. Vaginal exams should not be performed with active vaginal bleeding
      a. Possible placenta previa, placental abruption, fetal vessels may be lying over the cervical os
   4. Vaginal examinations are performed before analgesia and anesthesia, to determine the progress of labor, to determine whether second-stage pushing can begin.
   5. Cervical Assessment:
      a. Cervical dilation: Cervix opens from 0 to 10 cm.

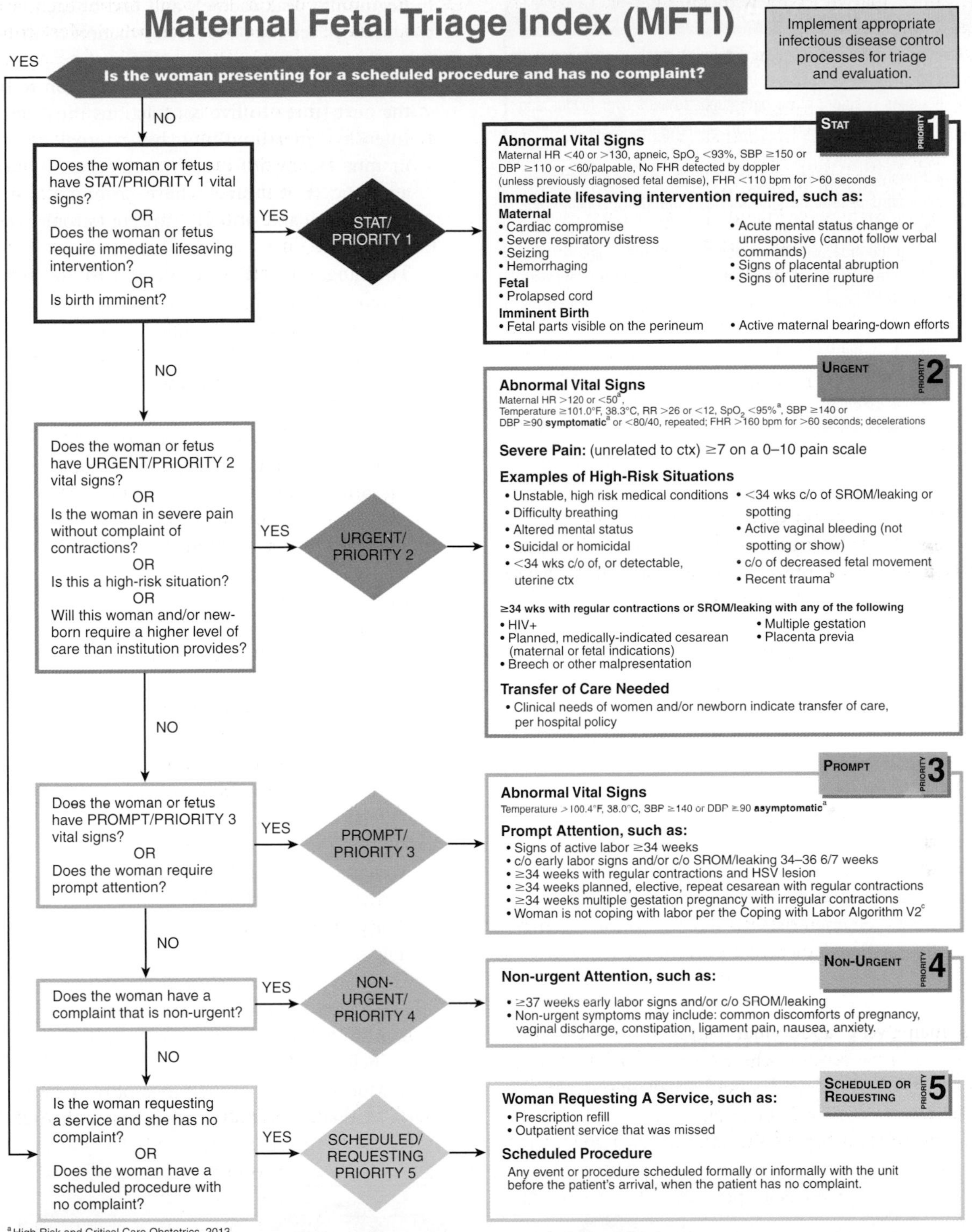

[a] High Risk and Critical Care Obstetrics, 2013
[b] Trauma may or may not include a direct assault on the abdomen. Examples are trauma from motor vehicle accidents, falls, and intimate partner violence.
[c] Coping with Labor Algorithm V2 used with permission.
The HFTI is exemplary and does not include all possible patient complaints or conditions. The MFTI is designed to guide clinical decision-making but does not replace clinical judgement. Vital signs in the MFTI are suggested values. Values appropriate for the population and geographic region should be determined by each clinical team, taking into account variables such as altitude.

Fig. 6.4 Maternal Fetal Triage Index (MFT) (Figure 19.3 in Lowdermilk). (From Reprinted with permission from the Association of Women's Health, Obstetric and Neonatal Nurses [AWHONN] [www.awhonn.org]. AWHONN Maternal Fetal Triage Index. Copyright AWHONN. To access the full PDF version of the MFTI Index for clinical use, email requests to permissions@awhonn.org.)

BOX 6.2 Leopold Maneuvers

Description: Abdominal palpations used to determine fetal presentation, lie, position, and engagement

A. With client in supine position, place both cupped hands over fundus and palpate to determine whether breech (soft, immovable, large) or vertex (hard, movable, small).
B. Place one hand firmly on side and palpate with other hand to determine presence of small parts or fetal back. (Fetal heart rate [FHR] is heard best through fetal back.)
C. Facing client, grasp the area over the symphysis with the thumb and fingers and press to determine the degree of descent of the presenting part. (A ballotable or floating head can be rocked back and forth between the thumb and fingers.)
D. Facing the client's feet, outline the fetal presenting part with the palmar surface of both hands to determine the degree of descent and attitude of the fetus. (If cephalic prominence is located on the same side as small parts, assume the head is flexed.)

b. Cervical effacement: Cervix is taken up into the upper uterine segment; expressed in percentages from 0% to 100%.
c. Cervical position: Cervix can be directly anterior and palpated easily, or can be posterior and difficult to palpate.
d. Cervical consistency: It is firm to soft.

6. Status of Membranes (ruptured, bulging, or intact)
   a. Determined by vaginal exam or obvious leaking of fluid
   b. Microscopic examination of vaginal fluid for ferning
   c. Nitrazine paper turns black or dark blue with presence of amniotic fluid.
   d. Chart time of rupture, fetal response, and any describing characteristics (color, odor, clarity) including evidence of meconium.

ELECTRONIC FETAL MONITORING

Variables Measured by Fetal Monitoring

A. Contractions
1. Beginning, peak (acme), and end of each contraction
2. Duration: length of each contraction from beginning to end
3. Frequency: beginning of one contraction to beginning of the next (three to five contractions must be measured)
4. Intensity: measured not by external monitoring but in mm Hg by internal (intrauterine) monitoring after amniotic membranes have ruptured; ranges from 30 mm Hg (mild) to 70 mm Hg (strong) at peak

B. Baseline FHR
1. The range of FHR (average 110 to 160 beats/min) between contractions, monitored over a 10-minute period. The baseline segment should be greater than 2 minutes of tracing.
2. The balance between parasympathetic and sympathetic impulses usually produces no observable changes in the FHR during uterine contractions (with a healthy fetus, a healthy placenta, and good uteroplacental perfusion; Fig. 6.10).

Clinical Judgment Measures Based on Fetal Heart Rate

A. Baseline FHR
1. Normal rhythmicity
2. Average FHR 110 to 160 beats/min
3. Description
   a. The FHR results from the balance between the parasympathetic and the sympathetic branches of the autonomic nervous system.
   b. It is the most important indicator of the health of the fetal CNS.

B. Variability
1. A characteristic of the baseline FHR and described as normal irregularity of the cardiac rhythm. Moderate variability signifies that the fetus does not have ischemia (Fig. 6.11).
2. There are four categories of variability.
   a. Absent: amplitude range undetectable
   b. Minimal: amplitude range detectable up to and including 5 beats/min
   c. Moderate: amplitude range of 6 to 25 beats/min
   d. Marked: amplitude range greater than 25 beats/min

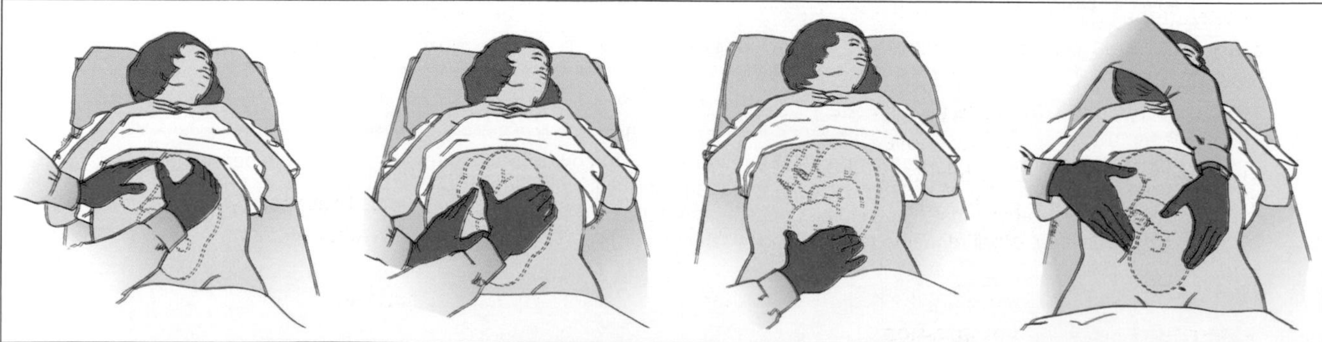

Fig. 6.5 **Leopold Maneuvers.** (From Lowdermilk, D. L., Perry, S. E., Cashion, K., Alden, K., & Olshansky, E. [2020]. *Maternity and women's health care* [12th ed.]. St. Louis: Elsevier.)

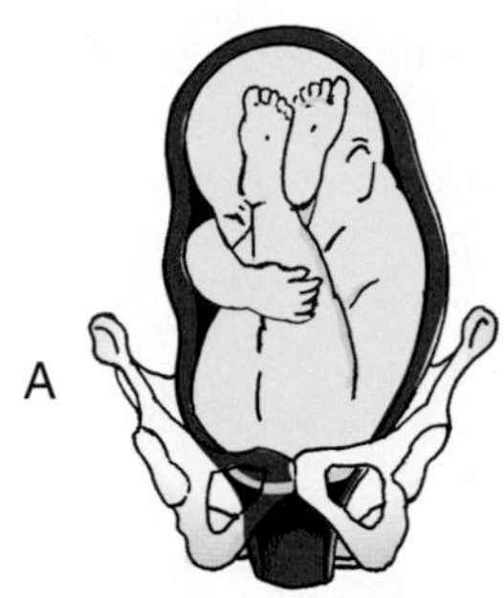

Frank breech

Lie: Longitudinal or vertical
Presentation: Breech (incomplete)
Presenting part: Sacrum
Attitude: Flexion, except for legs at knees

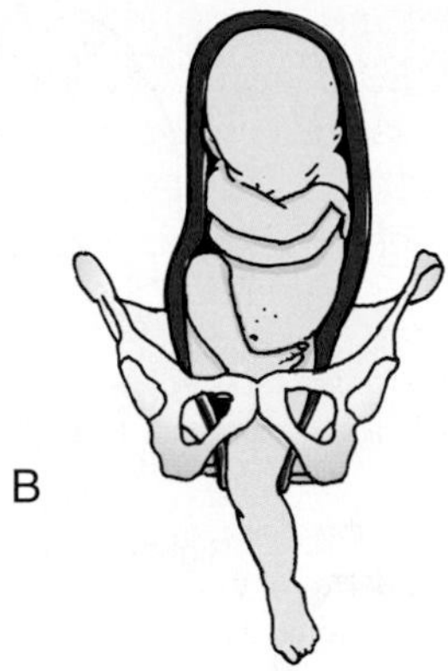

Single footling breech

Lie: Longitudinal or vertical
Presentation: Breech (incomplete)
Presenting part: Sacrum
Attitude: Flexion, except for one leg extended at hip and knee

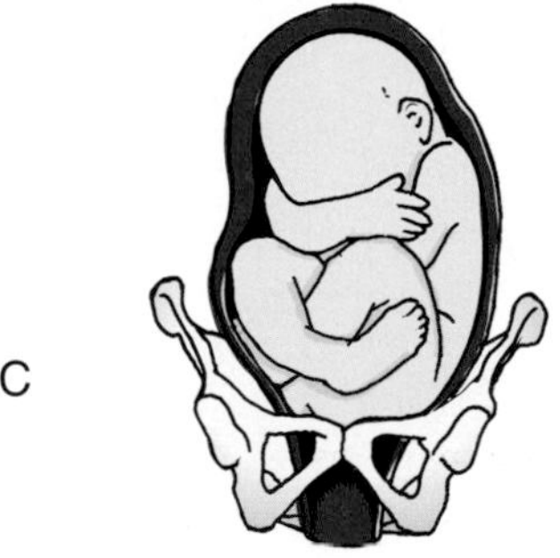

Complete breech

Lie: Longitudinal or vertical
Presentation: Breech (sacrum and feet presenting)
Presenting part: Sacrum (with feet)
Attitude: General flexion

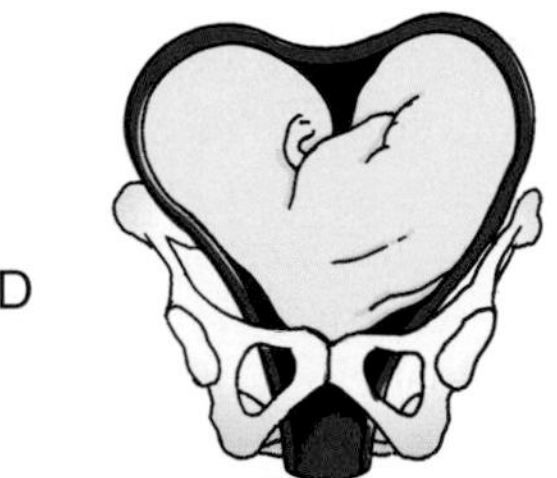

Shoulder presentation

Lie: Transverse or horizontal
Presentation: Shoulder
Presenting part: Scapula
Attitude: Flexion

Fig. 6.6 Fetal Presentations. (A–C) Breech (sacral) presentation. (D) Shoulder presentation.

C. Clinical Judgment Measures
   1. Assess contractions using monitor strip.
   2. Assess FHR for normal baseline range and variability.
D. Periodic changes
   1. FHR changes in relation to uterine contractions (Fig. 6.12)
   2. Description
      a. Accelerations: abrupt increase in FHR of at least 15 beats/min and lasting 15 seconds or more above baseline
         1) Caused by sympathetic fetal response
         2) Occur in response to fetal movement
         3) Indicative of a reactive, healthy fetus
      b. Early Decelerations: a gradual decrease in FHR, at least 30 seconds to lowest part of deceleration (nadir) (Fig. 6.13)
         1) Benign pattern caused by parasympathetic response, i.e., head compression
         2) Heart rate slowly and smoothly decelerates at beginning of contraction and returns to baseline at end of contraction.
         3) Often appear in active labor
   3. Nursing interventions for early decelerations
      a. No nursing interventions are required except to monitor the progress of labor.
      b. Document the processes of labor.

Fetal Heart Rate Patterns Requiring Clinical Judgment Measures

A. Decreased Variability
   1. Absent or minimal. Interpretation based on presence or absence of accelerations or recurrent decelerations
   2. Causes
      a. Hypoxia (asphyxia)
      b. Acidosis

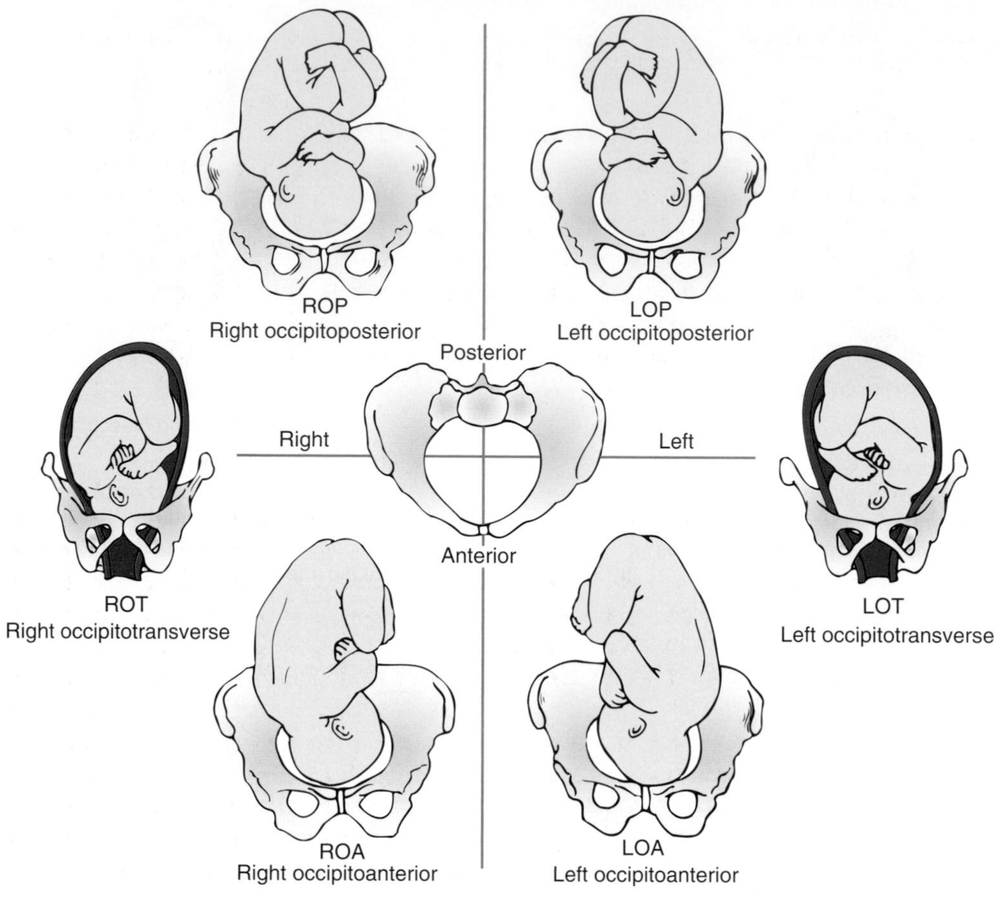

Lie: Longitudinal or vertical
Presentation: Vertex
Reference point: Occiput
Attitude: General flexion

Fig. 6.7 Fetal Positions.

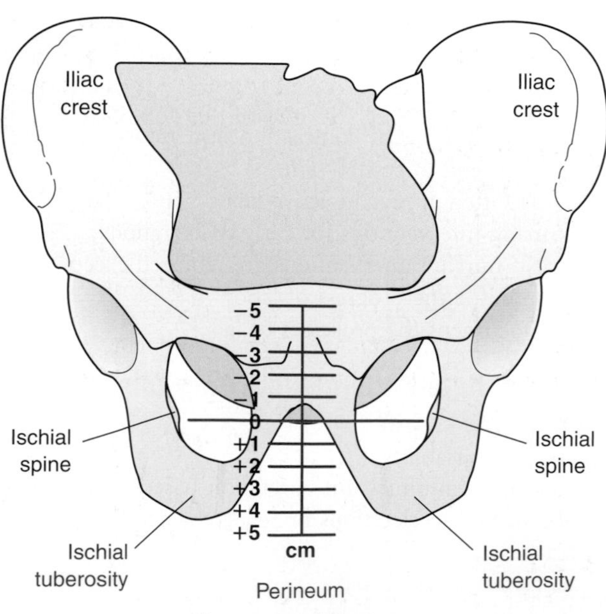

Fig. 6.8 Fetal Stations.

c. Maternal drug ingestion (opiates, CNS depressants such as magnesium sulfate, beta adrenergic agents [Terbutaline])
d. Fetal rest cycles; typically last 20 to 40 minutes

3. Nursing Intervention
   a. Change maternal position, left-lateral
   b. Stimulate fetal scalp if indicated.
   c. Discontinue oxytocin if infusing.
   d. Assist provider with application of scalp electrode for internal fetal monitoring.

B. Bradycardia
1. Baseline FHR is below 110 beats/min (assessed between contractions) for 10 minutes (as differentiated from a periodic change).
2. Causes
   a. Late manifestation of fetal hypoxia
   b. Fetal cardiac problems
   c. Maternal hypoglycemia, hypothermia
   d. Prolonged umbilical cord compression or head compression during rapid descent

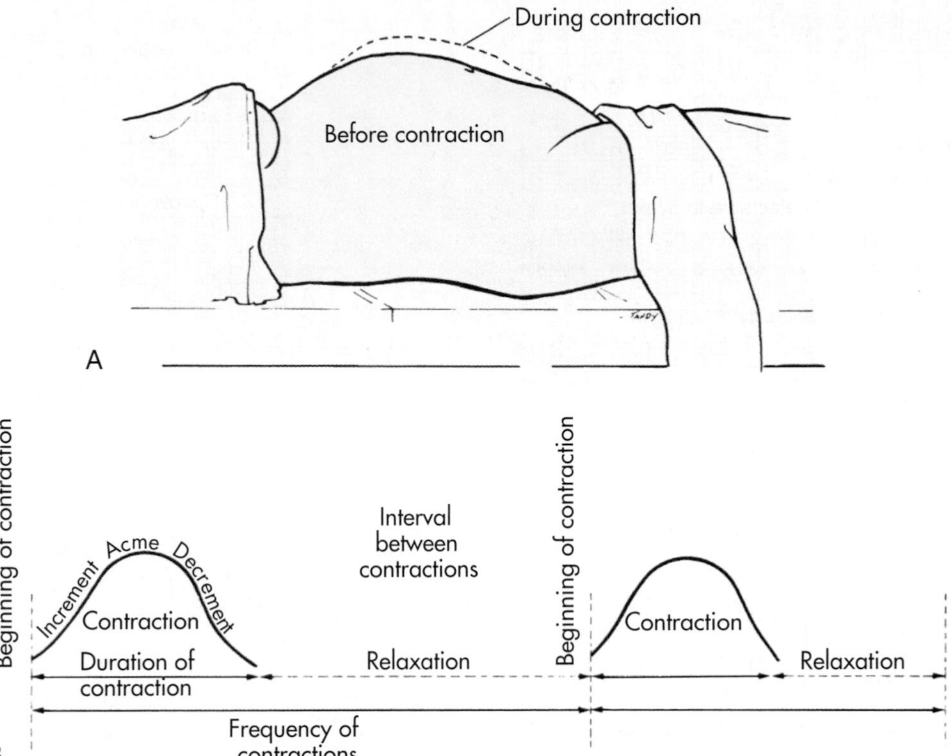

Fig. 6.9 Assessment of Uterine Contractions (A) Depiction of contraction at rest and during contraction (B) frequency of contraction. (From Lowdermilk, D. L., Perry, S. E., Cashion, K., Alden, K., & Olshansky, E. [2020]. *Maternity and women's health care* [12th ed., p. 388]. St. Louis: Elsevier, Courtesy Julie Perry Nelson, Loveland, CO.)

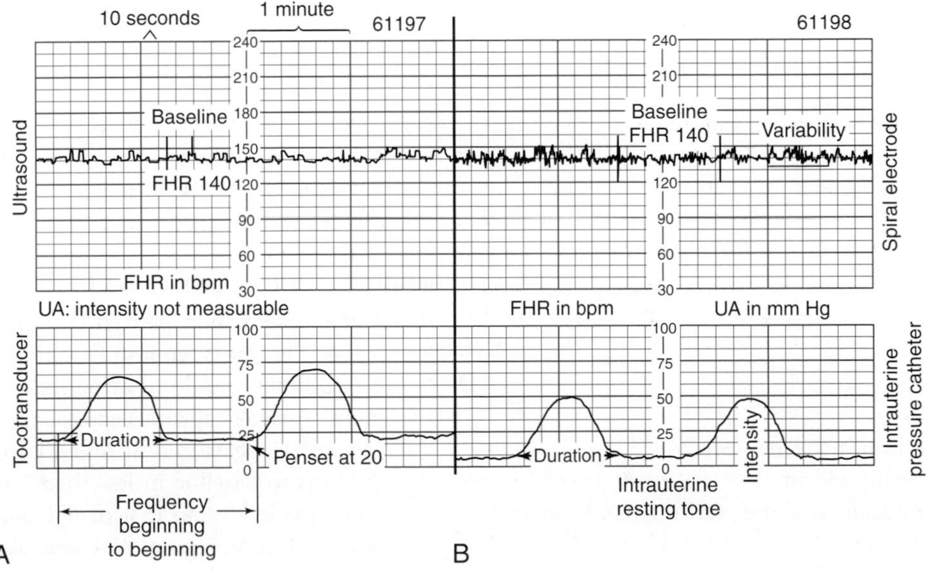

Fig. 6.10 Display of Fetal Heart Rate and Uterine Activity on Chart Paper. (A) External mode with ultrasound and tocotransducer as signal course. (B) Internal mode with spiral electrode and intrauterine catheter as signal source. Frequency of contractions is measured from the beginning of one contraction to the beginning of the next. Peak-to-peak measurement is sometimes used when electronic uterine activity monitoring is done. (From Miller, L., & Tucker, S. M. [2013]. *Pocket guide to fetal monitoring and assessment* [7th ed.]. St. Louis: Mosby.)

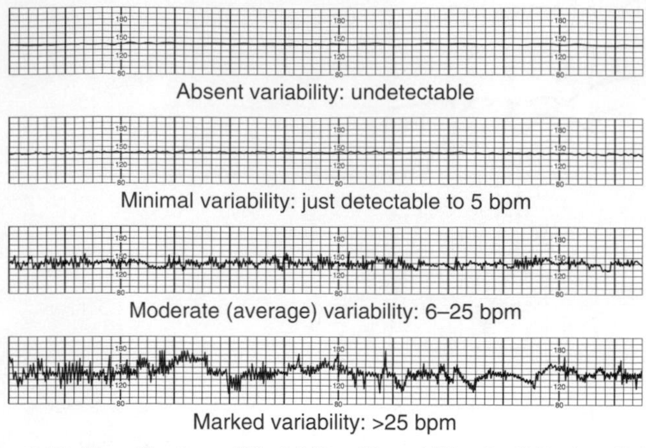

Fig. 6.11 Classification of Variability. (From Miller, L., & Tucker, S. M. [2013]. *Pocket guide to fetal monitoring and assessment* [7th ed.]. St. Louis: Mosby.)

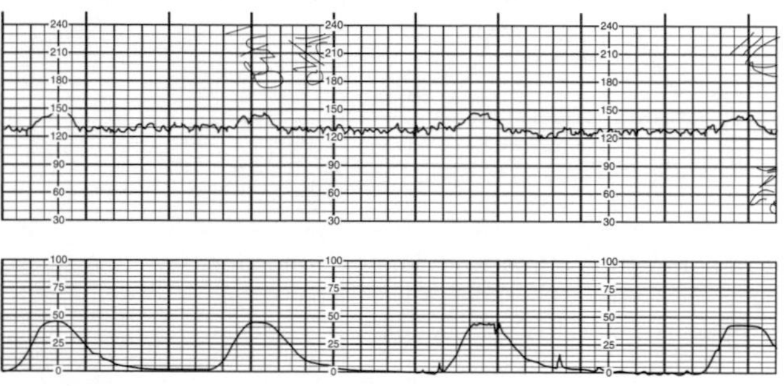

Fig. 6.12 Periodic Accelerations With Uterine Contractions. (From Miller, L., & Tucker, S. M. [2013]. *Pocket guide to fetal monitoring and assessment* [7th ed.]. St. Louis: Mosby.)

3. Nursing Interventions dependent on cause. Possible actions:
   a. Change maternal position to side-lying.
   b. Stop oxytocin (if being delivered).
   c. Administer maternal oxygen.
   d. Notify provider.

C. Tachycardia
   1. Baseline FHR is above 160 beats/min (assessed between contractions) for 10 minutes
   2. Causes
      a. Early sign of fetal hypoxia
      b. Fetal infection
      c. Maternal infection, maternal fever
      d. Maternal hyperthyroidism
      e. Medication induced (atropine, terbutaline, hydroxyzine) or illicit drugs
      f. Rare: fetal anemia, acute fetal blood loss (placental abruption)
      g. Mild tachycardia common in fetus less than 28 weeks gestation
   3. Nursing interventions dependent on cause. Possible actions:
      a. Reduce maternal fever; administer antipyretics as prescribed

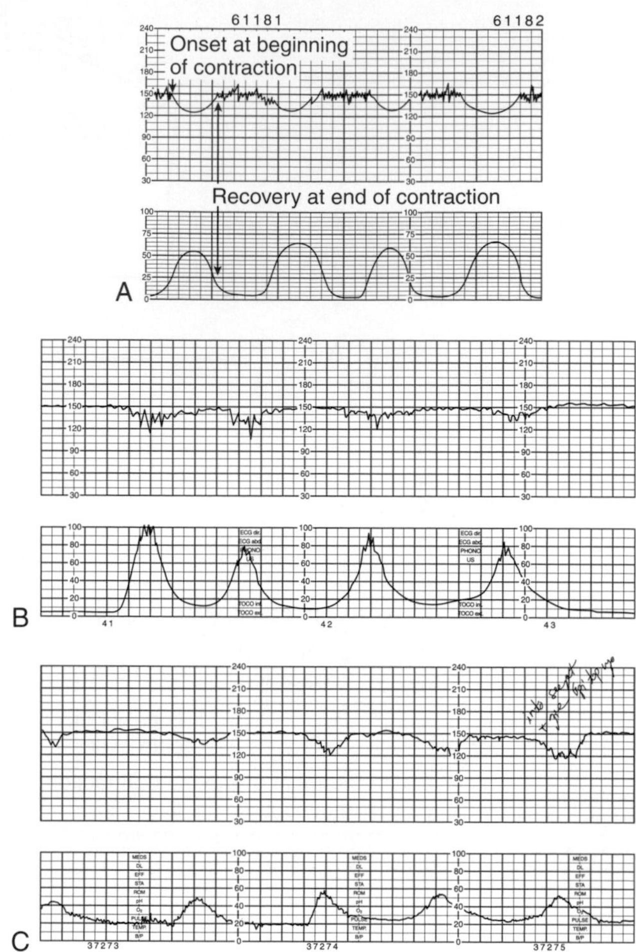

Fig. 6.13 (A) Early deceleration (illustration, with key points identified). (B and C) Early decelerations (actual tracings). (From Miller, L., & Tucker, S. M. [2013]. *Pocket guide to fetal monitoring and assessment* [7th ed.]. St. Louis: Mosby.)

      b. Administer maternal oxygen
      c. Consider IV fluid bolus
      d. Notify provider

Nonreassuring (Ominous) Signs

A. Variable deceleration pattern (Fig. 6.14)
   1. It is the most common variant pattern. May occur episodically (random) or periodically (with each contraction). Visually abrupt decrease in FHR below baseline of at least 15 beats/min or more, lasting at least 15 seconds, returns to baseline in less than 2 minutes from onset.
   2. It occurs in 45% to 75% of all labors and is caused mainly by cord compression but can also indicate rapid fetal descent, nuchal cord, or short cord.
   3. An occasional variable is usually benign. Variable decelerations that return to baseline in less than 60 seconds with associated normal baseline and moderate variability are not usually associated with fetal acidemia.
   4. If recurrent or if FHR below 70 beats/min lasting longer than 30 to 60 seconds, and accompanied by minimal or absent variability, indicates repeated interruption of fetal

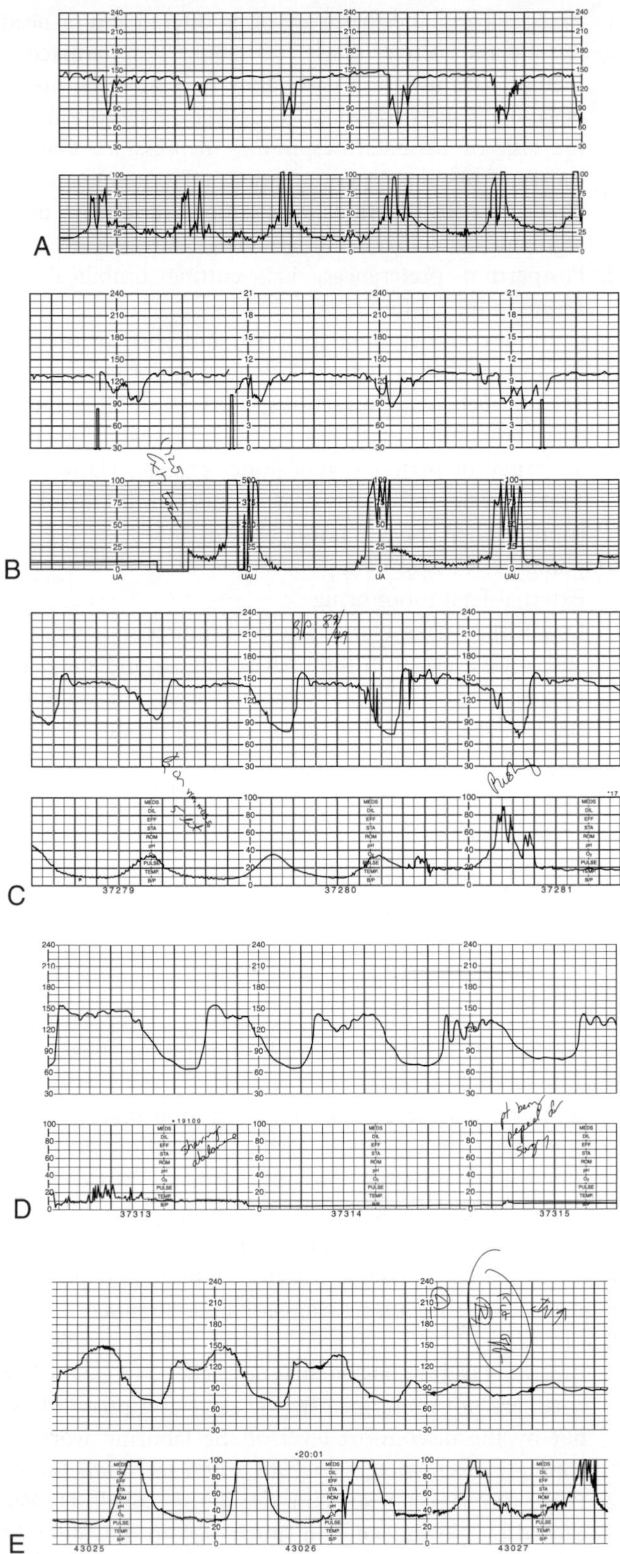

Fig. 6.14 **Variable Decelerations.** Note the progression in severity from panel (A) to panel (E), with overshoots and decreasing variability and eventually a prolonged and smooth deceleration (actual tracings). (From Miller, L., & Tucker, S. M. [2013]. *Pocket guide to fetal monitoring and assessment* [7th ed.]. St. Louis: Mosby.)

oxygen supply and requires urgent evaluation and consideration of action.

5. Clinical Judgment Measures for variable decelerations
   a. Discontinue oxytocin in infusing.
   b. Change maternal position.
   c. Administer oxygen at 10 L by facemask.
   d. Notify provider.
   e. Assist with vaginal or speculum examination.
   f. Assist with amnioinfusion if ordered.
   g. Prepare for delivery if pattern cannot be corrected.

B. Late decelerations (Fig. 6.15)

1. A visually apparent, gradual decrease in and return to baseline FHR. Associated with contractions. Deceleration begins after contraction starts and lowest point of deceleration occurs after contraction peak. Does not return to baseline until after contraction is over. The shape is uniform. The depth of the deceleration does not necessarily indicate severity; may become progressively deeper as fetal acidemia worsens.

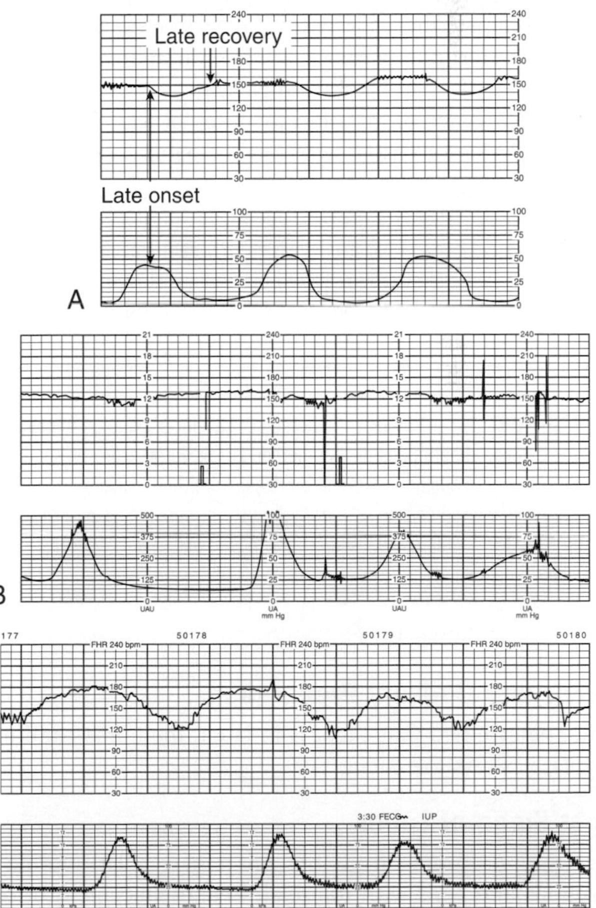

Fig. 6.15 (A) Late decelerations (illustration, with key points identified). (B and C) Late decelerations (actual tracings). (From Miller, L., & Tucker, S. M. [2013]. *Pocket guide to fetal monitoring and assessment* [7th ed.]. St. Louis: Mosby.)

a. The situation is ominous and requires immediate intervention when deceleration patterns are recurrent and associated with decreased or absent variability and tachycardia.
2. Indicative of UPI
a. Late decelerations indicate UPI and are associated with conditions such as postmaturity, uterine tachysystole, maternal supine hypotension, epidural or spinal anesthesia, placental previa or abruption, maternal hypertensive disorders, diabetes mellitus, cardiac disease, and intrauterine growth restriction (Fig. 6.16B).
b. A decrease in uteroplacental perfusion results in late decelerations with cord compression resulting in a pattern of variable decelerations (see Fig. 6.16C).
3. Clinical Judgment Measures
a. Discontinue oxytocin (Pitocin) if infusing.
b. Immediately turn client to lateral, side-lying position.
c. Administer oxygen at 10 L by nonrebreather facemask.
d. Correct maternal hypotension by elevating legs.
e. Maintain IV line, IV fluids.
f. Palpate uterus to assess for tachysystole.
g. Determine presence of FHR variability.
h. Notify health care provider.
i. Consider preparation for internal fetal monitoring.
j. Prepare to assist with birth if pattern cannot be corrected.

HESI HINT Check for labor progress if early decelerations are noted (see Fig. 6.13A). Early decelerations caused by head compression and fetal descent usually occur in the second stage of labor between 4 and 7 cm dilation.

HESI HINT If cord prolapse is detected, call for assistance immediately. The examiner should position the mother to relieve pressure on the cord (i.e., knee-chest position, extreme Trendelenburg) and using two gloved fingers (one on either side of the cord) push the presenting part off the cord to relieve compression and do not move hand. Notify obstetric provider immediately!

Labor and Delivery Preparation

Once determined that client is in labor, the nurse continues to regularly assess the client.

First Stage of Labor

Description: Begins from the onset of regular uterine contractions and ends with full dilation and effacement of cervix

Clinical Judgment Measures

A. Identify presence of support person.
B. Explain all activities and procedures to mother and support person.
C. Discuss Birth Plan.
1. Analgesia and anesthesia are often offered and or needed during the active phase of labor. If pharmacologic methods are used too early, they may slow the progress of labor; if used too close to delivery, narcotics increase the risk of neonatal respiratory depression. Common causes of first stage pain: dilation, effacement, stretching of cervix, contractions, distention of lower uterine segment
2. Postpartum preferences, i.e., cutting umbilical cord, rooming in, feeding choice
3. Cultural considerations for birth and postpartum care
D. Assess maternal vital signs (BP, P, Respirations)
1. Take BP *between* contractions, every 30 to 60 minutes in early labor and every 15 to 30 in active labor unless abnormal or maternal appearance changes (Lowd, 385).
2. Take temperature every 4 hours until membranes rupture, then every 2 hours (Lowd, 385).
E. Ongoing FHR assessment
1. External fetal monitoring
2. Low Risk: Assess FHR every 30 minutes in active phase and at least every 15 minutes during second stage.
3. Higher Risk: Assess FHR at least every 15 minutes in active phase and at least every 5 minutes during second stage.
4. Assess contractions when assessing FHR.
5. Vaginal exams as needed to identify labor progress

HESI HINT Meconium-stained fluid is yellow-green or gold-yellow and may indicate fetal stress.

F. Palpate for bladder distention and encourage regular voiding at least every 2 hours during labor (a full bladder can impede labor progress).
G. Oral intake: It is becoming more common practice for clients to have clear liquids during labor; however, nurses should follow obstetric provider orders. Provide mouth care as needed for dry mouth. Intravenous intake may be needed if client is not permitted oral intake during labor.
H. Assist woman with use of psychoprophylactic coping techniques, such as breathing exercises and effleurage (abdominal massage).
1. Breathing techniques, such as deep chest, accelerated, and cued, are not prescribed by the stage and phase of labor but by the discomfort level of the laboring woman. If coping is decreasing, switch to a new technique.
2. Hyperventilation results in respiratory alkalosis that is caused by blowing off too much carbon dioxide (CO_2). Symptoms include
a. Dizziness
b. Tingling of fingers
c. Stiff mouth
3. Have woman breathe into her cupped hands or a paper bag in order to rebreathe CO_2.
I. Encourage ambulation if membranes are intact, after ROM only if fetal presenting part is engaged and if client has

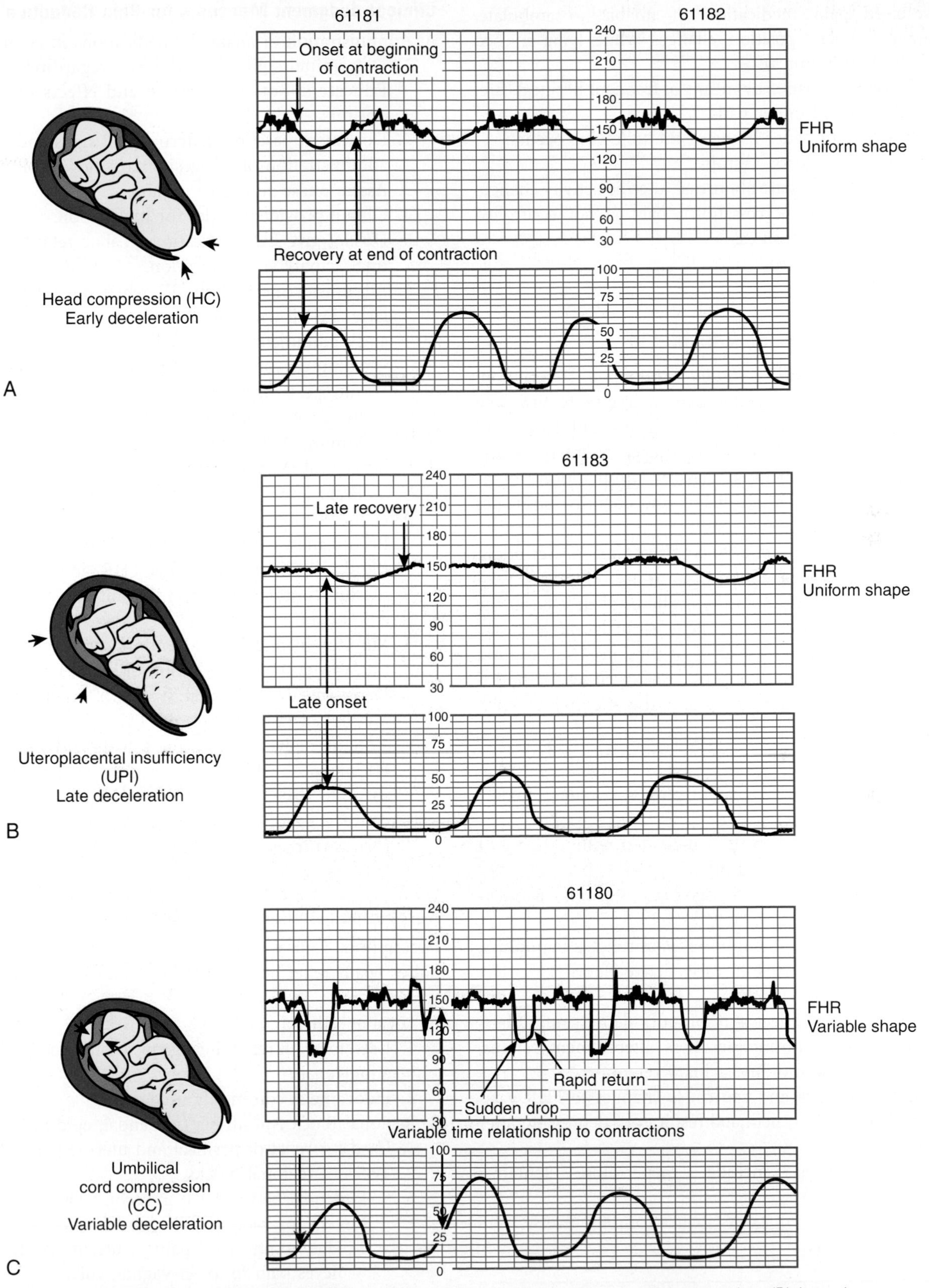

Fig. 6.16 Review of Fetal Variability. (A) Early decelerations caused by head compression. (B) Late decelerations caused by uteroplacental insufficiency. (C) Variable decelerations caused by cord compression. (From Miller, L., & Tucker, S. M. [2013]. *Pocket guide to fetal monitoring and assessment* [7th ed.]. St. Louis: Mosby.)

not received pain medication. If unable to ambulate, encourage frequent position changes while lying in bed (every 30 to 60 minutes).

J. Maintain asepsis in labor by means of frequent perineal care, changing linen and under pads.

K. Notify obstetric provider if any of the following occurs:
   1. Labor progress slows or stops.
   2. Maternal vital signs are abnormal, uterine activity changes (tachysystole, abrupt cessation), pain is not controlled with prescribed measures.
   3. Fetal distress is noted.

Labor With Analgesia or Anesthesia

Nonpharmacologic pain reduction strategies. Description. Methods are simple and inexpensive with rare to any side adverse reactions. They can be used throughout labor and include cutaneous stimulation (effleurage, counterpressure, walking, rocking, water therapy), sensory stimulation (aromatherapy, breathing techniques, music), and cognitive strategies (childbirth education and hypnosis).

Pharmacologic pain reduction strategies. Description: Pharmacologic pain management options are often used with nonpharmacologic strategies and typically implemented in the active phase of labor. Anesthesia includes analgesia, amnesia, relaxation, and reflex activity. Analgesia alleviates the sensation of pain without loss of consciousness. Use of either method is determined by the stage of labor and the method of birth planned by the woman

A. Sedatives (barbiturates)
   1. May be used in early or latent phases to relieve anxiety and help with sleep
   2. Should be avoided if birth anticipated within 12 to 24 hours, therefore not used often

B. Systemic analgesia (opioid agonists, opioids agonist-antagonists)
   1. Provides sedation and euphoria. Pain relief is temporary, generally more effective in early, active labor.
   2. Administered IM, IV, PCA
   3. Most serious side effect is respiratory depression. Others include nausea/vomiting, dizziness, altered mental status, decreased gastric motility, urinary retention.
   4. Cross the placenta and can cause changes to FHR variability during labor; neonatal respiratory depression after birth
   5. Common drugs include meperidine, fentanyl, nalbuphine.
   6. Naloxone (opioid antagonist) can promptly reverse CNS depressant effects.

> **HESI HINT** Opioid agonist-antagonist and antagonist analgesics should not be used in women with opioid dependence as they could precipitate withdrawal symptoms.

Clinical Judgment Measures for Pain Reduction

A. Administration of analgesic medications in labor
   1. Determine client's desires regarding analgesics. Educate about the purpose and effects of medication options.
   2. Document baseline maternal vital signs and FHR before administration of analgesics/narcotics (Table 6.12).
   3. Assess phase and stage of labor.
   4. Obtain provider's order for medication.
   5. Do *not* give PO medications. Labor retards gastrointestinal activity and absorption.
   6. Administer medications IV when possible, intramuscularly (IM) if necessary.
      a. IV administration of analgesics is preferred to IM administration for a client in labor because the onset and peak occur more quickly, and the duration of the drug is shorter. Typical IV administration: Onset: 5 minutes, Peak: 30 minutes
      b. Typical IM administration: Onset: within 30 minutes, Peak: 1 to 3 hours after injection

B. After medication administration
   1. Record the woman's response and level of pain relief.
   2. Monitor maternal vital signs, FHR, and characteristics of uterine contractions every 15 minutes for 1 hour after administration.
   3. Monitor bladder for distention and retention (medication can decrease perception of bladder filling).
   4. Decrease environmental stimuli: Darken room, reduce number of visitors, turn off TV.
   5. Note on delivery record the time between drug administration and birth. If delivery occurs during peak drug absorption time, notify pediatrician or neonatologist for delivery room assistance and possible use of naloxone (Narcan) for neonate (see Table 6.12).

Nerve Block Analgesia and Anesthesia

Description: Causes a temporary interruption of nerve impulses (pain relief and motor blockade) over a specific body area.

A. Local anesthesia
   1. Used for pain relief during episiotomy and perineal laceration repair
   2. Lidocaine is commonly used.

B. Regional Block Anesthesia (pudendal, epidural, spinal)
   1. Used for relief of perineal and uterine pain
   2. Types of regional blocks
      a. Pudendal block: given in second stage (episiotomy, forceps, or vacuum-assisted delivery)
         1) Has no effect on pain of uterine contractions, relieves pain in lower vagina, vulva, perineum.
      b. Epidural block: given in first or second stage of labor. Local anesthetic alone or in combination with opioid agonist analgesic. Common medications include bupivacaine, fentanyl. Injection between L4 & L5, re-

TABLE 6.12 **Analgesics**

Drugs	Indications	Adverse Reactions	Nursing Implications
• Fentanyl Citrate	• Opioid agonist analgesic used for moderate to severe labor pain, or post-operative pain (cesarean delivery)	• Sedation • Nausea and vomiting • Respiratory distress • Fetal distress • Hypotension	• Record use accurately. • Implement safety measures. • Have naloxone available as an antidote. • Monitor respirations, pulse, BP closely.
• Meperidine Hydrochloride	• Opioid agonist analgesic used for moderate to severe labor pain, or post-operative pain (cesarean delivery)	• Tachycardia • Sedation • Nausea and vomiting • Altered mental status • Decreased gastric motility, delayed gastric emptying • Urinary retention	• Implement safety measures. • Do not give if birth is expected to occur within 1–4 h after administration (may cause neonatal respiratory depression). • Monitor respirations, pulse.
• Nalbuphine Hydrochloride	• Opioid agonist-antagonist analgesic used for moderate to severe labor pain, or post-operative pain (cesarean delivery)	• Sedation • Nausea and vomiting • Dizziness • Respiratory depression • May cause temporary absent or minimal FHR variability	• May precipitate withdrawal symptoms in opioid-dependent woman and newborn. • Assess maternal vital signs, pain level, FHR, uterine activity prior to and after administration. • Observe for respiratory depression. • Encourage voiding, palpate for bladder distention.
• Naloxone Hydrochloride	• Opioid antagonist used to reverse opioid-induced respiratory depression in mother or newborn	• Maternal hypotension or hypertension • Tachycardia • Hyperventilation • Nausea and vomiting	• Do not administer if woman is opioid dependent as may cause abrupt withdrawal. • Duration of action is shorter than most opioids, monitor closely for return of opioid depression when effects of naloxone are gone, may need to readminister. • Pain may return suddenly.

lieves labor and vaginal birth pain through a block from T10 to S5. For cesarean birth, block form T8 to S1 needed.
   1) May be given in single dose or continuously through catheter threaded into epidural space
   2) Is moderately associated with hypotension, which can cause maternal and fetal distress
   3) Epidural block can be associated with prolonged second stage due to decreased effectiveness of pushing

c. Spinal block: given in second stage of labor. Local anesthetic alone or in combination with opioid agonist analgesic. Injection through L3, L4, or L5 lumbar interspace into subarachnoid space to relieve vaginal birth pain from T10 (hips) to feet. When used for cesarean birth, provides anesthesia from T6 (nipple) to feet.
   1) Rapid onset, but highly associated with maternal hypotension, which can cause maternal and fetal distress
   2) Client must remain flat for 6 to 8 hours after delivery.

d. Epidural block: injection of local anesthetic agent and opioid analgesic into epidural space to relieve pain from T10 to S5. Most common effective pharmacologic pain relief method in labor.

3. Contraindications to epidural and spinal blocks
   a. Client's refusal or fear
   b. Anticoagulant therapy or presence of bleeding disorder
   c. Presence of antepartum hemorrhage causing acute hypovolemia
   d. Infection or tumor at injection site
   e. Allergy to -caine medications
   f. CNS disorders, previous back surgery, or spinal anatomic abnormality

C. Clinical Judgment Measures for Nerve Block Analgesia and Anesthesia
   1. Ensure that the health care provider has explained the procedures, risks, benefits, and alternatives. Encourage woman to empty her bladder.
   2. Obtain maternal vital signs and a 20- to 30-minute electronic fetal monitoring strip to assess FHR and contractions prior to anesthesia. After anesthesia, maternal vital signs and FHR and pattern should be assessed and documented every 5 to 10 minutes.
   3. Fluid balance is assessed. Bolus of 500 to 1000 mL IV fluid (Lactated Ringers or normal saline) is infused 15 to 30 minutes before initiation of anesthetic. This IV fluid preload reduces the frequency of maternal hypotension after spinal anesthesia.
   4. The client sits or lies on her side with back curved to widen intervertebral space; head is flexed.

5. A test dose of medication may be given prior to administering a bolus dose or drip in epidurals. Ask client to describe symptoms after test dose.
   a. Metallic taste in mouth and ringing in ears denote possible injection of medication into bloodstream.
   b. Nausea and vomiting are among the first signs of hypotension.
   c. The first sign of a block's effectiveness is usually warmth and tingling in the buttocks or legs, feet, or toes.
6. Determine maternal vital signs every 5 minutes for the first half hour after administration of anesthetic drug and initiate continuous fetal monitoring. Maternal vitals should then be monitored every 10 minutes for the second half hour after administration and then every 30 minutes. Monitor for hypotension (20% decrease from preblock baseline level of ≤100 mm Hg systolic), fetal bradycardia, absent or minimal FHR variability.
7. If hypotension occurs:
   a. Immediately turn client onto lateral position.
   b. Maintain IV infusion rate as specified or increase per hospital protocol.
   c. Begin O_2 at 10 to 12 L/min by nonrebreather facemask.
   d. Elevate legs.
   e. Notify obstetric and anesthesia health care provider.
   f. Have vasopressor at bedside and administer per protocol if previous measures have been ineffective.
8. Assess maternal vital signs and FHR every 5 minutes until stable or per orders.
9. Assist client to keep bladder empty. Catheterization may be needed.
10. Assess level of pain relief.
11. Report return of pain sensation, incomplete anesthesia, or uneven anesthesia to anesthesiologist.
12. Because the woman is unable to sense contractions, assist client in the pushing technique once complete dilatation has been achieved.

D. General anesthesia is rarely used but may be needed because of a delivery complication, emergency delivery, or when regional block anesthesia is contraindicated.

E. Clinical Judgment Measures with general anesthesia
1. Make sure client is NPO.
2. Monitor maternal vital signs and FHR and pattern.
3. Ensure IV is in place.
4. Administer drugs to reduce gastric secretions (e.g., famotidine or clear [nonparticulate]), antacids to neutralize gastric acid.
5. Place wedge under one of client's hips; helps to displace uterus.
6. General anesthesia is associated with postpartum uterine atony. Assess closely for uterine atony; check fundal firmness and uterine contractions (Table 6.13).

Second Stage of Labor

Description: Begins with full cervical dilation (10 cm) and complete effacement (100%) and ends with the birth. The

TABLE 6.13 Clinical Judgment Measures: First Stage of Labor Pain Management

Clinical Judgment Measure	Assessment Characteristics
Recognize Cues	Note contraction pattern, frequency Note labor progress (cervical dilation, effacement, station) Review mother's birth plan; especially consider plan for pain management, analgesia, anesthesia
Analyze Cues	Determine mother's ability to manage pain without medication (breathing pattern, relaxation between contractions, activity with contractions, requests for pain medication) Identify effectiveness of support person during contractions Assess maternal vital signs (VS) Note fetal response to labor (heart rate decelerations, ominous fetal heart rate patterns)
Prioritize Cues	Note irregular BP, P, respirations, or temperature (dizziness, tingling of fingers), (resp. alkalosis), acute escalation of pain symptoms Report changes in fetal heart rate Report any stalling of labor progress to obstetric provider Report any changes in maternal pain tolerance (unable to relax between contractions, hyperventilation, verbal report of pain or request for additional pain management) Note any unusual vaginal bleeding, change in fetal presentation, cord prolapse
Solutions	Review birth plan; if mother and fetus are stable, and mother desires unmedicated birth, consider additional pain management options: Assist with position changes, walking if applicable, breathing techniques, use of tub (if applicable) to support non-medication pain management options as desired Assist support person with coaching during delivery If mother wishes to explore use of analgesia or anesthesia, discuss options Contact obstetric provider for orders

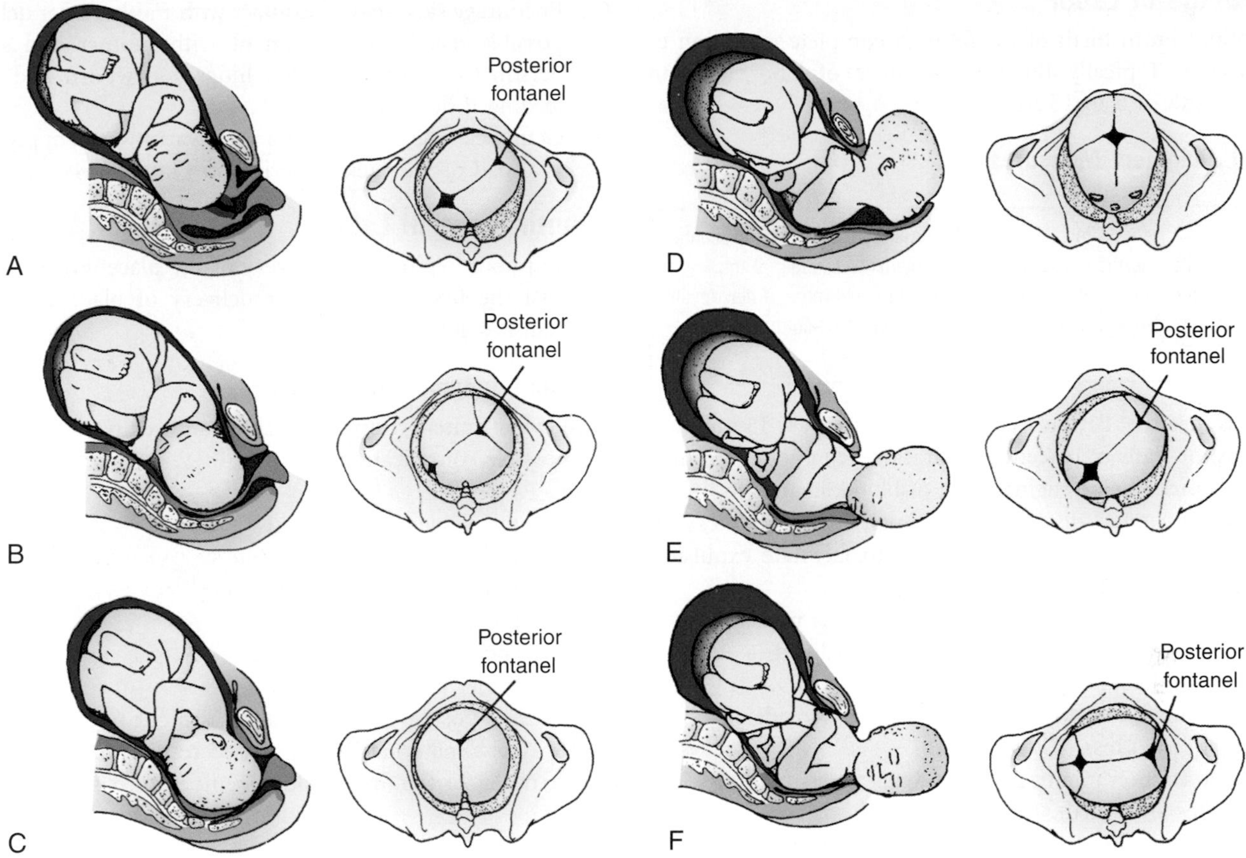

Fig. 6.17 Cardinal Movements of the Mechanism of Labor. Left occipitoanterior (LOA) position. Pelvic figures show the position of the fetal head as seen by the birth attendant. (A) Engagement and descent. (B) Flexion. (C) Internal rotation to occipitoanterior position (OA). (D) Extension. (E) External rotation beginning (restitution). (F) External rotation.

length of second stage varies and is affected by parity, use of epidural anesthesia, woman's age, BMI, emotional state and adequacy of support, level of fatigue, fetal size, position, and often presentation (Fig. 6.17). Second stage is comprised of the latent phase (passive descent) and the active pushing phase.

> **HESI HINT** The Ferguson reflex is activated when presenting part presses on stretch receptor of pelvic floor and triggers a strong, involuntary urge to bear down.

Clinical Judgment Measures

A. Assess and document maternal BP, pulse, respirations every 15 minutes between contractions.
B. Check FHR with each contraction or by continuous fetal monitoring.
   1. External fetal monitoring
      a. Low Risk: assess FHR and pattern at least every 15 minutes during second stage.
      b. Higher Risk: assess FHR and pattern at least every 5 minutes during second stage.
      c. Observe perineal area for increase in bloody show, signs of fetal descent (bulging perineum and anus, visibility of the presenting part).
      d. Palpate bladder for distention.
      e. Assess amniotic fluid for color and consistency.
      f. Comfort measures: continue mouth care, assist with position changes, help with pain relief, provide breathing instruction and support and positive reinforcement of pushing efforts.
      g. Teach mother positions for pushing such as squatting, side-lying, or high-Fowler/lithotomy and encourage open-glottis pushing (bearing down while exhaling) followed by a cleansing breath after each contraction.
      h. Set up delivery table, including bulb syringe, cord clamp, and sterile supplies.
      i. Perform perineal cleansing if directed.
      j. Make sure client and support person can visualize delivery if they desire. A mirror can be offered. If siblings are present, make sure they are closely attended to by support person explaining that their mom is all right.
      k. Record *exact* delivery time (complete delivery of baby).

Third Stage of Labor

Description: From birth of the fetus to complete expulsion of the placenta. Typically the shortest stage of labor with an average length of 5 to 15 minutes.

Clinical Judgment Measures

> **HESI HINT** Oxytocin (Pitocin) is typically administered after the placenta is delivered because the drug will cause the uterus to contract. If the oxytocic drug is administered before the placenta is delivered, it may result in a retained placenta, which predisposes the client to hemorrhage and infection.

1. Assess maternal BP, pulse, and respirations every 15 minutes.
2. Assess for signs of placental separation: lengthening of umbilical cord outside vagina, gush of blood, change in uterus shape from oval (discoid) to globular, vaginal fullness on exam. Assist mother to bear down to facilitate expulsion of placenta when directed to do so.
3. After placenta is expelled, uterine fundus is massaged, and oxytocic medication is administered as ordered.
4. Administer analgesics as ordered.
5. Observe for blood loss and ask obstetric provider for estimate of blood loss (EBL).
6. Dry and suction infant, perform Apgar assessment at 1 and 5 minutes after birth.
7. Encourage skin-to-skin contact with mother after delivery if possible. Facilitate attachment with mother and support person by encouraging touching of newborn and breastfeeding if desired.
8. Gently cleanse perineal area with warm water; apply a perineal pad or ice pack to perineum (Table 6.14).

Fourth Stage of Labor

Description: Begins after delivery of the placenta and includes at least the first 2 hours after delivery of placenta until the woman is stable.

Clinical Judgment Measures

A. Review antepartum and labor and delivery records for possible complications.
   1. PPH
   2. Uterine hyperstimulation
   3. Uterine overdistention
   4. Dystocia
   5. Antepartum hemorrhage
   6. Magnesium sulfate therapy
   7. Bladder distention

B. Routine postpartum physical assessment
   1. Assess maternal BP, pulse, and respirations every 15 minutes for the first 2 hours. Temperature is assessed at the

TABLE 6.14 Clinical Judgment Measures: Third Stage of Labor (Placental Expulsion)

Clinical Judgment Measure	Assessment Characteristics
Recognize Cues (after delivery of the fetus)	Vaginal bleeding Abdominal cramping Umbilical cord length Consistency of uterus
Analyze Cues	Determine where cramping is located and verify constitution of pain (cramping is typically the return of moderate to strong uterine contractions to facilitate placental expulsion) Determine the amount of vaginal bleeding present (trickle, gushing) Verify any lengthening of the umbilical cord (the portion of umbilical cord noted outside of the vagina) Verify consistency of uterus, i.e., firm and contracting or boggy
Prioritize Cues	Determine risk factors for retained placenta Determine if it has been longer than 15″ since delivery of the fetus Verify normalcy of third stage bleeding pattern; significant estimated blood loss, concern for immediate postpartum hemorrhage Verify apparent lengthening of umbilical cord as placenta descends to introitus Assess for any change in vital signs
Solutions	Teach clients about expectations for delivery of the placenta Be prepared for potential complications of retained placenta, immediate postpartum hemorrhage Assess vital signs every 15 min to observe for maternal stability Assess for early signs of placental separation Assist mother to push to facilitate expulsion of the placenta when appropriate
Actions	Monitor blood loss Provide uterine fundal massage as soon as the placenta is expelled Administer oxytocic medication as ordered to assist with uterine contraction and prevent hemorrhage Keep mother and partner informed of progress of third stage and answer any questions After placental expulsion, obtain blood sample from umbilical cord as ordered (used to determine baby's blood type, Rh status)

beginning of recovery and then every 4 hours for the first 8 hours after birth.

2. Assess fundal firmness and height, bladder, lochia, and perineum every 15 minutes for one hour, then as ordered.
   a. Fundus: firm, midline, at or below the umbilicus. Massage if soft or boggy to contract uterus and expel any clots prior to measuring. Suspect full bladder if above umbilicus and to the right side of abdomen. If the nurse finds the fundus soft, boggy, and displaced above and to the right of the umbilicus, the nurse should perform fundal massage, then have the client empty her bladder. Encourage frequent voiding.
   b. Lochia: rubra (red), moderate, and clots less than 2 to 3 cm. Amount similar to a heavy menstrual period. Suspect undetected laceration if fundus is firm and bright-red blood continues to trickle. Always check perineal pad *and* under buttocks.
   c. Perineum: Observe in good lighting. Should be intact or assess lacerations/episiotomy for redness, edema, ecchymosis, drainage, and approximation (REEDA). Suspect hematomas if very tender or discolored or if pain is disproportionate to vaginal delivery.

> **HESI HINT** A first-degree perineal laceration extends through skin and structures superficial to muscles. A second-degree laceration extends through muscles of perineal body. A third-degree laceration continues through external anal sphincter muscle. A fourth-degree laceration extends completely through anal sphincter and rectal mucosa. Tears cause pain and swelling and may impact voiding or bowel movements. Avoid rectal manipulations.

C. Monitor infusion of intravenous oxytocin (Pitocin) as ordered.
D. Administer analgesics as prescribed.
E. Report any abnormal vital signs, uterus not becoming firm with massage, second perineal pad soaked in 15 minutes, signs of hypovolemic shock: pale, clammy, tachycardic, lightheaded, hypotensive.
F. Support parental emotional needs and promote bonding with infant.
   1. Allow extended family time post-birth so family can hold and examine the newborn if status of mother and newborn allows. Encourage skin-to-skin contact.
   2. Encourage initiation of breastfeeding within 1 to 2 hours of birth if desired. In some cultures mothers may choose to delay initiation of breastfeeding.
   3. Provide a warm, darkened environment.
   4. Perform newborn admission and routine procedures in room with parents when possible (Table 6.15).

LABOR AND BIRTH COMPLICATIONS

Preterm Labor

Description: Regular contractions accompanied by a change in cervical status that occurs between 20 and 36 6/7 weeks' gestation. Predisposing factors include medical conditions (diabetes, cardiac disease, preeclampsia, and placenta previa), infections (UTI, STIs), overdistention of uterus (multifetal gestation, hydramnios), substance abuse, high levels of personal stress.

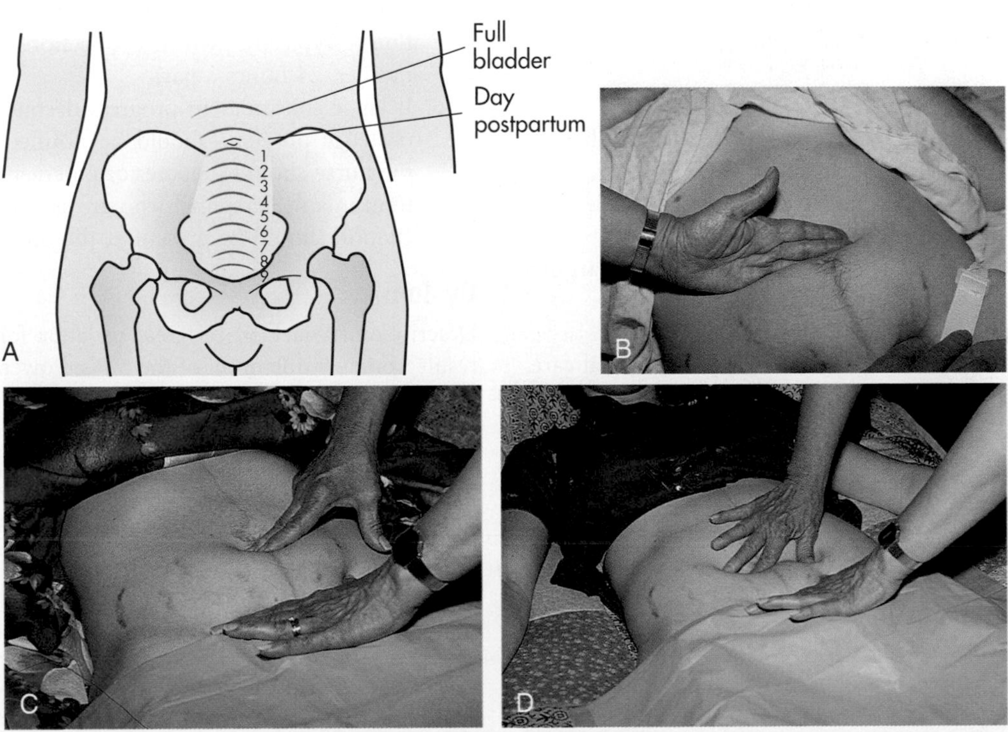

Fig. 6.18 Assessment of Involution of Uterus After Birth (A)Length of uterus (B) Measurement of fundud (C) Measurement of uterus to pubic bone (D) Uterine massage. (1) Normal progress, days 1 to 9 (2) Size and position of uterus (3) Two days after birth (4) Four days after birth. Note linea nigra and striae gravidarum ("stretch marks") in B-D. (From Lowdermilk DL, Perry SE, Cashion, K., Alden, K., & Olshansky, E. (2020). *Maternity and women's health care*, 12th ed, 10, St. Louis, MO, Elsevier. (Figure 20.1, p 418))

TABLE 6.15 Clinical Judgment Measures: Fourth Stage of Labor (Parental Attachment After Vaginal Birth)

Clinical Judgment Measure	Assessment Characteristics
Recognize Cues	Mother and support person are holding infant, making eye contact Mother is examining infant and verbalizing physical likeness to parents, counting fingers, toes, and commenting on hair, calling newborn by name Monitor attempts to feed infant, note mother's choice of feeding method
Analyze Cues	Recognize any circumstances that prohibit mother—infant contact, i.e., unstable infant needing NICU admission, mother is experiencing acute postpartum hemorrhage, VS are unstable If mother and infant are stable, note any skin-to-skin contact Note any verbal expression of exhaustion by mother, physical inability to hold infant Note engagement of support partner, other parent Note ability to comfort a crying infant Note any cultural considerations (some cultural practices may not be congruent with standard practices associated with the Anglo-American culture)
Prioritize Cues	Determine need to manage unstable maternal VS, control unusual vaginal bleeding, address maternal pain Determine if newborn is in need of additional interventions (suctioning, swaddling) Note any physical concerns that would prohibit early attachment (IVs in place, blood pressure cuff) Determine need to model early attachment behaviors (holding, eye contact, talking to infant)
Solutions	Assess mother and parents' comfort level in caring for a newborn (is this the first child for the family) Encourage skin-to-skin contact and assist with establishing this contact Teach clients about early newborn behavior Demonstrate newborn cares (diapering, umbilical cord care, bathing) Discuss and demonstrate newborn comfort techniques (swaddling, talking, rocking) Assist with feeding (positioning, burping, latch if breastfeeding) and discuss normal newborn feeding behaviors Discuss rooming-in options

A. Symptoms
   1. Frequent contractions with cervical changes occurring
   2. Menstrual-like cramps; low, dull backache; and pelvic pressure
   3. Urinary frequency
   4. Increase or change in vaginal discharge
   5. ROM

B. Labs
   1. Fetal fibronectin test obtained from a cervical swab indicates the client is at higher risk for preterm labor.
   2. CBC, urinalysis, and cervical cultures may be ordered

C. Diagnostics
   1. US may be ordered to check cervical length or as part of a BPP/NST to check on fetal well-being.

D. Clinical Judgment Measures
   1. Teach symptoms of preterm labor early in prenatal care.
   2. Educate on self-management of symptoms and when to notify obstetric provider.
   3. Select women may be managed at home with activity restriction, pelvic rest (avoidance of sexual activity), oral medications, adequate hydration.
      a. Teach about side effects and warning signs of medications.
   4. Many women will be admitted for observation, bed rest, and management with tocolytics (i.e., indomethacin, nifedipine, magnesium sulfate, terbutaline) to arrest labor after uterine contractions and cervical change has occurred.
      a. Follow protocols for continuous uterine and FHR monitoring, assessment of maternal vital signs.
   5. Glucocorticoids (betamethasone) may be administered to women between 24 and 34 weeks' gestation to accelerate fetal lung maturity (stimulates fetal surfactant production). Typically two IM injections are given to the mother, 24 hours a part.
   6. If labor continues to progress despite interventions, the obstetric provider should be notified immediately, and the nurse should prepare for emergent delivery of a preterm infant. Personnel who are skilled at neonatal resuscitation should be present at the birth (Table 6.16).

Dystocia

Description. A lack of progress in labor for any reason. May result from any one or all of the 5 P's: **P**owers (primary uterine contractions and secondary abdominal bearing-down efforts), **P**assage (maternal pelvis, uterus, cervix, vagina, perineum), **P**assenger (fetus and placenta), **P**syche (response to labor by woman), and **P**osition (position of the laboring woman).

A. Symptoms

   Dystocia is suspected when there is a

   1. Lack of progress in cervical dilatation
   2. Lack of fetal descent, or
   3. Uterine contractions become ineffective (hypertonic, hypotonic)
   4. Abnormal labor patterns

TABLE 6.16 Tocolytic Therapy for Preterm Labor

Medication and Action	Dosage and Route	Adverse Effects	Nursing Considerations
Magnesium Sulfate			
CNS depressant; relaxes smooth muscle, including uterus	IV fluid should contain 40 g in 1000 mL, piggyback to primary infusion, and administer using controller pump: Loading dose: 4–6 g over 20–30 min Maintenance dose: 1–4 g/h Use for stabilization only Discontinue within 24–48 h at the maintenance dose or if intolerable adverse effects occur	Maternal: • Hot flushes, sweating, burning at the IV insertion site, nausea and vomiting, dry mouth, drowsiness, blurred vision, diplopia, headache, ileus, generalized muscle weakness, lethargy, dizziness • Hypocalcemia • Dyspnea • Transient hypotension • Some reactions may subside when loading dose is completed. **Intolerable:** • Respiratory rate fewer than 12 breaths/min • Pulmonary edema • Absent DTRs • Chest pain • Severe hypotension • Altered level of consciousness • Extreme muscle weakness • Urine output <25–30 mL/h or <100 mL/4 h • Serum magnesium level of 10 mEq/L (9 mg/dL) or greater **Fetal (uncommon):** Decreased breathing movement Reduced FHR variability Nonreactive NST	Assess woman and fetus to obtain baseline before beginning therapy and then before and after each incremental change; follow frequency of agency protocol. Drug is almost always given IV but can also be administered IM. Monitor serum magnesium levels with higher doses; therapeutic range is 4–7.5 mEq/L or 5–8 mg/dL. Discontinue infusion and notify health care provider if intolerable adverse effects occur. Ensure that calcium gluconate is available for emergency administration to reverse magnesium sulfate toxicity. Do not give to women with myasthenia gravis. Total IV intake should be limited to 125 mL/h.
β-Adrenergic Agonist (β-Mimetic)			
Terbutaline (Brethine) relaxes smooth muscle, inhibiting uterine activity and causing bronchodilation.	Subcutaneous injection of 0.25 mg every 4 h Treatment should last no longer than 24 h Discontinue use if intolerable adverse effects occur	**Maternal (most are mild and of limited duration):** • Tachycardia, chest discomfort, palpitations, arrhythmias • Tremors, dizziness, nervousness • Headache • Nasal congestion • Nausea and vomiting • Hypokalemia • Hyperglycemia • Hypotension **Intolerable:** • Tachycardia >130 beats/min • BP <90/60 • Chest pain • Cardiac arrhythmias • Myocardial infarction • Pulmonary edema	Should not be used in women with known or suspected heart disease, pregestational or gestational diabetes, preeclampsia with severe features or eclampsia, hyperthyroidism, or with significant hemorrhage or possible chorioamnionitis. Myocardial infarction leading to death has been reported after use.
β-Adrenergic Agonist (β-Mimetic)—cont'd		Fetal: • Tachycardia • Hyperinsulinemia • Hyperglycemia	Assess woman and fetus according to agency protocol, being alert for adverse effects. Assess maternal glucose and potassium levels before treatment is initiated and periodically during treatment. Significant hyperglycemia (>180 mg/dL) and hypokalemia (<2.5 mEq/L) may occur.

Continued

TABLE 6.16 Tocolytic Therapy for Preterm Labor—cont'd

Medication and Action	Dosage and Route	Adverse Effects	Nursing Considerations
			Notify health care provider if the following are noted: Maternal heart rate >130 beats/min; arrhythmias, chest pain BP <90/60 mm Hg Signs of pulmonary edema (e.g., dyspnea, crackles, decreased SaO_2) Fetal heart rate >180 beats/min. Hyperglycemia occurs more frequently in women who are being treated simultaneously with corticosteroids. Ensure that propranolol (Inderal) is available to reverse adverse effects related to cardiovascular function.
Prostaglandin Synthetase Inhibitors (NSAIDs)			
1. Indomethacin (Indocin) relaxes uterine smooth muscle by inhibiting prostaglandins.	Loading dose: 50 mg orally, then 25–50 mg orally every 6 h for 48 h	Maternal (common): • Nausea and vomiting • Heartburn **(Less common but more serious):** a. GI bleeding b. Prolonged bleeding time c. Thrombocytopenia d. Asthma in aspirin-sensitive clients **Fetal:** a. Constriction of ductus arteriosus b. Oligohydramnios, caused by reduced fetal urine production c. Neonatal pulmonary hypertension	a. The long-acting formulations decrease the incidence of adverse effects. b. Used only if gestational age is <32 weeks. c. Administer for 48 h or less. d. Do not use in women with renal or hepatic disease, active peptic ulcer disease, poorly controlled hypertension, asthma, or coagulation disorders. e. Can mask maternal fever. f. Assess woman and fetus according to agency policy, being alert for adverse effects. g. Determine amniotic fluid volume and function of fetal ductus arteriosus before initiating therapy and within 48 h of discontinuing therapy; assessment is critical if therapy continues for more than 48 h. h. Administer with food to decrease GI distress. i. Monitor for signs of postpartum hemorrhage.
Calcium Channel Blockers			
Nifedipine (Adalat, Procardia) relaxes smooth muscle including the uterus by blocking calcium entry.	Initial dose: 10–20 mg, orally, every 3–6 h until contractions are rare, followed by long-acting formulations of 30 or 60 mg every 8–12 h for 48 h while corticosteroids are being given (however, the ideal dose has not been established)	Maternal (most effects are mild): • Hypotension • Headache • Flushing • Dizziness • Nausea **Fetal:** • Hypotension (questionable)	Avoid concurrent use with magnesium sulfate because skeletal muscle blockade can result. Should not be given simultaneously with or immediately after terbutaline because of effects on heart rate and blood pressure. Assess woman and fetus according to agency protocol, being alert for adverse effects. Do not use sublingual route of administration.

NOTE: There are variations in recommended administration protocols; always consult agency protocol, which should be evidence based.
BP, Blood pressure; *CNS,* central nervous system; *DTRs,* deep tendon reflexes; *FHR,* fetal heart rate; *GI,* gastrointestinal; *IM,* intramuscular; *IV,* intravenous; *NSAIDs,* nonsteroidal anti-inflammatory drugs; *NST,* nonstress test; *SaO_2,* arterial oxygen saturation; *SOB,* shortness of breath.
Adapted from Lowdermilk, D. L., Perry, S. E., Cashion, K., Alden, K., & Olshansky, E. (2020). *Maternity and women's health care* (12th ed.). St. Louis: Elsevier.

B. Clinical Judgment Measures
1. Continuous uterine and fetal monitoring; notify obstetric provider if abnormal labor patterns occur
   a. Assist with placement of intrauterine pressure catheter, fetal scalp electrode.
2. Assist with diagnostic procedures (ultrasound, pelvimetry, vaginal examination) to rule out CPD.
3. Assist with amniotomy. Artificial rupture of membranes (AROM) may enhance labor forces.
   a. Explain procedure.

b. Assess FHR.
c. Assess fluid for color, odor, and consistency (blood, meconium, or vernix particles).

4. Administer oxytocin infusion for induction (initiation) or augmentation (stimulation) of labor as ordered (Box 6.3).

REVIEW OF INTRAPARTUM NURSING CARE

1. List five prodromal signs of labor the nurse might teach the client.
2. How is true labor discriminated from false labor?
3. State two ways to determine whether the membranes have truly ruptured.
4. Hyperventilation often occurs in the laboring client. What results from hyperventilation, and what actions should the nurse take to relieve the condition?
5. Describe the maternal changes that characterize the transition phase of labor.
6. When should a laboring client be examined vaginally?
7. Define cervical effacement.
8. Where is the FHR best heard?
9. Normal FHR during labor is _____.
10. Normal maternal BP during labor is _____.
11. Normal maternal pulse during labor is _____.
12. Normal maternal temperature during labor is _____.
13. List three signs of placental separation.
14. When should the postpartum dosage of oxytocin be administered? Why is it administered?
15. What is the danger associated with regional blocks?
16. Why are PO medications avoided in labor?
17. When is it dangerous to administer an agonist/antagonist narcotic to a woman in labor?
18. Hypotension commonly occurs after the laboring client receives a regional block. What is one of the first signs the nurse might observe?
19. State three actions the nurse should take when hypotension occurs in a laboring client.
20. How is the fourth stage of labor defined?
21. What actions can the nurse take to assist in preventing postpartum hemorrhage?
22. What nursing interventions are used to enhance maternal–infant bonding during the fourth stage of labor?
23. List the symptoms of a full bladder that might occur in the fourth stage of labor.
24. What action should the nurse take first when a soft, boggy uterus is palpated?
25. What are the symptoms of hypovolemic shock?
26. How often should the nurse check the fundus during the fourth stage of labor?

See Answer Key at the end of this text for suggested responses.

BOX 6.3 Medication Guide: Oxytocin

Medication	Action	Adverse Reactions	Nursing Implications
Oxytocin (Pitocin)	Used for labor induction and augmentation, also used to control postpartum bleeding	Uterine tachysystole Placental abruption Uterine rupture Water intoxication, severe hyponatremia Abnormal FHR pattern, fetal hypoxia Unplanned cesarean birth secondary to adverse effects	This is a high-alert medication. Assess maternal and fetal vital signs prior to administration and frequently during administration. A primary IV infusion line is started first and oxytocin is administered through a secondary line. Assess I & O. Monitor contraction pattern and uterine tone frequently and per institutional protocol. Discontinue oxytocin if uterine tachysystole occurs.

FHR, Fetal heart rate

Adapted from Lowdermilk, D. L., Perry, S. E., Cashion, K., Alden, K., & Olshansky, E. (2020). *Maternity and women's health care* (12th ed.). St. Louis: Elsevier. (Medication Guide: Oxytocin, p. 703) Data from American College of Obstetricians and Gynecologists. (2009, reaffirmed 2019). Practice Bulletin No. 107: Induction of labor. *Obstetrics & Gynecology, 114*(2, pt 1), 386–397; Clark, S., Simpson, K., Knox, G., & Garite, T. J. (2009). Oxytocin: New perspectives on an old drug. *American Journal of Obstetrics and Gynecology, 200*(1), 35.e1–35.e6; Hill, W., & Harvey, C. (2013). Induction of labor. In N. Troiano, C. Harvey, & B. Chez (Eds.), *AWHONN's high risk and critical care obstetrics* (3rd ed.). Philadelphia: Wolters Kluwer/Lippincott Williams & Wilkins; Mahlmeister, L. (2008). Best practices in perinatal care: Evidence-based management of oxytocin induction and augmentation of labor. *Journal of Perinatal and Neonatal Nursing, 22*(4), 259–263; Simpson, K. R., & O'Brien-Abel, N. (2014). Labor and birth. In K. R. Simpson & P. Creehan (Eds.), *AWHONN's perinatal nursing* (4th ed.). Philadelphia: Lippincott; and Simpson, K., & Knox, G. (2009). Oxytocin as a high-alert medication: Implications for perinatal patient safety. *American Journal of Maternal/Child Nursing, 34*(1), 8–15.

NORMAL PUERPERIUM (POSTPARTUM)

Description: The interval between birth and return of reproductive organs to normal nonpregnant state. It is sometimes called the fourth trimester. This has traditionally been considered to last 6 weeks; however, physiological and emotional recovery varies for every woman, and the entire first year after delivery is considered to be the postpartum period.

A. Care during this period is focused on recovery and wellness.
B. Teaching must be initiated early to cover the physical self-care needs and the emotional needs of the mother, infant, and family.

Normal Puerperium Physiologic Changes

A. Maternal Adaptations
 1. Vital Signs
  a. Temperature: Slight risk in first 24 hours, then afebrile
  b. Pulse: Slightly elevated in first 24 hours, then decreases over 48 hours; puerperal bradycardia (40 to 50 beats/min) can temporarily occur.
  c. Respirations: Should be within normal
  d. Blood pressure: Transient increase over first few days after birth but should return to normal within a few days. Orthostatic hypotension can develop in first 48 hours.
   1) Increases greater than 140/90, measured on 2 occasions at least 4 hours apart, can indicate gestational HTN or preeclampsia
   2) About half of women may experience "shivering" during first hour after birth; exact cause unknown.
 2. Uterus
  a. Uterine contractions occur for several days after delivery. During the first 2 hours postdelivery they may decrease in intensity and become uncoordinated. Therefore, exogenous oxytocin is usually administered IV or IM immediately after delivery of the placenta to help the uterus remain firm and well contracted. Endogenous oxytocin also helps strengthen and coordinate uterine contractions. Breastfeeding increases the release of endogenous oxytocin. Primiparous women may perceive only minimal contractions but afterpains are more common in subsequent pregnancies and may be experienced for 3 to 7 days after birth.
  b. Involution (return of uterus to nonpregnant state). Occurs (1 to 2 cm/day).
   1) End of third stage: uterus is midline, about 2 cm below level of umbilicus
   2) Within 12 hours, fundus can rise to about 1 cm above umbilicus.
   3) Over the next few days, the fundus descends 1 to 2 cm every 24 hours.
   4) By 2 weeks postpartum, the uterus should not be palpable abdominally.
  c. Uterine placenta site contracts and heals without scarring secondary to endometrial growth and sloughing of necrotic tissue. Endometrial regeneration begins within 3 days after birth and regeneration of placental site is complete by week 6.
  d. Lochia (post-birth uterine discharge, vaginal bleeding)
   1) Lochia rubra: blood-tinged discharge, including shreds of tissue and decidua; lochia rubra lasts 1 to 3 days postpartum
   2) Lochia serosa: pale pinkish to brownish discharge lasting up to 10 days postpartum
   3) Lochia alba: thicker, whitish-yellowish discharge with leukocytes and degenerated cells; lochia alba can last up to 6 weeks postpartum.
 3. Cervix
  a. Bruised and edematous immediately after birth. By 3 days postpartum, shortens, becomes firm, and regains form. The cervical os closes gradually and is about 1 cm dilated by 1 week post-birth. External os never regains pre-pregnancy appearance and appears as a transverse slit. Typically healed within 6 weeks
 4. Vagina
  a. Rugae (folds) reappear within 3 weeks but are more flattened. Walls are atrophic and can have localized dryness until ovarian function and menstruation resumes. Mucosa may remain atrophic during lactation, and vaginal dryness is common in breastfeeding mothers.
  b. Introitus is edematous and erythematous after birth. Episiotomy and laceration repairs may be present. Initial healing of repairs occurs within 2 to 3 weeks but full healing may take 4 to 6 months.
 5. Breasts

Both breastfeeding and non-breastfeeding women should be educated about symptoms of engorgement (breasts are distended, firm, tender to touch secondary to milk production, temporary venous congestions, lymphatic circulation for 24 to 48 hours) and encouraged to observe for erythema, cracked nipples, indications of mastitis (infection in milk duct with accompanying fever, erythema, flu-like symptoms).

  a. Non-breastfeeding
   1) Nodules may be palpable, bilateral, and diffuse.
   2) Colostrum is present. Engorgement may occur 3 to 5 days postpartum but will spontaneously resolve without milk expression. Lactation will typically cease within about 1 week. Ice bags and supportive bra may help with discomfort.
  b. Breastfeeding
   1) Milk sinuses (lumps) are palpable.
   2) Colostrum (yellowish fluid) is present. Thick yellow fluid. Breasts gradually become fuller, tender, may feel warm. Colostrum color transitions to whiter appearance, eventually becoming mature milk that is bluish-white.
   3) Encourage frequent breastfeeding to help establish milk supply.
 6. Cardiovascular system

a. At delivery maternal blood volume can decrease secondary to blood loss during delivery. Average blood loss for vaginal birth: 300 to 500 mL (10% blood volume). Average blood loss for cesarean birth: 500 to 1000 mL (15% to 30% blood volume)
b. Over the first 72 hours, cardiac output increases slightly over first hours after birth by 60% to 80% over pre-labor values; returns to prepregnant levels in 2 to 3 weeks.

7. Hematologic system
   a. Hct level drops moderately for 3 to 4 days after birth, then increases to nonpregnant levels by 8 weeks postpartum.
   b. WBC count is elevated (up to 30,000 mm^3).
   c. Blood-clotting factors remain elevated immediately postpartum; increases risk for thromboembolism.
8. Urinary system
   a. Diuresis of tissue fluid accumulated during pregnancy occurs within 12 hours after birth; woman excretes up to 3000 mL/day of urine during first 2 to 3 days after birth. Diaphoresis also frequently occurs and can be especially heavy at night.
   b. Bladder distention and incomplete emptying are common and may occur due to birth trauma, increased bladder capacity after birth, effects of anesthesia. With adequate emptying, tone is generally restored within 1 week.
   c. Dilation of ureter and renal pelvis return to nonpregnant state in 6 to 8 weeks; persistent dilation of urinary tract for 3 months or longer can increase risk for UTI.
9. Gastrointestinal system
   a. Excess analgesia and anesthesia may decrease peristalsis. Mothers often feel very hungry after full recovery from analgesia, anesthesia.
   b. Bowel movements can be delayed for 2 to 3 days.
10. Integumentary system
    a. Melasma (Chloasma or "mask of pregnancy") and hyperpigmentation areas (linea nigra, areolae) regress; some areas may remain permanently darker in about 30% of women.
    b. Striae gravidarum (stretch marks) may fade but usually do not fully disappear.
    c. Palmar erythema declines quickly.
    d. Spider nevi fade; some in legs may remain.
    e. Hair loss may occur over first 3 months postpartum.
11. Musculoskeletal system
    a. Pelvic muscles regain tone in 3 to 6 weeks.
    b. Abdominal muscles regain tone in 6 weeks. Persistence of diastasis recti (separation of rectus abdominis muscles) can occur but becomes less apparent over time.
    c. Relaxation and subsequent hypermobility of joints as well as change in maternal center of gravity that occurred during pregnancy generally resolve in a few weeks to months after birth.
12. Neurologic system
    a. Postpartum headaches can be common but must be evaluated for postpartum onset of preeclampsia, stress, leaking of cerebrospinal fluid into extradural space with epidural or spinal anesthesia.
13. Psychosocial system
    a. A variety of emotions secondary to hormonal changes, fatigue, and transition to parenthood are common.
    b. Postpartum blues can occur in the first 10 to 14 days postpartum and include symptoms of decreased appetite, sleep interference, emotional lability.

> **HESI HINT** Client and family teaching is a common subject of NCLEX-RN questions. Remember that, when teaching, the first step is to assess the clients' (parents') level of knowledge and to identify their readiness to learn. Client teaching regarding lochia changes, perineal care, breastfeeding, and sore nipples are subjects that are commonly tested.

B. Clinical Judgment Measures
1. Review prenatal, antepartum, labor and delivery (L&D), and early postpartum records for status, laboratory data, and possible complications.
2. Review newborn's record for Apgar scores, sex, possible complications, and relevant psychosocial information (adoption, single parent, etc.).
3. Assess maternal postpartum status.
   a. Vital signs. Monitor blood pressure and pulse every 15 minutes for the first 2 hours after birth. Assess temperature every 4 hours for the first 8 hours after birth and then at least every 8 hours.
   b. Fundal height. Check fundal height and firmness. Massage the fundus if it is soft or boggy by stabilizing the bottom of the uterus before applying pressure. Teach about the normalcy of afterpains.
   c. Lochia. Frequently assess and document lochia saturation on perineal pad; check under buttocks.
      1) Scant: (<2.5 cm)
      2) Light: (<10 cm)
      3) Moderate: (>10cm)
      4) Heavy: saturated pad within 2 hours
      5) A perineal pad saturated in 15 minutes or less and pooling under buttocks requires immediate intervention; notify obstetric provider
      6) Clots:
      7) Odor: fleshy, not foul
   d. Perineum. Assess perineum and episiotomy site.
      1) Place woman in lateral position, wear gloves, and use flashlight to increase accuracy of visualization.
      2) Check for redness, edema, intactness, and presence of hematomas; teach self-inspection with mirror.
      3) Teach hygiene and comfort and healing measures.
         a) Instruct to change pad as needed and with every voiding and defecation.
         b) Instruct to wipe perineum front to back.
         c) Instruct to use good handwashing technique.

d) Teach about use of ice packs, sitz baths, using a squeeze bottle for perineal lavage, and topical application of anesthetic spray and pads.
e) Breasts.
   (1) Assess nipples for cracks, fissures, redness, and tenderness.
   (2) Palpate breasts for lumps and nodules.
   (3) Determine mother's desired feeding method: breastfeeding or bottle feeding.
      (a) For breastfeeding mothers
         1. Assess breasts for engorgement.
         2. Teach mothers how to prevent engorgement.
         3. Assist mother and infant with breastfeeding.
      (b) If not breastfeeding, teach woman nonpharmacologic measures of milk suppression: supportive bra or soft binder, ice packs, and avoiding breast stimulation.
   (4) Teach breast self-examination.
f) Bladder and urine output.
   (1) Palpate for spongy, full feeling over symphysis.
   (2) Check urge to void when bladder is palpated.
   (3) Assist client to ambulate for first void (orthostatic hypotension may occur); measure if possible.
      (a) Client should void within 4 hours of delivery.
      (b) Monitor client closely for urine retention. Suspect retention if voiding is frequent and less than 100 mL per voiding.
      (c) Run warm water over perineum or place spirit of peppermint in bedpan to relax urethra if necessary.
      (d) Catheterize only if necessary.
      (e) Teach symptoms of UTI: dysuria, frequency, and urgency.
      (g) Bowel and anal area:
         1. Inspect for hemorrhoids; describe size and number.
         2. Auscultate bowel sounds; check abdominal distention.
         3. Document flatus and bowel movement.
         4. Encourage early ambulation.
         5. Encourage increased fluids and use of roughage and bulk in diet.
         6. Administer stool softeners as prescribed. Rectal suppositories and enemas should not be administered to women with third- or fourth-degree perineal lacerations and repairs as they can cause hemorrhage or damage to sutures and predispose women to infection.
   (4) Assess maternal–infant bonding and identify teaching needs of mother and family.
      (a) Assess mother–infant bonding behaviors:
         1. Eye contact between mother and neonate
         2. Exploration of infant from head to toe
         3. Stroking, kissing, and fondling the neonate
         4. Smiling, talking, singing to the neonate
         5. Absence of negative statements, such as, "She just doesn't like me."
      (b) Promote bonding opportunities
         1. Ensure mother is comfortable; provide pain relief, hygiene, adequate rest.
         2. If possible, have baby room-in; include family in teaching; praise and reinforce positive parenting behaviors.
         3. Teach about neonatal behavioral traits.
         4. Teach responses to cues from the baby.
   (5) Maintain safety.
      (a) Women may feel lightheaded or have a syncopal (fainting) episode on the first ambulation after delivery (usually related to vasomotor changes, orthostatic hypotension).
   (6) Prevent venous thromboembolism (VTE).
      (a) Encourage early ambulation.
      (b) Encourage flexion and extension of feet and legs. Rotate ankles in circular motion.
      (c) Examine legs of postpartum client frequently for pain, warmth, and tenderness or a swollen vein that is tender to the touch.
   (7) Prevent Rh isoimmunization
      (a) Determine the need for Rh immune globulin within 72 hours after birth for Rh-negative clients who have newborns who are Rh-positive (RhoGAM).
      (b) Determine the need for vaccinations.
         1. Rubella vaccination for women who are serologically nonimmune, Rubella titer of $\leq$1.10 or enzyme immunoassay (EIA) of $\leq$0.10. Vaccine should be administered prior to discharge. Caution to avoid pregnancy for at least 28 days after receiving vaccination.
         2. Varicella vaccination for postpartum women who have no immunity. Should be administered

prior to discharge. A second dose will be given at 4 to 8 weeks postpartum. Caution to avoid pregnancy for at least 28 days after receiving each varicella vaccination.
3. Tetanus-diphtheria-acellular pertussis vaccination (Tdap) is recommended for clients who have not previously had this vaccine or did not receive this vaccine during pregnancy (ideally between 27 and 36 weeks of pregnancy). Breastfeeding is not contraindicated. Advise that other adults and children who will be around the newborn should be vaccinated with Tdap if they have previously not received the vaccine.

(8) Assess maternal psychological adaptation.
   (a) Review effects of birth experience.
   (b) Assess for signs of potential psychosocial concerns (Box 6.4).
   (c) Consider family structure, cultural beliefs, and practices.
   (d) Encourage verbalization of feelings; offer support in nonjudgmental manner.

HESI HINT Informed consent should be obtained for vaccinations in the postpartum period and include information about possible side effects. Women should understand that they should not become pregnant for 28 days after rubella and varicella vaccinations.

C. Discharge teaching
1. Instruct client to notify obstetric provider promptly of
   a. Heavy vaginal bleeding with clots
   b. Temperature of 38°C or higher lasting 24 hours or longer
   c. A red, warm lump in breast
   d. Pain on urination
   e. Tenderness in calf
   f. Symptoms of preeclampsia
2. Teach self-care.
   a. Instruct to continue perineal care and regular pad changes.
   b. Encourage balanced diet and fluid intake.
   c. Encourage client to rest or nap when newborn does.
   d. Educate about signs of baby blues and postpartum depression (Box 6.5).
3. Discuss sexual activity and contraception
   a. Encourage to abstain from sexual intercourse until bleeding has stopped and perineum is healed. Most couples can resume sexual intercourse by 4 to 6 weeks after birth unless directed otherwise but this will vary for every couple.
   b. Inform that first sexual experience may be uncomfortable because of vaginal dryness, perineal repairs, fear of pain with intercourse.
   c. Discuss contraceptive options before discharge. Include partner in discussion if client desires. Discuss use, risks, side effects, and available options postpartum and with breastfeeding (Tables 6.17 and 6.18).

BOX 6.4 Signs of Potential Complications: Postpartum Psychosocial Concerns

The following signs suggest potentially serious complications and should be reported to the health care provider or clinic (these may be noticed by the partner or other family members):
- Unable or unwilling to discuss labor and birth experience
- Refers to self as ugly and useless
- Excessively preoccupied with self (body image)
- Markedly depressed
- Lacks a support system
- Partner or other family members react negatively to the baby
- Refuses to interact with or care for baby; for example, does not name baby, does not want to hold or feed baby, is upset by vomiting and wet or soiled diapers (cultural appropriateness of actions must be considered)
- Expresses disappointment over baby's sex
- Sees baby as messy or unattractive
- Baby reminds mother of family member or friend she does not like
- Has difficulty sleeping
- Experiences loss of appetite

BOX 6.5 Signs of Postpartum Blues, Depression, and Psychosis

- Signs of baby blues (these should go away in a few days or a week):
  - Sad, anxious, or overwhelmed feelings
  - Crying spells
  - Loss of appetite
  - Difficulty sleeping
- Signs of postpartum depression (can begin any time in the first year):
  - Same signs as baby blues, but they last longer and are more severe
  - Thoughts of harming yourself or your baby
  - Not having any interest in the baby
- Signs of postpartum psychosis:
  - Seeing or hearing things that are not there
  - Feelings of confusion
  - Rapid mood swings
  - Trying to hurt yourself or your baby
- When to call your health care provider:
  - The baby blues continue for more than 2 weeks
  - Symptoms of depression get worse
  - Difficulty performing tasks at home or at work
  - Inability to care for yourself or your baby
  - Thoughts of harming yourself or your baby

From Lowdermilk, D. L., Perry, S. E., Cashion, K., Alden, K., & Olshansky, E. (2020). *Maternity and women's health care* (12th ed.). St. Louis: Elsevier. Data from US Department of Health and Human Services Office of Women's Health. (2018). *Depression during and after* pregnancy *fact sheet.* Retrieved from http://www.womenshealth.gov/publications/our-publications/fact-sheet/depression-pregnancy.html

TABLE 6.17 Nonhormonal Methods of Contraception

Method	Considerations
Barrier Methods • Diaphragm • Cervical caps • Condoms (male and internal) • Contraceptive sponge	• All barrier methods must be applied near the time of sexual intercourse. • Barrier methods are less effective than hormonal methods. • Diaphragms and cervical caps should be used with spermicide; some condoms are lubricated with a spermicide. • Diaphragms, cervical caps must be fitted by a health care provider; not recommended for use immediately postpartum (cervix should be healed) and woman's weight should be stabilized (diaphragm must be refitted if excessive weight gain or loss occurs). • Condoms and sponges are single use only. • Ideally, diaphragms, cervical caps, and sponges should not be left in the vagina for more than 24 h. • Only condoms protect against STIs.
Fertility • Awareness-Based Methods (FABM). • Determines when a woman is most fertile during each month and uses abstinence or barrier contraception during that time to prevent pregnancy • Calendar methods, basal body temperature charting • CycleBeads • Postovulation method, cervical mucus assessment	• Most women will benefit from detailed education about FABM • It can be more difficult for women to identify their fertile window if ovulation is impacted by the postpartum recovery period (irregular menses) or by breastfeeding (absence of menses).
Lactational Amenorrhea Method • The act of infant suckling during breastfeeding increases maternal prolactin levels, which inhibits ovulation	• Three conditions should be present to increase the effectiveness of this method: (a) amenorrhea (no vaginal bleeding after 56 days postpartum), (b) exclusive or near-exclusive breastfeeding, and (c) infant younger than 6 months
Permanent Contraception (Sterilization) • May be chosen when the woman and/or the couple decides they no longer want children • Tubal Occlusion • Vasectomy	• Tubal occlusion may be done in the hospital after delivery and prior to discharge; should be discussed with provider prior to the birth • Both methods are highly effective in preventing pregnancy.

Adapted from Current NCLEX-RN Examination (2021) Philadelphia: Elsevier and Schuiling, K., & Likis, F. (2022) *Gynecologic health care* (4th ed.). Burlington, MA: Jones & Bartlett Learning.

TABLE 6.18 Hormonal Contraception

Composition	Route of Administration	Duration of Effect
Combination estrogen and progestin (synthetic estrogens and progestins in varying doses and formulations)	Oral Transdermal Vaginal ring insertion	24 h; extended cycle 12 weeks 7 days 3 weeks
Progestin only		
Norethindrone, norgestrel	Oral	24 h
Medroxyprogesterone acetate	Intramuscular injection; subcutaneous injection	3 months
Progestin, etonogestrel	Subdermal implant	Up to 3 years
Levonorgestrel	Intrauterine device	Up to 5 years

From Lowdermilk, D. L., Perry, S. E., Cashion, K., Alden, K., & Olshansky, E. (2020). *Maternity and women's health care* (12th ed.). St. Louis: Elsevier.

Nonhormonal Methods of Contraception

There are several options for nonhormonal contraception. All require commitment to use with each act of sexual intercourse if preventing pregnancy is the goal. These options do not have systemic adverse effects. Nonhormonal methods may fit within many cultural beliefs (see Table 6.18).

Hormonal Methods of Contraception

There are several hormonal options of contraception available to the woman. They may contain both progestin and estrogen (combined) or progestin only. The primary mechanism of action is to prevent ovulation, however, progestin-only products can also thicken cervical mucus and alter the endometrium. Long-acting reversible contraception (LARC) methods like intrauterine contraception (copper IUD or progestin IUDs containing levonorgestrel) and emergency contraceptive options are also available.

Hormonal contraceptives are very effective in preventing pregnancy but may have adverse side effects like headache, nausea, breast pain, mood changes, and metabolic effects. Increased risk of VTE is primarily a concern with combined methods. Initiation of combined hormonal methods are contraindicated until 21 days postpartum and preferably delayed until after 42 days postpartum (elevated risk for VTE). Most progestin-only methods can be initiated within the first month postpartum.

Women who are breastfeeding should also be aware that estrogen-containing products may affect milk supply. Combined methods are typically delayed until breastfeeding is well established. Some women may choose to initiate combined methods when they wean from breastfeeding. Progestin-only methods may typically be initiated within the first month postpartum without known adverse effects on breastfeeding (see Table 6.18).

4. Review Schedule of Postpartum Care
   a. All women should have contact with obstetric care provider within first 3 weeks after delivery. This may vary for women with chronic medical conditions, hypertensive disorders, high risk of mood or anxiety disorders, or breastfeeding mothers with lactation concerns.
   b. Breastfeeding newborns should be seen by a pediatric provider within 3 to 5 days after birth or 48 to 72 hours after hospital discharge to assess feeding adequacy and weight loss.
   c. Encourage client to contact obstetric provider sooner if complications arise or she has questions or concerns.
   d. A comprehensive well woman visit and exam should occur no later than 12 weeks after delivery.
5. Offer information and referral information for community resources.

REVIEW OF NORMAL PUERPERIUM (POSTPARTUM)

A nurse discovers a postpartum client with a boggy uterus that is displaced above and to the right of the umbilicus. What nursing action is indicated?

1. Which women experience afterpains more than others?
2. Upon admission to the postpartum room, 3 hours after delivery, a client has a temperature of 37.5°C. What nursing actions are indicated?
3. A client feels faint on the way to the bathroom. What nursing assessments should be made?
4. What factor places the postpartum client at risk for thromboembolism?
5. A breastfeeding mother complains of very tender nipples. What nursing actions should be taken?
6. Three days postpartum, a lactating mother has full, warm, taut, tender breasts. What nursing actions should be taken?
7. What information should be given to a client regarding resumption of sexual intercourse after delivery?
8. A woman asks why she is urinating so much in the postpartum period. The nurse bases the response on what information?
9. A woman's WBC count is 17,000 mm^3; she is afebrile and has no symptoms of infection. What nursing action is indicated?
10. What is the most common cause of uterine atony in the first 24 hours postpartum?
11. What is the purpose of giving docusate sodium to the postpartum client?
12. What should the fundal height be at 3 days postpartum for a woman who has had a vaginal delivery?
13. List three signs of positive bonding between parents and newborn.

See Answer Key at the end of this text for suggested responses.

POSTPARTUM COMPLICATIONS

Postpartum Infections

Description: Any clinical infection that occurs within 28 days of delivery, after spontaneous or induced abortion. The presence of a fever (38°C or higher) on two successive days of the first 10 days postpartum. Typical sites of infection include the vagina, perineum, uterus, bladder, or breasts. Risk factors include prolonged ROM, any lacerations, or operative incisions (forceps, episiotomy, or cesarean section), hemorrhage, intrauterine manipulation, manual removal of placenta, retained placental fragments, anemia.

A. Symptoms

1. Wound (abdomen, perineum)
   a. Fever
   b. Red, swollen, very tender
   c. Purulent and/or foul-smelling drainage, induration
2. Endometritis (infection of lining of uterus)
   a. Fever
   b. Chills
   c. Increased pulse
   d. Malaise, anorexia
   e. Excess fundal tenderness long after it is expected, pelvic pain
   f. Uterine subinvolution

g. Lochia returning to rubra from serosa
h. Foul-smelling lochia
3. UTI (can progress to pyelonephritis if not identified and treated)
a. Slight or no fever
b. May have chills
c. Dysuria, frequency, urgency, suprapubic tenderness
d. Hematuria, bacteriuria
e. Cloudy urine
f. Development of flank pain or costovertebral-angle tenderness, nausea or vomiting may indicate progression to pyelonephritis
4. Mastitis (secondary to breast engorgement, blocked ducts, trauma, improper latch with breastfeeding, infrequent breastfeeding)
a. Nipple fissures
b. Fatigue
c. Flulike symptoms: malaise, chills, and fever
d. Red, warm, hard lump in breast (typically unilateral)

B. Clinical Judgment Measures
Implement general care pertinent to any client with a diagnosed infection.

1. Use and teach good hygiene techniques, aseptic technique with wound care.
2. Frequently assess and record vital signs, including pain.
3. Manage fever by increasing fluids, providing comfort measures. Administer fever-reducing medications as ordered.
4. Analgesics as ordered.
5. Emphasize adherence to medication regimen.
a. Broad-spectrum antibiotics. Administer IV as directed if client is hospitalized.
b. Educate about proper antibiotic use, need to complete entire course, side effects, directions for home use (Table 6.19).
6. Site-specific interventions:
a. Perineal: assist with sitz bath, cool compresses, encourage meticulous perineal care.
b. Endometritis: assess lochia, obtain vaginal cultures if ordered
c. Mastitis: Encourage frequent breastfeeding, educate on breastfeeding technique, well-fitting bra (no underwire), use of breast pads (frequent changing, cleanliness), monitor for abscess formation or worsening symptoms, educate on when to contact obstetric provider (Table 6.20)

C. Labs
1. Collect specimens for cultures as indicated
2. CBC if applicable

HESI HINT Remember, the risk for postpartum infections is higher in clients who experienced problems during pregnancy (e.g., anemia, diabetes) and who experienced trauma during labor and delivery.

Postpartum Hemorrhage

Description: Obstetric emergency. It is a leading cause of maternal mortality that demands prompt recognition and intervention. The definition of acute PPH, also known as early or primary PPH, is a cumulative blood loss of greater than or equal to 1000 mL or bleeding associated with signs/symptoms of hypovolemia within 24 hours of birth, regardless of type of birth. Contributing factors for hemorrhage include uterine atony (overdistention of the uterus: polyhydramnios, multiple gestation, large neonate), lacerations of the genital tract, hematomas, placental complications (retained fragments, placenta accrete syndrome, abruption, previa), high parity, dystocia, prolonged labor, operative delivery (cesarean or forceps delivery, intrauterine manipulation), and previous history. Late, or secondary, PPH is possible but less common. The

TABLE 6.19 Antibiotics

Drugs	Indications	Adverse Reactions	Nursing Implications
Clindamycin	Broad-spectrum antibiotic used to treat postpartum endometritis	• Nausea, vomiting • GI irritation • Diarrhea	• Must be used in combination with gentamicin
• Ampicillin-sulbactam	• Broad-spectrum antibiotic used to treat postpartum endometritis	• Rash, dermatitis • Nausea, vomiting • GI irritation	• Do not administer to clients with penicillin sensitivity. • Alternative to clindamycin and gentamicin combination
• Gentamicin sulfate	• Aminoglycoside antibiotic used for serious puerperal infections	• GI irritation • Nephrotoxicity • Ototoxicity • Neurotoxicity • Possible hypersensitivity	• Do not mix with any other drug. • Observe for ototoxicity: ataxia, tinnitus, headache. • Observe for nephrotoxicity: elevated BUN and creatinine levels. • Observe for neurotoxicity: paresthesia, muscle weakness. • Monitor I&O closely.
• Cephalexin	• Broad-spectrum antibiotic used to treat lactational mastitis	• Rash, dermatitis • Nausea, vomiting	• Do not administer to clients with penicillin allergy.

GI, Gastrointestinal

TABLE 6.20 Clinical Judgment Measures: Mastitis in a Breastfeeding Mother

Clinical Judgment Measure	Assessment Characteristics
Recognize Cues	Choice of newborn feeding method (breastfeeding or non-breastfeeding mother) Number of days postpartum (most cases of mastitis occur 2–4 weeks postpartum, but can occur at any time) Breast pain, areas of redness, warmth Sudden onset of influenza-like symptoms (fever, chills, malaise, body aches, headache, nausea, vomiting)
Analyze Cues	Determine where breast pain is located (mastitis typically presents unilaterally in the upper outer quadrant of the breast) Assess vital signs (especially temperature) Assess for signs of engorgement Assess for axillary lymphadenopathy Assess for cracked, sore, reddened nipples Observe integrity of breast tissue for signs of abscess or open areas, areas of warmth, redness Determine frequency of breastfeeding episodes daily, i.e., feeding every 2–3 h vs. feeding every 6 h; any pumping Determine if mother is still able to breastfeed (since onset of symptoms), is pumping only, or has stopped breastfeeding completely
Prioritize Cues	Determine need for any surgical intervention (abscess requiring I & D, aspiration) Determine if newborn is receiving adequate, uninterrupted nutrition
Solutions	Teach clients about symptoms of mastitis before discharge from birthing facility and when to notify health care provider Encourage prevention measures: frequent breastfeeding on both breasts, adequate rest and nutrition for mother, appropriate breast hygiene, and handwashing Advise to avoid use of underwire bras
Actions	Warm compresses for discomfort Take antibiotics (complete entire course) and analgesics as ordered Teach mother to contact provider if symptoms are not relieved with antibiotic therapy or worsen Review proper breastfeeding technique, latch Refer to lactation consultant for assistance as appropriate Educate on safety of continued breastfeeding, safety of breastmilk when mastitis is present; safety of breastfeeding with antibiotic therapy Educate about mastitis and answer any questions

definition of a late PPH is a hemorrhage that occurs more than 24 hours but less than 6 weeks after the birth.

A. Symptoms
   1. Increase in lochia
      a. Perineal pad is soaked within 15 minutes
      b. Bleeding may be a continuous trickle or spurts
   2. Large blood clots may be present (larger than a quarter in size)
   3. Hypotonic (boggy) uterus
      a. Fundus that does not firm up with massage
   4. Change in vital signs: hypotension, increased pulse
   5. Pallor, cool, clammy skin

B. Clinical Judgment Measures

Acute PPH

1. Review chart for predisposing factors.
2. Monitor vital signs, fundus, lochia frequently and according to institution's policy.
   a. Count pads saturated and time required to saturate.
3. Monitor level of consciousness.
4. Keep the bladder empty.
5. Contact obstetric provider if atony or bleeding continues despite massage.
6. Anticipate administering uterine stimulant medication as ordered (Table 6.21).
7. Monitor I&O (at least 30 mL/h output); maintain fluid replacement.

Late Postpartum Hemorrhage

Anticipate hospitalization, pelvic examination/labs/diagnostics to determine cause of bleeding and subsequent treatment. Subinvolution (uterus remains enlarged, often from placental fragments or pelvic infection) is a common cause of late PPH. Lochia persists and may have irregular patterns or become excessive with brisk periods of lochia rubra. A dilation and curettage (D&C) may be necessary.

1. Frequent vital signs
2. Initiate IV access.
3. Type and crossmatch for possible blood transfusion.
4. Obtain cultures if ordered.
5. Administer antibiotics as prescribed.
6. Keep the client warm and be alert for symptoms of shock.
7. Prepare client for possible surgical repair of laceration, evacuation of hematomas, or curettage for removal of placental fragments.

C. Labs
   1. CBC
   2. Blood type and crossmatch

TABLE 6.21 Uterotonic Drugs to Manage Postpartum Hemorrhage

Drug	Side Effects	Contraindications	Nursing Considerations
Oxytocin (Pitocin)	Infrequent: water intoxication, nausea and vomiting	None for PPH	Continue to monitor vaginal bleeding and uterine tone.
Misoprostol (Cytotec)	Headache, nausea, vomiting, diarrhea, fever, chills	None	Continue to monitor vaginal bleeding and uterine tone.
Methylergonovine (Methergine)	Hypertension, hypotension, nausea, vomiting, headache	Hypertension, preeclampsia, cardiac disease	Check blood pressure before giving, and do not give if >140/90 mm Hg; continue monitoring vaginal bleeding and uterine tone.
15-Methylprostaglandin $F_2\alpha$ (Prostin/15 m; Carboprost, Hemabate)	Headache, nausea and vomiting, fever, chills, tachycardia, hypertension, diarrhea	Avoid with asthma or hypertension	Continue to monitor vaginal bleeding and uterine tone.
Dinoprostone (Prostin E_2)	Headache, nausea and vomiting, fever, chills, diarrhea	Use with caution with history of asthma, hypertension, or hypotension	Continue to monitor vaginal bleeding and uterine tone.

IM, Intramuscular; *IV,* intravenous; *PO,* by mouth; *PPH,* postpartum hemorrhage.
Adapted from Lowdermilk, D. L., Perry, S. E., Cashion, K., Alden, K., & Olshansky, E. (2020). *Maternity and women's health care* (12th ed.). St. Louis: Elsevier. Data from Francois, K. E., & Foley, M. R. (2017). Antepartum and postpartum hemorrhage. In S. G. Gabbe, J. R. Niebyl, J. L. Simpson, et al. (Eds.), *Obstetrics: Normal and problem pregnancies* (7th ed.). Philadelphia: Elsevier; and Lyndon, A., Lagrew, D., Shields, L., et al. (Eds.). (2015). *California maternal quality care collaborative toolkit to transform maternity care: Improving health care response to obstetric hemorrhage version 2.0.* Stanford, CA: California Maternal Quality Care Collaborative (CMQCC). Retrieved from https://www.cmqcc.org/ob_hemorrhage

3. Coagulation studies

D. Diagnostics
1. US may be ordered

HESI HINT During medical emergencies such as bleeding episodes, clients need calm, direct explanations, and assurance that everything possible is being done to care for the woman. If possible, allow support person at bedside.

Cesarean Birth

Description: The birth of the fetus or fetuses through a transabdominal uterine incision. This may be scheduled or unplanned and may be the choice of birth when maternal and/or fetal complications arise. A woman may have a vaginal birth after cesarean (VBAC) if she has no contraindications, is at low risk for uterine rupture, and she desires to do this after consultation with her obstetric provider. A trial of labor (TOL) to observe the mother and fetus for a reasonable period of spontaneous labor may be required before proceeding with a VBAC. Preparations must be in place for any emergent needs like an immediate cesarean birth.

A. Symptoms
1. Planned
2. Maternal or fetal complications requiring immediate operative delivery

B. Clinical Judgment Measures
1. Obtain informed consent; explain procedure
2. Provide emotional support
3. Monitor vital signs
4. Assess fetal well-being (FHR)
5. Establish IV access, initiate IV fluids as ordered
6. Assist with anesthesia
7. Administer preoperative medications if prescribed
8. Maintain safety
9. Intraoperative care: Place client in supine position with wedge under one hip to displace uterus laterally and prevent compression of vena cava; monitor vital signs, I & O, IV fluids, FHR, assist per institutional protocol.
10. Post-surgical care: Review complete surgery report, conduct standard postpartum assessments for vital signs, I & O, fundal height, lochia, signs of infection, excessive bleeding. Administer pain medications as prescribed.
11. Encourage early ambulation.
12. Encourage participation in infant care as soon as possible, including initiation of breastfeeding.

C. Labs
1. Blood type, Rh, and crossmatch
2. CBC, may be repeated post-op
3. Chemistry panel

D. Discharge
1. Provide discharge instructions and follow-up care as ordered.
   a. Information about PPH, preeclampsia, infection, pulmonary embolism, deep vein thrombosis, thrombophlebitis, postpartum depression

REVIEW OF POSTPARTUM COMPLICATIONS

1. May women with a positive HIV antibody try to breastfeed?
2. What are the common side effects of antibiotics used to treat puerperal infection?
3. How does the nurse differentiate the symptomatology of cystitis from that of pyelonephritis?
4. What are the signs of endometritis?

5. State four risk factors for or predisposing factors to postpartum infection.
6. State four risk factors for or predisposing factors to postpartum hemorrhage.
7. What immediate nursing actions should be taken when a postpartum hemorrhage is detected?
8. Must women diagnosed with mastitis stop breastfeeding?

See Answer Key at the end of this text for suggested responses.

THE NORMAL NEWBORN

Description: During the immediate transitional period (first 6 to 8 hours of life) and the early newborn period (first few days of life), the nurse assesses, plans, and provides nursing interventions based on the outcomes of the individual newborn's examination.

Newborn Transition to Extrauterine Life

The newborn should be carefully observed during the initial 6 to 8 hours after birth for adaptation of key systems to extrauterine life.

A. Respiratory
   1. Establishment of respirations after umbilical cord is clamped and cut (clamping causes a rise in BP which increases circulation and lung perfusion)
   2. Initiation of respirations occurs because of chemical, mechanical, thermal, and sensory factors

B. Cardiovascular
   1. Cord clamping and cutting causes changes in pressures of cardiovascular system triggering functional closure of the foramen ovale, ductus arteriosus, and ductus venosus.
   2. BP range: 60 to 80 mm Hg systolic/40 to 50 mm Hg diastolic

C. Thermogenic
   1. Heat regulation is critical to survival.
   2. Newborns have only a thin layer of subcutaneous fat, blood vessels are close to the skin's surface, and they have a larger body surface-to-body weight (mass) ratio.
   3. Thermoregulation is the balance between heat loss and heat production. Hypothermia (heat loss) leads to depletion of glucose and, therefore, to the use of brown fat (special fat deposits fetus develops in last trimester; they are important to thermoregulation) for energy (Table 6.22).

Immediate Care of Newborn After Delivery

Description: Nursing care provided to the newborn immediately after birth that includes a brief, initial assessment of systems and identification of any abnormalities requiring emergency interventions. If possible, the assessment should be completed while skin-to-skin contact is maintained with the mother.

A. Brief initial exam
   1. Observe for life-threatening abnormalities (poor muscle tone, not crying, not breathing or respiratory distress), need for resuscitation, birth injuries.
   2. Immediately dry infant, place cap on head, and establish skin-to-skin contact with mother by laying infant on mother's chest or abdomen. Infant may alternatively be placed on radiant warmer.
   3. Nasal and oral secretions should be wiped away; suction mouth and nose with bulb syringe if needed; keep head slightly lower than body; and assess airway status.
   4. Place identity bands on neonate and mother.

HESI HINT Suction the mouth first and then the nose. Stimulating the nares can initiate inspiration, which could cause aspiration of mucus in oral pharynx.

B. Apar Score
   1. Obtain Apgar score at 1 and 5 minutes (Table 6.23).

C. Physical Assessment
   1. General physical assessment should be completed as soon as possible after birth. Check for gross anomalies, including no back lesions and a patent anus.

TABLE 6.22 Newborn Vital Sign Norms

Vital sign	Normal	Nursing Implications

Respirations	Rate: 30–60 breaths/min	• Remember the ABCs (airway, breathing, circulation).
		• Count 1 full minute by observing abdomen or auscultating breath sounds.
		• Note five symptoms of respiratory distress
		  • Tachypnea
		  • Cyanosis
		  • Flaring nares
		  • Expiratory grunt
		  • abdominal breathing
		Retractions

Heart rate	110–160 beats/min; may decrease as low as 100 during sleep; may increase as high as 180 during crying	• Auscultate for 1 full minute at the PMI (point of maximal impulse): third to fourth intercostal space.
Temperature	Range: 36.5°C–37.5°C	• Rectal approach may perforate rectum; if taken rectally, insert only ¼ to ½ inch for 5 min and hold legs firmly to prevent trauma.
Blood pressure	Average 80/50 mm Hg	• Not usually measured unless problems in circulation have been assessed.

TABLE 6.23 Apgar Assessment

Performed at exactly 1 and 5 min after birth.
Cannot adjust eyeball; must have hands-on examination. Score:
- 7–10: good
- 4–6: needs moderate resuscitative efforts
- 0–3: severe need for resuscitation

Heart rate	Absent = 0; <100 = 1; ≥100 = 2
Respiratory effort	No cry = 0; weak cry = 1; vigorous cry = 2
Muscle tone	Flaccid = 0; some flexion = 1; total flexion = 2
Reflex irritability	No response to foot tap = 0; slight response to foot tap (grimace) = 1; quick foot removal = 2
Color	Dusky, cyanotic = 0; acrocyanotic = 1; totally pink = 2

2. Encourage parent's presence during exam.
3. Assess vital signs, including body length, weight, and head circumference (Table 6.24).
4. Collect cord blood and capillary stick for lab analysis as ordered
   a. Blood type and Rh status
   b. CBC
   c. Glucose
   d. Bilirubin
5. Examine cord clamp for closure, absence of blood oozing from cord; check for presence of three vessels (Table 6.25).

Ongoing Newborn Assessment

A. History
1. Review L&D report of neonatal history to determine risks during newborn transition caused by medical and obstetric complications.
   a. Cesarean delivery
   b. Prematurity or postmaturity
   c. Medical conditions of the mother (GDM, HTN)
   d. Prolonged ROM greater than 24 hours: sepsis workup
   e. Rh+ isoimmunization (positive direct Coombs test)
   f. Traumatic (forceps or vacuum suction) delivery
2. Review L&D report of neonatal history to determine risks during newborn transition caused by analgesia and anesthesia during labor and delivery.
   a. Magnesium sulfate during labor: Hypermagnesemia in neonate causes depressed respirations, hypocalcemia, and hypotonia.
   b. Late administration of narcotic analgesics; causes decreased respirations and hypotonia.
   c. Epidural or spinal anesthesia
   d. General anesthesia
3. Review L&D report of neonatal history to determine risks during newborn transition caused by degree of birth asphyxia.
   a. Potential asphyxia events during labor: documented late decelerations, decreased variability, severe variable decelerations
4. Review significant maternal social history: partner and support system, infections (TORCH, STDs), cultural influences (language, preferences for newborn care), maternal substance use.

B. Clinical Judgment Measures

The nurse is responsible for monitoring the newborn whether the infant is rooming-in or in the nursery. Parent–infant attachment and bonding should be encouraged.
1. Maintain oxygen supply.
2. Maintain body temperature.
   a. Keep newborn warm and dry.
   b. If newborn's temperature falls below 36.4°C, place in radiant warmer and apply skin temperature probe to regulate isolette temperature. May also double-wrap or put skin to skin (kangaroo) with mother.
3. Assess for neonatal pain.
   a. Every neonate should have an initial pain assessment and pain management plan.
      1) Physiologic pain responses may be noted by a change in vital signs, decreased oxygenation, skin pallor or sweating, increased muscle tone, or dilated pupils.
      2) Behavioral pain responses may be noted by crying, whimpering, grimace, furrowed brows, chin quivering, thrashing, rigidity or flaccidity, fist clenching, irritability.
4. Document the infant's elimination pattern daily.
   a. Stool progression: meconium (black, tarry, sticky) stool within the first 24 hours to transitional (yellowish-green) to milk stool (yellow). Report if no stool within 24 hours.

TABLE 6.24 Physical Measurements

Assessment	Normal	Nursing Implications
Weight	• Majority weigh between 2700 and 4000 g (6–9 lb)	• Weigh at birth and daily, with neonate completely naked. • Normally lose 5%–15% (average 10%) of birth weight in first week of life; weight should be documented carefully.
Length	• Average range: 46–52.5 cm	• Measured from crown to rump and rump to heel, or from crown to heel at birth
Head circumference	• Average range: 33–35 cm (normally, 2 cm larger than chest circumference)	• Tape measure placed above eyebrows and stretched around fullest part of occiput, at posterior fontanel (frontal-occipital circumference [FOC])
Chest circumference	• Average range: 31–33 cm	• Tape measure is stretched around scapulae and over nipple line.

TABLE 6.25 **Physical Examination of Newborn**

Normal	Abnormal	Rationale
General Appearance		
• Awake • Flexed extremities • Moves all extremities • Strong, lusty cry • Obvious presence of subcutaneous fat • No obvious anomalies	• Little subcutaneous fat	• Intrauterine growth problems • Fetal stress
	• Frog position	• Prematurity
	• Flaccid	• Asphyxia • Prematurity
	• Hard to arouse	• Sepsis • CNS problems • Asphyxia
	• High-pitched cry	• CNS damage or anomalies • Hypoglycemia • Drug withdrawal
Integument		
• Smooth, elastic turgor and subcutaneous fat, superficial peeling after 24 h; veins rarely visible • Milia, vernix increases • Lanugo, mottling • Harlequin sign (pink-red skin on one side of body) • Erythema toxicum (pink papular rash is normal) • Mongolian spots • Telangiectatic nevi (stork bites)	• Extreme desquamation	• Postmaturity
	• Many visible veins	• Prematurity
	• Meconium staining	• Fetal distress
	• Cyanosis	• Heart disease • Asphyxia
	• Jaundice (within 24 h)	• Blood incompatibilities • Sepsis • Drug reactions
	• Vesicle	• Herpes, syphilis
	• Café-au-lait spots	• Neurofibromatosis
Head		
• Round or slightly molded • Caput succedaneum (edema over occiput) • Open, flat anterior and posterior fontanels, sutures slightly separated or overlapping due to molding	• Bulging fontanel	• Increased ICP
	• Crosses suture line, present at birth	
	• Sunken fontanel	• Dehydration
	• Widely separated sutures	• Hydrocephalus
	• Premature suture closure	• Genetic disorders
	• Cephalohematoma	• Blood under periosteum due to trauma; can cause hyperbilirubinemia
Eyes		
• Symmetrically placed • Pseudostrabismus • Chemical conjunctivitis (from eye prophylaxis) • Clear cornea • White-blue sclera • Subconjunctival hemorrhage from pressure • Absence of tears • Doll's eye movement (slight nystagmus)	• Purulent discharge	• Gonorrhea or chlamydia
	• Brushfield spots in iris	• Down syndrome
	• Absence of red reflex	• Congenital cataracts
	• Epicanthal folds	• Down syndrome
	• Setting-sun sign	• CNS disorders
	• Absent glabellar reflex (blink)	• CNS or neuromuscular problem
Ears		
• Pinna at or above level of line drawn from outer canthus of eye • Well-formed and firm with instant recoil if folded against head	• Low set	• Down syndrome
	• Unformed, soft	• Prematurity
	• Preauricular sinus	• Possible renal anomaly

Continued

TABLE 6.25 **Physical Examination of Newborn—cont'd**

Normal	Abnormal	Rationale
Nose		
• In midline • Appears flattened • Is being used for breathing • Occasional sneezing	• Short, upturned, small philtrum (creases under nose)	• Fetal alcohol syndrome
	• Nasal flaring	• Respiratory distress
	• Grunting	• Respiratory distress • Choanal atresia (obstruction between nares and pharynx)
	• Snuffles	• Syphilis
	• Excessive sneezing	• Drug withdrawal
Mouth and Chin		
• Symmetrical movement • Intact lip and palate • Epstein pearls • Mobile tongue • Sucking pads in cheeks • Presence of rooting, sucking, swallowing, and gagging reflexes	• Asymmetry	• Facial nerve injury (Bell palsy)
	• Cleft lip	• Genetic disorder
	• White plaques on cheeks, tongue	• Monilia infection/thrush
	• Absence of protective reflexes	• Prematurity • CNS disorders
	• Excessive drooling	• Esophageal atresia
Neck		
• Short • Range of motion • Nonpalpable thyroid • Ability to lift head momentarily	• Limited range of motion	• Torticollis (wry neck)
	• Nuchal rigidity	• Meningitis
	• Enlarged thyroid	• Hyperthyroidism
	• Crepitus over clavicle	• Fractured clavicle
Chest		
• Symmetrical excursion • Breath sounds clear and equal • Transient rales at birth • Round • Breast engorgement (hormonal) • Transient murmurs	• Persistent murmur	• Patent ductus arteriosus
	• Visible activity over precordium	• Congenital heart anomaly • Heart failure
	• Retractions	• Respiratory distress
	• Asymmetrical chest	• Pneumothorax
Back, Hips, Buttocks, and Anus		
• Spine intact • Symmetrical gluteal folds • Equal limb lengths • Patent anus	• Pilonidal dimple or sinus (at base of sacrum)	• CNS anomaly • Covert spina bifida
	• Hip click • Unequal limb lengths • Asymmetrical gluteal folds	• Congenital hip dislocation
	• Absence of stools after 24 h	• Imperforate anus • GI obstruction
Abdomen		
• Full, rounded, soft • Present bowel sounds • Palpable liver 1–2 cm below right costal margin • Two arteries, one vein in cord; white cord with Wharton jelly	• Scaphoid	• Diaphragmatic hernia
	• Distention	• Meconium ileus • GI obstruction • Hirschsprung disease
	• Hepatosplenomegaly	• Sepsis
	• Purulent discharge at base of cord, foul odor	• Omphalitis (cord infection)
	• One artery	• Renal or heart anomalies
	• Omphalocele	• Abdominal contents in umbilicus (anomaly)
	• Gastroschisis	• Abdominal contents outside of abdomen (anomaly)

Continued

Genitals		
Female	• Labia minora and clitoris visible	• Prematurity
• Slightly edematous labia covering clitoris and labia minora • Pseudomenstruation • Visible hymenal tag		
Male	• Undescended testes	• Prematurity
• Penis with foreskin intact	• Meatus on dorsal surface penis	• Epispadias
• Meatus in middle at tip of penis • Descended testes	• Meatus on ventral surface penis	• Hypospadias
• Slight edema of scrotum	• Fluid in testes	• Hydrocele
• Rugae on scrotum	• Intestine in inguinal canal	• Inguinal hernia
Extremities		
• Arms, hands, fingers, legs, feet, toes	• Incurving little finger	• Down syndrome
• Flexion	• Simian crease	• Drug withdrawal
• Symmetrical movement	• Flapping tremors	• Extra digit (family trait)
• Palpable brachial and radial pulses	• Polydactyly	• Webbed digit (family trait)
• Palmar and plantar grasp reflex present	• Syndactyly	• Coarctation of aorta
• Strong grasp reflex • Multiple palmar and plantar creases	• Difference in pulses between upper and lower extremities	
• Slightly bowed legs • Femoral pulses present	• Absence of plantar creases	• Prematurity
• Positive Babinski reflex	• Rigid fixation of ankle	• Club feet (talipes)
	• Absent Babinski reflex	• CNS injury

   b. Infant should void within 4 to 6 hours of birth; then should use one diaper for each day of life, minimum, until day 6. On day 6 and beyond infant should use a minimum of six to eight diapers per day. Report if there is no urination within 24 hours. There may be brick-red "dust" in the first voidings (uric acid crystals).
   c. To evaluate exact urine output, weigh dry diaper before applying. Weigh the wet diaper after infant has voided. Calculate and record each gram of added weight as 1 mL urine.
5. Document nutrition intake and calculate nutrition needs.
   a. Demand feeding (bottle or breast) is preferred.
   b. Most bottle-fed newborns eat every 3 to 4 hours; breastfed infants eat every 1 to 3 hours (the breast milk is digested more quickly).
   c. After the initial weight loss period, the infant should gain approximately 1 oz (30 g) per day.
   d. An infant needs about 50 calories/lb or 108 calories/kg of body weight for the first 6 months.

C. Medications
1. Eye prophylaxis
   a. Recommended to prevent ophthalmia neonatorum
   b. Erythromycin ophthalmic ointment 0.5% is recommended.
   c. Administer within first hour of birth. If parents desire an open-eye bonding period, may delay eye prophylaxis for up to 2 hours.
2. Vitamin K prophylaxis
   a. Neonates have low vitamin K levels at birth.
   b. Recommended to prevent vitamin K–dependent hemorrhagic disease of the newborn
   c. Administer phytonadione 0.5 to 1 mg IM soon after birth.
   d. May be delayed until after first breastfeeding
3. Hepatitis B vaccination
   a. Recommended for all newborns before discharge
   b. If mother is positive for Hepatitis B, infant should receive HepB vaccine and HepB immune globulin (HBIG) within 12 hours of birth.

D. Gestational assessment

Description: Assessment of the gestational age of the infant examines six physical and six neuromuscular signs. A frequently used method is the New Ballard Score. The initial examination should be performed in the first 48 hours of life (Fig. 6.19, Tables 6.26 and 6.27).

E. Labs and Diagnostic Tests
1. Universal newborn screening (usually completed in the first 24 hours of life). Screens for core disorders (hemoglobinopathies, inborn errors of metabolism [Phenylketonuria (PKU)], galactosemia) and secondary disorders. State laws differ regarding informed consent newborn screening.
2. Hearing screening. Early detection of hearing loss allows for early intervention and treatment.
3. Critical congenital heart disease (CCHD) screening. Uses pulse oximetry testing at 24 and 48 hours of age to detect critical congenital heart defects that present with hypoxemia.
4. Monitor laboratory values (Table 6.28).

E. Assessment of Physiologic Problems

NEUROMUSCULAR MATURITY

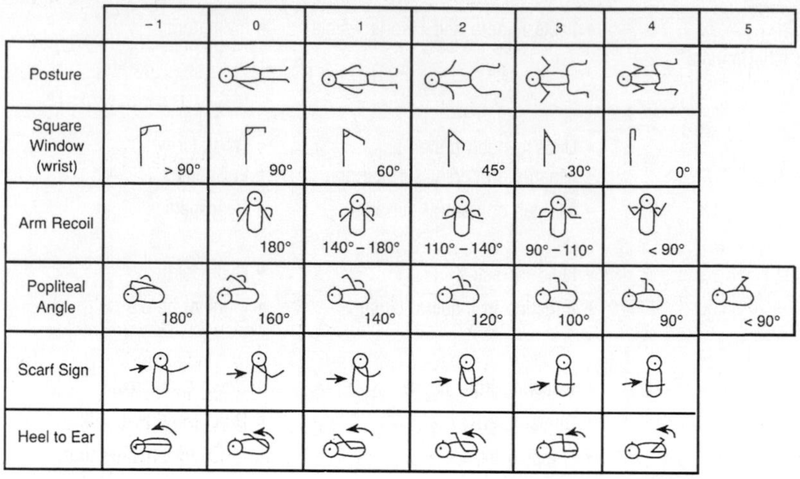

	−1	0	1	2	3	4	5
Posture							
Square Window (wrist)	> 90°	90°	60°	45°	30°	0°	
Arm Recoil		180°	140°–180°	110°–140°	90°–110°	< 90°	
Popliteal Angle	180°	160°	140°	120°	100°	90°	< 90°
Scarf Sign							
Heel to Ear							

PHYSICAL MATURITY

Skin	sticky friable transparent	gelatinous red, translucent	smooth pink, visible veins	superficial peeling or rash, few veins	cracking pale areas rare veins	parchment deep cracking no vessels	leathery cracked wrinkled
Lanugo	none	sparse	abundant	thinning	bald areas	mostly bald	
Plantar Surface	heel-toe 40–50 mm: −1 <40 mm: −2	>50 mm no crease	faint red marks	anterior transverse crease only	creases ant. 2/3	creases over entire sole	
Breast	imperceptible	barely perceptible	flat areola no bud	stippled areola 1–2 mm bud	raised areola 3–4 mm bud	full areola 5–10 mm bud	
Eye/Ear	lids fused loosely: −1 tightly: −2	lids open pinna flat stays folded	sl. curved pinna; soft; slow recoil	well-curved pinna; soft but ready recoil	formed & firm instant recoil	thick cartilage ear stiff	
Genitals (male)	scrotum flat, smooth	scrotum empty faint rugae	testes in upper canal rare rugae	testes descending few rugae	testes down good rugae	testes pendulous deep rugae	
Genitals (female)	clitoris prominent labia flat	prominent clitoris small labia minora	prominent clitoris enlarging minora	majora & minora equally prominent	majora large minora small	majora cover clitoris & minora	

MATURITY RATING

score	weeks
-10	20
-5	22
0	24
5	26
10	28
15	30
20	32
25	34
30	36
35	38
40	40
45	42
50	44

Fig. 6.19 Estimation of Gestational Age. New Ballard scale for newborn maturity rating. Expanded scale includes extremely premature infants and has been refined to improve accuracy in more mature infants. (From Ballard, J., Khoury, J. C., Wedig, K. L., Wang, L., Eilers-Walsman, B. L., & Lipp, R. [1991]. New Ballard score, expanded to include extremely premature infants. *The Journal of Pediatrics, 119*[3], 4177.)

TABLE 6.26 Neuromuscular Assessment

Reflex	Normal Response	Lasts Until
Rooting	Baby turns toward stimulus when cheek or corner of lip is touched.	3–4 months (possibly 1 year)
Moro	When startled, baby symmetrically extends and abducts all extremities. Forefingers form a C shape.	3–4 months
Tonic neck	When neck is turned to side, baby assumes fencing posture.	3–4 months
Babinski	When sole of foot is stroked from heel to ball, toes hyperextend and fan apart from big toe.	1 year—18 months
Palmar grasp	When examiner's finger is placed in the infant's palm, the newborn will curl his or her fingers around the examiner's finger.	Lessens by 3–4 months
Plantar	A finger at base of toes causes them to curl downward.	8 months
Stepping	When infant is held in upright position with feet touching a hard surface, walking motions are made.	3–4 months

TABLE 6.27 Gestational Age Assessment

By Date	By Weight
Preterm: 20–37 weeks gestation	Small for gestational age (SGA): Weight below the tenth percentile for estimated weeks of gestation
Term: 38–42 weeks gestation	Average for gestational age (AGA): Weight between the tenth and ninetieth percentiles for estimated weeks of gestation
Postterm: >42 weeks gestation	Large for gestational age (LGA): Weight above the ninetieth percentile for estimated weeks of gestation

TABLE 6.28 Standard Laboratory Values in a Term Neonate

Hematology	Values
Hemoglobin (g/dL)	15–24
Hematocrit (%)	44–70
Red blood cells (RBCs)/μL	4.8 × 106 to 7.1 × 106
Reticulocytes (%)	1.8–4.6
Fetal hemoglobin (% of total)	50–70
Platelet Count/mm^3	
≤1 week	84,000–478,000
>1 week	150,000–300,000
White blood cells (WBCs)/μL	9000–30,000
Bilirubin, Total (mg/dL)[a]	
24 h	2–6
48 h	6–7
3–5 days	4–6
Serum Glucose (mg/dL)	
<1 day	40–60
>1 day	50–90
Arterial Blood Gases	
pH	7.35–7.45
Pco_2	35–45 mm Hg
Po_2	60–80 mm Hg
HCO_3	18–26 mEq/L
Base excess	(−5) to (+5)
O_2 saturation	92%–94%

[a]Bilirubin levels should be interpreted according to the hour-specific nomogram (AAP Subcommittee on Hyperbilirubinemia, 2004).

dL, Deciliter; *μL*, microliter; *Pco_2*, partial pressure of carbon dioxide; *Po_2*, partial pressure of oxygen.

Data from American Academy of Pediatrics [AAP] Subcommittee on Hyperbilirubinemia. (2004). Clinical practice guideline: Management of hyperbilirubinemia in the newborn infant 35 or more weeks of gestation. *Pediatrics, 114*(1), 297–316; Blackburn, S. T. (2018). *Maternal, fetal, and neonatal physiology* (5th ed.). St. Louis: Elsevier; Kliegman, R. M., Stanton, B. F., St. Geme III, et al. (Eds.), (2016). *Nelson textbook of pediatrics* (20th ed.). Philadelphia: Elsevier; Pagana, K. D., & Pagana, T. J. (2014). *Mosby's manual of diagnostic and laboratory tests* (5th ed.). St. Louis: Elsevier; Barry, J. S., Deacon, J., Hernández, C., et al. (2016). Acid-base homeostasis and oxygenation. In: S. L. Gardner, B. S. Carter, M. Enzman-Hines, et al. (Eds.), *Merenstein & Gardner's handbook of neonatal intensive care* (8th ed.). St. Louis: Elsevier.

Hypoglycemia

Description: Blood glucose level inadequate to support the newborn. At-risk infants include those born preterm or late preterm, small-for-gestational-age (SGA), large-for-gestational-age (LGA), low birth weight, infants born to mothers with diabetes, infants who experienced respiratory, asphyxia, or cold stress.

1. Perform a heelstick blood glucose assessment on all SGA or LGA babies, on infants of diabetic mothers (IDMs), on jittery babies, and on babies with high-pitched cries (Box 6.6).
1. Report any blood glucose levels under 40 mg/dL. Normal serum glucose is 40 to 80 mg/dL. Administer glucose gel if ordered and per institution protocol.
2. Feed the baby early (breast milk or formula) if a low glucose level is detected. In addition, review orders and institution protocol to apply glucose gel for infants with a blood glucose level under 40 mg/dL. Notify provider.
3. Prevent cold stress, which leads to hypoglycemia.

Hyperbilirubinemia

A. Description: Elevation of serum bilirubin. Most newborns will experience some level of jaundice. Physiologic jaundice is caused by increased levels of unconjugated bilirubin, is usually self-limiting, and often requires no treatment. Evaluate for Rh isoimmunization (Rh+ newborn, Rh− mother; maternal Rh+ antibodies are passed to the fetus and cause RBC hemolysis) and for ABO incompatibility (mother blood type O, newborn blood type A or B; maternal anti-A or anti-B antibodies are passed to newborn and cause less-severe hemolysis).

BOX 6.6 Heelstick Procedure for Newborns

- Wash hands and put on gloves.
- Clean heel with alcohol and dry with a gauze pad.
- Choose a site for puncture that avoids the plantar artery in the middle of the heel.
- Use only the lateral surfaces of the heel.
- Puncture deep enough to trigger a free flow of blood. Wipe away first drop with sterile gauze pad.
- Collect blood in appropriate tube, on card, or on glucose "stick."

B. Promote stooling by early feedings of milk. (Bilirubin, a byproduct of RBC destruction, binds to protein for excretion or metabolism.)
C. Assess at birth and at least every 8 to 12 hours for presence of jaundice.
   1. Visual assessment to look for yellowish skin color, sclera, and mucous membranes; jaundice tends to proceed cephalocaudally (relationship between the head and the base of the spine).
      a. Assess skin for jaundice: apply pressure with thumb over bony prominences to blanch skin. After the thumb is removed, the area will look yellow before normal skin color reappears.
      b. The best areas for assessment are the nose, forehead, and sternum. In dark-skinned infants, observe conjunctival sac and oral mucosa.
      c. Visual assessment alone does not provide an accurate assessment. Also follow POC transcutaneous bilirubin level (TcB) protocols.
   2. Measurements for total serum bilirubin level (TSB) or (TcB) should be conducted as ordered. Repeat testing is based on risk level, age of neonate, and progression of jaundice.
D. Assist with phototherapy if ordered (Table 6.29).

HESI HINT Physiologic jaundice, which occurs after 24 hours of age, peaks at about 3 to 5 days in term infants, and resolves after 1–2 weeks. It is due to the immature liver's normal inability to keep up with RBC destruction and to bind bilirubin. Remember that unconjugated bilirubin is the culprit.

HESI HINT When phototherapy is used, the infant's eyes must be protected by a special opaque mask designed to prevent retinal damage, and no ointments, creams, or lotions should be applied to the newborn's skin to prevent burns.

TABLE 6.29 Clinical Judgment Measures: Pathologic Jaundice in Newborn

Clinical Judgment Measure	Assessment Characteristics
Recognize Cues	Jaundice appearing before 24 h of age usually indicates a pathologic condition TSB levels increase by more than 0.2 mg/dL per hour; TSB is >95th percentile for age in hours Direct serum bilirubin levels exceed 1.5–2 mg/dL
Analyze Cues	Review maternal history and labor/birth record for potential risk factors a. Rh incompatibility; ABO incompatibility; other hemolytic disease (G6PD deficiency) b. Prematurity c. Sepsis d. Maternal diabetes, intrauterine infections e. Native American or Asian race f. Birth trauma (including vacuum or forceps assisted delivery); cephalohematoma g. Previous sibling who received phototherapy Monitor serum bilirubin levels closely; repeat testing as ordered Review other labs as ordered (direct Coombs test, reticulocyte count, Hgb, Hct) Monitor urine and stools Document visual assessment of jaundice (in addition to serum levels) Observe and document changes in infant behavior
Prioritize Cues	The time of onset of jaundice is a key factor in evaluating its cause and determining needed treatment; increasing levels of unconjugated bilirubin that are left untreated can quickly result in a. Acute bilirubin encephalopathy with symptoms of lethargy, hypotonia, irritability, seizures, coma, death b. Kernicterus (irreversible, long-term consequences of bilirubin toxicity (hypotonia, delayed motor skills, hearing loss, cerebral palsy)
Solutions	Encourage frequent and adequate feedings Assess for risk factors prior to delivery Closely observe infant in the first 24 h of life for signs of jaundice Teach parents about the differences between physiologic and pathologic jaundice; answer questions
Actions	Treatment will depend on TSB levels, infant's gestational age, presence of risk factors; goal is to reduce the newborn's serum levels of unconjugated bilirubin Phototherapy or exchange infusion may be needed to reduce unconjugated bilirubin levels Teach parents the importance of follow-up care and clearly review discharge instructions
Evaluate Outcomes	The overall status of the newborn will be determined by decreasing TSB levels, behavior, and reduction in visible jaundice Early identification and treatment will prevent acute bilirubin encephalopathy and kernicterus

TSB, Total serum bilirubin.

E. Newborn Discharge Teaching
1. Provide parent and family with teaching plan for newborn care.
   a. Bathing. Teach *not* to submerge infant in water until cord falls off (10 to 14 days); continue cord care and keep diaper off cord.
   b. Diapering. Teach to use warm water to clean infant after voiding; use mild soap and water with stools (remember, cleanse female perineum front to back); dry completely before applying next diaper.
   c. Crying. Teach that all infants cry. Instruct on strategies to calm a crying or fussy baby. Encourage picking the baby up.
   d. Comfort. Encourage parents to implement swaddling, back massage, rhythmic movement such as rocking to help with calming infant.
2. Teach to recognize signs and symptoms of a sick newborn who needs medical attention.
   a. Lethargy or difficulty waking
   b. Temperature above 37.8°C
   c. Vomiting (large emesis, not spitting up)
   d. Green, liquid stools
   e. Refusal of two feedings in a row
   f. Presence of fever
3. Review follow-up care. Most infants will have an appointment with a healthcare provider within 48 to 72 hours of discharge. This is especially important for breastfed infants to monitor weight and hydration status.

HESI HINT Teach parents to take infant's temperature, both axillary and rectal. Axillary is recommended, but some pediatricians request a rectal (core) temperature.

REVIEW OF NEWBORN

1. The newborn transitional period consists of the first _____ of life.
2. The nurse anticipates which newborns will be at greater risk for problems in the transitional period. State three factors that predispose to respiratory depression in the newborn.
3. What is the danger to the newborn of heat loss in the first few hours of life?
4. Normal newborn temperature is _____. Normal newborn heart rate is _____. Normal newborn respiratory rate is ___. Normal newborn BP is ____.
5. The nurse records a temperature below 36.1°C on admission of the newborn. What nursing actions should be taken?
6. True or false: The newborn's head is usually smaller than the chest.
7. During the physical examination of the newborn, the nurse notes the cry is shrill, high-pitched, and weak. What are the possible causes?
8. The nurse notes a swelling over the back part of the newborn's head. Is this a normal newborn variation?
9. Should the normal newborn have a positive or negative Babinski reflex?
10. When suctioning the newborn with a bulb syringe, which should be suctioned first, the mouth or the nose?
11. A new mother asks the nurse whether circumcision is medically indicated in the newborn. How should the nurse respond?
12. Normal blood glucose in the term neonate is _____.
13. Why does the newborn need vitamin K in the first hour after birth?
14. Physiologic jaundice in the newborn occurs _____. It is caused by _____.
15. When is the screening test for PKU done?
16. A term newborn needs to take in _____ calories per pound per day. After the initial weight loss is sustained, the newborn should gain _____ per day.
17. List five signs and symptoms new parents should be taught to report immediately to a health care provider or clinic.

See Answer Key at the end of this text for suggested responses.

NEWBORN COMPLICATIONS

Neonatal Sepsis

Description: One of most significant causes of neonatal mortality and morbidity. Classified into either early-onset (within first 7 days of life) or late-onset (occurring 7 to 30 days of age) sepsis. Neonatal infections may be bacterial, viral, or fungal.

A. General Symptoms (may vary with causative agent)
1. Earliest symptoms are often nonspecific and include lethargy, poor feeding, and temperature instability.
2. Subtle color changes: mottling, duskiness
3. Subtle changes in behavior
4. Respiratory distress, apnea

Example: Group B Streptococcus (GBS)

Description: GBS lives in human GI and genitourinary tracts. It is a leading cause of perinatal infections. In the newborn it can cause focal or systemic disease. Women who are GBS positive during pregnancy can pass the infection on to the newborn; however, the practice of providing prophylactic intrapartum antibiotics to women with GBS has greatly reduced the incidence in newborns. GBS disease in the newborn can be early onset (within the first 7 days of birth, usually from vertical transmission during birth) or late onset (from 7 days of life to 3 months of age).

Risk factors include preterm birth, ROM greater than 18 hours before birth, intrapartum maternal fever, maternal GBS bacteriuria during current pregnancy.

A. GBS Symptoms
   1. Early-onset typically presents with severe respiratory distress (rapid breathing, grunting, apnea), being fussy, lethargic, change in blood pressure.
   2. Late-onset disease associated with meningitis, osteomyelitis, musculoskeletal pain, or decreased movement
B. Clinical Judgment Measures for neonates with sepsis
   1. Prevent infection in the newborn
      a. Meticulous handwashing
      b. Maintain sterile technique during procedures.
      c. Universal precautions. Wear gloves; clean environment and equipment, change linens.
   2. Review maternal chart for risk factors.
   3. Monitor vital signs.
   4. Monitor daily weights.
   5. Monitor I & O, fluid status.
   6. Maintain adequate nutrition: Calculate calorie, protein, and fluid needs according to weight.
   7. Administer antibiotics, antivirals, antifungals as prescribed.
      a. Dosage is typically based on the neonate's weight in kilograms.
C. Labs
   1. Blood, urine, CSF cultures
   2. CBC with differential
   3. C-reactive protein/Procalcitonin
   4. Chemistry panel
D. Discharge Instructions
   1. Provide emotional support to parents.
   2. Provide instructions for medication use, follow-up care.

> **HESI HINT** Sepsis can be indicated by both a temperature increase and a temperature decrease.

PRETERM NEWBORN

Description: Infants born after 20 weeks gestation and before the completion of 37 weeks gestation. Additional classifications include late preterm infants, born from 34 (0/7) weeks' through 36 (6/7) weeks' gestation, and early term infants, born from 37 (0/7) weeks' through 38 (6/7) weeks' gestation. Supportive care for the neonate born at less than 38 weeks' gestation is based on the level of immaturity identified by gestational age and physical assessment.

A. Symptoms will vary according to system response to prematurity
   1. Respiratory system. Signs of distress (apnea, tachypnea, flaring nares, retractions, seesaw breathing, grunting, abnormal blood gases) due to
      a. Lung immaturity
      b. Deficient surfactant levels
      c. Immaturity of respiratory center in brain causing apnea and bradycardia
   2. Cardiovascular system. Signs of distress include abnormal rate and rhythm; persistent murmurs; differentials in pulse, dusky skin color; circumoral cyanosis.
   3. Thermoregulation. Temperature instability related to
      a. Insufficient subcutaneous fat
      b. Larger ratio of body surface area to body weight
      c. Extended, open body position
      d. Immature hypothalamus
   4. CNS System. Function is dependent on gestational age. Clinical signs may include
      a. Lethargy
      b. High-pitched cry or weak cry
      c. Hyperirritability, seizure activity
      d. Increased intracranial pressure
      e. Hypotonia
   5. Nutrition problems related to intake and metabolism.
      a. Weak or absent suck, swallow, gag reflexes
      b. Difficulty coordinating suck and swallow
      c. Small stomach capacity
      d. Immature digestion process: lacks some gastric and pancreatic enzymes, decreased gastric emptying time
   6. Immunity
      a. Shortage of stored maternal immunoglobulins
      b. Impaired ability to make antibodies
      c. Increased risk for a thin skin barrier
B. Clinical Judgment Measures
   1. Conduct initial, rapid assessment at birth, perform resuscitation measures if needed, and transfer infant to NICU for advanced care.
   2. Promote growth and development through an extrauterine environment that approximates that of the fetus.
   3. Continual assessment of physiologic status of each system
   4. Monitor vital signs.
   5. Provide and monitor O_2 therapy.
   6. Monitor thermoregulation.
      a. Place infant under radiant warmer.
      b. Infants may be placed in polyethylene bag to reduce heat and insensible water loss as applicable.
      c. Warm all things that touch newborn: hands, equipment, O_2, and surfaces.
   7. Monitor fluid and electrolytes. Observe for signs of
      a. Hypoglycemia: jitteriness, tremors, lethargy, hypotonia, apnea, weak or high-pitched cry, eye rolling, and seizures
      b. Overhydration: edema, tachycardia, bulging fontanels, crackles in lungs, increased weight gain

BOX 6.7 Procedure for Inserting a Gavage Feeding Tube

Equipment

- Infant feeding tube
  - For infants less than 1 kg (2.2 lb), size 4 Fr
  - For infants more than 1 kg (2.2 lb), size 5 to 6 Fr
- Stethoscope
- Sterile water (lubricant)
- Syringe: 5–10 mL
- Tape, optional transparent dressing
- Gloves

Procedure

- Measure the length of the gavage tube from the tip of the nose to the earlobe to the midpoint between the xiphoid process and the umbilicus. Mark the tube with indelible ink or a piece of tape.
- Lubricate the tip of the tube with sterile water and insert gently through the nose or mouth until the predetermined mark is reached. Placement of the tube in the trachea will cause the infant to gag, cough, or become cyanotic.
- Check correct placement of the tube by:
  a. Pulling back on the plunger to aspirate stomach contents. Lack of stomach aspirate or fluid is not necessarily evidence of improper placement. Aspiration of respiratory secretions can be mistaken for stomach contents; however, the pH of the stomach contents is much lower (more acidic) than the pH of respiratory secretions.
  b. Injecting a small amount of air (1–3 mL) into the tube while listening for gurgling by using a stethoscope placed over the stomach. Ensure that the tube is inserted to the mark; air entering the stomach can be heard even if the tube is positioned above the gastroesophageal (cardiac) sphincter.
  c. Abdominal or chest radiography. This is the only definitive way to verify tube placement.
- Using tape or a transparent dressing, secure the tube in place and tape it to the cheek to prevent accidental dislodgment and incorrect positioning
  a. Assess the infant's skin integrity before taping the tube.
  b. Edematous or very preterm infants should have a pectin barrier placed under the tape to prevent abrasions, or a hydrocolloid adhesive should be used to prevent epidermal stripping.
- Tube placement *must* be assessed before each feeding.

From Lowdermilk, D. L., Perry, S. E., Cashion, K., Alden, K., & Olshansky, E. (2020). *Maternity and women's health care* (12th ed.). St. Louis: Elsevier.

c. Dehydration: sunken fontanels, poor skin turgor, and dry mucous membranes, weight loss, decreased urine output
d. Maintain urine output of 1 mL/kg/h and specific gravity of 1.005 to 1.012.

8. Maintain nutrition: Human milk is the best source of nutrition.
   a. Administer nutrition (parental or enteral) as prescribed; infant may need IV or gavage feedings (see Box 6.7, Fig. 6.20).
   b. Once infant is able to tolerate oral nipple feedings, observe for coordinated suck-swallow ability and gag reflex as well as signs of fatigue or tachycardia.
   c. Provide options for non-nutritive sucking as applicable; i.e., pacifier.

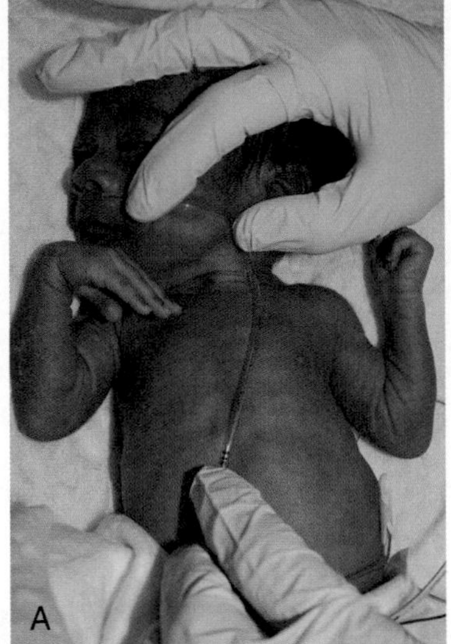

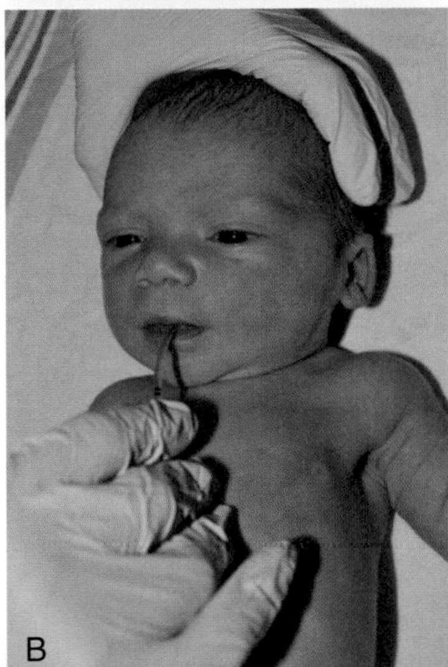

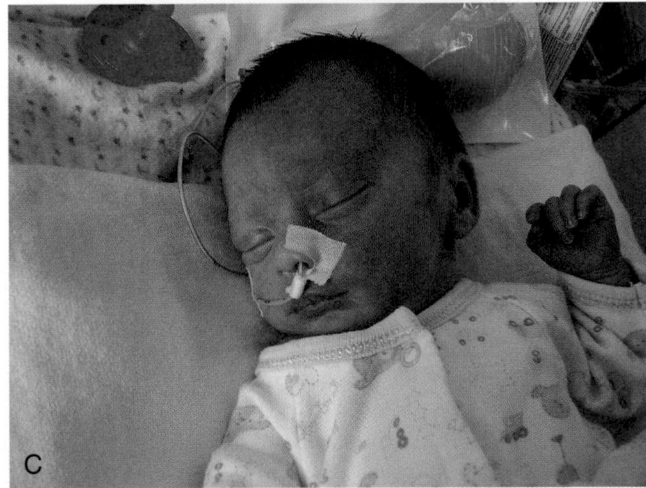

Fig. 6.20 Gavage Feeding. (A) Measurement of gavage feeding tube from tip of nose to earlobe and to midpoint between end of xiphoid process and umbilicus. Tape may be used to mark correct length on tube. For accurate measure the infant should be facing up. (B) Insertion of gavage tube using orogastric route. (C) Indwelling gavage tube, nasogastric route. After feeding by orogastric or nasogastric tube, infant is propped on right side or placed prone (preterm infant) for 1 hour to facilitate emptying of stomach into small intestine. (From Lowdermilk, D. L., Perry, S. E., Cashion, K., Alden, K., & Olshansky, E. [2020]. *Maternity and women's health care* [12th ed.]. St. Louis: Elsevier. A and B, Courtesy Cheryl Briggs, RNC, Annapolis, MD. C, Courtesy Randi and Jacob Wills, Clayton, NC.)

9. Support family and parental adjustment.
   a. Initiate early visitation and accompany parents on visits to the neonatal intensive care unit (NICU).
   b. Provide information to parents daily.
   c. Teach caregiving skills.
   d. Continue to enhance parent–infant bonding. Physical contact is important to establish bonding.
   e. Expect that some parents may experience anticipatory grief over potential loss of a preterm infant or the loss of the delivery of a healthy, full-term infant. Provide ongoing support.
10. Plan for discharge using multidisciplinary approach.

RESPIRATORY DISTRESS SYNDROME

Description: Lung disorder that is caused by a lack of pulmonary surfactant. Complications include progressive atelectasis, respiratory acidosis, infection, intraventricular hemorrhage (IVH). The incidence and severity of respiratory distress syndrome (RDS) increase as gestational age decreases. Risk factors include prematurity, perinatal asphyxia (meconium aspiration, nuchal cord or cord prolapse), maternal diabetes, familial predisposition, cesarean birth without labor.

A. Symptoms
   1. Usually appear immediately after or within 6 hours of birth but clinical course is variable
   2. Lung sounds: crackles, poor air exchange
   3. Pallor; cyanosis
   4. Use of accessory muscles (retractions)
   5. Nasal flaring, grunting
   6. Apnea
B. Clinical Judgment Measures
   1. Immediate initial assessment of respiratory status at birth and frequently thereafter
      a. Prepare for newborn resuscitation measures if needed.
   2. Supportive measures
      a. Establish and maintain ventilation, oxygenation (may include positive-pressure ventilation, nasal CPAP, oxygen therapy).
      b. Monitor pulse oximetry and arterial blood gases (ABGs).
   3. Administer exogenous surfactant as ordered.
   4. Monitor thermoregulation.
   5. Maintain nutrition, fluids, electrolytes.
   6. Monitor I & O.
   7. Provide emotional support to parents and educate about ongoing interventions.
C. Labs
   1. ABGs/CBC
   2. CBC with differential; cultures (blood and urine) if sepsis suspected
   3. Lumbar puncture may be considered.
D. Diagnostics
   1. Chest x-ray
E. Discharge
   1. Educate on signs of respiratory distress.
   2. Teach parents importance of follow-up care.

Effects Substance Abuse on the Neonate

Description: Maternal substance use and abuse can greatly impact the developing fetus. Polysubstance use is common and includes alcohol, tobacco, illicit drugs, and prescription drugs. In recent years, the opioid crisis has brought more attention to prescription opioid misuse and opioid use disorders. The effects of individual drugs as well as collective use may vary according to dose, route of administration, genotype of the mother or fetus, and timing of the drug exposure.

The newborn can experience withdrawal symptoms at birth or several hours or even days after birth. Neonatal abstinence syndrome (NAS) refers to the clinical signs that can be associated with withdrawal from any substance (Box 6.8). Neonatal opioid withdrawal syndrome (NOWS) refers to the clinical signs associated specifically with withdrawal from opioids.

A. Symptoms of NAS
B. Consequences of maternal substance misuse and abuse
   1. Many drugs have vasoconstrictive effects which cause hypoxemia and contribute to fetal growth delays (small size, IUGR) and fetal distress.
   2. Increased risk for spontaneous abortion, preterm labor and birth, placental abruption.
   3. Cognitive and developmental delays; often not fully recognized until childhood.

BOX 6.8 Signs of Neonatal Abstinence Syndrome

Acute Signs and Symptoms That May Persist for Several Weeks

Restlessness
Tremors (disturbed at first to undisturbed)
High-pitched cry
Increased muscle tone
Irritability and inconsolability
Increased deep tendon reflexes
Exaggerated Moro reflex
Seizures in approximately 1%–2% of heroin-exposed neonates and approximately 7% of methadone-exposed neonates

Subacute Signs and Symptoms That May Persist for 4–6 months

- Irritability
- Sleep pattern disturbance
- Hyperactivity
- Feeding problems
- Hypertonia

From Lowdermilk, D. L., Perry, S. E., Cashion, K., Alden, K., & Olshansky, E. (2020). *Maternity and women's health care* (12th ed.). St. Louis: Elsevier. Data from Weiner, S. M., & Finnegan, L. P. (2016). Drug withdrawal in the neonate. In S. L. Gardner, B. S. Carter, M. Enzman-Hines, & J. A. Hernandez (Eds.), *Merenstein & Gardner's handbook of neonatal intensive care* (8th ed.). St. Louis: Mosby.

4. Alcohol is specifically causative for an umbrella of fetal alcohol spectrum disorders (FASDs) that include fetal alcohol syndrome (FAS), partial FAS, alcohol-related neurodevelopmental disorder (ARND), alcohol-related birth defects (ARBDs), and neurobehavioral disorder associated with prenatal alcohol exposure.
   a. FAS is the most severe FASD and criteria for diagnosis include specific dysmorphic facial features, growth deficiency, and CNS abnormalities (Fig. 6.21).

C. Clinical Judgment Measures
   1. Review maternal prenatal record and history noting documentation of any substance use.
   2. Conduct a thorough assessment of the newborn, including gestational age, maturity, and behavior.
      a. Nurses typically document an additional, ongoing neonatal abstinence scoring system assessment to monitor changes in withdrawal symptoms and guide nonpharmacologic and pharmacologic treatment regimens. Two of the most common systems in use are the Finnegan Neonatal Abstinence Scoring System and the Eat, Sleep, Console (ESC) approach.
   3. Monitor vital signs.
   4. Monitor fluids and electrolytes.
   5. Nonpharmacologic interventions include swaddling, gentle handling, decreasing environmental stimuli, providing nonnutritive suckling with a pacifier.
   6. Administer pharmacologic agents as ordered. Pharmacotherapy is usually based on severity of withdrawal symptoms.
   7. Provide education and support to parents.

D. Labs
   1. Drug screen of urine, meconium, or umbilical cord testing may be ordered

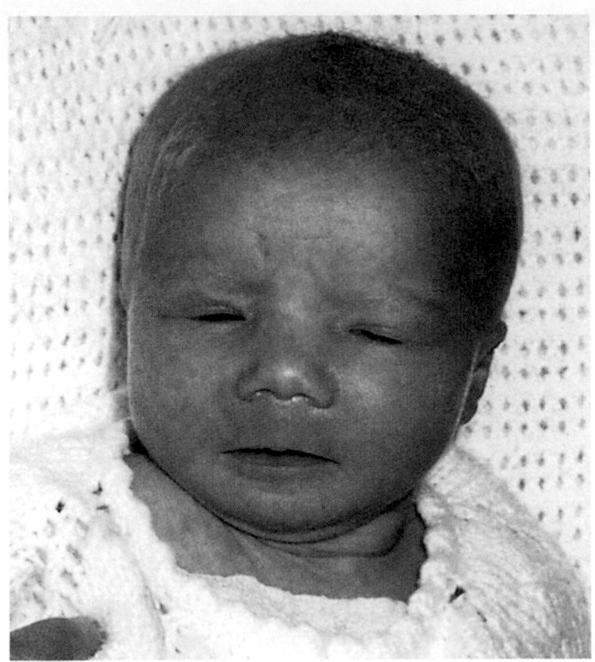

Fig. 6.21 Infant With Fetal Alcohol Syndrome. (From Lowdermilk, D. L., Perry, S. E., Cashion, K., Alden, K., & Olshansky, E. [2020]. *Maternity and women's health care* [12th ed., p. 777]. St. Louis: Elsevier.)

   2. Possible labs:
      a. CBC
      b. Chemistry panel

E. Discharge
   1. Teach parents about importance of ongoing follow-up care.
   2. Provide community resources for referrals for addiction services, social services as indicated and desired.

REVIEW OF SUBSTANCE ABUSE DISORDER

1. List the major CNS danger signals that occur in the neonate.
2. A baby is delivered blue, limp, has a heart rate less than 100, and is gasping. The nurse dries the infant, suctions the oropharynx, and gently stimulates the infant while blowing O_2 over the face. The infant still does not respond. What is the next nursing action?
3. What conditions make oxygenation of the newborn more difficult?
4. What are the cardinal symptoms of sepsis in a newborn?
5. A premature baby is born and develops hypothermia. State the major nursing interventions to treat hypothermia.
6. What factors does a nurse look for in determining a newborn's ability to take in nourishment by nipple and mouth?
7. List four nursing interventions to enhance family and parent adjustment to a high-risk newborn.
8. List the risk factors for hyperbilirubinemia.
9. List the symptoms of hyperbilirubinemia in the neonate.
10. List three nursing interventions for the neonate undergoing phototherapy.
11. List the symptoms of neonatal abstinence syndrome.
12. Neonates with complications may receive too much stimulation in the form of invasive procedures and handling and too little developmentally appropriate stimulation and affection. How might such an infant respond?
13. How should a nurse determine the length of a tube needed for the oral gavage feeding of a newborn?
14. What are the two best ways to test for correct placement of the gavage tube in the infant's stomach?
15. What characteristics would the nurse expect to see in a neonate with FAS?

See Answer Key at the end of this text for suggested responses.

For more review, go to http://evolve.elsevier.com/HESI/RN for HESI's online study examinations.

NEXT-GENERATION NCLEX (NGN) EXAMINATION-STYLE QUESTION: BOWTIE QUESTION

Prenatal Record

Ms. Betty is a 34yo Caucasian woman (G5T3P1A0L4). She entered into prenatal care at 32 weeks gestation. Obstetric history was significant for opioid use disorder currently being treated with methadone and intimate partner violence. Ms. Betty reported contractions at 36 4/7 weeks gestation and was directed to the ER for further evaluation.

Labor and Delivery Record

Ms. Betty presented to the ER in active labor and had a precipitous birth at 36 4/7 weeks gestation. She was admitted to the postpartum floor and the infant boy was admitted to the NICU for observation.

Orders

Begin assessment using Neonatal Abstinence Scoring System, Vital signs, monitor lab values, IV fluids, I & O

Instructions

Complete the diagram by selecting from the choices below to specify which potential condition the client is most likely experiencing, 2 actions to take, and 2 parameters the nurse would monitor to assess the client's progress.

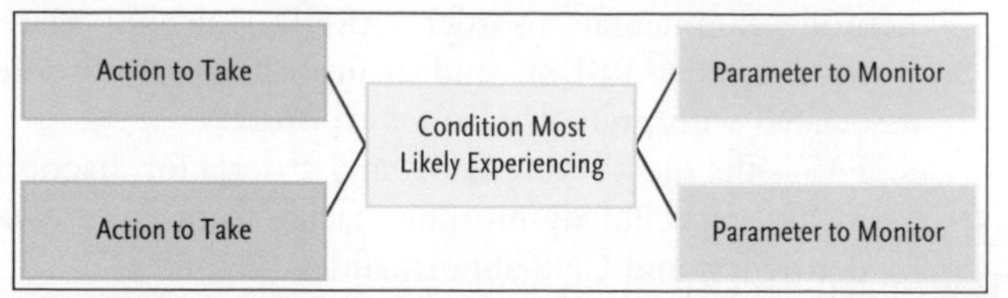

Actions to Take	Potential Conditions	Parameters to Monitor
Gestational Assessment	Seizures	Feeding
Use of bright lights to enhance physical assessment skills	Excessive sleep patterns	Temperature
Increase stimuli (talking, frequent handling) to enhance newborn adaptation to extra-uterine life	Lethargy	Eye Contact
Swaddle infant with legs flexed	Neonatal hyperglycemia	Output
Provide bottle to infant		Group therapy

Answers highlighted in Answer Key at the end of this text

BIBLIOGRAPHY

American College of Obstetricians and Gynecologists (ACOG). (2019). ACOG Practice Bulletin No. 202: Gestational Hypertension and Preeclampsia. *Obstetrics & Gynecology, 133*(1), e1–e25.

American College of Obstetricians and Gynecologists (ACOG). (2020). *Nutrition during pregnancy.* Retrieved from https://www.acog.org/womens-health/faqs/nutrition-during-pregnancy

King, T., Brucker, M., Osborne, K., & Jevitt, C. (2019). *Varney's midwifery* (6th ed.). Jones & Bartlett Learning.

Lowdermilk, D. L., Perry, S. E., Cashion, K., Alden, K., & Olshansky, E. (2020). *Maternity and women's health care* (12th ed.). St. Louis: Elsevier.

Murray SS, & McKinny ES. (2010). Foundations of Maternal Newborn and Women's Health Nursing (5th ed.). Philadelphia: Saunders.

Schuiling, K., & Likis, F. (2022). *Gynecologic health care* (4th ed.). Jones & Bartlett Learning.

7

Psychiatric Nursing

The United States is in the midst of a national mental health dilemma. More than 50% of all Americans experience some form of mental illness in their lifetime (The National Alliance on Mental Illness (NAMI), is the nation's largest grassroots mental health organization dedicated to building bette, 2021), and over 20% of adults experience a mental illness each year (NAMI, 2021). Of those, only about 50% receive treatment. Nonetheless, many opportunities exist for nurses to intervene to improve the outcomes of patients who seek mental health services. Psychiatric-mental health (PMH) nurses are ideally suited for the identification and management of mental illness (Rice, 2018).

Psychiatric nurses focus their attention primarily on individuals with chronic or major mental illnesses and have assumed case management roles with multidisciplinary teams. Developments in psychopharmacology have changed treatment for mental illness. Consequently, the use of psychotropic medications to treat mental illness and manage symptoms and behaviors through psychopharmacology has led to a decrease in overall hospitalization and institutionalization, earlier discharges and return of patients to community-dwelling status. This change has led to a major shift away from less-invasive forms of therapy, such as counseling, as the main psychiatric treatment to treatment with medications (Whitaker, 2011). Although many nurses are trained in the use of psychosocial interventions, the potential for nurses to deliver cognitive—behavioral therapy to those with common mental disorders has not been fully realized (Gournay, 2018), yet the need for cognitive-behavioral therapies has not declined. The phenomenon of briefer in-patient stays and fewer patient-nurse interactions has led to an ever-growing need for nurses to provide short patient-nurse encounters. Nurses conduct brief meetings providing short-term interventions that screen, identify, and prioritize individual care along the health care continuum from in-patient to community-based settings. Such interventions focus on safe and secure therapeutic environments of care, psychotropic psychoeducational administration and management, and promote self-care and self-management for individuals with mental health conditions.

Nurses perform necessary roles in caring for individuals in need of psychiatric care and supporting patients in the management of their mental health and well-being (Delaney, Shattell, & Johnson, 2017). A number of nursing roles include providing patients with *safe*, therapeutic, and recovery-oriented treatment by means of *structure, support, and self-management* which provides the framework for the clinical judgment measures for psychiatric nursing (Shattell & Delaney, 2015).

SAFETY

At the most basic level, inpatient treatment environments must be safe. A fundamental nursing responsibility is to ensure that staff and patients are free from harm (Delaney et al. 2015). Safety is connected to the reduction of aggression, violence, and avoiding of coercive interventions such as seclusion and restraints. Principles of safety also include the techniques that nurses and other health care workers employ to avoid such confrontations or events and to offer patients choices in difficult situations. With an increased emphasis on and initiating measures to engage, anticipate risk, and intervene early prior to an escalating situation, safety has taken a broader meaning beyond preventing physical aggression, violence, or harm to include maintaining both the physical *and* trauma-informed care approach of psychological safety (Bryson et al., 2017). This requires nurses to promote positive interactions in patient settings and maintain supportive environments that promote healing and recovery (Delaney et al. 2015).

Fundamentally, safety demands creating a physical environment that is free of any object that could be used for self-harm or that could easily harm others. Nurses and other staff members must consistently follow policies and protocols surrounding sharp objects (sharps) and other potentially dangerous items. Safety plans should include unit safety checks for contraband and for tracking incidents of safety breaches. Units must also have a system of precautions for monitoring aggression or suicide risks that determine the frequency of monitoring commensurate with the risk (Delaney et al. 2018).

Nurses must be aware of less obvious measures that ensure safety, such as adequate staffing and ensuring that nurses and staff are appropriately trained. Training needs to be consistent with in-patient psychiatric assessment, early intervention, restraint reduction techniques, and the use of noncoercive interventions and less-restrictive measures (Scanlan, 2009). Nurses should evaluate their interventions by using debriefing techniques and reviewing data that improves patient outcomes and improve their practice (Azeem, Aujla, Rammerth, Binsfeld, & Jones, 2011).

STRUCTURE

Structure encompasses a unit's rules and expectations. Many episodes of aggression occur following interactions where staff impose unit rules when dealing with a specific patient request (Bowers, 2014). In maintaining structure, staff constantly balance the need for consistency while avoiding infringements on the individual's sense of personal control (Voogt, Goossens, Nugter, & van Achterberg, 2014). To achieve this, balance demands that structure depends on nurses and other staff members' assessment skills, clinical judgment measures, and critical thinking.

These moment-to-moment decisions around rules and subsequent responses to an individual's behaviors also set the culture of the unit. A unit culture can easily slip into a rule-driven mindset and the staff's role becomes enforcing expectations. Alternately, a unit can adopt a flexible interpretation of rules/norms prioritizing how to use structure to meet individual needs. The latter approach helps to develop coping skills and begin to see caregivers as helpful to remain organized and in control.

SUPPORT

The culture of caring is an important psychiatric nursing role. Providing support also demands that nurses and staff interact with patients and engage with the individual (Polacek et al., 2015). Engagement that operates at the interpersonal level involves empathy, adjustment to the individual's experience, and understanding what is meaningful to them (Salamone-Violi, Chur-Hansen, & Winefield, 2015) while maintaining boundaries (Ward et al. 2014). Nurses attempt to engage with patients by interacting at the interpersonal level, directing attention to establishing a presence, and tailoring responses based on the patients' individual experiences (Delaney et al., 2017). Patients may lack insight into connecting events to behaviors and emotions and/or they may be unable to articulate emotions and distress in a manner of behavior that is inappropriate (Foster & Smedley, 2019). For example, patients on inpatient units struggle with maintaining control of their behaviors or managing emotions such as anger and frustration (Delaney, 2006). Nurses must recognize expressions of distress through behaviors and emotions and then interpret the underlying meaning of the behaviors (Geanellos, 2002).

SELF-MANAGEMENT

The final important aspect of engagement is related to activities that foster self-management among patients. This includes educating patients on health and/or management of symptoms associated with an illness (Delaney et al., 2000). Typically, nurses should employ a collaborative problem-solving approach (Bobier, Dowell, & Swadi, 2009; Pollastri, Epstein, Heath, & Ablon, 2013) when developing strategies to manage psychiatric patients.

Self-management strategies should be geared to the population of clients being treated on the unit. For instance, for children hospitalized secondary to suicidal ideations, interventions should be geared toward teaching coping behaviors but delivered in the context of a supportive, collaborative approach (Montreuil, Butler, Stachura, & Pugnaire Gros, 2015). For adolescents, specific strategies to address suicidal thoughts may include family interventions and individual skills training around emotional regulation and problem solving (Glenn, Franklin, & Nock, 2014).

THERAPEUTIC MODALITIES

Nurses should make themselves aware of the current treatment modalities that they or their patients may encounter in mental health and psychiatric treatment. These may include a range of options such as electroconvulsive therapy (ECT) or individual and group therapy. Most of these options strive to assist individuals with the promotion of mental health for individuals, social and family functioning.

Electroconvulsive therapy (ECT). ECT involves the use of electrically induced seizures for psychiatric purposes. It is used for the severely depressed clients who do not respond to antidepressant medications and therapy. Nurses play an essential role in ECT, because of their close involvement with patients before and after the procedure. Although ECT has been found to be one of the most robust and rapid treatments for severe depression, it is widely underused partly because of negative perceptions and inaccurate knowledge about the treatment (Tsai et al., 2021). Nurses must apprise themselves of the knowledge and attitude of the nursing staff working in ECT rooms can have a direct impact on the quality of their nursing practice.

1. Client care prior to ECT
   a. Prepare client by teaching about ECT
   b. Avoid using the word "shock"
   c. Administer medication before and after procedure
   d. Provide an emergency cart, suction equipment, and oxygen available in the room.
2. Client care post ECT
   a. Maintain patent airway; the client is unconscious immediately after ECT.
   b. Check vital signs frequently according to institutional policy
   c. Reorient client after ECT
   d. Common complaints that often occur after anesthesia is administered may include modest headache, mild muscle soreness, moderate nausea, retrograde pain.

HESI HINT Vomiting by an unconscious post-ECT client can lead to aspiration. Remember to maintain a patent airway in these clients.

REVIEW OF THERAPEUTIC COMMUNICATION AND TREATMENT MODALITIES

1. A nurse plans to teach a patient about a new diagnosis of bipolar disorder so that the patient can be more aware of fluctuating moods over time. This would be best be described as
   a. Self-management
   b. Safety
   c. Structure
   d. Therapy
2. On an inpatient psychiatric unit, clients are expected to get up at a certain time, attend breakfast at a certain time, and arrive for their medications at the correct time. What form of therapy is incorporated into this unit?
3. The wife of a man killed in a motor vehicle accident has just arrived at the emergency department and is told of her husband's death. What nursing actions are appropriate for dealing with this crisis?
4. A 66-year-old client is admitted to the psychiatric unit with agitated depression. The client has not responded to antidepressants in the past. What would be the medical treatment of choice for this client?
5. Describe the nursing interventions used to care for a client during and after ECT.

See Answer Key at the end of this text for suggested responses.

COMMON MENTAL HEALTH TREATMENTS AND INTERVENTIONS

Although nurses do not typically participate or conduct therapy, they should be aware that individuals they encounter or care for may be participating in therapy. Nurses who possess an understanding of the basic goals and structures of therapies can help patients by showing empathy for the challenges that patients face. Nurses can identify patient problems and concerns or can make recommendations to health providers for referral or treatment. Moreover, nurses are expected to provide brief clinical interventions when interacting with individuals in their care. Knowledge of the types of interventions available can help nurses to remain consistent with the patients' therapy and assist in the delivery of nurse-driven brief clinical interventions.

Group therapy: Group therapy is a form of treatment that is reserved for individuals with various issues, and may include addiction, anger management, depression, and anxiety. An important aspect of group therapy is that it brings people together and creates a dynamic of support and inclusion. Because each participant is present for a similar purpose, participants can feel comfortable about sharing problems and struggles with the group. In addition to togetherness and support, group therapy provides an excellent opportunity for its participants to learn and listen. Hearing about others' challenges can be insightful and help the participant to gain alternative perspectives. The benefits and flexibility that come along with group therapy are one of the many reasons why group therapy is commonly used. Groups may be closed (a predetermined group) or open (members may join and leave) and focus on psychoeducation, providing support, psychotherapy, or self-help. The advantages associated with groups include the development of socializing techniques, proving opportunities for feedback, and promotion of a feeling of universality (not being alone in experiencing a problem).

Interpersonal therapy: Interpersonal therapy is a brief, attachment-focused form of therapy that aims to help patients address challenges in managing relationships and ultimately improve the symptoms of mood disorders, such as depression (Van Hees, Rotter, Ellermann, & Evers, 2013). This type of therapy is commonly used because healthy relationships with other people are extremely conducive to an individual's success and opportunities in life. Someone who struggles to get along with other people will experience difficulties in the workplace and other critical aspects of life.

Interpersonal therapy largely focuses on relationship stressors and the root cause of the issues which impact the patient's ability to maintain healthy relationships with those around them. The underlying cause can vary depending on a series of factors; however, once the root cause of the problem is identified and addressed, the patient can begin to heal and learn appropriate methods for developing healthy, positive relationships.

Family therapy: While family therapy is common, it does share a separate distinction from other types of individual psychological treatment. Family therapy can help members of a family to define or explain problems in relational networks (Colapinto, 2019) or terms of family structures, boundaries, hierarchies, roles, rules, and patterns of interaction and coalitions (Tadros & Finney, 2018). One important goal of family therapy is to strengthen family interactions and to improve behavioral outcomes (Collyer & Eisler, 2020).

BRIEF INTERVENTIONS

Brief interventions are typically face-to-face sessions, with or without the addition of written materials such as self-help manuals, workbooks, or self-monitoring diaries with the purpose of addressing specific problems (Heather, 1995, p. 287). The primary goal of brief interventions is to raise awareness of problems such as (alcohol and substance use) and then to recommend a specific change or activity or motivate the client to change (Miller and Munoz, 1982; Miller and Rollnick, 1991). The brevity and lower delivery costs of these brief approaches make them ideal mechanisms for use in settings where cost and time constraints are a consideration. The person delivering the brief intervention is usually trained to be empathic, warm, encouraging, and non-confrontational. Brief interventions ranged from relatively unstructured counseling and feedback to more formal, structured therapy (Miller and Hester, 1986;

Miller and Taylor, 1980). Brief interventions may be delivered by treatment staff or other professionals, and do not require extensive training, making it suitable for nurses at various levels of experience and education. A nurse may identify a problem and ask how much the problems interfere with daily functioning and then make suggestions for further treatment, self-help, or to continue to focus on the problem as opportunities arise on the unit.

HESI HINT A nurse may use any private interaction with a patient as an opportunity for a properly executed brief intervention.

A nurse may identify clients who may benefit from particular types of therapies. The nurse can arrange for therapy and schedule an appropriately trained therapist and encourage and provide support for attendance.

PSYCHIATRIC REVIEW QUESTIONS

Nurses have assessed clients on a unit and have viewed each as an individual that would benefit from tailored interventions that address personal, emotional, mental health, and family needs. This contrasts with a "fits-all" approach.

1. A client arrives at a busy emergency department smelling of alcohol after an altercation with his significant other. The client states this has happened before while drinking. The nurse asks, "How often is alcohol a factor in arguments?" What is this an example of?
2. Describe the nurse's role in preparing a client for ECT.
3. A client has been provided with an individualized plan in the morning describing scheduled therapies and activities for the entire day. What is the proposed purpose of such an intervention?
4. A 55-year-old client arrives at an inpatient unit angry and verbally abusive to staff. How should a nurse approach and manage this situation?
5. A 24-year-old was admitted after a suicide attempt. The client expresses lots of problems getting along with friends. What types of therapies might be appropriate for this client and why?
6. A 61-year-old client with schizophrenia states "I never could trust anyone in my life, including you." Describe how a nurse may explore distortions in thinking.

PSYCHIATRIC ASSESSMENT STRATEGIES FOR INPATIENTS: RESOURCES WITH A PURPOSE

Adults with psychiatric conditions who are admitted as inpatients need to be assessed carefully to ensure they receive the best possible care. Although staff nurses do not diagnose, a nurse's observations and assessment can help providers in the formulation of diagnoses and treatment plans. Nurses should observe and record pertinent information based on the patient's statement, behaviors, family history, chief complaint, and other information such as circumstances surrounding admission. Clinical assessment is enhanced by having a breadth of knowledge about psychiatric diagnoses and their presentation and psychopathology.

Schizophrenia and Schizoaffective Disorder

Clinicians consider five domains when assessing patients for schizophrenia or schizoaffective disorder—delusions, hallucinations, disorganized thinking and speech, grossly disorganized or abnormal motor behavior (including catatonia), and negative symptoms.

HESI HINT Catonia occurs across several categories of disorders and can be present in depressive, bipolar, and psychotic disorders.

Delusions are fixed beliefs not amenable to change even in light of conflicting evidence (excluding religious beliefs commonly held in the community).

Examples include:

- delusions of persecution ("someone is out to get me")
- nihilistic delusions ("something bad is going to happen")
- somatic delusions ("something is terribly wrong with me")
- control delusions ("someone is making me do something")
- thought-withdrawal delusions ("aliens are stealing my thoughts")
- thought-insertion delusions ("aliens are putting thoughts into my head")
- thought-broadcasting delusions ("everyone can hear my thoughts")
- referential delusions ("people are talking about me")
- delusions of grandeur (for instance, a patient thinks she's royalty and should be treated as such)
- erotomania (a false belief that others are in love with the patient).

Hallucinations are perception-like experiences that occur without an external stimulus. In schizophrenics, auditory hallucinations (AHs) are more common than visual or other hallucinations. Visual hallucinations (VHs) may be illusions (misinterpretation of visual stimuli; for instance, a shadow becomes a menacing black dog). VHs can occur with other medical conditions, such as alcohol withdrawal, or may manifest as an aura with a seizure or brain injury. AHs and VHs rarely occur at the same time.

Disorganized thinking and speech may include:

- circumstantiality (verbalization of concrete details that's slow in getting to the point)
- concrete thinking (making literal rather than figurative interpretations; for instance, the patient answers "I took the bus" when asked how he or she ended up in the hospital)

- clang associations (rhyming words and not completing sentences)
- loose associations (sentences or phrases not logically connected to those coming before or after)
- tangentiality (going from topic to topic without making a point)
- neologisms (making up words that have meaning only to the patient)
- "word salad" (a stream of unconnected words).

Grossly disorganized and abnormal motor behavior may manifest as:

- unpredictable behavior that interferes with task completion or causes agitation
- failure to follow instructions to move
- holding a fixed bizarre position
    - lack of verbal or physical response
- purposeless or repetitive movements
- staring at staff
- catatonic stupor not caused by a physical problem
- negative symptoms refer to lack of something, including:
- lack of emotional expressions
- avolition (lack of motivation for goal-oriented tasks)
- alogia (decreased speech)
- anhedonia (lack of pleasure from activities previously enjoyed)
- asociality (lack of interest in others).

A schizophrenic patient with negative symptoms seems to lack personality.

Clinical signs and symptoms of schizoaffective disorder include:

- a major mood episode of either major depression or mania for at least 1 month
- at least 2 weeks of delusions or hallucinations that don't occur at the same time as a major mood episode

> **HESI HINT** When evaluating client behaviors, consider when the client is receiving or not receiving medications and whether any changes preceded or followed medication therapy.

Clinical Assessment tips

If your patient seems to be hearing voices, observe him or her to determine the following:

- Is the patient talking to a wall or an empty space?
- Is he or she mumbling or yelling? If so, can you make out words or themes?
- Is the patient's eyes darting, staring, or frightened?
- Does the patient seem to be lost in thought?
- Is the patient thought blocking (stopping talking abruptly)?
- What is the patient's affect (nonverbal expression of feelings, including posture, facial expression, and tone of voice)?

Try to determine if the patient seems internally preoccupied or is behaving in a way that's consistent with AHs. Once you've formed general impressions, ask the patient questions such as the following:

TABLE 7.1 Clinical Judgment Measures: Spectrum of Schizophrenia

Clinical Judgment Measure	Assessment Characteristics
Recognize Cues	Delusions Hallucinations Disorganized speech Disorganized behavior
Analyze Cues	Assess disturbance in perceptions Assess affect Assess interpersonal relationships
Prioritize Cues	Establish trust Provide assistance with physical hygiene and activities of daily living (ADL) Use clear, simple concrete terms when talking to the client Set limits on behavior Avoid stressful situations
Solutions	Encourage client to identify positive characteristics related to self Praise socially acceptable behavior
Actions	Provide safe environment Establish Trust
Evaluate Outcomes	Determine ability to return to ADL Communication is linear, organized, rational, and logical.

- Are the voices frightening?
- What are they saying?
- Are they telling you to do something?
- Are they loud?
- Do you believe the voices?
- How often do you hear them?

Keep in mind that paranoid patients may not admit to hearing voices until they have developed trust in you or until antipsychotic medications start to take effect. Try to identify a theme to what the voices are saying, for example, are they worried something bad will happen? Unfortunately, voices rarely go away completely even when the patient is well managed on medications (Table 7.1).

Bipolar I Disorder

Bipolar I disorder involves manic episodes that last at least 1 week or manic symptoms severe enough to require immediate hospital care. Mixed episodes (mania and depression at the same time) may occur as well. Some patients also experience episodes of hypomania (similar to mania but less intense). The episodes do not stem from a medical condition or substance use.

Clinical signs and symptoms of bipolar I disorder include:

- Persistently elevated mood, including high energy output, expansiveness, persistence, task and goal orientation, or marked irritability
- Significant behavior changes, such as grandiose behavior, constantly moving without purpose, taking part in high-risk activities, such as sex with strangers, or incessant rapid speech.

In many cases, patients with bipolar disorder require hospitalization to protect themselves from their own behavior.

Clinical Assessment tips

When assessing the patient, ask yourself these questions:

- What is the patient's mood? (Document this in the patient's own words.)
- What is the patient's affect? (How does the patient appear to be feeling?)
- What is the quality and content of the patient's behavior and speech?

Documentation tips: Describe specific risks of the patient's manic behavior, including sexual risks, antagonizing others, making intrusive phone calls, making life-defining decisions, or losing weight because the patient can't sit long enough to eat a meal. Keep in mind that a patient with bipolar I disorder may be in the depressed phase of the condition, so be sure to assess for depression, suicide risk, and marked shifts in mood or affect. When documenting the quality and content of the patient's behavior and speech, be as specific as possible.

Major Depressive Disorder

Major depressive disorder causes severe symptoms that affect how the patient thinks and feels. It also may affect such activities as sleeping, eating, and working. The patient must have signs or symptoms for at least 2 weeks. In 2014, an estimated 15.7 million adults aged 18 or older in the United States had at least one major depressive episode in the past year, making it one of the most common mental health disorders.

Essential information to communicate during care transitions includes:

- Pain management history
- Pain assessment tools and scales used
- Complementary and pharmacologic interventions tried and shown to be either effective or ineffective
- Patient goals for pain outcomes

Clinical decision-making tools, such as alerts in the electronic health record regarding inappropriate or high-alert medications, flag alerts for frail elders, and embedded standard communication and pain assessment tools, may promote effective communication and documentation.

Clinical Signs and Symptoms

Patients with a major depressive disorder have a depressed mood or loss of pleasure or interest in activities that usually provide pleasure. Other signs and symptoms include:

- unintentional weight loss or gain (5% or more in 1 month)
- insomnia or hypersomnia
- psychomotor agitation
- fatigue
- feelings of worthlessness or excessive guilt
- decreased ability to concentrate
- suicidal thoughts or a suicide attempt

Be aware that depression differs from dementia and delirium. Dementia is a gradual neurocognitive decline involving decreased logic and memory; for instance, patients try to answer questions but give the wrong answer. Delirium is marked by the sudden onset of rapid fluctuations in behavior and level of consciousness; it stems from medication, substance use, or a medical condition. Delirium usually is a medical emergency.

Clinical **assessment tips:** When assessing patients with a suspected major depressive disorder, start by evaluating their risk for suicidal ideation or behavior. See Table 7.2.

Ask the patient how he or she is feeling and document the answer in the patient's own words; for instance, "Patient states that mood is sad or depressed." Also ask the patient to rate his or her mood on a scale of 1 to 10, with 10 indicating the most severe feelings of depression. Note the patient's affect (how he or she appears to be feeling) and determine if it matches the stated mood. Next, assess the amount and pattern of the patient's sleep, fluid and food intake, recent weight changes, activity and behavior level, and self-care (noting how much prompting or assistance the patient

TABLE 7.2 Columbia-Suicide Severity Rating Scale

		Past 1 Month
1. Have you wished you were dead or wished you could go to sleep and not wake up?		
2. Have you actually had any thoughts about killing yourself?		
If **YES** to 2, answer questions 3, 4, 5, and 6 If **NO** to 2, go directly to question 6		
3. Have you thought about how you might do this?		
4. Have you had any intention of acting on these thoughts of killing yourself, as opposed to you having the thoughts but you definitely would not act on them?		**High Risk**
5. Have you started to work out or worked out the details of how to kill yourself? Did you intend to carry out this plan?		**High Risk**
Always Ask Question 6	**Life-time**	**Past 3 Months**
6. Have you done anything, started to do anything, or prepared to do anything to end your life? *Examples*: Collected pills, obtained a gun, gave away valuables, wrote a will or suicide note, held a gun but changed your mind, cut yourself, tried to hang yourself, etc.		**High Risk**

From Posner, K., Brown, G. K., Stanley, B., Brent, D. A., Yershova, K. V., Oquendo, M. A., et al. (2011). The Columbia-suicide severity rating scale: Initial validity and internal consistency findings from three multisite studies with adolescents and adults. *American Journal of Psychiatry, 168*(12), 1266–1277.

needs). Keep in mind that depressed patients typically give brief answers or may say they don't care or don't know the answer. Also, patients with depression who have an unknown history of manic or hypomanic episodes may be tipped into a manic phase when they begin antidepressants without also taking mood-stabilizing medication.

Evaluation of Suicide Intent

1. Directly ask the patient their intent to harm themselves.
2. Offer the patient hope such as "we have medication that can help you through your bad times."
3. Identify the method chosen: the more lethal the method the higher the probability that an attempt may occur. Ask: "What is your plan to harm yourself?" For example, they may mention a shotgun.
4. Determine the availability of the method chosen. For example, is a gun readily available?

Clinical Judgment Measures

A. Maintain client's physical health. Provide nutrition, rest, and hygiene.
B. Provide a safe environment.
C. Decrease environmental stimulation.
D. Implement suicide precautions.
E. Use a consistent approach to minimize manipulative behavior.
F. Use frequent, brief contacts to decrease anxiety.
G. Implement constructive limit setting.
H. Avoid giving attention to bizarre behavior.
I. Try to meet needs as soon as possible to keep client from becoming aggressive.
J. Provide small frequent feedings of food.
K. Engage in simple, active, noncompetitive activities.
L. Avoid distracting or stimulating activities in the evening to help promote sleep and rest.
M. Praise self-control, acceptable behavior.
N. Promote family involvement in therapy, teaching, and medication compliance
O. Administer lithium, sedatives, and antipsychotics as prescribed (Table 7.3).
P. Redirect negative behavior or verbal abuse in a calm, firm, nonjudgmental, nondefensive manner.
   1. Suggest a walk or another physical activity.
   2. Set limits on intrusive behavior.
   3. If a client becomes totally out of control, administer medication or use seclusion if the client is a danger to self or others.

HESI HINT Clients who are experiencing mania can be very caustic toward authority figures. Be prepared for personal putdowns. Avoid arguing or becoming defensive.

TABLE 7.3 Mood-Stabilizing Drugs

Drugs	Indications	Adverse Reactions	Nursing Implications
• Lithium carbonate	• Bipolar disorders, especially the manic phase	• Nausea, fatigue, thirst, polyuria, and fine hand tremors • Weight gain • Hypothyroidism • Early signs of toxicity: diarrhea, vomiting, drowsiness, muscle weakness, lack of coordination • Possible renal impairment	• Lithium is excreted by the kidney. Maintain adequate serum levels. • Assess electrolytes, especially sodium. • Baseline studies of renal, cardiac, and thyroid status must be obtained before lithium therapy is begun. • Teach client early symptoms of lithium toxicity. If the drug is continued, coma, convulsions, and death may occur. • Instruct client to keep salt usage consistent. • Use with diuretics is contraindicated. Diuretic-induced sodium depletion can increase lithium levels, causing toxicity.
Anticonvulsant Mood Stabilizers			
• Valproic acid	• Used in bipolar disorder alone or with lithium	• GI distress: nausea, anorexia, vomiting • Hepatotoxicity • Neurologic symptoms: tremor, sedation, headache, dizziness	• Administer with food. • Monitor blood levels. • Maintain serum levels 50–125 μg/mL.
• Carbamazepine	• Used in bipolar disorders • Used as an alternative to lithium	• Dizziness • Ataxia • Blood dyscrasias	• Maintain serum levels at 8–12 g/mL. • Stop drug if WBC drops below 3000/mm^3 or neutrophil count goes below 1500/mm^3. • Monitor hepatic and renal function.
• Lamotrigine	• Used in bipolar disorder alone or with other mood stabilizers	• Headache • Dizziness • Double vision • Rash (Stevens-Johnson syndrome)	• To minimize the risk of severe rash, give low dose, 25–50 mg/day initially, then gradually increase to a maintenance dose of 200 mg/day (used alone) or 100 mg/day (with valproate) or 400 mg/day (with carbamazepine).

REVIEW OF MOOD DISORDERS

1. Identify the physiologic changes that commonly occur with depression.
2. A client who has been withdrawn and tearful comes to breakfast one morning smiling and interacting with peers. Before breakfast, the client gave a roommate a favorite possession. What actions should the nurse take and why?
3. Name the components of a suicide assessment.
4. A client on your unit refuses to go to group therapy. What is the most appropriate nursing intervention?
5. A client is standing on a table loudly singing "The Star-Spangled Banner" and is encircled by sheets, which have been set afire. In order of priority, describe appropriate nursing actions.

See Answer Key at the end of this text for suggested responses.

ALCOHOL WITHDRAWAL SYNDROME

Alcohol withdrawal syndrome occurs when a person reduces or stops consuming alcohol, especially after a period of heavy or prolonged drinking. Severe withdrawal symptoms require medical attention and possibly hospitalization for detoxification.

Clinical Signs and Symptoms

- Autonomic hyperactivity (diaphoresis, increased pulse)
- Tremor (usually of the hands)
- Insomnia
- Nausea and vomiting
- Hallucinations or illusions typically start as sensitivity (for instance, the patient complains that lights are too bright, or sounds are too loud) and then develop into hallucinations (usually tactile or visual). Other signs and symptoms include anxiety, general tonic-clonic seizures, inability to sit still, and constant purposeless movement or fidgeting. (For more information on alcohol, opioid, and stimulant withdrawal, see Substance withdrawal assessment.)

Clinical Judgment Measures

- Maintain safety, nutrition, hygiene, and rest
- Obtain a blood alcohol level on admission or when the client appears intoxicated
- Monitor vital signs
- Intake (I)&output (O)
- Observe for delirium tremors (DTs)
- Prevent aspiration: implement seizure precautions
- Reduce environment stimuli
- Medicate with antianxiety medication, see Table 7.4
- Provide a high-protein diet and adequate fluid intake
- Provide vitamin supplements (B1 and B complex)
- Provide emotional support
- Provide care during withdrawal:
  - Use a direct, nonjudgmental attitude
  - Confront denial and rationalization (main coping styles used by alcoholics)
  - Confront any manipulation
  - Set short-term realistic goals
  - Help increase self-esteem
  - Explore ways to increase frustration tolerance without alcohol
  - Identify ways to decrease loneliness
  - Identify support groups (AA)
  - Identify friendships not related to drinking
  - Provide group and family therapy (family AA groups)
  - Provide patient and family teaching regarding the side effects of disulfiram (Anabuse)

TABLE 7.4 Alcohol Deterrents

Drugs	Indications	Adverse Reactions	Nursing Implications
• Disulfiram	• Treatment of alcoholism; aversion therapy • Interferes with the breakdown of alcohol, causing an accumulation of acetaldehyde (a byproduct of alcohol in the body)	• Severe side effects occur if alcohol is consumed: • Nausea and vomiting • Hypotension, headaches • Rapid pulse and respirations • Flushed face and bloodshot eyes • Confusion • Chest pain • Weakness, dizziness	• Teach the client what to expect if alcohol is consumed while taking the drug. • Be aware that some alcoholic clients use the side effects as a means of "punishing" themselves or as a form of masochism, and if a client repeatedly consumes alcohol while taking the drug, the health care provider should be notified. • Persons with serious heart disease, diabetes, epilepsy, liver impairment, or mental illness should not take Antabuse. • Use in motivated clients who have shown the ability to stay sober.
• Acamprosate	• Treatment of alcohol dependence by reducing anxiety and unpleasant effects that trigger resuming drinking • Balances Gamma-aminobutyric acid (GABA) (GABA, 2021) and glutamate neurotransmitters	• Headache • Nausea and diarrhea	• Helps reduce cravings • Does not reduce or eliminate withdrawal symptoms

• Encourage an outpatient day center or AA when the patient is discharged.

OPIOID WITHDRAWAL

Opioids include heroin, methadone, oxycodone, hydrocodone, and certain other substances. Heavy opioid use over several weeks, changes brain chemistry. Opioid withdrawal occurs when the person stops using opioids.

Clinical Signs and symptoms: Patients with opioid withdrawal may have insomnia or a sad or depressed mood. Physiologic signs and symptoms may include:

- nausea and vomiting
- muscle ache
- lacrimation (tearing eyes)
- rhinorrhea (running nose)
- pupil dilation
- piloerection
- diaphoresis
- diarrhea
- yawning
- fever

Clinical Judgment measures include the following:

A. Assess the level of consciousness and vital signs. (Rapid withdrawal can be fatal for persons addicted to barbiturates and antianxiety medications and hypnotics.)
B. Monitor I&O and electrolytes.
C. Implement suicide precautions if assessment indicates risk.
D. Provide adequate nutrition, hydration, and rest.
E. Administer medications according to detoxification protocol of medical unit.
F. Phenothiazines, benzodiazepines, beta-blockers, clonidine, and anticonvulsants may be used to decrease the discomfort of withdrawal.
G. Confront denial
   1. Focus on the substance abuse problem
   2. Confront the placing of blame on external problems.
H. Reinforce reality in simple, concrete terms.
I. Encourage verbal expressions of anger and depression.

Stimulant withdrawal: Stimulants include amphetamine, methylphenidate (Ritalin), amphetamine with dextroamphetamine (Adderall), cocaine, and certain other substances. They cause changes in brain chemistry after short periods of use and have a short half-life. Withdrawal occurs after the person stops using stimulants.

Clinical Signs and symptoms: Patients with stimulant withdrawal may have a dysphoric mood along with:

- vivid and scary dreams
- insomnia or hypersomnia
- increased appetite
- psychomotor retardation
- inability to sit still
- constant purposeless movement or fidgeting

Key points to remember: When assessing patients for mental illness or substance withdrawal, always assess the risk for suicidal and aggressive behavior, regardless of the patient's specific diagnosis. Also, be aware that a patient may not admit to experiencing certain symptoms until he or she trusts you. Finally, be sure to fully document your observations in the health record so psychiatric physicians and nurse practitioners can more easily diagnose the patient's specific problem using the *Diagnostic and Statistical Manual of Mental Disorders*, 5th Edition (DSM-5).

REVIEW OF SUBSTANCE ABUSE DISORDER

1. Three days ago, a client was admitted to the medical unit for a gastrointestinal (GI) bleed. The client's blood pressure (BP) and pulse rate gradually increased, and the client developed a low-grade fever. What assessment data should the nurse obtain? What kind of anticipatory planning should the nurse develop?
2. What physical signs might indicate that a client is abusing intravenous medications?
3. What behaviors would indicate to the nurse manager that an employee has a possible substance abuse problem?
4. A client becomes extremely agitated, abusive, and very suspicious. He is currently being detoxification from alcohol with chlordiazepoxide (Librium) 15 mg every 6 hours. What nursing actions are indicated?
5. A client in the third week of a cocaine rehabilitation program returns from an unsupervised pass. The nurse notices that the client is euphoric and is socializing with the other clients more than in the past. What nursing actions are indicated?

See Answer Key at the end of this text for suggested responses.

NEXT-GENERATION NCLEX EXAMINATION-STYLE QUESTION: BOWTIE QUESTION

Medical Record

Carrie Smith, a 29-year old woman, is admitted to the emergency room with feelings of being on a high. She has had grandiose feelings for 2 weeks and today she was brought in by her son because she was talking constantly and had a bizarre and severe dress that did not match her other clothes. She was screaming in pain stating that her doctor told her to come to the E.R. Additionally, Ms. CS was extremely talkative and kept fighting with her hair.

Orders

Admit to Psy. Ward. Monitor I&O, daily weights, suicide precautions, administer lithium, sedatives and antipsychotics, obtain routine blood work, and provide a safe environment.

Instructions

Complete the diagram by selecting from the choices below to specify which potential condition the client is most likely experiencing, 2 actions to take, and 2 parameters the nurse would monitor to assess the client's progress.

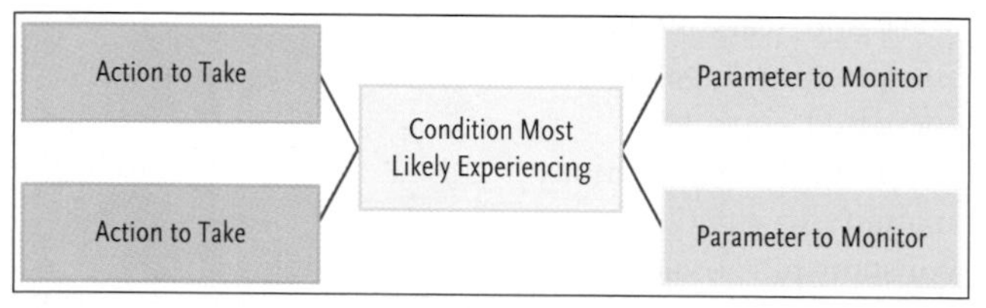

Actions to Take	Potential Conditions	Parameters to Monitor
Praise self-control, acceptable behavior.	Attention-Deficit Disorder	Increase conversations with the client to establish more attention.
Restrain the individual for own safety.	Bipolar disorder or manic-depressive illness	Provide small, frequent, feedings, record I&O.
Provide frequent stimulation such as playing physical games.	Delirium	Monitor physical activity/ over-stimulation.
Monitor I&O	Over-use of amphetamines	Use a variety of approaches to maximize manipulative behavior.
Give prescribed medication		Monitor vital signs for changes related to stress

Answers highlighted in Answer Key at the end of this text

BIBLIOGRAPHY

American Psychiatric Association. (2013). *Diagnostic and statistical manual of mental disorders: DSM-5* (5th ed.). Washington, DC: American Psychiatric Publishing.

Azeem, M. W., Aujla, A., Rammerth, M., Binsfeld, G., & Jones, R. B. (2011). Effectiveness of six core strategies based on trauma informed care in reducing seclusions and restraints at a child and adolescent psychiatric hospital. *Journal of Child and Adolescent Psychiatric Nursing, 24*(1), 11–15.

Biering, P., & Jensen, V. H. (2011). The concept of patient satisfaction in adolescent psychiatric care: A qualitative study. *Journal of Child and Adolescent Psychiatric Nursing, 24*(1), 3–10.

Bobier, C., Dowell, J., & Swadi, H. (2009). An examination of frequent nursing interventions and outcomes in an adolescent psychiatric inpatient unit. *International Journal of Mental Health Nursing, 18*(5), 301–309.

Bowers, L. (2014). Safewards: A new model of conflict and containment on psychiatric wards. *Journal of Psychiatric and Mental Health Nursing, 21*(6), 499–508.

Colapinto, J. (2019). Structural family therapy. In B. H. Fiese, M. Celano, K. Deater-Deckard, E. N. Jouriles, & M. A. Whisman (Eds.), *APA handbook of contemporary family psychology: Family therapy and training* (pp. 107–121). American Psychological Association. https://doi.org/10.1037/0000101-007.

Collyer, H., et al. (2019). Systematic literature review and meta-analysis of the relationship between adherence, competence and outcome in psychotherapy for children and adolescents. https://doi.org/10.1007/s00787-018-1265-2.

Coombs, T., Curtis, J., & Crookes, P. (2013). What is the process of a comprehensive mental health nursing assessment? Results from a qualitative study. *International Nursing Review, 60*(1), 96–102.

Delaney, K., Johnson, M., et al. (2015). Development and testing of the combined assessment of psychiatric environments: A patient-centered quality measure for inpatient psychiatric treatment. *Journal of the American Psychiatric Nurses Association, 21*(2), 134–147. https://doi.org/10.1177/1078390315581338.

Delaney, K.R., & Naegle, M.A., et al. (2018). *The Journal of Behavioral Health Services & Research 45*, 300–309.

Delaney, K. R., et al. (2000). Psychiatric hospitalization and process description: What will nursing add? *Journal of Psychosocial Nursing and Mental Health Services, 38*(3), 7–13. https://doi.org/10.3928/0279-3695-20000301-08. PMID: 10779939.

Delaney, K. R. (2006). Learning to observe in context: Child and adolescent inpatient mental health assessment. *Journal of Child and Adolescent Psychiatric Nursing, 19*(4), 170–174. https://doi.org/10.1111/j.1744-6171.2006.00068.x. PMID: 17118051 Review.

Delaney, K. R., Shattell, M., & Johnson, M. E. (2017). Capturing the interpersonal process of psychiatric nurses: A model for engagement. *Archives of Psychiatric Nursing, 31*(6), 634–640.

Drummond, D. C. (1997). Alcohol interventions: Do the best things come in small packages? *Addiction, 92*(4), 375–379.

Ercole-Fricke, E., Fritz, P., Hill, L. E., & Snelders, J. (2016). Effects of a collaborative problem-solving approach on an inpatient adolescent psychiatric unit. *Journal of Child and Adolescent Psychiatric Nursing, 29*(3), 127–134.

Foster, C., & Smedley, K. (2019). Understanding the nature of mental health nursing within CAMHS PICU: 2. Staff experience and support needs. *Journal of Psychiatric Intensive Care, 15*(2), 103–115.

GABA (2021) retrieved from https://my.clevelandclinic.org/health/articles/22857-gamma-aminobutyric-acid-gaba.

Geanellos, R. (2002). Exploring the therapeutic potential of friendliness and friendship in nurse—client relationships. *Contemporary Nurse, 12*(3), 235–245.

Gerace, A., Oster, C., O'Kane, D., Hayman, C. L., & Muir-Cochrane, E. (2018). Empathic processes during nurse-consumer conflict situations in psychiatric inpatient units: A qualitative study. *International Journal of Mental Health Nursing, 27*(1), 92–105.

Gill, F., Butler, S., & Pistrang, N. (2016). The experience of adolescent inpatient care and the anticipated transition to the community: Young people's perspectives. *Journal of Adolescence, 46*, 57–65.

Gournay, K., Winstanley, K., Mancey-Johnson, A., & Tracey, N. (2018). *British Journal of Mental Health Nursing*, 161–166. https://doi.org/10.12968/bjmh.2019.0034.

Glenn, C. R., Franklin, J. C., & Nock, M. K. (2014). Evidence-based psychosocial treatments for self-injurious thoughts and behaviors in youth. *Journal of Clinical Child and Adolescent Psychology, 44*(1), 1–29.

Heather. (1995). *Brief Interventions and Brief Therapies For Substance Abuse Treatment Improvement Protocol (TIP) Series 34*. U.S. Department of Health and Human Services Substance Abuse and Mental Health Services Administration (1995). Retrieved: https://store.samhsa.gov/sites/default/files/d7/priv/sma12-3952.pdf.

Hodgson, R. (1983b). How to control your drinking. W. Miller and R. Munoz, London: Sheldon press, 1982, £3.95. *Behavioural and Cognitive Psychotherapy, 11*(3), 279–280.

Huckshorn, K. A. (2004). Reducing seclusion & restraint use in mental health settings: Core strategies for prevention. *Journal of Psychosocial Nursing and Mental Health Services, 42*(9), 22–33.

Hutchinson, K. (2015). In *Psychiatric-mental health nursing: Nursing review and resource manual* (5th ed.). American Nurses Credentialing Center.

Jacobsen, F. (2012). Type II workplace violence in an urban acute hospital: How do we know if we are creating a safer environment for patients and staff? *Journal of Safety Management and Disrupt Assault Behaviour, 20*(2), 4–8.

Jacobsen, F., Adler, J., & Ortega, J. S. (2012). *CIWA-Ar training*. San Francisco, CA: CPMC Sutter Psychiatry.

MacPherson, H. A., Cheavens, J. S., & Fristad, M. A. (2012). Dialectical behavior therapy for adolescents: Theory, treatment adaptations, and empirical outcomes. *Clinical Child and Family Psychology Review, 16*(1), 59–80.

Makki, M., Hill, J. F., Bounds, D. T., McCammon, S., Mc Fall johnsen, M., & Delaney, K. R. (2018). Implementation of an ACT curriculum on an adolescent inpatient psychiatric unit: A quality improvement project. *Journal of Child and Family Studies, 27*(9), 2918–2924.

Miller, W. R., & Hester, R. K. (1986). The effectiveness of alcoholism treatment. *Treating Addictive Behaviors*, 121–174.

Miller, W. R., & Muñoz, R. F. (1982). *How to control your drinking*. Albuquerque, NM: University of New Mexico Press.

Miller, W. R., & Rollnick, S. (1991). Motivational interviewing: Preparing people to change addictive behavior. *Psychology of Addictive Behaviors, 4*, 82–90.

Miller, W. R., & Taylor, C. A. (1980). Relative effectiveness of bibliotherapy, individual and group self-control training in the treatment of problem drinkers. *Addictive Behaviors, 5*(1), 13–24.

Montreuil, M., Butler, K. J. D., Stachura, M., & Pugnaire Gros, C. (2015). Exploring helpful nursing care in pediatric mental health settings: The perceptions of children with suicide risk factors and their parents. *Issues in Mental Health Nursing, 36*(11), 849–859.

National Institute of Mental Health. Major depression among adults.

National Institute for Health and care excellence, 2015; richter 2006; Roberton *et al.* 2012

Pederson, D. D. (2013). *PsychNotes: Clinical pocket guide* (4th ed., p. 2013). Philadelphia: F.A. Davis Company.

Polacek, M. J., Allen, D. E., Damin-Moss, R. S., Schwartz, A. J. A., Sharp, D., Shattell, M., et al. (2015). Engagement as an element of safe inpatient psychiatric environments. *Journal of the American Psychiatric Nurses Association, 21*(3), 181–190.

Pollastri, A. R., Epstein, L. D., Heath, G. H., & Ablon, J. S. (2013). The collaborative problem solving approach: Outcomes across settings. *Harvard Review of Psychiatry, 21*(4), 188–199.

Posner, K., Brown, G. K., Stanley, B., Brent, D. A., Yershova, K. V., Oquendo, M. A., et al. (2011). The Columbia-Suicide Severity Rating Scale: Initial validity and internal consistency findings from three multisite studies with adolescents and adults. *American Journal of Psychiatry, 168*(12), 1266–1277.

Rice, S. M., Purcell, R., & McGorry, P. D. (2018). Adolescent and young adult male mental health: Transforming system failures into proactive models of engagement. *Journal of Adolescent Health, 62*(Suppl. 3), S9–S17. https://doi.org/10.1016/j.jadohealth.2017.07.024.

Richter, D., Berger, K., et al. (2009). *Psychological consequences of patient assaults on mental health staff.* Prospective and retrospective data. EuropePMC.

Salamone-Violi, G. M., Chur-Hansen, A., & Winefield, H. R. (2015). "I don't want to be here but I feel safe": Referral and admission to a child and adolescent psychiatric inpatient unit: The young person's perspective. *International Journal of Mental Health Nursing, 24*(6), 569–576.

Scanlan, J. N. (2009). Interventions to reduce the use of seclusion and restraint in inpatient psychiatric settings: What we know so far a review of the literature. *International Journal of Social Psychiatry, 56*(4), 412–423.

Shattell, M., Delaney, S., Bartlett, R., Southard, K., Beres, K., Judge, C., et al. (2015). How patients and nurses experience an open versus enclosed nursing station on an inpatient psychiatric unit. *Journal of the American Psychiatric Nurses Association, 21*(6), 398–405. https://doi.org/10.1177/1078390315617038.

Stringaris, A., Maughan, B., Copeland, W. S., Costello, E. J., & Angold, A. (2013). Irritable mood as a symptom of depression in youth: Prevalence, developmental, and clinical correlates in the great smoky mountains study. *Journal of the American Academy of Child & Adolescent Psychiatry, 52*(8), 831–840.

Tadros, E., & Finney, N. (2018). Structural family therapy with incarcerated families: A clinical case study. *The Family Journal, 26*(2), 253–261. https://doi.org/10.1177/1066480718777409.

Torio, C. M., Encinosa, W., Berdahl, T., McCormick, M. C., & Simpson, L. A. (2015). Annual report on health care for children and youth in the United States: National estimates of cost, utilization and expenditures for children with mental health conditions. *Academic Pediatrics, 15*(1), 19–35.

Townsend, M. C. (2015). *Psychiatric mental health care: Concepts of care in evidenced-based practice* (8th ed.). Philadelphia, PA: F.A. Davis.

Tsai, J., et al. (2021). Twenty-year trends in use of electroconvulsive therapy among homeless and domiciled veterans with mental illness. *CNS Spectrums, 1–7*. https://doi.org/10.1017/S1092852921001061.

Twohig, M. P., Woidneck, M. R., & Crosby, J. M. (2013). Newer generations of CBT for anxiety disorders. *CBT for Anxiety Disorders*, 225–250.

Van Hees, L. J. M., et al. (2013). The effectiveness of individual interpersonal psychotherapy as a treatment for major depressive disorder in asdult outpatients: A systematic review. *BMC Psychiatry, 13*, 22. https://doi.org/10.1186/1471-244X-13-22.

Voogt, L. A., Goossens, P. J. J., Nugter, A., & van Achterberg, T. (2013). An observational study of providing structure as a psychiatric nursing intervention. *Perspectives in Psychiatric Care, 50*(1), 7–18.

Ward, M. C., DeJaun, T., et al. (2014). A meta-review of lifestyle interventions for cardiovascular risk factors in the general medical population: lessons for individuals with serious mental illness. *The Journal of Clinical Psychology*, 18–22.

Whitaker, R. (2011). *Anatomy of an Epidemic: Magic Bullets, Psychiatric Drugs, and the Astonishing Rise of Mental Illness in America* (pp. 53–57). Crown publications.

Wilk, A. I., Jensen, N. M., & Havighurst, T. C. (1997). Meta-analysis of randomized control trials addressing brief interventions in heavy alcohol drinkers. *Journal of General Internal Medicine, 12*(5), 274–283.

8

Gerontologic Nursing

In 2019, the number of people aged 60 years and older was 1 billion. This number will increase to 1.4 billion by 2030 and 2.1 billion by 2050. In 2018, World Health Organization (WHO, 2018) has made recommendations for healthy aging and has designed actions that are evidence-based policies for older persons. In the United States, the number of people 65 and older has increased steadily and the life expectancy of older people continues to increase to more than 600,000 by 2060 or 1% of the total population ("Aging & Health...," 2019).

The concept of aging has been defined as young-old (65 to 74), middle-old (75 to 84), old-old (over 85), elite-old (over 90), centenarian (100+), and super-centenarian (110+). Because the aging process is inevitable, most older people have one or more chronic diseases. As a result, there is a high prevalence of somatic diseases, behavioral health problems, cognitive, and other functional limitations that impact the older population, not to mention geriatric syndromes such as falls and frailty. To fully address these challenges and improve the lives of older adults, the nursing community plays a key role in providing healthcare to this population.

THEORIES OF AGING

Psychosocial Theories

A. Disengagement theory: Progressive social disengagement occurs naturally with aging and is accepted by the older adult. Variation in disengagement across older populations is related to cultural style and behaviors in different geographic regions.
B. Activity theory: Successful aging requires a high level of activity and involvement to maintain life satisfaction and positive self-esteem.

Biologic Theories

A. Pacemaker theory: A programmed decline or cessation of many components occurs in the nervous and endocrine systems.
B. Immunity theory: A programmed accumulation of damage and decline of the immune system's function (immunosenescence) takes place due to oxidative stress.
C. Wear-and-tear theory: After repeated use, damaged cells in the body structures wear out from the harmful effects of internal and external stressors, now known as *free radicals.*

> **HESI HINT** The concept of aging is shifting from viewing older adults as frail and dependent to being able to engage in healthy living. Clinical judgment to differentiate the majority of those aged 65 and older regard their health as good or excellent. The clinical judgment model differentiates the ability of an older person to perform activities of daily living (ADLs) is a more accurate measure of an older person's age than chronological age.

Developmental Theories

A. Erik Erikson's theory: Theory identifies eight stages of developmental tasks throughout the life span; the eighth stage is integrity versus despair.
B. Maslow's theory: Maslow's hierarchy of needs ranks an individual's needs from the most basic to the most complex. Maslow uses the terms *physiologic, safety and security, belonging, self-esteem,* and *self-actualization* needs to describe the process that generally motivates individuals to move through life.

Physiologic Changes

A. Aging affects every cell in every organ of the body, but not at the same rate.
B. Three physiologic changes are clinically significant in making older adults vulnerable to injury and disease.
   1. Loss in compensatory reserve
   2. Progressive loss in the efficiency of the body to repair damaged tissue
   3. Decreased functioning of the immune system processes
C. Diseases in older adults do not always present with classic signs and symptoms.
D. Physiologic changes increase more rapidly with increasing age.
E. Aging changes are influenced by genetic makeup and environment.

COMMUNICATION

> **HESI HINT** Clinical judgment measures may include the development of preventive care such as exercise, teaching about good nutrition, and rehabilitation programs for the older adult. Keep in mind that the type of prevention programs should be tailored to the age of the person as well as diagnosis of the chronic disease.

Communicating With Older Adults

Communication is the beginning of understanding. Older adults often have difficulty in hearing or speech. As a result, the role of the nurse is not only to observe verbal and nonverbal behaviors but also to be able to listen, interpret, and provide effective communication skills during an initial assessment of a patient.

A. Address client with respect: "Good morning, Mrs. Jones."
B. Orient the client to the purpose and length of the interview.
C. Give the older adult time to respond because verbal response slows with age.
D. Choose words based on the client's sociocultural background and formal education; do not use slang or jargon (Fig. 8.1).
E. Keep questions short and to the point.
F. Give nonverbal cues and responses such as nodding and direct eye contact; avoid patting or stroking the client.
G. Active listening validates the older person. Reminiscence is an excellent way to obtain data about the client's current health problems and support systems (Fig. 8.2).
H. To help cognitive losses due to alcohol consumption, smoking, and breathing polluted air, the nurse should teach older clients to shop during less-crowded times in stores that are familiar to them, slow down well in advance of traffic signals, stay in the slower lane of the freeway, avoid freeways during rush hours, and leave for appointments well ahead of time.
I. Discuss the problems family members have in dealing with clients with Alzheimer disease in relation to the following disease manifestations:
   1. Depression
   2. Night wandering
   3. Aggressiveness or passiveness
   4. Inability to recognize family members

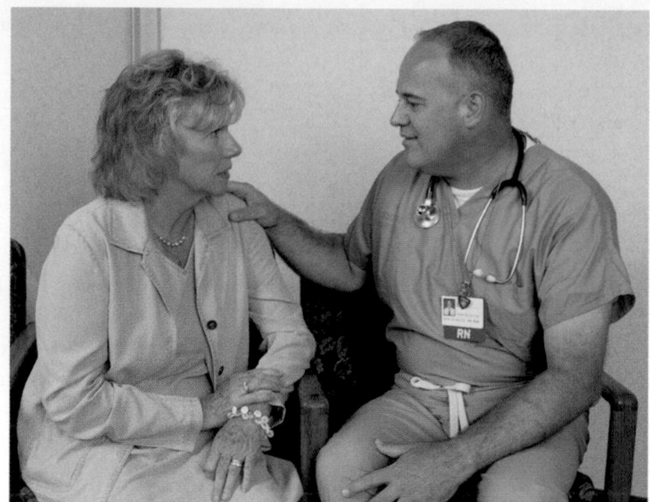

Fig. 8.2 Body Language and Communication. (From Potter, P., Perry, A. G., Stockert, P., & Hall, A. [2013]. *Basic nursing, multimedia enhanced version* [7th ed., 9. 529]. St. Louis: Mosby.)

Clinical Judgment Measures

Clinical judgment measures (CJM) refers to a systematic method of reflecting on a clinical issue. It consists of six levels of critical thinking: recognizing cues, analyzing cues, prioritization, solutions, actions, and evaluation of outcomes. For each of the psychosocial and physiologic changes that occur during aging, it is important to systematically review the CJM associated with each of these systems. For example, each system that will be presented will provide a table that will list the identified clinical measure and the assessment characteristics associated with each. The essential content will be systematically presented to facilitate a comprehensive review of the essential content needed to understand the overall concept. This will facilitate an understanding as to how to prioritize the nursing care associated with the older adult. It is essential to be able to accurately use CJM when providing the nursing care needs of the older adult.

Other issues that will be reviewed include content associated with the health and preventive care for older adults, health care maintenance, and interventions associated with end-of-life care. The overall nursing care needs of the older adult not only includes their psychological and physiological needs but includes their ability toward healthy aging and safe environments.

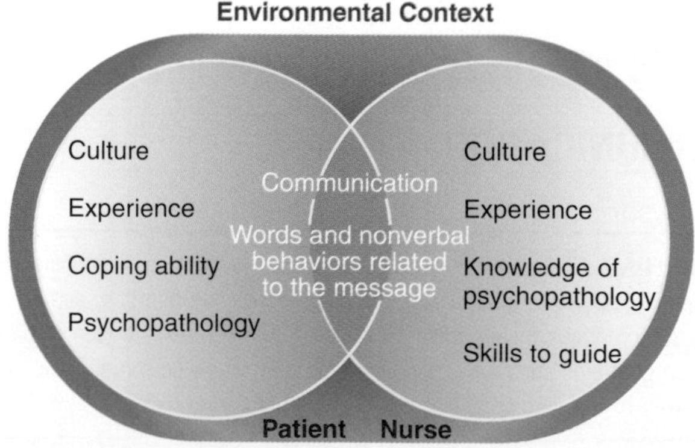

Fig. 8.1 Variables in the Therapeutic Communication Environment. (From Keltner, N., & Steele, D. [2014]. *Psychiatric nursing* [7th ed., pp. 77–78]. St. Louis: Mosby.)

Integumentary System

Description: Skin, hair, and nail changes occur with aging and can cause problems concerning discomfort and self-esteem.

A. Thin skin provides a less effective barrier to trauma due to a loss of subcutaneous tissue.
   1. Increased risk for dehydration due to decline in lean mass and loss of body water
   2. Decreased ability of the skin to detect and regulate temperature
   3. Dry skin resulting from a decrease in endocrine secretion
   4. Loss of elastin and increased vascular fragility
B. Keratinocytes become smaller and regeneration slows; wound healing is slower.
C. Hair loss occurs; women have increased facial hair.

D. Vascular hyperplasia causes more varicosities (brown or blue discolorations).
E. Increased appearance of "age spots" and/or "liver spots" and raised lesions (seborrheic keratosis).
F. Nails become brittle and thick.

Table 8.1 provides an example of a clinical judgment checklist applicable to the Integumentary System.

HESI HINT The NCLEX will test your clinical judgment to differentiate between normal and pathologic causes of skin and hair conditions, for example, the differences between seborrheic keratosis and melanoma.

Musculoskeletal System

Description: Age-related changes in the musculoskeletal system are gradual but have a significant impact on levels of mobility, which puts older adults at risk for falls and fractures.

A. The musculoskeletal system is composed of bones, joints, tendons, ligaments, and muscles.
B. Age-related changes are not life threatening but can affect function and quality of life.
C. Bone loss begins around age 40 and is more common in women than in men; thus, osteoporosis occurs more often in women.
D. There is a shortening of the trunk due to thinning of vertebral disks.
E. Loss of bone calcium, atrophic cartilage, and muscle occurs.
F. Bone mineral density (BMD) decreases, resulting in osteopenia and osteoporosis.
G. Range of motion (ROM) of joints decreases.
H. Progressive loss of cartilage occurs, resulting in osteoarthritis.
I. Muscle cells are lost and not replaced.
J. Lean body mass decreases with increased body fat.

Table 8.2 provides an example of a clinical judgment checklist applicable to the Musculoskeletal System.

HESI HINT Clinical judgment differentials include impaired mobility, impaired skin integrity, decreased peripheral circulation, and a lack of physical activity, all of which place the older adults at risk for the development of pressure injuries.

Cardiovascular System

A. Age-related changes in the cardiovascular system predispose the older person to the development of dysrhythmias and other cardiac problems.
B. Cardiac output decreases as a result of a decrease in heart rate and stroke volume.
C. Cardiac output decreases because vessels lose elasticity. The heart's contractility decreases in response to increased demands.
D. Diastolic murmurs are present in more than one-half of older adults because the mitral and aortic valves become thick and rigid.

TABLE 8.1 Clinical Judgment Measures: Integumentary System

Clinical Judgment Measure	Assessment Characteristics
Recognize Cues	Skin dryness and tears Nails for changes in shape, color, and brittleness Lesions to differentiate normal from abnormal Bony prominences for signs of pressure ulcers
Analyze Cues	Determine types of skin (open wound, infection) Potential skin integrity issues that impact on assessment
Prioritize Cues	Determine if a problem is emergent. Determine wound scale measurement score (Braden's scale 9–23, lower score = higher risk). Determine the impact of the problem on the patient's overall health status.
Solutions	Encourage the use of oils or lubricants on the skin at least twice a day. Discourage the use of powder, which can be drying. Teach to avoid overexposure to sunlight. Encourage balanced nutrition and increased fluid intake. Teach to maintain adequate humidity in the environment. Teach to avoid temperature extremes. Teach good foot care. Observe bony prominences for signs of pressure. Teach that poor peripheral circulation may slow the healing of foot and hand lesions.
Actions	Apply topical moisturizing non-allergic lubricant to skin every morning and evening. Measure humidity in the room so that it is within normal limits (below 30%–60%, Wolkoff, P, 2018). Perform foot care and have patient demonstrate understanding back to you
Evaluate Outcomes	The overall status of the patient's skin has improved from the first to the second visit (improved skin turgor, no signs or symptoms of skin tears or wounds). Height and weight is normal for age.

TABLE 8.2 Clinical Judgment Measures: Musculoskeletal System

Clinical Judgment Measure	Assessment Characteristics
Recognize Cues	Dietary intake of calcium and vitamin D Weight; underweight or overweight Height Lifestyle habits; inappropriate nutrition, smoking, and inadequate exercise History of fractures ROM Pain and chronic pain management strategies
Analyze Cues	Determine type of diet for adequate intake. Verify lifestyle habits (smoking, exercise). Ascertain ability to functionally move (ROM, walk without limp or pain).
Prioritize Cues	Determine risk factors for fractures (emergent versus non-emergent) Clarify nutritional factors. Establish weight parameters.
Solutions	Teach that adequate calcium intake may help lessen osteoporotic changes. Establish muscle-strengthening program (small weights, aquatic therapy). Prevent accidents by ensuring a clutter-free, safe environment. Provide adequate lighting day and night to prevent falls. Teach clients not to back up but to turn around to move in the direction they wish to go. Teach clients to walk looking straight ahead instead of looking down at their feet to optimize balance. Encourage regular exercise inclusive of balance, weight-bearing, and low-resistance training. Teach to avoid excessive joint strain. Teach that medications (diuretics and sedatives) may contribute to falls. The following are ways to help prevent or decrease the occurrence of falls: • Install adequate lighting. • Install grab bars in bathtubs. • Wear proper footwear that supports the foot and contributes to balance; shoes should be made of non-slippery materials. • Place a bell on any resident cats; cats move quickly and can get underfoot. • Paint the edges of stairs a bright color. **Discourage excessive alcohol intake and encourage smoking cessation.** Encourage older people to change positions slowly to prevent orthostatic hypotension.
Actions	Provide patient with nutritionist appointment. Communicate which exercise programs are available. Enroll patient into fall prevention class. Educate patient about healthy lifestyle (cessation of smoking, overeating, immobility).
Evaluate Outcomes	The overall status of the patient's musculoskeletal system has improved from the first to the second visit (improved balance, walking without cane, no signs or symptoms of joint injuries). Weight is improved (loss or added).

ROM, Range of motion.

E. Dysrhythmias (bradycardia, tachycardia, atrial fibrillation, and heart block) become more common as one ages, in part because of higher systolic blood pressure (BP) and increased size of the atria.
   1. Dysrhythmias in older adults are particularly serious because older people cannot tolerate decreased cardiac output, which can result in syncope, falls, and transient ischemic attacks (TIAs). The pulse may be rapid, slow, or irregular in this population.

F. Significant increases in systolic BP occur as a result of the altered distribution of blood flow and increased peripheral resistance.

G. Arteriosclerosis increases with age and can cause cardiovascular problems.
   1. Peripheral vascular disease
   2. Edema
   3. Coronary artery disease: acute coronary insufficiency, myocardial infarction, dysrhythmias, heart failure (HF)

H. Much heart disease is preventable.

Table 8.3 provides an example of a clinical judgment checklist applicable to the Cardiovascular System.

> **HESI HINT** Clinical judgment differentials for angina include myocardial infarction, esophagitis, or musculoskeletal disorders, all of which must be investigated in older adults.

Respiratory System

A. Older adults have increased demands for oxygen. The life span of an older adult increases the chance for exposure to toxic or infectious agents. Due to the aging process,

TABLE 8.3 Clinical Judgment Measures: Cardiovascular System

Clinical Judgment Measure	Assessment Characteristics
Recognize Cues	BP and vital signs History of dizziness or blackouts with sudden position change (orthostatic hypotension) Diuresis after lying down Feelings of heart palpitations Angina 1. Angina symptoms may be absent in older adults. 2. They can also be confused with gastrointestinal (GI) symptoms. Swelling in hands and feet (rings and shoes have become tight) Weight gain without changes in eating pattern Difficulty breathing at night (without elevation of the head of the bed). Confusion and personality changes can result from oxygen deficit.
Analyze Cues	BP and vital signs are consistent with age and diagnosis of patient. Neuro status is stable (no dizziness, movement). Breathing patterns are regular for age and diagnosis of patient. Mini-mental exam reliable for patient status
Prioritize Cues	Keep in mind any emergent issue related to airway, breathing, or circulation (A, B, C's). Mentation intact measured by mini-mental exam (confusion, speech, responses)
Solutions	Monitor BP in lying, sitting, and standing positions. Encourage frequent rest periods to avoid fatigue. Encourage regular, low-impact exercise. Teach to change positions slowly to avoid falls and injuries. Take apical and radial pulse; note deficits or rhythm abnormalities. Teach to avoid extreme hot and cold because of decreased peripheral sensation. Teach to avoid sitting with feet in a dependent position. Assess edema: Weigh daily if indicated. Encourage strict adherence to medication regimen. Teach not to stop medications without prior approval from the health care provider.
Actions	Check vital signs for the normalcy of the patient's age. List up-coming doctor appointments. Evaluate patient's understanding of current cardiac medications. Examine patient's ability to understand changes in cardiac status (when to call 911, when to contact doctor). Reassess patient's overall ability to ambulate and do routine ADLs.
Evaluate Outcomes	The patient's overall cardiac status is stable for health condition. Patient or caregiver demonstrates an understanding of cardiac medications and follow-up health visits. Patient's functional status is intact (ADL).

ADL, Activities of daily living; *BP*, blood pressure; *GI*, gastrointestinal.

multiple exposures over time can be damaging to the lungs and even life threatening.

B. Major age-related changes to the respiratory system.
   1. Breathing mechanics: Lungs lose elasticity; muscles become rigid and lose muscle mass and strength.
      a. Declining muscle strength may impair cough efficiency. This fact makes older people more susceptible to chronic bronchitis, emphysema, and pneumonia.
   2. Oxygenation: Increased ventilation and perfusion are imbalanced; increased dead space in the lungs and a decrease of alveolar surface area
   3. Ventilation control: decreased reaction of peripheral and central chemoreceptors to hypoxia and hypercapnia
   4. Immune response: decrease of cilia; decreased ability to clear mucus secretions, decreased ability to cough and deep breathe, and a decreased immune response
   5. Exercise capability: decrease of strength and muscle mass in the body
   6. Breathing ability: decreased reaction to hypoxemia and hypercapnia

Table 8.4 provides an example of a clinical judgment checklist applicable to the Respiratory System.

HESI HINT Chronic obstructive pulmonary disease is the major cause of respiratory disability in older adults. Aspiration pneumonia is one of the major clinical judgment diagnoses that must be considered in older adults because it accounts for an overall rate of 21% and a 29.7% rate for "in-hospital" deaths (Gamache and Hoo, 2018).

Gastrointestinal System

A. Age-related changes are bothersome and can affect comfort, function, and quality of life, but are rarely a direct cause of death.

B. Decreased saliva and dry mouth (xerostomia) are common.

TABLE 8.4 Clinical Judgment Measures: Respiratory System

Clinical Judgment Measure	Assessment Characteristics
Recognize Cues	Confusion (may be the first sign of respiratory infection) Vital signs for elevated temperature, BP, or elevated/decreased respiratory rate Lungs for congestion or atelectasis vital capacity Dyspnea and fatigue Cough reflex and sputum production
Analyze Cues	Breathing patterns are consistent with age of patient without shortness of breath (SOB), confusion, orthopnea. Respiratory rate, BP, and other vital signs are consistent with age and diagnosis of patients. Productive/non-productive cough
Prioritize Cues	Keep in mind any emergent issue related to airway, breathing, or circulation (A, B, C). Mentation is what is expected for age and diagnosis without confusion in speech, or wrong responses to questions. Change in skin color (pale, cyanosis)
Solutions	Encourage clients to receive an influenza vaccine yearly. Encourage clients to receive the pneumonia vaccine after age 65 (a second dose may be given one additional time after about 5 years). Remember that hypoxia can manifest as confusion. If the client is a smoker, encourage him or her to stop. (Regardless of age, cardiovascular and respiratory status improve with smoking cessation and exercise.) For older postoperative clients, turning, deep breathing, and use of incentive spirometer are imperative to prevent complications. Encourage deep breathing. Teach breathing techniques such as pursed-lip breathing to facilitate respiration.
Actions	Test mental status (date, time, place). Check vital signs for normalcy of patient's age. Note that respiratory rate is within normal limits. Review medications for respiratory system (have patient recite medication, dosage, and routine). Auscultate lungs for consolidation. Reassess patient's overall ability to ambulate and do routine ADLs.
Evaluate Outcomes	Respiratory status has improved (respiratory rate normal, color good, use of oxygen properly if ordered for age and patient's diagnosis). Mentation within normal limits (recites date, time, mini-mental exam) Respiratory rate consistent with activity (walking, ADL) Patient is able to recite the list of respiratory medications and dosage.

ADL, Activities of daily living; *BP*, blood pressure

C. Dental caries (tooth decay) and loss of teeth increase, resulting in decreased ability to chew food.
D. Hunger sensations decrease due to diminishing taste buds.
E. Relaxation of the lower esophageal sphincter or a sliding hiatal hernia increase the risk for gastroesophageal reflux disease and aspiration.
F. The production of pepsin and hydrochloric acid decreases.
G. Delayed gastric emptying makes digestion of large amounts of food difficult.
H. Decreased peristalsis and decreased absorption in the small intestine of protein, fats, minerals (calcium), vitamins B_1 and B_2, and carbohydrates contribute to constipation problems. Decreased muscle tone of the colon also causes constipation.
I. Decreased enzyme production in the liver affects drug metabolism and detoxification processes.
J. Weight changes, especially weight loss, can be early indicators of health problems.

Table 8.5 provides an example of a clinical judgment checklist applicable to the Gastrointestinal System.

> **HESI HINT** Older people may appear to eat small quantities of food at mealtimes. This is because the digestive system of older people features a decrease in the contraction time of the muscles, resulting in more time needed for the cardiac sphincter to open. It takes more time for the food to be transmitted to the stomach; thus, the sensation of fullness may occur before the entire meal is consumed (Dumic et al., 2019).

Genitourinary System

There are functional and structural changes, as well as psychosocial changes, in the older adult pertaining to the urinary system. The urinary system consists of the kidney and bladder.

Kidney

A. Size and weight of the kidney decrease due to reduced renal tissue growth.

TABLE 8.5 **Clinical Judgment Measures: Gastrointestinal (GI) System**

Clinical Judgment Measure	Assessment Characteristics
Recognize Cues	Brittle teeth due to thinning enamel Receding gums resulting from periodontal disease (the major cause of tooth loss after the age of 30) Decrease in taste sensation and appetite Dry mouth due to a decrease in saliva production Elimination pattern for evidence of constipation or diarrhea Use of pain medications that may cause constipation Poor tolerance of high-fat meals and poor absorption of fat-soluble vitamins Decreased glucose tolerance Fluid intake Weight change
Analyze Cues	Condition of teeth consistent with age (repairs, dentures, gums) Taste, appetite, and eating patterns suitable for age Bowel habits acceptable for age Food tolerance (regular, soft, portion size) consistent with age
Prioritize Cues	Nutritional status (gain or loss of weight) proper for age Fluid intake of 7–8 (8 oz./day) Picetti et al. (2017). Vitamin intake consistent with recommendations for people over 51 (https://www.nia.nih.gov/health/vitamins-and-minerals-older-adults)
Solutions	Encourage good oral hygiene (the use of a soft tooth, dental floss, and regular dental visits). Assess dentures for proper fit. Educate older clients about hidden sodium (canned soups, antacids, over-the-counter medications). Promote adequate bowel functioning. • Determine what is normal GI functioning for each individual. • Encourage the client to increase fiber and bulk in the diet. • Provide adequate hydration. • Encourage regular exercise. • Encourage eating small, frequent meals. • Discourage the use of laxatives and enemas. • Document bowel movements: frequency and consistency.
Actions	Verify nutritional status (nutrition for age and weight). Provide vitamins for any deficiency. Check height and weight. Provide a list of community services for seniors (food banks, meals on wheels, community lunches).
Evaluate Outcomes	Patient maintains a healthy weight for age. Annual or semi-annual dental visits. Patient is engaged in senior lunch programs.

B. Glomerular filtration rate decreases due to a decrease in renal blood flow resulting from the lower cardiac output. Decreased renal clearance of drugs is the result.
C. Tubular function diminishes.
D. Increased risk for reflux of urine into the ureters.
E. Chronic diseases such as atherosclerosis and hypertension also decrease renal functioning in older adults.

Bladder

A. The capacity of the bladder decreases by one-half, resulting in urinary frequency and nocturia.
B. Emptying the bladder may become difficult because of a weakening of the bladder and perineal muscles and because of a decrease in the sensation of urge to void. (This sets up a propensity for urinary tract infections [UTIs] due to residual urine in the bladder.)
C. Increased frequency and dribbling may occur in men because of a weakened bladder and an enlarged prostate.
D. Prostatic enlargement may cause urinary retention and bladder infection in men.
E. Women may experience stress incontinence.
F. The nurse should monitor intake and output to assess renal function.
G. A decrease in the filtration efficiency of the kidneys has grave implications for people who are taking medication, particularly penicillin, tetracycline, and digoxin, which are cleared from the bloodstream primarily by the kidneys.
   1. These drugs remain active longer in an older person's system.
   2. As people age, the total number of functioning glomeruli decreases until renal function has been reduced by nearly 50%.
   3. Drug levels may be more potent, indicating a need to adjust/reduce the dose and frequency of administration.

Table 8.6 provides an example of a clinical judgment checklist applicable to the Genitourinary System.

HESI HINT Clinical judgment measures include psychosocial effects since older adults may be embarrassed because they have become incontinent. They may seek isolation or become depressed, thereby predisposing themselves to loneliness.

TABLE 8.6 Clinical Judgment Measures: Genitourinary System

Clinical Judgment Measure	Assessment Characteristics
Recognize Cues	
Kidney	Signs of dehydration or electrolyte imbalance • Decreased skin turgor (tenting) • Intake/output • Confusion • Concentrated urine • Medications such as diuretics Laboratory values • Proteinuria • Increased blood urea nitrogen (BUN) and creatinine • Presence of blood in urine
Bladder	Signs of UTI • Urinary elimination patterns: normal voiding patterns and symptoms such as burning, urgency, and frequency • Mental status (knowledge of name, date, time, place)
Analyze Cues	
Kidney	Laboratory values assessed for the development of acute kidney insufficiency (an elevated BUN level, an elevation in serum creatinine, and a decrease in creatinine clearance accompanied by a decrease in urine output)
Bladder	Urinary output consistent for age (urinary output measured 800–2400 mL/day (Corder et al., 2020)
Prioritize Cues	
Kidney	Keep in mind acute renal failure issues (BP changes, laboratory value changes) for age and diagnosis Changes in heart rate (heart failure) Impaired cognition (disorientation) Immune function (infection/sepsis)
Bladder	Monitor symptoms: • Lower UTI: dysuria, urgency, frequency, and hematuria • Upper UTI: chills, fever, flank pain, mentation changes (septicemia)
Solutions	
Kidney	Encourage an intake of at least 2–3 L of fluid daily, if not contraindicated. Instruct client about signs and symptoms of dehydration and to contact health care provider immediately. Instruct client about the importance of completing antibiotics until the entire prescription is gone, even if symptoms go away. Write out antibiotic schedule, including any special instructions. Print in large letters.
Bladder	Initiate a bladder-training program if indicated. Encourage older women to void at first urge when possible. Initiate a skin-care program if incontinence is present. Provide methods of dealing with incontinence. Kegel exercises can help. Kegel exercises consist of tightening and relaxing the vaginal and urinary meatus muscles. • Teach to avoid sleeping pills and sedation, which may cause nocturnal incontinence. • Teach to avoid caffeine because it promotes diuresis. • Caffeine inhibits the production of antidiuretic hormone (ADH).
Actions	
Kidney	Monitor vital signs Monitor fluid intake and urinary output Monitor laboratory values Determine suitable mentation for age and diagnosis
Bladder	Monitor fluid intake and urinary output Monitor vital signs Provide mini-mental health score Monitor sleep patterns (waking up to urinate, frequency, odor)
Evaluate Outcomes	
Kidney	Quality of life report is good for age and patient's condition Renal function is stable (levels of BUN, creatinine, hematocrit, fluid, and electrolytes are normal for age)
Bladder	Vital signs, functional status, ADLs for age, and health condition is fitting

ADH, Antidiuretic hormone; *ADL*, activities of daily living; *BP*, blood pressure; *BUN*, blood urea nitrogen; *UTI*, urinary tract infections.

Reproductive System

Age-related changes are related to hormonal and nervous system control for both men and women.

Women

A. Physiologic changes include changes related to the vaginal walls becoming thinner, dryer, less elastic, and sometimes irritated.
   1. Women's ovarian function decreases; breast tissue involutes.
   2. Ovaries and the uterus slowly atrophy, and neither may be palpable.
   3. muscle weakness and atrophy of the vulva occur with age.
   4. Vaginal mucous membrane becomes dry, elasticity of tissue decreases, surface becomes smooth, and secretions become reduced and more alkaline. May lead to dyspareunia (painful intercourse).
   5. Risk of vaginal yeast infection increases.

B. Lower estrogen levels due to menopause may cause cardiovascular changes, reduce cholesterol, or increase the risk of osteoporosis.

C. Libido may or may not decline.
   1. Many older adults are sexually active or maintain an interest in sexual activities; therefore, nurses should obtain a sexual assessment among older women in the acute care, community, and long-term care settings.
   2. Lower sex drive (libido) and sexual response may occur.

Men

A. Physiologic changes in the male reproductive system occur gradually because of the decrease in testosterone. Age-related changes include:
   1. Testes atrophy, lose weight, and soften.
   2. Erectile dysfunction (less frequent erections, inability to have an erection).
   3. Erection changes are seen.
   4. Prostate enlargement due to changes in testosterone levels.

B. Normal aging does not prevent older men from being able to enjoy sexual relationships. Older men may still experience orgasmic pleasure, or their libido may not decline. For older men, the most common physiologic changes during intercourse may include:
   1. An erection that is less firm
   2. Shorter duration of erection
   3. Diminished force of ejaculation

C. The term for male menopause is *andropause.* Diminished testosterone is believed to be the cause of androgen decline in the aging male (ADAM).

Table 8.7 provides an example of a clinical judgment checklist applicable to the Reproductive System in Women and Men.

> **HESI HINT** Sexually active older adults are at risk for sexually transmitted diseases if they seek sexual relations with different partners. An important clinical judgment measure is to ascertain the number of sexual partners and knowledge of HIV infection among older adults (Ekong et al., 2020).

Neurologic System

Neurocognitive disorders (NCDs; DSM-5) are the major cause of disability in older adults. Dementia, cerebrovascular disorders, and movement disorders (e.g., Parkinson's disease) are the major disorders in this category

A. The nervous system is the most complex of all systems and functions alone and in conjunction with many systems.

B. There is a decrease of neurons and neurotransmitters in the brain, which do not regenerate.

C. The neurologic system consists of two main components: the central nervous system (CNS) and the peripheral nervous system (PNS): decrease in both CNS and PNS functioning.

D. Intelligence remains constant in the healthy older adult.

E. Central processing decreases: performance of tasks is slower.

F. PNS changes in aging people may include the following:
   1. Significantly lower or nonexistent vibratory senses in the lower extremities
   2. Decrease of tactile sensitivity
   3. Loss of connection in nerve endings in the skin
   4. Loss of proprioception, affecting balance

G. Sleep disturbances
   1. Shorter stages of sleep, particularly shorter cycles in stages 3 and 4 and rapid-eye-movement sleep (stage 4 is deep sleep).
   2. Easily awakened by environmental stimuli. Older adults often compensate by napping during the day, which leads to further disruptions of night sleep.
      a. A common response is the use of prescription sleeping pills, which can create still further problems of disorientation, etc.

Table 8.8 provides an example of a clinical judgment checklist applicable to the neurologic system.

> **HESI HINT** The most common neurological disorders in the older adult include: cognitive disorders, behavioral changes, and alterations in physical abilities. Clinical judgment measures are most crucial to differentiate the signs and symptoms that the older adult may exhibit during the assessment phase.

Endocrine System

In the older adult, glands atrophy and decrease the rate of secretion. The impact is unclear, except it is more prevalent in women than in men due to the decline of estrogen, which causes menopause.

A. Consists of the thyroid, parathyroid, pituitary, adrenal, and pineal glands; the thymus; and the endocrine pancreas.

B. Thyroid activity decreases (see "Hypothyroidism (Hashimoto Disease, Myxedema)" in Chapter 4: Medical-Surgical Nursing). Symptoms are commonly undiagnosed in the older adult because they are attributed to being "normal for age."

C. Metabolic rate slows.

D. Estrogen production ceases with menopause; ovaries, uterus, and vaginal tissue atrophy.

E. Gonadal secretion of progesterone and testosterone decreases.

TABLE 8.7 Clinical Judgment Measures: Reproductive System Women and Men

Clinical Judgment Measure	Assessment Characteristics
Recognize Cues	
Women	Vital signs (temperature), discharge, or labial or vulvar redness and pruritus for possible infections (vaginitis) Complaints of hot flashes, mood swings, or night sweat Dyspareunia (painful intercourse)
Men	Complaints of urinary problems (dribbling, incontinence, frequent waking up at night to urinate), prostate enlargement Testosterone hormone levels
Analyze Cues	
Women	All vital signs are consistent for age of patient. Loss of pubic muscle tone may cause the bladder to fall (prolapse) of the uterus.
Men	Benign prostatic hyperplasia (BPH) can cause slowed urine or ejaculation. Medication (antihypertensives) use may decrease libido.
Prioritize Cues	
Women	Monitor changes in vital signs (increased temperature) Changes in discharge (infection, vaginitis)
Men	Monitor vital signs (increase in temperature) Prostatitis risk (greater in men over 50)
Solutions	
Women	Teach client signs of vaginitis; report and treat if present. Promote perineal care as needed. Prescription creams can help with vaginal dryness. Encourage client to obtain mammogram per guidelines.
Men	Encourage annual digital examination for early identification of prostate cancer.
Actions	
Women	Monitor vital signs for normalcy for age. List signs and symptoms of vaginitis. Promote creams that help with vaginal dryness. Encourage wellness plan: annual mammogram and annual physical
Men	Monitor vital signs for normalcy for age. Encourage annual physical exam following prostate guidelines.
Evaluate Outcomes	
Women	Stable vital signs during annual physical exam No pain during sexual encounters
Men	Stable vital signs during annual physical exam Signs and symptoms of prostatitis are negative.

BPH, Benign prostatic hyperplasia.

F. Insulin production decreases or insulin resistance increases.
G. Thyroxine (T_4) and triiodothyronine (T_3) secreted by the thyroid gland remain unchanged with aging; however, their metabolic clearance rate is decreased. Production of parathyroid hormone decreases, which is made evident by osteoporosis.
H. Adrenal changes may affect circadian patterns of adrenocorticotropic hormone (ACTH).

Table 8.9 provides an example of a clinical judgment checklist applicable to the Neurologic System.

HESI HINT Clinical judgment measures that differentiation between thyroid dysfunction and type 2 diabetes is important since both disorders are common endocrine syndromes of the older adult.

Sensory System

The sensory system consists of vision, hearing, taste, touch, and smell. Changes in the sensory system, including balance, occur gradually and are often unnoticed.

A. A loss of cells in the olfactory bulb of the brain and a decrease in sensory cells in the nasal lining occur.
B. Sensitivity to smells declines.
C. Taste perception decreases due to the loss of taste buds on the tongue.
D. Tear production decreases.
E. Abnormal, progressive clouding or opacity of the lens in the eyes occurs (cataracts).
F. A partial or complete white ring encircles the periphery of the cornea (arcus senilis).

TABLE 8.8 Clinical Judgment Measures: Neurologic System

Clinical Judgment Measure	Assessment Characteristics
Recognize Cues	Comprehensive functional assessment; weaknesses, tremors, and gait disturbances
	History of falls
	Pain, headaches, ROM, and neuropathies in extremities
	Sudden changes in vision, cognition, and muscle weakness
	Depression
	Sleep patterns
Analyze Cues	Sleep disorders (sleep-wake cycle) consistent for age
	Answers related to old and new information dependable for age, memory reliable
	Hearing, smell, vibratory sensations, taste consistent for age
	Balance steady for age
	Mini cog—screens for cognitive impairment, consistent for age
	Mental status assessment: attention, memory, orientation, etc. intact for age and diagnosis
	Neurologic assessment: cranial nerves, gait, balance, distal deep tendon reflexes, plantar responses, primary sensory modalities in lower extremities, and cerebrovascular integrity intact for age
	Functional assessment: Dementia Severity Rating Scale (DSRS) normal score 4 or less (increases with age), consistent for age
	Mini cog—screens for cognitive impairment, consistent for age
	Screen for age-associated issues: The three *D*s: depression, delirium, and dementia: consistent for age
Prioritize Cues	Keep in mind acute changes with patient: changes in vital signs, stroke assessment (headaches, vomiting, seizures, mental status changes (including coma), fevers, and electrocardiogram (ECG) changes mentation, slurred speech, ABC's.
	Cognitive changes, outbursts, disorientation, emotional or sensory overload, confusion, agitation
Solutions	Perform a complete mental status examination.
	Screen for depression.
	Screen for cognitive impairment.
	Monitor for conditions caused by lack of sleep.
	• Fatigue, confusion, disorientation
	Monitor blood pressure and hydration status.
	Request physical and occupational service evaluations, if indicated.
	Provide assistive devices as needed for ambulation.
	Encourage walking, ROM, and balance exercises.
	Teach individual relaxation techniques, stress management, and adaptive self-care management.
	Minimize potential sources of injury in the environment.
	Educate family and caregivers about support groups and other resources (agencies).
Actions	Vital signs assess and normal for age
	Mini-mental status exam intact
	Functional status exam stable for age
	Judgment, home activities, personal care, speech and language recognition, feeding, incontinence, and mobility or walking consistent for age
	Physical activities consistent for age (ROM, balance, gait) and appraised by the care provider
Evaluate Outcomes	Check vital signs for normalcy for age
	Behavioral changes (mood, sleep patterns, fatigue, confusion, orientation) consistent for age and diagnosis of the patient as reported by the care provider and/or patient
	No gait or balance issues, no falls in home environment
	Effectiveness of health teaching evident in patient's ability to effectively balance when walking and report by the caregiver about community senior support groups

DSRS, Dementia severity rating scale; *ECG*, electrocardiogram; *ROM*, range of motion.

G. Increased intraocular pressure (IOP), usually bilaterally, leads to optic nerve damage (glaucoma).

H. Hearing of high pitches diminishes first; the ability to discriminate tones is lost (presbycusis).

Table 8.10 provides an example of a clinical judgment checklist applicable to the Sensory System.

HESI HINT Clinical judgment measures associated with changes in the sensory system are important to determine the overall functional status of older adults.

Neurocognitive Disorder: Dementia

Dementia is the permanent, progressive impairment in cognitive functioning manifested by memory loss (both long term and short term) and accompanied by impairment in judgment, abstract thinking, and social behavior.

A. Dementia is characterized by the following:
   1. Personality changes
   2. Confusion
   3. Disorientation

TABLE 8.9 Clinical Judgment Measures: Endocrine System

Clinical Judgment Measure	Assessment Characteristics
Recognize Cues	Signs and symptoms of diabetes in older adults; dehydration and confusion History of recurrent infections, fatigue, and nausea; delayed wound healing; paresthesia Weight loss or gain without change in eating pattern Laboratory values; hemoglobin A_{1C}, aldosterone, and cortisol levels Bone density testing Sleeping pattern Depression
Analyze Cues	Vital signs are consistent for age of patient Laboratory values are normal (Hemoglobin A_{1C} in normal limits) No sleepiness, no changes in mentation
Prioritize Cues	Concentrate on vital signs, changes in mental status (mini-mental test) Keep in mind changes in blood sugar (sleepiness, cognitive responses, slurred speech)
Solutions	Encourage thyroid testing for older clients who seem depressed. Hypothyroidism is often dismissed as depression. Refer to "Hypothyroidism (Hashimoto Disease, Myxedema)" in Chapter 4: Medical-Surgical Nursing. Older clients may have difficulty with lifelong medication regimens. Develop memory cues for medications and caution against abrupt withdrawal. See "Diabetes Mellitus (DM)" in Chapter 4: Medical-Surgical Nursing. Encourage annual physical examination with routine laboratory tests. Encourage annual eye examinations. Teach daily foot care and monthly toenail care.
Actions	Vital signs assessed for normalcy for age Mini-mental status exam intact Functional status exam stable for age Judgment intact for ADLs
Evaluate Outcomes	Check vital signs for normalcy for age Functional status exam normal for age as reported by caregiver Behavioral changes not evident (sleep patterns, no fatigue, or confusion).

ADL, Activities of daily living; *DM*, diabetes Mellitus.

4. Deterioration of intellectual functioning, loss of memory
5. Decline of appropriate judgment and ADLs
6. Difficulty performing familiar tasks
7. Misplacing things
8. Problems with abstract thinking
9. Changes in mood or behavior

B. The four A's of cognitive impairment are agnosia, amnesia, apraxia, and aphasia.

C. Types of dementia
1. Alzheimer disease: The brains of individuals with Alzheimer disease have an abundance of beta-amyloid plaques, neurofibrillary tangles, and atrophic brain cells and tissue. Alzheimer's disease is the most common brain disorder and is one of the leading causes of death in the older adult.
2. Vascular or multifocal dementia: Ischemic brain lesions develop as a result of a history of hyperlipidemia, hypertension, smoking, or obesity.
3. Dementia with Lewy bodies (DLB): Microscopic deposits develop in the brain that damage nerve cells.
4. Frontotemporal dementia (Pick disease): The frontal and temporal lobes of the brain degenerate.

Table 8.11 provides an example of a clinical judgment checklist applicable to the Neurocognitive Disorder: Dementia.

Psychosocial Changes

Loss.

A. Loss includes loss of functional ability, decreased self-image, and death of significant others (family members, friends, or pets).

B. Loss is a universal, incontestable event of the human experience.

C. Regardless of the loss, each event has the potential to cause grief and the process called *bereavement* or *mourning*.

D. Grief is an individual response and is different depending on social and cultural norms.

E. Losses may be compounded (e.g., relocation, loss of support network, economic changes, and/or role changes), causing bereavement overload.
1. Losses can make the older adult prone to emotional and mental stress, depression, and substance abuse.

Table 8.13 provides an example of a clinical judgment checklist applicable to Psychosocial changes: Loss.

HESI HINT Think about the clinical judgment measures for each of the following situations. How can the client's life be affected? Discuss the nursing care priorities for each:
- A nursing supervisor has a stroke and is sent to a long-term facility for rehabilitation.
- An oil company executive retires after 42 years with the company and travels in his recreational vehicle with his wife and dog.
- Shortly after their 60th wedding anniversary, a man's wife has a cerebrovascular accident and is paralyzed.

TABLE 8.10 Clinical Judgment Measures: Sensory System

Clinical Judgment Measure	Assessment Characteristics
Recognize Cues	Assess visual and hearing acuity, as well as glasses and/or hearing aids used Eyes for cloudiness or opacity Ears for wax and hearing loss Evaluate dietary intake for unplanned weight loss and salt and sugar intake
Analyze Cues	Vital signs are consistent for age of patient Able to clearly read (patient reads simple list, assess for accuracy). Understands simple directions (responds to health care provider without increasing voice) Weight consistent for age
Prioritize Cues	Concentrate on vital signs, mentation changes (acute disorientation) Acute pain in eyes, ears, nose, or mouth
Solutions	Provide interventions to supplement the loss of sensory input. Encourage social interaction. Make the client's environment as safe as possible to increase orientation and decrease confusion. Maximize visual and nonvisual aids, such as bright colors, large print for written material, recorded books, lighted mirror, and glasses, if applicable. Encourage the use of hearing aids with frequent battery changes, if applicable. 1. The nurse should use a lower tone of voice when talking to an older person who is hearing impaired. a. High-pitched tones (e.g., women's voices) are the first to become difficult to hear. Encourage the use of glasses and frequent cleaning, if applicable. 1. Diminished eyesight results in the following: a. A loss of independence (driving and the ability to perform ADLs) b. A lack of stimulation c. The inability to read (recommend audiotapes) d. The fear of blindness 2. Decreased independence due to fear of not being able to clearly see Encourage the use of artificial tears; teach to avoid rubbing and touching of the eyes (increases risk for infection). Encourage regular eye examinations. Directly face hearing-impaired clients so they may read lips and view facial expressions. Adapt ethnic favorites to dietary and taste limitations. Use frequent touch to compensate for visual and auditory sensory loss and decrease the sense of isolation 1. The nurse should make the older adult aware that he or she is going to be touched and should therefore ask permission before touching the client. The nurse should be cognizant of cultural differences with direct eye contact, touch, and taste. 2. The nurse should teach the caregiver or patient to carefully use sharp kitchen utensils since the patient may unintentionally injure themselves. Educate the client's support system about interventions to maintain a safe and comfortable environment.
Actions	Vital signs normal for age Mini-mental status exam intact Functional exam for vision, hearing, and taste stable for age (use of glasses, hearing aids, diet recall) Judgment intact for ADLs
Evaluate Outcomes	Check vital signs for consistency for age Functional status exam normal for age related to vision (screen with Simple eye chart to check vision (SNELLEN exam), screen for hearing ADLs as reported by caregiver (able to eat and feed self, smell intact)

ADL, Activities of daily living.

Health Maintenance and Preventive Care: Nursing Plans and Interventions

A. Encourage periodic health appraisal and counseling to prevent illness.
   1. Electrocardiogram to detect subtle heart abnormalities.
   2. Chest radiograph to detect tuberculosis or lung cancer.
   3. Pulmonary function tests to detect chronic bronchitis and emphysema.
   4. Tonometer test to measure IOP as a test for glaucoma.
   5. Blood glucose to detect diabetes mellitus.
   6. Pap smear to detect cancer of the cervix; digital rectal examination to detect cancer of the prostate.
   7. Hearing and vision testing to detect sensory deprivation.
   8. Breast self-examination and mammogram, if indicated.
   9. Serum cholesterol as indicated by health status.
   10. Screen at-risk older adults for bone density, thyroid functioning, and abdominal aneurysm (in males).
   11. Screen for depression and cognitive impairment.
   12. Screen for BP as indicated by health status.

TABLE 8.11 Clinical Judgment Measures: Neurocognitive Disorder: Dementia

Clinical Judgment Measure	Assessment Characteristics
Recognize Cues	Memory complaints: short term/long term; recognition of family, friends, or environment Impaired physical functioning: shuffling, difficulty swallowing, and inability to perform ADLs Conditions that mimic dementia Unrecognized medical conditions 1. Acute infection (UTI), dehydration (electrolyte imbalance), medication, pain, and metabolic disorder. 2. Medications, adverse reactions & nursing implications (Table 8.12)
Analyze Cues	Vital signs are normal for age Mini-mental score is normal (cognitive assessment score is not elevated, able to complete a clock drawing test with number spacing that is correct) Laboratory values normal (WBC count normal) No nausea or vomiting associated with medications
Prioritize Cues	Vital signs normal for age Acute cognitive changes (delirium, no recognition of family or caregiver) Headache, dizziness, or GI distress
Solutions	Administer screening tools for depression and cognitive impairment. Keep the client functioning and actively involved in social and family activities for as long as possible. Maintain an orderly, almost ritualistic, schedule to promote a sense of security. Maintain a regularly scheduled reality orientation on a daily basis. 1. Keep the client oriented as to time, place, and person (repeatedly). 2. Keep a calendar and clock within sight at all times. a. Display a calendar and clock that can be read by the older person (i.e., a clock with large numbers and a calendar that can be read by those with deteriorating vision). b. Be sure the date and time are accurate (i.e., keep the calendar current and the clock in working order). Keep familiar objects, such as family pictures, in the older adult's environment to promote a sense of continuity and security. Administer prescribed drugs to reduce emotional lability, agitation, and irritability or prescribed antidepressant, as indicated. Speak in a slow, calm voice; avoid excitement. Redirect the client who exhibits combative behavior. Educate family and caregivers on a safe home environment. Provide support and education to family and long-term caregivers. Encourage end-of-life planning, including a will, do not resuscitate status, power of attorney, and funeral arrangements.
Actions	Vital signs normal for age Oriented to place, time, environment Mini-mental status exam intact ADLs intact (teach family/caregiver changes in the ability to complete daily activities: eating, bathing) Medication regime adequate for diagnosis Teach family/caregiver to take medications with meals to avoid GI upset
Evaluate Outcomes	Check vital signs for consistency for age Mini-mental status exam intact for age ADLs as reported by caregiver (able to eat, feed self, and bathe self) Medication compliance adherence as reported by family or caregiver

ADL, Activities of daily living; *GI*, gastrointestinal; *UTI*, urinary tract infections.

TABLE 8.12 Alzheimer Medications

Drugs	Adverse Reactions	Nursing Implications
Acetylcholinesterase Inhibitors		
• Tacrine HCl • Donepezil HCl • Rivastigmine • Galantamine	• Overall—nausea and diarrhea • Cognex: considerable GI distress, elevated liver enzymes	• Teach clients that they should take *no* anticholinergic medication. • Medications should not be used in cases of severe liver impairment. • Take with meals to avoid GI upset. • Do not discontinue abruptly. • For early to moderate stage disease.
N-Methyl-D-Aspartate (NMDA) Antagonist		
• Memantine	• Headaches, dizziness, and constipation	• Add to acetylcholinesterase inhibitors in moderate to severe Alzheimer disease.

TABLE 8.13 Clinical Judgment Measures: Psychosocial changes: Loss

Clinical Judgment Measure	Assessment Characteristics
Recognize Cues	Any loss or losses The older adult's day-to-day functioning (e.g., eating and sleeping and work or social patterns) Level of depression and suicide risk The support system in place to assist with loss Ability to express emotions related to the loss or losses Any feelings of uselessness and nonparticipation in social events Any loss of income that affects health care needs and quality of life New or increased alcohol consumption on a daily or weekly basis Past coping styles used with past losses
Analyze Cues	Scores on the Geriatric Depression Scale (GDS) are within normal limits (no indication of symptoms related to loss, self-image, or late-life depression). ADLs within normal limits (no change in sleeping or eating patterns).
Prioritize Cues	Vital signs normal for age. Keep in mind symptoms associated with loss (recent spouse, child) feelings of uselessness, loneliness Changes in income status (retirement, social security).
Solutions	If needed, offer or refer to grief counseling or a support group. Encourage activities that allow the individual to use past coping strategies that will promote a feeling of self-worth and increased self-esteem. Encourage the individual to share his or her feelings. Encourage socialization with family peers and reminiscing about significant life experiences.
Actions	Vital signs normal for age. Oral responses consistent without evidence of depression, loneliness during examination. Evidence of social support by family members and friends.
Evaluate Outcomes	Vital signs normal for age. GDS scores normal (no evidence of depression) ADLs normal for age (no evidence of changes in eating or sleep patterns).

ADL, Activities of daily living; *GDS*, geriatric depression scale.

13. Screen for obesity.
14. Screen for substance abuse.
15. Screen for physical or emotional abuse.

B. Promote accident prevention.
1. Educate about safety measures to take to prevent falls.
2. Encourage physical and mental activities to promote mobility and confidence.
3. Encourage regular muscle-strengthening and balance-training exercises.
4. Encourage the use of assistive devices when needed (e.g., cane, walker, glasses, hearing aids).
5. Monitor driving skills; encourage American Association of Retired Persons (AARP) driving evaluation and training.

C. Protect against infectious diseases.
1. Encourage handwashing.
2. Educate older adults to avoid individuals who are ill.
3. Encourage immunization for influenza, pneumonia, and Td/Tdap.
4. Recommend herpes zoster (shingles); hepatitis A and B; and measles, mumps, rubella, and varicella immunizations if risk factors are present.

D. Avoid temperature extremes; prevent hypothermia.
E. Encourage the older person to stop smoking and discourage excessive alcohol intake.
F. Educate clients about proper foot care.
G. Encourage proper nutrition and weight control.
H. Encourage social interaction and use of support services (e.g., Meals on Wheels) and support groups (e.g., church).
I. Discourage the use of over-the-counter medications.
J. Review all medications yearly and encourage the client to throw away outdated drugs and prescriptions.
K. Diseases and conditions that affect older adults are the same as those that affect younger adults. However, in older adults, the signs and symptoms of pathology may be subtle, slow to develop, and quite different from those seen in younger people (Table 8.14).

Maintenance and Preventive Care: End-of-Life Care

End-of-life care shifts care from invasive interventions aimed at prolonging life to supportive interventions that focus on control of symptoms. Insurance and hospice entities view the end-of-life stage as 6 months before death. However, a major problem with this definition is the difficulty in predicting the period of client survival. Health care providers may overestimate or underestimate survival time. Care includes the following:

A. Pain management is a priority in end-of-life care because untreated or undertreated pain consumes energy; interferes with function; affects quality of life and social interactions; and contributes to sleep disturbances, hopelessness, and loss of control.

TABLE 8.14 Diseases and Conditions in Older Adults

Disease or Condition	Description in Terms of the Older Adult	Nursing Implications
Delirium	• Acute confused state with rapid onset, usually the result of systemic illness or medication. • Decreased level of consciousness.	• Establish a meaningful environment. • Help maintain body awareness. • Help client cope with confusion, delusions, and illusions. • Review medications for synergistic effects.
Dementia	• Slow onset of symptoms. • Level of consciousness may be intact.	• See "Nursing Plans and Interventions" for "Neurocognitive Disorder: Dementia."
Cardiac dysrhythmias	• Incidence increases with age. • More serious in older adults because of lower tolerance of decreased cardiac output (can result in syncope, falls, TIAs, and confusion). • Symptoms result from compromised circulation and oxygen deficit.	• Assess, prevent, and manage dysrhythmias. • Advise smoking cessation. • Encourage exercise and weight control.
Cataracts	• Often a result of normal aging changes. • Most common pathologic problem affecting the eyesight of older adults. • Treatment is surgical removal.	• Teach instillation of eye drops. • Reduce glare in environment. • Assistance is required postoperatively because affected eye is covered, and disorientation may occur.
Glaucoma	• Risk of acquiring increases with age.	• Loss of sensory input can result in confusion.
Macular degeneration	• Principal cause of blindness.	• Loss of sensory input can result in confusion. • Yearly examination important.
Cerebrovascular accident	• Interruption of cerebral circulation, caused by occlusion or hemorrhage in the brain. • Risk increases with age.	• Prevent deterioration of client's condition. • Maximize functional abilities (occupational therapy). • Assist client in accepting physical deficits. • Check gag reflex before the client receives food or fluids. • Prevent injuries to paralyzed limbs.
Pressure ulcer	• Immobility puts older adults at risk.	• Reposition frequently. • Massage bony prominences. • Provide adequate nutrition.
Hypothyroidism	• Usually occurs after age 50. • Symptoms are often similar to normal aging changes and have an insidious onset, making it difficult to detect in older adults. • Older adults are at greater risk for the development of myxedema coma, which is life threatening.	• Often diagnosed as depression; with treatment, signs of depression disappear. • Caution against abruptly discontinuing medication.
Thyrotoxicosis (Graves disease)	• Symptoms may be absent or attributed to other, more common diseases in older adults. • Weight loss and heart failure may be predominant symptoms.	• It is precipitated by stressful events such as trauma, surgery, or infection. Be alert for signs and symptoms. • Can be fatal if untreated.
Chronic obstructive pulmonary disease	• A major cause of respiratory disability in older adults • Most older people exhibit both chronic bronchitis and chronic emphysema. • Fatigue is a common result because of the increased work required to breathe (dyspnea).	• Encourage to stop smoking. • Keep in mind an older person's state of confusion when teaching about treatment regimen. • Plan rest periods to allow the patient to maintain oxygen levels.
Urinary tract infections (UTIs)	• Their incidence increases with age. • Older people are often asymptomatic or exhibit vague, ill-defined symptoms. • With infections, older people often become confused.	• Suspect UTI when client's voiding habits change.

NCD, Neurocognitive disorder; *UTI*, urinary tract infections.

B. Alleviating dyspnea can contribute to the client's comfort and decrease the family's anxiety. Dyspnea (distressing shortness of breath) may be related to pulmonary, cardiac, neuromuscular, or metabolic disorders; obesity; anxiety; and spiritual distress. Families need support, in particular when the gurgling sound ("death rattle") occurs close to the end of life.

C. Listening, reassuring, and reinforcing nonpharmacologic interventions to help manage anxiety (a mild to severe subjective feeling of apprehension, tension, insecurity, and uneasiness) may need to be followed by pharmacologic agents.

D. Managing gastrointestinal (GI) symptoms of nausea, vomiting, gastritis, constipation, and diarrhea ensures comfort and quality of life.

E. Assessing for psychiatric symptoms of depression and delirium common at the end of life and providing care as needed. If unrecognized, they can rob clients of quality of life and quality of care.

F. Recognizing the spiritual needs of older adults can help them come to terms with their illness and the end of their life. *Spirituality* is a broad concept that encompasses the search for meaning in life experiences, relationships with others, and a sense of connectedness to a personal deity. Recognition of spiritual distress is important to help the dying client come to terms with the end of life.

G. Supporting family caregivers is important because family caregivers may do everything for the client, from assisting with ADLs to giving medications and managing medical equipment and treatments. Often, they are the ones who serve as go-betweens for the client and health care providers. Although caregivers may find great satisfaction in their role, they often experience stress and diminished physical health.

H. Family bereavement support is essential because survivors are at an increased risk for illness or death. Normal responses to grief can be physical, psychological, cognitive, and/or spiritual. Uncomplicated grief is a dynamic, pervasive, and highly individualized process. Individuals who are overwhelmed or remain interminably in the state of grief without progression through the mourning process to completion may be experiencing complicated grief. When the nurse identifies complicated grief, it should be reported so that a referral for help can be made to the correct provider, such as a bereavement counselor.

REVIEW OF GERONTOLOGIC NURSING

1. What are the normal memory changes that occur as one ages?
2. What three physiologic changes are clinically significant in older adults?
3. Why can the BP of older adults be expected to increase?
4. What is the major cause of respiratory disability in older adults?
5. List five nursing interventions to promote adequate bowel functioning for older people.
6. What lifestyle factors negatively affect nearly every system in the older adult's body?
7. What visual problem most commonly occurs in older adults?
8. What are the three most common disorders that result from changes in the neurologic system?
9. What is the difference between delirium and NCD?
10. Falls are the result of what physiologic changes?
11. What are two factors that cause a decrease in the excretion of drugs by the kidneys?
12. What areas are important for end-of-life care?

See Answer Key at the end of this text for suggested responses.

For more review, go to http://evolve.elsevier.com/HESI/RN for HESI's online study examinations.

NEXT-GENERATION NCLEX (NGN) EXAMINATION-STYLE QUESTION: BOWTIE QUESTION

Medical Record

Mr. James, a 76-year-old male, lives in a long-term care facility and has dementia.

Mr. Woods is dependent on nursing and support staff for assistance with bathing, dressing, ambulation, and meals. He is able to feed himself but requires supervision and prompting because he forgets why he is sitting at the table. His urine is concentrated and malodorous and his skin is dry.

Orders

Daily I & O, weekly laboratory, ambulate, safety parameters, daily vital signs.

Instructions

Complete the diagram by selecting from the choices below to specify which potential condition the client is most likely experiencing, 2 actions to take, and 2 parameters the nurse would monitor to assess the client's progress.

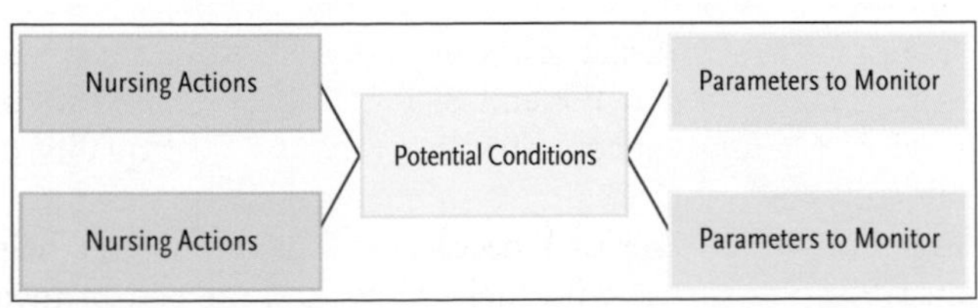

Actions to Take	Potential Conditions	Parameters to Monitor
Administer oxygen 2 L/min NC	Stroke	Pain Level
Assist in feeding patient	Constipation	Oriented to time, person, and place
Initiate fall precautions	Hypotension	Pulse oximetry
Monitor I & O	Infection	>1000 cc fluid intake per day
Increase activity		Check respiratory rate q4hr.

Answers highlighted in Answer Key at the end of this text

BIBLIOGRAPHY

Aging and Health: Improving Care for Older Adults. (2019). *Health Affairs event*. National Press Club. https://doi.org/10.1377/he20190829.971169

Corder, C. J., Rathi, B. M., Sharif, S., & Leslie, S. W. (2020). 24-Hour urine collection. Updated 2020, October 27. In *StatPearls [Internet]*. StatPearls Publishing. https://www.ncbi.nlm.nih.gov/books/NBK482482/

Dumic, I., Nordin, T., Jecmenica, M., Lalosevic, M. S., Milosavljevic, T., & Milovanovic, T. (2019). Gastrointestinal tract disorders in older age. *Canadian Journal of Gastroenterology and Hepatology*, 6757524. https://doi.org/10.1155/2019/6757524. Published online January 17, 2019.

Ekong, N., Curtis, H., Ong, E., Sabin, C. A., & Chadwick, D. (2020). British HIV Association (BHIVA) Audit and Standards Sub-Committee. Monitoring of older HIV-1-positive adults by HIV clinics in the United Kingdom: A national quality improvement initiative. *HIV Medicine, 21*(7), 409–417. https://doi.org/10.1111/hiv.12842. PMID 32125760.

Gamache, J., & Hoo, G. S. (2018). What is the mortality rate of aspiration pneumonia? Aspiration pneumonitis and pneumonia. *Medscape*. https://www.medscape.com/answers/296198-38080/what-is-the-mortality-rate-of-aspiration-pneumonia (accessed February 13, 2021).

Heidari, S. (2016). Sexuality and older people: A neglected issue. *Reproductive Health Matters, 24*(48), 1–5. https://doi.org/10.1016/j.rhm.2016.11.011

Picetti, D., Foster, S., Pangle, A. K., Schrader, A., George, M., Wei, J. Y., et al. (2017). Hydration health literacy in the elderly. *Nutrition and Healthy Aging, 4*(3), 227–237. https://doi.org/10.3233/NHA-170026

Wolkoff, P. (2018). Indoor air humidity, air quality and health—an overview. *International Journal of Hygiene and Environmental Health, 221*(3), 376–390. https://doi.org/10.1016/j.ijheh.2018.01.015 Get rights and content.

World Health Organization. (2018). *Aging and health*. https://www.who.int/news-room/fact-sheets/detail/ageing-and-health (accessed February 14, 2021).

ANSWER KEY TO REVIEW QUESTIONS

CHAPTER 2

Legal Aspects of Nursing

1. Sterile or invasive procedures.
2. Would a reasonable and prudent nurse act in the same manner under the same circumstances?
3. Duty: Failure to protect the client against unreasonable risk. Breach of duty: Failure to perform according to established standards. Causation: A connection exists between the conduct of the nurse and the resulting damage. Damages: Damage is done to the client, whether physical or mental.
4. Conduct causing damage to another person in a *willful* or *intentional* way *without* just cause. Example: Hitting a client out of anger, not in a manner of self-protection.
5. Voluntary: Client admits self to an institution for treatment and retains his or her civil rights; he or she may leave at any time. Involuntary: Someone other than the client applies for the client's admission to an institution (a relative, a friend, or the state); requires certification by one or two health care providers that the person is a danger to self or others; the person has a right to a legal hearing (habeas corpus) to try to be released, and the court determines the justification for holding the person.
6. Vote, make contracts or wills, drive a car, sue or be sued, hold a professional license.
7. Voluntary, informed, written.
8. Alert, coherent, or otherwise competent adults; a parent or legal guardian; a person in loco parentis of minors or incompetent adults.
9. The Good Samaritan Act.
10. Inform the health care provider; record that the health care provider was informed and the health care provider's response to such information; inform the nursing supervisor; refuse to carry out the prescription.
11. Inform the health care provider or person asking the nurse to perform the task that he or she is unprepared to carry out the task; refuse to perform the task.
12. Apply restraints properly; check restraints frequently to see that they are not causing injury and *record* such monitoring; remove restraints as soon as possible; use restraints *only* as a last resort.
13. A patient must give written consent before health care providers can use or disclose personal health information; health care providers must give patients notice about providers' responsibilities regarding patient confidentiality; patients must have access to their medical records; providers who restrict access must explain why and must offer patients a description of the complaint process; patients have the right to request that changes be made in their medical records to correct inaccuracies; health care providers must follow specific tracking procedures for any disclosures made that ensure accountability for maintenance of patient confidentiality; patients have the right to request that health care providers restrict the use and disclosure of their personal health information, although the provider may decline to do so.

Leadership and Management

1. State Nurse Practice Act
2. Implementation
3. Assertive communication skills
4. Right task, right circumstance, right person, right direction or communication, and right supervision
5. Delegation is as follows:
   A. Is a sterile invasive procedure and should not be delegated to a UAP.
   B. Falls within the implementation phase of the nursing process and does not require nursing judgment. Evaluation of I&O must be done by the nurse.
   C. Client teaching requires the abilities of a nurse and should not be delegated. The UAP may be instructed to report anything unusual that is observed and any symptoms reported by the client, but this does not replace assessment by the nurse.
   D. Assessment must be performed by the nurse and should not be delegated. The UAP may be instructed to report anything unusual that is observed or any symptoms reported by the client, but this does not replace assessment by the nurse.
6. Direction, evaluation, and follow-up
7. Examples
   A. This is an aggressive communication, which causes anger, hostility, and a defensive attitude.
   B. Assertive communication begins with "I" rather than "you" and clearly states the problem.
8. Common signs of substance are clients complaining that pain medication does not relieve pain when administered by a certain nurse, frequent inaccuracies of controlled medication counts for a specific nurse, and client reports not taking pain medications but several doses are signed out for that client.
9. Common characteristics of incivility/bullying are refusing to work with others, yelling or cursing at peers, making degrading comments, and verbal abuse. Workplace violence contributes to high staff turnover rate and decline in client care.

Disaster Nursing

1. Disaster preparedness, disaster response, disaster recovery
2. Primary: develop plan, train and educate personnel and public; secondary: triage, treatment-shelter supervision; tertiary: follow-up, recovery assistance, prevention of future disasters

3. To sort or categorize
4. Anthrax, pneumonic plague, botulism, smallpox, inhalation tularemia, viral hemorrhagic fever, ricin, sarin, radiation
5. Three infection control measures for Ebola include the following:
   A. Place the client in a single-patient room with a private bathroom.
   B. Wear full personal protective equipment (PPE).
   C. When there are copious amounts of blood and other body fluids, caregivers should wear additional PPE, including double gloves, disposable shoe covers, and leg coverings.
6. Notify appropriate health care providers, supervisors, and the CDC of clients with a suspected diagnosis of the Ebola virus.

Next-Generation NCLEX (NGN) Examination-Style Question: Bowtie Question

Case Record

Sarah Lee, a 32-year-old emergency room nurse was on her way home from the hospital when a major hurricane began to hit her hometown. Her car was pushed into the oncoming lane; however, she did not hit another victim, rather she waited at the side of the road until most of the wind and rain receded. Because of her experience as a triage nurse, she immediately checked for her own injuries and began to assess her surroundings. She noted that several other people were walking around and were injured while others were laying in the middle of the road. Sara began to review her disaster training to initiate assistance to others in the area.

Disaster principles: Invoke disaster training protocol.

Correct answers are highlighted

Actions to Take	Potential Conditions	Parameters to Monitor
Disaster preparedness, response, recovery	Blunt chest injuries	Infection control principles should be used
Monitor vital signs	Hypotension	Note any frank bleeding on any person
Initiate CPR	Infection disease exposure	Monitor individuals who are treatable
Render first aid to injured	Constipation	Assess pain and monitor response
Provide water to the injured		Monitor bowel movements

CHAPTER 3

Respiratory Failure

1. PO_2 below 60 mm Hg
2. PCO_2 above 45 mm Hg
3. Acute Respiratory Failure
4. Dyspnea/tachypnea; intercostal and sternal retractions; cyanosis
5. Congenital heart disease; infection or sepsis; respiratory distress syndrome; aspiration; fluid overload or dehydration
6. 100%

Shock and DIC

1. Widespread, serious reduction of tissue perfusion, which leads to generalized impairment of cellular function.
2. Hypovolemia.
3. Release of endotoxins by bacteria, which act on nerves in vascular spaces in the periphery, causing vascular pooling, reduced venous return, and decreased cardiac output and result in poor systemic perfusion.
4. Quick restoration of cardiac output and tissue perfusion.
5. Rapid infusion of volume-expanding fluids.
6. History of MI with left ventricular failure or possible cardiomyopathy, with symptoms of pulmonary edema.
7. Pulmonary edema; administer medications to manage preload, contractility, and/or afterload. For example, to decrease afterload, nitroprusside may be administered.
8. Tachycardia; tachypnea; hypotension; cool, clammy skin; decrease in urinary output.
9. Epinephrine, dopamine, dobutamine, norepinephrine, or isoproterenol.
10. 30 mL/h.
11. BP mean of 80 to 90 mm Hg; Po_2 greater than 50 mm Hg; CVP 2 to 6 mm HG H_2O; urine output at least 30 mL/h.
12. A coagulation disorder in which there is paradoxical thrombosis and hemorrhage.
13. PT, prolonged; PTT, prolonged; platelets, decreased; FSPs, increased.
14. Heparin.
15. Gently provide oral care with mouth swabs. Minimize needle sticks and use the smallest gauge needle possible when injections are necessary. Eliminate pressure by turning the client frequently. Minimize the number of BP measurements taken by cuff. Use gentle suction to prevent trauma to mucosa. Apply pressure to any oozing site.

Review of Resuscitation

1. Call 9-1-1 (or send someone to do that) and begin CPR by pushing hard and fast in the center of the chest.
2. Necrosis of the heart muscle due to poor perfusion of the heart.
3. Unrelieved chest pain after nitroglycerin.
4. For adults, check carotid pulse and, if no pulse, deliver CPR.
5. False. Palpate for no more than 10 seconds, recognizing that arrhythmias or bradycardia could be occurring.
6. Adults 30:2, use chest compression rate of ~100 to 120/min for infants and children. Single rescuers compression to ventilation rate 30:2; two rescuers 15:2.
7. Epinephrine.
8. Defibrillation.

9. Check for a carotid or femoral pulse. Watch for chest excursion and auscultate bilaterally for breath sounds.
10. When the person points to his or her throat and can no longer cough, talk, or make sounds.
11. Because the object might be pushed farther down into the throat.

Fluid and Electrolyte Balance

1. GI causes: vomiting, diarrhea, GI suctioning; decrease in fluid intake; increase in fluid output such as sweating, massive edema, ascites
2. Heart failure, renal failure; cirrhosis; excess ingestion of table salt or overhydration with sodium-containing fluids
3. Ringer's lactate; normal saline
4. Lungs; kidneys; chemical buffers
5. Normal values
   A. 7.35 to 7.45 pH
   B. 35 to 45 mm Hg PCO_2
   C. 21 to 28 mEq/L HCO_3
6. Disorders
   A. Respiratory alkalosis
   B. Metabolic acidosis
   C. Metabolic alkalosis
   D. Respiratory acidosis

Electrocardiogram (ECG)

1. P wave, QRS complex, T wave, ST segment, PR interval
2. Represented by the P wave
3. QRS complex
4. The time required for the impulse to travel from the atria through the AV node
5. Hypokalemia
6. Count the number of RR intervals in the 30 large squares and multiply by 10 to determine the heart rate for 1 minute
7. Ability of the client to tolerate the arrhythmia
8. 80 beats/min

Perioperative Care

1. Age: very young and very old, obesity and malnutrition, preoperative dehydration/hypovolemia, preoperative infection, use of anticoagulants (aspirin) preoperatively
2. Impairs ability to detoxify medications used during surgery; impairs ability to produce prothrombin to reduce hemorrhage
3. Respiratory activities: coughing, breathing, use of spirometer; exercises: ROM, leg exercises, turning; pain management: medications, splinting; dietary restrictions: NPO evolving to progressive diet; dressings and drains; orientation to recovery room environment
4. Contact lenses, glasses, dentures, partial plates, wigs, jewelry, prostheses, makeup, and nail polish
5. Usually on the side or with head to side to prevent aspiration of any emesis
6. Teaching client to splint incision when coughing; encouraging coughing and deep breathing in early postoperative period when sutures are strong; monitoring for signs of infection, malnutrition, and dehydration; encouraging high-protein diet
7. Avoiding postoperative catheterization; increasing oral fluid intake; emptying bladder every 4 to 6 hours; early ambulation
8. Early ambulation; limiting the use of narcotic analgesics; NG tube decompression
9. Teaching performance of in-bed leg exercises; encouraging early ambulation; applying antiembolus stockings; teaching avoidance of positions and pressures that obstruct venous flow
10. Ascertain correct sponge, needle, and instrument count; position client to avoid injury; apply ground during electrocautery use; apply strict use of surgical asepsis
11. Answer SBAR (Situation-Background-Assessment-Recommendation) technique provides a framework for communication between members of the health care team about a patient's condition. S = Situation (a concise statement of the problem) B = Background (pertinent and brief information related to the situation) A = Assessment (analysis and considerations of options—what you found/think) R = Recommendation (action requested / recommendation) answer is correct

HIV Infection

1. HIV is transmitted through blood and body fluids—for example, unprotected sexual contact with an infected person, sharing needles with drug-abusing persons, infected blood products (rare), breast milk (mother-to-fetus transmission), and breaks in universal precautions (needle sticks or similar occurrences).
2. Vertical transmission occurs 30% to 50% of the time.
3. Protection from blood and body fluids is the goal of standard precautions. Standard precautions initiate barrier protection between caregiver and client through handwashing; using gloves; using gowns and masks; using eye protection as indicated, depending on activity of care and the likelihood of exposure; preventing needle sticks by not recapping needles.
4. CD4 T-cell count describes the number of infection-fighting lymphocytes the person has.
5. CD4 T-cell count drops because the virus destroys CD4 T cells as it invades them and replicates.
6. Pediatric acquisition may occur through infected blood products, through sexual abuse, and through breast milk.

Pain

1. Massage, heat and cold, acupuncture, TENS

2. The more pain experienced in childhood, the greater is the perception of pain in adulthood or with the current pain experience
3. Acupuncture, administration of placebos, TENS
4. Location, intensity, comfort measures, quality, chronology, and subjective view of pain
5. NSAIDs act via a peripheral mechanism at the level of damaged tissue by inhibiting prostaglandin synthesis and other chemical mediators involved in pain transmission
6. Initiation of withdrawal symptoms
7. Nausea/vomiting; constipation; CNS depression; respiratory depression
8. Narcan
9. Decreased duration of drug effectiveness
10. Intravenous push, or bolus
11. Heat and cold applications; TENS; massage; distraction; relaxation techniques; biofeedback techniques

Death and Grief

1. Denial, anger, bargaining, depression, acceptance.
2. Denial.
3. Gently point out both the positive and negative aspects of her relationship with her father. Try to minimize the idealization of the deceased.
4. This is a normal expression of the anger and guilt that occur. Try to minimize rumination on these thoughts.
5. This is a dysfunctional grief reaction. Mrs. Green has never moved out of the denial stage of her grief work.

Next-Generation NCLEX (NGN) Examination-Style Question: Bowtie Questions

Medical Record: Mrs. Nicholas, 65-year-old female, brought in to emergency department for difficulty breathing new onset. Grandson visiting and is positive for COVID-19. She has been living independently and providing all self-care.
Mrs. Nicholas is now on oxygen saturations are 82%. Her rapid test is COVID positive.

Orders: Stat Computerized tomography with angiogram, ABG, IV Fluids

Correct answers are highlighted

Actions to Take	Potential Conditions	Parameters to Monitor
Administer oxygen to increase saturation	Allergic response	Pain Level
Check musculoskeletal integrity	Hypoxemia	Lab values
Initiate fall precautions	Hypertension	Pulse oximetry
Evaluate for agitation/ restlessness	Infection	Nutritional status
Assess for hyperactive bowel sounds		Check for bleeding

Medical Record: Jamie Medina, 45-year-old LGBTQ pronoun She/Her/Hers, brought in to emergency department for malnutrition, weakness, confusion, and depression. Daughter found her on the floor at home and called an ambulance for concern due to confusion. Jaime has been living independently and providing all self-care. Jaime has a past history of being HIV positive with a T-cell count greater than 200 over 2 months ago.

Orders: IV Fluids, Laboratory Data, Stroke Evaluation

Actions to Take	Potential Conditions	Parameters to Monitor
Evaluate for infection	Infection	Monitor EKG
Evaluate pulses	Hypercapnea	Lab values T-cell count
Initiate fall precautions	Hypotension	Pulse oximetry
Evaluate for agitation/ restlessness	Constipation	Nutritional status
Evaluate for stroke		Record temperature every 4 hr.

CHAPTER 4

Respiratory System

1. Tachypnea, fever with chills, productive cough, bronchial breath sounds.
2. Encourage deep breathing; increase fluid intake to 3 L/day; use humidity to loosen secretions; suction airway to stimulate coughing.
3. Confusion, lethargy, anorexia, rapid respiratory rate.
4. Deliver 100% O_2 (hyperinflating) before and after each endotracheal suctioning.
5. Monitor client's respiratory status and secure connections; establish a communication mechanism with the client; keep airway clear by coughing and suctioning.
6. Barrel chest, dry or productive cough, decreased breath sounds, dyspnea, crackles in lung fields.
7. Smoking (cigarettes and/or marijuana).
8. Involve family and client in the manipulation of tracheostomy equipment before surgery; plan acceptable communication methods; refer to speech pathologist; discuss rehabilitation program.
9. Maintain a dry occlusive dressing on chest tube. Keep all tubing connections tight and taped. Monitor client's clinical status. Encourage the client to breathe deeply periodically. Monitor the fluid drainage, and mark the time of measurement and the fluid level.
10. Place the end of the tube in a sterile water container at a 2-cm level. Apply an occlusive dressing and notify health care provider stat.
11. Do not wash off lines; wear soft cotton garments; avoid the use of powders and creams on radiation site.

12. A mask for anyone entering the room; private room; client must wear a mask if leaving the room.
13. Cough into tissues and dispose of immediately in special bags. Long-term need for daily medication. Good handwashing technique. Report symptoms of deterioration, such as blood in secretions.

Renal System

1. Acute renal failure: often reversible, abrupt deterioration of kidney function. Chronic renal failure: irreversible, slow deterioration of kidney function characterized by increasing BUN and creatinine. Eventually dialysis is required.
2. Toxic metabolites that accumulate in the blood (urea, creatinine) are derived mainly from protein catabolism.
3. Do not take BP or perform venipuncture on the arm with the AV shunt, fistula, or graft. Assess access site for thrill and bruit.
4. Calcium and aluminum antacids bind phosphates and help keep phosphates from being absorbed into bloodstream, thereby preventing rising phosphate levels; must be taken with meals.
5. Fluid intake 3 L/day; good handwashing; void every 2 to 3 hours during waking hours; take all prescribed medications; wear cotton undergarments.
6. Straining all urine is the most important intervention. Other interventions include accurate I&O documentation and administering analgesics as needed.
7. Maintain high fluid intake of 3 to 4 L/day. Pursue follow-up care (stones tend to recur). Follow prescribed diet based on calculi content. Avoid supine position.
8. The fourth day.
9. Continued strict I&O. Continued observations for hematuria. Inform client burning and frequency is a possible outcome and may last for up to a week.
10. Respiratory status (breathing is guarded because of pain); circulatory status (the kidney is very vascular and excessive bleeding can occur); pain assessment; urinary assessment (most important, assessment of urinary output).

Cardiovascular System

1. Described as squeezing, heavy, burning, radiates to left arm or shoulder, transient or prolonged.
2. Take at first sign of anginal pain. Take no more than three, 5 minutes apart. Call for emergency attention if no relief in 10 minutes.
3. Less than 140/90.
4. Essential HTN has no known cause; secondary HTN develops in response to an identifiable mechanism.
5. Explain how and when to take medication, reason for medication, necessity of compliance, need for follow-up visits while on medication, need for certain laboratory tests, and vital sign parameters while initiating therapy.
6. Pain related to PVD; the pain occurs with exercise and disappears with rest.
7. Keep extremities elevated when sitting, rest at first sign of pain, keep extremities warm (but do not use heating pad), change position often, avoid crossing legs, wear unrestrictive clothing.
8. Atherosclerosis.
9. PTT, PT, Hgb, Hct, platelets.
10. When they begin to occur more often than once in 10 beats, occur in twos or threes, land near the T wave, or take on multiple configurations.
11. Left-sided failure results in pulmonary congestion due to backup of circulation in the left ventricle. Right-sided failure results in peripheral congestion due to backup of circulation in the right ventricle.
12. Dysrhythmias, headache, nausea, and vomiting.
13. Hypokalemia (which is more common when diuretics and digitalis preparations are given together).
14. Cease cigarette smoking, if applicable; control weight; exercise regularly; and maintain a low-fat, low-cholesterol diet.
15. Administer O_2 by nasal cannula at 2 to 5 L/min; ensure patent IV or start an IV to deliver emergency medication; take measures to alleviate pain and anxiety (administer PRN pain medications and antianxiety medications); place the client on immediate strict bed rest to lower O_2 demands on heart.
16. Dry mouth and thirst, drowsiness and lethargy, muscle weakness and aches, and tachycardia.
17. 60 beats/min; 100 beats/min.
18. Take prophylactic antibiotics.

Gastrointestinal System

1. Sit up while eating and for 1 hour after eating. Eat frequent, small meals. Eliminate foods that are problematic.
2. Antacids, H2 receptor blockers, mucosal healing agents, proton pump inhibitors.
3. Upper GI: melena, hematemesis, tarry stools; lower GI: bloody stools, tarry stools; common to both: tarry stools.
4. Early mechanical obstruction: high-pitched sounds; late mechanical obstruction: diminished or absent bowel sounds.
5. Irrigate daily at same time; use warm water for irrigations; wash around stoma with mild soap and water after each ostomy bag change; ensure that pouch opening extends at least ⅛ inch around the stoma.
6. Scleral icterus (yellow sclera), dark urine, chalky or clay-colored stools.
7. Fried, spicy, and fatty foods.
8. Rectal bleeding, change in bowel habits, sense of incomplete evacuation, abdominal pain with nausea, weight loss.
9. Avoid injections; use small-bore needles for IV insertion; maintain pressure for 5 minutes on all venipuncture sites; use electric razor; use soft-bristle toothbrush for mouth care; check stools and emesis for occult blood.
10. Diarrhea.
11. Homosexual males, IV drug users, those who have had recent ear piercing or tattooing, and health care workers.

12. Give with meals or snacks. Powder forms should be mixed with fruit juices.

Endocrine System

1. T3, T4
2. Hypothyroidism, requiring thyroid replacement
3. Hyperthyroidism: weight loss, heat intolerance, diarrhea; hypothyroidism: fatigue, cold intolerance, weight gain
4. Continue medication until weaning plan is begun by the physician; monitor serum potassium, glucose, and sodium frequently; weigh daily, and report gain of greater than 5 lb/week; monitor BP and pulse closely; teach symptoms of Cushing syndrome
5. Moon face, obesity in trunk, buffalo hump in back, muscle atrophy, and thin skin
6. Type 1
7. Type 2
8. Polydipsia, polyuria, polyphagia, weakness, weight loss
9. Hunger, lethargy, confusion, tremors or shakes, sweating
10. The underlying pathophysiology of the disease; its management and treatment regimen; meal planning; exercise program; insulin administration; sick-day management; symptoms of hyperglycemia (not enough insulin); symptoms of hypoglycemia (too much insulin, too much exercise, not enough food); foot care
11. Identify the prescribed dose and type of insulin per physician order; store unopened insulin in a refrigerator. Opened insulin vials may be kept at room temperature. Draw up regular insulin first; rotate injection sites; may reuse syringe by recapping and storing in a refrigerator
12. Rapid-acting regular insulin: 2 to 4 hours; immediate-acting insulin: 6 to 12 hours; long-acting insulin: 14 to 20 hours
13. Stress and stress hormones usually increase glucose production and increase insulin need. Conversely, exercise may increase the chance of a hypoglycemic reaction; therefore, the client should always carry a fast-acting source of carbohydrate, such as glucose tablets or hard candies, when exercising
14. Hypoglycemia/insulin reaction
15. Check feet daily, and report any breaks, sores, or blisters to health care provider; wear well-fitting shoes; never go barefoot or wear sandals; never personally remove corns or calluses; cut or file nails straight across; wash feet daily with mild soap and warm water

Musculoskeletal System

1. Rheumatoid arthritis occurs bilaterally. OA occurs asymmetrically.
2. NSAIDs, of which salicylates are the cornerstone of treatment, and corticosteroids (used when arthritic symptoms are severe).
3. Warm, moist heat (compresses, baths, showers); diversionary activities (imaging, distraction, self-hypnosis, biofeedback); and medications.
4. Possible estrogen replacement after menopause, high calcium and vitamin D intake beginning in early adulthood, calcium supplements after menopause, and weight-bearing exercise.
5. GI irritation, tinnitus, thrombocytopenia, mild liver enzyme elevation.
6. Administer or teach client to take drugs with food or milk.
7. Hip, knee, finger.
8. Elevate residual limb (stump) for first 24 hours. Do not elevate residual limb (stump) after 48 hours. Keep residual limb (stump) in extended position, and turn client to prone position three times a day to prevent flexion contracture.
9. Be aware that phantom pain is real and will eventually disappear. Administer pain medication; phantom pain responds to medication.
10. A fat embolism, which is characterized by hypoxemia, respiratory distress, irritability, restlessness, fever, and petechiae.
11. Notify physician stat, draw blood gases, administer O_2 according to blood gas results, assist with endotracheal intubation, and treatment of respiratory failure.
12. Venous thrombosis, urinary calculi, skin integrity problems.
13. Passive ROM exercises, elastic stockings, and elevation of foot of bed 25 degrees to increase venous return.

Neurologic System

1. Parasympathomimetic for pupillary constriction; beta-adrenergic receptor-blocking agents to inhibit the formation of aqueous humor; carbonic anhydrase inhibitors to reduce aqueous humor production; and prostaglandin agonists to increase aqueous humor outflow.
2. Conductive (transmission of sound to the inner ear is blocked) and sensorineural (damage to the eighth cranial nerve).
3. Care of blind: announce presence clearly, call by name, orient carefully to surroundings, guide by walking in front of the client with his or her hand in your elbow. Care of deaf: reduce distraction before beginning conversation, look and listen to the client, give client full attention if he or she is a lip reader, face client directly.
4. An objective assessment of the level of consciousness based on a score of 3 to 15, with scores of 7 or less indicative of coma.
5. Position for maximum ventilation (prone or semi-prone and slightly to one side); insert airway if tongue is obstructing; suction airway efficiently; monitor arterial PO_2 and PCO_2; and hyperventilate with 100% O_2 before suctioning.

6. Persons with histories of HTN, previous TIAs, cardiac disease (atrial flutter or fibrillation), diabetes, or oral contraceptive use; and older adults.
7. Frequent ROM exercises, frequent (every 2 hours) position changes, and avoidance of positions that decrease venous return.
8. Anoxia, distended bladder, covert bleeding, or a return to consciousness.
9. Irrigation of eyes PRN with sterile prescribed solution, application of ophthalmic ointment every 8 hours, close assessment for corneal ulceration or drying.
10. When peristalsis resumes as evidenced by active bowel sounds, passage of flatus or bowel movement.
11. Establishment of regularity.
12. A disruption of blood supply to a part of the brain, which results in sudden loss of brain function.
13. Left.
14. Hypotension, bladder and bowel distention, total paralysis, lack of sensation below lesion.
15. HTN, bladder and bowel distention, exaggerated autonomic responses, headache, sweating, goose bumps, and bradycardia.
16. A change in the level of responsiveness.
17. Increased BP, widening pulse pressure, increased or decreased pulse, respiratory irregularities, and temperature increase.
18. Call his physician now and inform him or her of the fall. Symptoms needing medical attention would include vertigo, confusion or any subtle behavioral change, headache, vomiting, ataxia (imbalance), or seizure.
19. Change in-bed position, extreme hip flexion, endotracheal suctioning, compression of jugular veins, coughing, vomiting, and straining of any kind.
20. They dehydrate the brain and reduce cerebral edema by holding water in the renal tubules to prevent reabsorption and by drawing fluid from the extravascular spaces into the plasma.
21. Narcotics mask the level of responsiveness and pupillary responses.
22. Headache that is more severe upon awakening, and vomiting not associated with nausea are symptoms of a brain tumor.
23. Supratentorial: elevated; infratentorial: flat.
24. Yes.
25. No.
26. Anticholinesterase drugs, which inhibit the action of cholinesterase at the nerve endings to promote the accumulation of acetylcholine at receptor sites; this should improve neuronal transmission to muscles.

Hematology and Oncology

1. Diet lacking in iron, folate, or vitamin B_{12}; use of salicylates, thiazides, diuretics; exposure to toxic agents, such as lead or insecticides.
2. Normal saline.
3. Turn off transfusion. Infuse normal saline using a new bag and new tubing. Take temperature. Send blood being transfused to a laboratory. Obtain urine sample. Keep vein patent with normal saline.
4. Use a soft toothbrush, avoid salicylates, do not use suppositories.
5. Oral cavity and genital area.
6. Glandular meats (liver), milk, green leafy vegetables.
7. Use strict aseptic technique. Change dressings two or three times per week or when soiled. Use caution when piggybacking drugs; check purpose of line and drug to be infused. When possible, use lines to obtain blood samples to avoid "sticking" client.
8. Double check order with another nurse. Check for blood return before administration to ensure that medication does not go into tissue. Use a new IV site daily for peripheral chemotherapy. Wear gloves when handling the drugs and dispose of waste in special containers to avoid contact with toxic substances.
9. Leucovorin is used as an antidote with methotrexate to prevent toxic reactions.
10. Collection of trough: Draw blood 30 minutes before administration of antibiotic; collection of peak: Draw blood 30 minutes after administration of antibiotic.
11. Protect from infection. Observe for anemia. Encourage high-nutrient foods. Provide emotional support to client and family.
12. Handwashing technique. Avoid infected persons. Avoid crowds. Maintain daily hygiene to prevent spread of microorganisms.

Reproductive System

1. Severe menorrhagia leading to anemia, severe dysmenorrhea requiring narcotic analgesics, severe uterine enlargement causing pressure on other organs, severe low back and pelvic pain.
2. Symptoms include incontinence or stress incontinence, urinary retention, and recurrent bladder infections. Conditions associated with cystocele include multiparity, trauma in childbirth, and aging.
3. Avoid taking rectal temperatures and rectal manipulation; manage pain; and encourage early ambulation.
4. Do not permit pregnant visitors or pregnant caretakers in room. Discourage visits by small children. Confine client to room. Nurse must wear radiation badge. Nurse limits time in room. Keep supplies and equipment within client's reach.
5. Females under the age of 21 should not have Pap smear screenings.
6. Women should report any changes in their breasts to the health care provider. A baseline mammography should be performed for women between 35 and 40 years of age with a mammogram every 1 to 2 years for women between ages 40 and 44. An annual mammogram should be performed for women between ages 45 and 54.

7. Position arm on operative side on pillow. Avoid BP measurements, injections, and venipunctures in operative arm. Encourage hand activity and use.
8. Arrange for Reach to Recovery visit. Discuss the grief process with the client. Have physician discuss with client the reconstruction options.
9. Chlamydia trachomatis.
10. Treponema pallidum (spirochete bacteria).
11. Trichomonas vaginalis.
12. Herpes simplex type II.
13. Signs and symptoms of STD; mode of transmission; avoiding sex while infected; providing concise written instructions regarding treatment, and requesting a return verbalization to ensure that the client understands; teaching safer sex practices.

Burns

1. Thermal, radiation, chemical, electrical.
2. Superficial partial-thickness, first degree: pink to red skin (e.g., sunburn), slight edema, and pain relieved by cooling; deep partial-thickness, second degree: destruction of epidermis and upper layers of dermis; white or red, very edematous, sensitive to touch and cold air, hair does not pull out easily. Full-thickness, third degree: total destruction of dermis and epidermis; reddened areas do not blanch with pressure; not painful; inelastic; waxy white skin to brown, leathery eschar.
3. Stage I (emergent phase): Replacement of fluids is titrated to urine output. Stage II (acute phase): Patent infusion site is maintained in case supplemental IV fluids are needed; saline lock is helpful; colloids may be used. Stage III (rehabilitation phase): No extra fluids are needed, but high-protein drinks are recommended.
4. Administer pain medication, especially before dressing wound. Teach distraction and relaxation techniques. Teach use of guided imagery.
5. Provide a patent airway because intubation may be necessary. Determine baseline data. Initiate fluid and electrolyte therapy. Administer pain medication. Determine depth and extent of burn. Administer tetanus toxoid. Insert NG tube.
6. High-calorie, high-protein, high-carbohydrate diet; medications with juice or milk; no "free" water; tube feeding at night. Maintain accurate, daily calorie counts. Weigh client daily.
7. Thermal: Remove clothing, immerse in tepid water. Chemical: Flush with water or saline. Electrical: Separate client from electrical source.
8. Singed nasal hairs, circumoral burns; sooty or bloody sputum, hoarseness, and pulmonary signs, including asymmetry of respirations, rales, or wheezing.
9. Water may interfere with electrolyte balance. Client needs to ingest food products with highest biologic value.
10. Use of client's own skin for grafting.

Next-Generation NCLEX (NGN) Examination-Style Question: Bowtie Question

The nurse in the emergency department is caring for an 82-year-old client.

Nurse's Notes

1600: Client is accompanied by spouse. Left-sided ptosis with facial drooping and slurred speech is noted. Left-sided weakness is noted in extremities. Client is alert but having difficulty answering questions. Spouse reports client had similar symptoms a few days earlier, but they went away after a few hours. These symptoms started at 0600 and not improved and believes the leg weakness is worse since the client cannot stand on the leg. Spouse also reports that the client is not eating well and has not voided in 24 hours. Lung sounds are clear. Pupils are reactive but the right is smaller. Bowel sounds are present in all quadrants, skin is warm and dry. Vital signs: & 98.4 F, P 130, RR 18, BP 190/94 pulse oximetry 92% on room air.

The nurse is reviewing the client's assessment to start a plan of care.

Correct Answers are highlighted

Action to take	Potential Conditions	Parameters to monitor
Obtain a blood glucose	Dehydration	Electrocardiogram (EKG)
Obtain a urine sample for analysis	Hypoglycemia	Neurologic status
Request an order for Normal Saline to be administered intravenously	TIA/Stroke	Intake and Output
Request an order for an antihypertensive	Migraine	Fall precautions
Start range of motion exercises on the affected side		Serum glucose level

CHAPTER 5

Child Health Promotion

1. Immunocompromised child or a child in a household with an immunocompromised individual.
2. Use a pain rating scale appropriate for the child's age and developmental level. Also, observe for physiologic responses to pain, such as increased heart rate, increased respiratory rate, diaphoresis, and decreased oxygen levels.
3. Look for Patterns of Injury: Bruises, burns, welts, cuts, history of broken bones.
4. Liver, sweet potatoes, carrots, spinach, peaches, and apricots.
5. Anemia; pale conjunctiva; pale skin color; atrophy of papillae on tongue; brittle, ridged, or spoon-shaped nails; and thyroid edema Weight, skinfold thickness, and arm circumference.

6. Poor skin turgor, absence of tears, dry mucous membranes, weight loss, depressed fontanel, and decreased urinary output.
7. Loss of bicarbonate/decreased serum pH, loss of sodium (hyponatremia), loss of potassium (hypokalemia), elevated Hct, and elevated BUN.
8. By using the Lund–Browder chart, which takes into account the changing proportions of the child's body.
9. By monitoring urine output.
10. By being taught to lock all cabinets, to safely store all toxic household items in locked cabinets, and to examine the house from the child's point of view.
11. Assessment of the child's respiratory, cardiac, and neurologic status.
12. Anemia, acute cramping, abdominal pain, vomiting, constipation, anorexia, headache, lethargy, hyperactivity, aggression, impulsiveness, decreased interest in play, irritability, short attention span.

Respiratory Disorders

1. To help open the airways by relaxing the bronchial muscles
2. Expiratory wheezing, rales, tight cough, and signs of altered blood gases
3. Pancreatic enzyme replacement; fat-soluble vitamins; and a moderate- to low-carbohydrate, high-protein, moderate- to high-fat diet
4. Because the disease is autosomal recessive in its genetic pattern
5. Restlessness, tachycardia, tachypnea, diaphoresis, flaring nostrils, retractions, and grunting
6. Upright sitting, with chin out and tongue protruding ("tripod position")
7. The child is at risk for dehydration and acid-base imbalance
8. Hearing loss
9. Hemorrhage; frequent swallowing, vomiting fresh blood, and clearing throat

Cardiovascular Disorders

1. A right-to-left shunt bypasses the lungs and delivers unoxygenated blood to the systemic circulation, causing cyanosis. A left-to-right shunt moves oxygenated blood back through the pulmonary circulation.
2. VSD, overriding aorta, pulmonary stenosis, and right ventricular hypertrophy.
3. Poor feeding, poor weight gain, respiratory distress and infections, edema, and cyanosis.
4. Reduce the workload of the heart and increase cardiac output.
5. Give small, frequent feedings or gavage feedings. Plan frequent rest periods. Maintain a neutral thermal environment. Organize activities to disturb child only as indicated.
6. Aortic valve stenosis and mitral valve stenosis.
7. Penicillin, erythromycin, and aspirin.

Neuromuscular Disorders

1. Simian creases in palms, hypotonia, protruding tongue, and upward–outward slant of eyes
2. A common characteristic of spastic CP in infants; legs are extended and crossed over each other; feet are plantar flexed
3. Prevention of infection of the sac and monitoring for hydrocephalus (measure head circumference, check fontanel, assess neurologic functioning)
4. Irritability, change in LOC, motor dysfunction, headache, vomiting, unequal pupil response, and seizures
5. Information about signs of infection and increased ICP; understanding that shunt should not be pumped, and that child will need revisions with growth; guidance concerning growth and development
6. Maintain patent airway, protect from injury, and observe carefully
7. Gingival hyperplasia, dermatitis, ataxia, GI distress
8. Fever, irritability, vomiting, neck stiffness, opisthotonos, positive Kernig sign, positive Brudzinski sign; infant may not show all classic signs even though very ill
9. Ampicillin, ceftriaxone, or chloramphenicol
10. Flat or on either side
11. Osmotic diuretics remove water from the CNS to reduce cerebral edema
12. Suctioning and positioning, turning
13. Duchenne muscular dystrophy is inherited as an X-linked recessive trait
14. Gowers sign is an indicator of muscular dystrophy; the child experiences difficulty rising from a squatting position; has to use arms and hands to "walk" up legs, to stand erect.

Renal Disorders

1. AGN: gross hematuria, recent strep infection, hypertension, and mild edema; nephrosis: severe edema, massive proteinuria, frothy-appearing urine, anorexia.
2. Beta-hemolytic streptococcal infection.
3. AGN: low-sodium diet with no added salt; nephrosis: high-protein, low-salt diet.
4. Hypoproteinemia occurs because the glomeruli are permeable to serum proteins.
5. Long-term prednisone should be given every other day. Signs of edema, mood changes, and GI distress should be noted and reported. The drug should be tapered, not discontinued suddenly.
6. Avoid bubble baths; void frequently; drink adequate fluids, especially acidic fluids such as apple or cranberry juice; and clean genital area from front to back.
7. A malfunction of the valves at the end of the ureters, allowing urine to reflux out of the bladder into the ureters and possibly into the kidneys.
8. Protect the child from injury to the encapsulated tumor. Prepare the family and child for surgery.

9. Preschoolers fear castration, achieving sexual identity, and acquiring independent toileting skills.

Gastrointestinal Disorders

1. Use lamb's nipple or prosthesis. Feed child upright, with frequent bubbling.
2. Choking, coughing, cyanosis, and excess salivation.
3. Maintain NPO immediately and suction secretions.
4. Maintain IV hydration, and provide small, frequent oral feedings of glucose or electrolyte solutions or both within 4 to 6 hours. Gradually increase to full-strength formula. Position infant on right side in semi-Fowler position after feeding.
5. A barium enema reduces the telescoping of the intestine through hydrostatic pressure without surgical intervention.
6. Check vital signs and take axillary temperatures. Provide bowel cleansing program and teach about colostomy. Observe for bowel perforation, measure abdominal girth.
7. Family needs education about skin care and appliances. Referral to an enterostomal therapist is appropriate.
8. A newborn who does not pass meconium within 24 hours; meconium appearing through a fistula or in the urine; an unusual-appearing anal dimple.
9. Maintain fluid balance (I&O, nasogastric suction, monitor electrolytes); monitor vital signs; care for drains, if present; assess bowel function; prevent infection of incisional area and other postoperative complications; and support child and family with appropriate teaching.

Hematologic Disorders

1. Give oral iron on an empty stomach and with vitamin C. Use straws to avoid discoloring teeth. Tarry stools are normal. Increase dietary sources of iron.
2. Meat, green leafy vegetables, fish, liver, whole grains, legumes.
3. It is an X-linked recessive chromosomal disorder transmitted by the mother and expressed in male children.
4. A vasoocclusive crisis is caused by the clumping of RBCs, which blocks small blood vessels; therefore, the cells cannot get through the capillaries, causing pain and tissue and organ ischemia. Lowered oxygen tension affects HgbS, which causes sickling of the cells.
5. Hydration promotes hemodilution and circulation of the RBCs through the blood vessels.
6. Keep child well hydrated. Avoid known sources of infections. Avoid high altitudes. Avoid strenuous exercise.
7. Anemia (decreased erythrocytes); infection (neutropenia); bleeding thrombocytopenia (decreased platelets).
8. The nursing interventions and medical treatment are dependent on the type of treatment. Children with inherited blastoma need to be screened throughout their lives for development of other forms of cancer.

Metabolic and Endocrine Disorders

1. Newborn screening revealing a low T4 and a high TSH
2. Large, protruding tongue; coarse hair; lethargy; sleepiness; and constipation
3. Mental retardation and growth failure
4. CNS damage, mental retardation, and decreased melanin
5. Lofenalac and Phenex-1
6. Meat, milk, dairy products, and eggs
7. Polydipsia, polyphagia, and polyuria
8. Hypoglycemia: tremors, sweating, headache, hunger, nausea, lethargy, confusion, slurred speech, anxiety, tingling around mouth, nightmares. Hyperglycemia: polydipsia, polyuria, polyphagia, blurred vision, weakness, weight loss, and syncope
9. Provide care for an unconscious child, administer regular insulin IV in normal saline, monitor blood gas values, and maintain strict I&O
10. Need to be like peers; assuming responsibility for own care; modification of diet; snacks and exercise in school
11. During exercise, insulin uptake is increased and the risk for hypoglycemia occurs.

Skeletal Disorders

1. Warm extremity, brisk capillary refill, free movement, normal sensation of the affected extremity, and equal pulses.
2. Damage to nerves and vasculature of an extremity due to compression.
3. Abnormal neurovascular assessment: cold extremity, severe pain, inability to move the extremity, and poor capillary refill.
4. Fractures of the epiphyseal plate (growth plate) may affect the growth of the limb.
5. Skeletal traction is maintained by pins or wires applied to the distal fragment of the fracture.
6. Check child's circulation. Keep cast dry. Do not place anything under cast. Prevent cast soilage during toileting or diapering. Do not turn child using an abductor bar.
7. Unequal skin folds of the buttocks, Ortolani sign, limited abduction of the affected hip, and unequal leg lengths.
8. Ask the child to bend forward from the hips, with arms hanging free. Examine the child for a curve in the spine, a rib hump, and hip asymmetry.
9. The child should be instructed to wear the brace 23 hours per day; wear a T-shirt under brace; check skin for irritation; perform back and abdominal exercises; and modify clothing. The child should be encouraged to maintain normal activities as able.
10. Prescribed exercise to maintain mobility; splinting of affected joints; and teaching about medication management and side effects of drugs.

Next-Generation NCLEX (NGN) Examination-Style Question: Bowtie Question

Medical Record: Jamie Smith, a 15-year-old adolescent woman, is admitted to the emergency room with joint pain, nausea, and vomiting. Jamie loves track and was at track practice when she had excruciating pain in her joints and fell on the track. She had difficulty getting up from the track and trying to walk. She was brought to the emergency room with shortness of breath, pain, and a possible sprained ankle. Jamie told the doctor that she was diagnosed with sickle cell anemia since she was 5 years old. She has very aware of her symptoms and tries to avoid being hospitalized. Unfortunately, today she was running, fell on the track, and was extremely fatigued.

Orders: Oxygen at 2L, Toradal 40 mg q.3–4 h; IV 1000 NS @ 100 cc/h. routine laboratory, daily I & O, ambulate, safety parameters.

Actions to Take	Potential Conditions	Parameters to Monitor
Administer oxygen 2 L/min NC	Fracture to Right Ankle	Pulse oximetry
Administer pain medication	Exacerbated flu syndrome	>1000 cc fluid intake per day
Initiate fall precautions	Sickle cell crisis	Oriented to time, person, and place
Monitor I & O	Acute appendicitis	Check bowel sounds
Obtain daily weights		Monitor skin for breakdown

Medical Record: Baby Carlos Mejaho is a 6-month-old infant who is admitted to the pediatric medical floor with difficulty eating, coughing and vomiting, mild nasal flaring, retractions, and grunting. Carlos is usually happy and breastfeeds regularly. He is having trouble with sucking and swallowing and trying to latch due to difficulty with breathing. His mother brought him to the hospital due to dry diapers and increasing lethargy. He is being admitted with viral syndrome and his past medical history has no known allergies or birth history of concern. Her concern was worsened today due to his dry diapers and his lack of interest in eating including his increasing ability to suck, swallow, and breathe while seemingly fatigued.

- Weight (17 lb 8 oz [7.9 kg])
- Vaccines (CDC, https://www.cdc.gov/vaccines/parents/by-age/months-6.html)
- Diphtheria, tetanus, and whooping cough (pertussis) (DTaP) (3rd dose)
- Haemophilus influenzae type b disease (Hib) (3rd dose)
- Polio (IPV) (3rd dose)
- Pneumococcal disease (PCV13) (3rd dose)
- Rotavirus (RV) (3rd dose)

Orders: O_2 oxygen 2–6 L high flow, Tylenol 15 mL/kg/dose every 6 hours prn for comfort, report all temperatures; IV D5 0.45 NS with 10 meq/L at 150 mL/kg/day. Routine laboratory, Hourly I & O, safety parameters.

Actions to Take	Potential Conditions	Parameters to Monitor
Administer oxygen 2–6 L/min NC		Pulse oximetry
Administer pain medication	Viral syndrome	Pain Level
	Vaccine hesitancy	Need of catch up vaccines
Obtain MRI	< 50% percentile	Percentile in growth chart
Initiate safety precautions	Falls	Fatigue and lethargy
Monitor strict I & O		

CHAPTER 6

Anatomy and Physiology of Reproduction and Antepartum Nursing Care

1. Abundant, thin, clear cervical mucus; Spinnbarkeit (egg-white stretchiness) of cervical mucus; open cervical os; slight drop in basal body temperature and then 0.5° to 1°F rise; ferning under the microscope.
2. 14 days.
3. 10 lunar months; 9 calendar months consisting of three trimesters of 3 months each; 40 weeks; 280 days.
4. Nausea and vomiting: crackers before rising; fatigue: rest periods and naps and 7 to 8 hours of sleep at night.
5. At the umbilicus; 200 to 400 g; a baby—with hair, lanugo, and vernix, but without any subcutaneous fat.
6. Total gain should average 11.3 to 15.9 kg (25 to 35 lb.). Gain should be consistent throughout pregnancy. An average of 1 lb/week should be gained in the second and third trimesters.
7. 10 to 12.
8. Once every 4 weeks until 28 weeks; every 2 weeks from 28 to 36 weeks; then once a week until delivery.

Fetal and Maternal Assessment Techniques

1. Diagnosis of preeclampsia, diabetes mellitus, or cardiac disease; less than 3 months between pregnancies; maternal age (under 17 or over 34 years of age); parity (over 5)
2. Fetal well-being.
3. Have client fill bladder. Do not allow client to void. Position client supine with a uterine wedge.
4. Can be done between 8 and 12 weeks' gestation, with results returned within 1 week, which allows for decision about termination while still in first trimester.

5. To determine AFP levels: elevated AFP may indicate the presence of neural tube defects; or low AFP levels may indicate trisomy 21.
6. L/S ratio (lung maturity, lung surfactant development).
7. FHR acceleration of 15 beats/min for 15 seconds in response to fetal movement.
8. The inability to control oxytocin "dosage" and the chance of tetany/hyperstimulation.

Intrapartum Nursing Care

1. Lightening, Braxton Hicks contractions, increased bloody show, loss of mucous plug, burst of energy, and nesting behaviors.
2. True labor: regular, rhythmic contractions that intensify with ambulation, pain in the abdomen sweeping around from the back, and cervical changes. False labor: irregular rhythm, abdominal pain (not in back) that decreases with ambulation.
3. Nitrazine testing: Paper turns dark blue or black. Demonstration of fluid ferning under microscope.
4. Respiratory alkalosis occurs; it is caused by blowing off CO_2 and is relieved by breathing into a paper bag or cupped hands.
5. Irritability and unwillingness to be touched but does not want to be left alone; nausea, vomiting, and hiccupping.
6. Vaginal examinations should be done before analgesia and anesthesia to rule out cord prolapse, to determine labor progress if it is questioned, and to determine when pushing can begin.
7. The taking up of the lower cervical segment into the upper segment; the shortening of the cervix expressed in percentages from 0% to 100%, or complete effacement.
8. Through the fetal back in vertex, OA positions.
9. 110 to 160 beats/min.
10. Less than 140/90
11. Less than 100 beats/min
12. 38° C.
13. Gush of blood, lengthening of cord, and globular shape of uterus.
14. Give immediately after placenta is delivered to prevent postpartum hemorrhage and atony.
15. Hypotension resulting from vasodilatation below the block, which pools blood in the periphery, reducing venous return.
16. Gastric activity slows or stops in labor, decreasing absorption from PO route; it may cause vomiting.
17. When the client is an undiagnosed drug abuser of narcotics, it can cause immediate withdrawal symptoms.
18. Nausea.
19. Turn client to left side. Administer O_2 by mask at 10 L/min. Increase speed of intravenous infusion (if it does not contain medication).
20. The first 1 to 4 hours after delivery of placenta.
21. Massage the fundus (gently) and keep the bladder emptied.
22. Withhold eye prophylaxis for up to 1 hour. Perform newborn admission and routine procedures in room with parents. Encourage early initiation of breastfeeding. Darken room to encourage newborn to open eyes.
23. Fundus above umbilicus, dextroverted (to the right side of abdomen), increased bleeding (uterine atony)
24. Perform fundal massage.
25. Pallor, clammy skin, tachycardia, lightheadedness, and hypotension.
26. Every 15 minutes for 1 hour; every 30 minutes for 2 hours if normal.

Normal Puerperium (Postpartum)

1. Perform immediate fundal massage. Ambulate to the bathroom or use bedpan to empty bladder because cardinal signs of bladder distention are present.
2. Breastfeeding women, multiparas, and women who experienced overdistention of the uterus.
3. Temperature is probably elevated due to dehydration and work of labor; force fluids and retake temperature in an hour; notify physician if above 38°C.
4. Assess BP sitting and lying; assess Hgb and Hct for anemia.
5. Increased clotting factors.
6. Have her demonstrate infant position on breast (incorrect positioning often causes tenderness). Leave bra open to air-dry nipples for 15 minutes three times daily. Express colostrum and rub on nipples.
7. She is engorged; have newborn suckle frequently; take measures to increase milk flow: warm water, breast massage, and supportive bra.
8. Avoid until postpartum examination. Use water-soluble jelly. Expect slight discomfort due to vaginal changes.
9. Up to 3000 mL/day can be voided because of the reduction in the 40% plasma volume increase during pregnancy.
10. Continue routine assessments; normal leukocytosis occurs during postpartal period because of placental site healing.
11. A full bladder.
12. To soften the stool in mothers with third- or fourth-degree episiotomies, hemorrhoids, or cesarean section delivery.
13. Three fingerbreadths/cm below the umbilicus.
14. Calling infant by name, exploring newborn head to toe, using end face position.

Normal Newborn

1. 6 to 8 hours.
2. Cesarean section delivery; magnesium sulfate given to mother in labor; asphyxia or fetal distress during labor.
3. It leads to depletion of glucose (there is very little glycogen storage in immature liver); body begins to use brown fat for energy, producing ketones and causing subsequent ketoacidosis and shock.
4. 36.5° to 37.4° C; 110 to 160 beats/min; 30 to 60; 80/50.
5. Place newborn in isolette or under radiant warmer and attach a temperature skin probe to regulate temperature in isolette or radiant warmer. Double-wrap newborn if

no isolette or warmer is available and put cap on head. Watch for signs of hypothermia and hypoglycemia.

6. False: The head is usually 2 cm larger unless severe molding occurred.
7. CNS anomalies, brain damage, hypoglycemia, drug withdrawal.
8. It depends on the finding. If it crosses suture lines and is a caput (edema), it is normal. If it does not cross suture lines, it is a cephalohematoma with bleeding between the skull and periosteum. This could cause hyperbilirubinemia. This is an abnormal variation.
9. Positive; the transient reflex is present until 12 to 18 months of age.
10. The mouth; stimulating the nares can initiate inspiration, which could cause aspiration of mucus in the oral pharynx.
11. There is controversy concerning this issue, but we do know it causes pain and trauma to the newborn, and the medical indications (prevention of penile and cervical cancer) may be unfounded.
12. 40 to 80 mg/dL.
13. The sterile gut at delivery lacks intestinal bacteria necessary for the synthesis of vitamin K; vitamin K is needed in the clotting cascade to prevent hemorrhagic disorders.
14. Jaundice occurs at 2 to 3 days of life and is caused by immature liver's inability to keep up with the bilirubin production resulting from normal RBC destruction.
15. At 2 to 3 days of life, or after enough breast milk or formula, usually after 24 hours, is ingested to allow for determination of body's ability to metabolize amino acid phenylalanine.
16. 50; 1 oz, or 30 g.
17. Lethargy, temperature greater than 37.7° C, vomiting, green stools, refusal of two feeds in a row.

High-Risk Disorders

1. Maintain strict bed rest for 24 to 48 hours. Avoid sexual intercourse for 2 weeks.
2. Weigh daily; check urine ketone three times daily; give progressive diet; check FHR every 8 hours; monitor for electrolyte imbalances.
3. Prevent pregnancy for 1 year. Return to clinic or doctor for monthly HCG levels for 1 year. Postoperative D&C instructions: Call if bright-red vaginal bleeding or foul-smelling vaginal discharge occurs or temperature spikes over 38° C.
4. Ectopic pregnancy.
5. Abruptio placentae: fetal distress; rigid, boardlike abdomen; pain; dark-red or absent bleeding. Previa: pain-free; bright-red vaginal bleeding; normal FHR; soft uterus.
6. More than five contractions per hour; cramps; low, dull backache; pelvic pressure; change in vaginal discharge.
7. Urinary tract infection; overdistention of uterus; diabetes; preeclampsia; cardiac disease; placenta previa, psychosocial factors such as stress.
8. Answers are as follows:
   A. To prevent seizures by decreasing CNS irritability
   B. CNS depression (seizure prevention)
   C. Calcium gluconate
   D. Reduced urinary output, reduced respiratory rate, and decreased reflexes
9. Systolic blood pressure of 160 mm Hg or more, or diastolic blood pressure of 110 mm Hg or more on two occasions at least 4 hours apart (unless antihypertensive therapy is initiated before this time).
10. No. Oral hypoglycemic medications are teratogenic to the fetus. Insulin will be used.
11. Maternal: hypoglycemia, hyperglycemia, ketoacidosis. Fetal: macrosomia, hypoglycemia at birth, fetal anomalies.
12. When the client's respirations are less than 12/min, DTRs are absent, or urinary output is less than 100 mL/4 h.
13. Monitor for signs of blood loss. Continue to assess BP and DTRs every 4 hours. Monitor for uterine atony.
14. Late in the third trimester and in the postpartum period, when insulin needs drop sharply (the diabetogenic effects of pregnancy drop precipitously).
15. It is short acting, predictable, can be infused intravenously, and can be discontinued quickly if necessary.
16. Preeclampsia, hydramnios, infection.

Postpartum High-Risk Disorders

1. No, HIV has been found in breast milk.
2. GI adverse reactions: nausea, vomiting, diarrhea, and cramping. Hypersensitivity reactions: rashes, urticaria, and hives.
3. Pyelonephritis has the same symptoms as cystitis (dysuria, frequency, and urgency) with the addition of flank pain, fever, and pain at a costovertebral angle.
4. Subinvolution (boggy, high uterus); lochia returning to rubra with possible foul smell; temperature 38.0° C or higher; unusual fundal tenderness.
5. Operative delivery, intrauterine manipulation, anemia or poor physical health, traumatic delivery, and hemorrhage.
6. Dystocia or prolonged labor, overdistention of the uterus, abruptio placentae, and infection.
7. Fundal massage. Notify health care provider if massage does not firm fundus. Count pads to estimate blood loss. Assess and record vital signs. Increase IV fluids and administer oxytocin infusion as prescribed.
8. No, women who stop breastfeeding abruptly may make the situation worse by increasing congestion and engorgement and providing further media for bacterial growth. Client may have to discontinue breastfeeding if pus is present or if antibiotics are contraindicated for neonate.

Newborn High-Risk Disorders

1. Lethargy, high-pitched cry, jitteriness, seizures, and bulging fontanels.
2. Begin oxygenation by bag and mask at 30 to 50 breaths/min. If heart rate is <60, start cardiac massage at 120 events per

minute (30 breaths and 90 compressions). Assist health care provider in setting up for intubation procedure.

3. RDS: alveolar prematurity and lack of surfactant; anemia; and polycythemia.
4. Lethargy, temperature instability, difficulty feeding, subtle color changes, subtle behavioral changes, and hyperbilirubinemia.
5. Place under radiant warmer or in incubator with temperature skin probe over liver. Warm all items touching newborn. Place plastic wrap over neonate.
6. Infant has good suck, has coordinated suck—swallow, takes less than 20 minutes to feed, gains 20 to 30 g/day.
7. Initiate early visitation at ICU. Provide daily information to family. Encourage participation in a support group for parents. Encourage all attempts at caregiving (enhances bonding).
8. Rh incompatibility, ABO incompatibility, prematurity, sepsis, perinatal asphyxia.
9. Bilirubin levels rising 5 mg/day, jaundice, dark urine, anemia, high reticulocyte (RBC) count, and dark stools.
10. Apply opaque mask over eyes. Leave diaper loose so stools and urine can be monitored but cover genitalia. Turn every 2 hours. Watch for dehydration.
11. Irritability, hyperactivity, high-pitched cry, frantic sucking, coarse flapping tremors, and poor feeding.
12. Failure to thrive, absence of crying.
13. Measure from the bridge of the nose to the earlobe and then to a point halfway between the xiphoid and the umbilicus.
14. Aspiration of stomach contents and pH testing; auscultation of an air bubble injected into the stomach.
15. Microcephaly, strabismus, growth retardation, short palpebral fissures, maxillary hypoplasia, abnormal palmar creases, irregular hair, whorls, poor suck, cleft lip, cleft palate, small teeth.

Next-Generation NCLEX (NGN) Examination-Style Question: Bowtie Question

Correct Answers are highlighted

Actions to Take	Potential Conditions	Parameters to Monitor
Gestational Assessment	Seizures	Feeding
Use of bright lights to enhance physical assessment skills	Excessive sleep patterns	Temperature
Increase stimuli (talking, frequent handling) to enhance newborn adaptation to extrauterine life	Lethargy	Eye Contact
Swaddle infant with legs flexed	Neonatal hyperglycemia	Output
Provide bottle to infant		Group therapy

CHAPTER 7

Review of Therapeutic Communication and Treatment Modalities

1. Self-management.
2. Structure.
3. Support, assist the wife with immediate needs, engage with the patient by interacting at an interpersonal level.
4. Electroconvulsive therapy (ECT) would be the medical treatment of choice for this client.
5. **Client care prior to ECT**.
   - Prepare client by teaching about ECT
   - Avoid using the word "shock"
   - Administer medication before and after procedure
   - Provide an emergency cart, suction equipment, and oxygen available in the room.

Client care post-ECT

- Maintain patent airway; the client is unconscious immediately after ECT.
- Check vital signs frequently according to institutional policy
- Reorient client after ECT

Common complaints that often occur after anesthesia is administered may include modest headache, mild muscle soreness, moderate nausea, retrograde pain.

Psychiatric Review Questions

1. Brief intervention inquiring about the use of alcohol.
2. The nurse's role prior to an ECT includes assisting individuals with the promotion of mental health for individuals and family members. Additionally, the nurse teaches the patient about the use of ECT for depression.
3. Structuring one's therapy helps to develop a routine and assists them in balancing their life.
4. Provide a brief intervention that includes understanding their situation but being firm in expectations.
5. Individual therapy initially to investigate their own behavior, then group therapy to help him see his/her view through others eyes.
6. Understand what is meaningful to them but set boundaries.

Review of Mood Disorders

1. Weight change, constipation, fatigue, and decreased sexual desire.
2. Suicidal precautions because the client changed her/his mood abruptly, was giving away their possessions and may decide to commit suicide.
3. Risk assessment should include: Asking about giving possessions away, telling you that they have a plan, determine if they have the means of fulfilling their intent, gun availability.
4. Accompany client to the group; do not give an option, patient needs to be mobilized.
5. Remove the patient and others in the area to a safe area, and have someone activate the fire plan. When the area is safe place, the patient in a quiet environment with low stimulation and medicate as necessary.

Review of Substance Abuse Disorder

1. Obtain a drug and alcohol assessment including type, frequency, and time of last dose or drink. Call the health care provider and report the findings. Anticipate withdrawal and DTs. Provide a quiet, safe environment. Place on seizure precautions. Anticipate giving a medication such as chlordiazepoxide (Librium).
2. Needle track marks; cellulitis at puncture sites, poor nutritional status.
3. Change in work performance, withdrawal, increase in absences (Monday—Friday), increase in number of times tardy, long breaks, lateness returning from lunch.
4. Notify healthcare provider and anticipate an increase in dose or frequency of Librium to 50 mg. Provide a quiet, safe environment. Approach in a quiet, calm manner. Avoid touching client.
5. Notify health care provider of observed behavior change. Get a urine drug screen as prescribed. Confront client with observed behavior change.

Next-Generation NCLEX (NGN) Examination-Style Question: Bowtie Question

Medical Record: Carrie Smith, a 29-year-old woman, is admitted to the emergency room with feelings of being on a high. She has had grandiose feelings for 2 weeks and today she was brought in by her son because she was talking constantly, and had a bizarre and severe dress that did not match her other clothes. She was screaming in pain stating that her doctor told her to come to the E.R. Additionally, Ms. CS was extremely talkative and kept fighting with her hair.

Orders: Admit to Psy. Ward. Monitor I & O, daily weights, suicide precautions; administer lithium, sedatives, and antipsychotics; obtain routine blood work; and provide a safe environment

Correct Answers are highlighted

Actions to Take	Potential Conditions	Parameters to Monitor
Praise self-control, acceptable behavior	Attention-Deficit Disorder	Increase conversations with client to establish more attention
Restrain individual for own safety.	Bipolar disorder or manic-depressive illness	Provide small, frequent, feedings, record I & O
Provide frequent stimulation such as playing physical games.	Delirium	Monitor physical activity/ over-stimulation
Monitor I & O	Over-use of amphetamines	Use a variety of approaches to maximize manipulative behavior.
Give prescribed medication		Monitor vital signs for changes related to stress

CHAPTER 8

Gerontologic Nursing

1. Short-term memory declines, whereas long-term memory stays the same.
2. Loss in compensatory reserve, progressive loss in efficiency of the body to repair damaged tissue, and decreased functioning of the immune system processes.
3. The heart's work increases in response to increased peripheral resistance.
4. COPD.
5. Determine what is "normal" GI functioning for each individual, increase fiber and bulk in the diet, provide adequate hydration, encourage regular exercise, and encourage eating small meals frequently.
6. Smoking, excessive alcohol intake, sedentary lifestyle (inactivity), and excessive dietary intake versus energy output.
7. Cataracts.
8. Dementia disorders, cerebrovascular disorders, and movement disorders (e.g., Parkinson disease).
9. Delirium has a sudden onset and is reversible; NCD is a slowly progressive, irreversible disease.
10. Falls are the result of cardiovascular changes, musculoskeletal system changes, and neurologic system changes.
11. Decrease in glomerular filtration and slowed organ functioning.
12. Pain, dyspnea, anxiety, GI symptoms, psychiatric symptoms, spirituality, support for family caregivers, and family support during the bereavement period are important for end-of-life care.

Next-Generation NCLEX (NGN) Examination-Style Question: Bowtie Question

Medical Record: Mr. James, 76-year-old male, lives in a long-term care facility and has dementia.

Mr. Woods is dependent on nursing and support staff for assistance with bathing, dressing, ambulation, and meals. He is able to feed himself but requires supervision and prompting because he forgets why he is sitting at the table. His urine is concentrated and malodorous and his skin is dry.

Orders: Daily I & O, weekly laboratory, ambulate, safety parameters, daily vital signs.

Correct answers are highlighted

Actions to Take	Potential Conditions	Parameters to Monitor
Administer oxygen 2 L/min NC	Stroke	Pain Level
Assist in feeding patient	Constipation	Oriented to time, person, and place
Initiate fall precautions	Hypotension	Pulse oximetry
Monitor I & O	Infection	> 1000 cc fluid intake per day
Increase activity		Check respiratory rate q4hr.

Common Laboratory Tests

Test	Purpose	Significance
Blood grouping with Rh factor and antibody screen	To determine blood type screen for possible maternal-fetal blood incompatibility	Identifies possible causes of maternal-fetal blood incompatibility. If father is Rh positive and mother is Rh negative and unsensitized, $Rh_o(D)$ immune globulin will be given during pregnancy and after birth
Complete blood count (CBC)	To identify infection, anemia, or cell abnormalities	More than $15,000/mm^3$ white blood cells or decreased platelets require follow-up
Hemoglobin (Hgb) or hematocrit (Hct)	To detect anemia; often checked several times during pregnancy	Low Hgb or Hct may indicate a need for added iron supplementation
Venereal Disease Research Laboratory (VDRL) or rapid plasma reagin (RPR)	To screen for syphilis	Treat if positive. Retest if indicated
Rubella titer	To determine immunity	If titer is 1:8 or less, mother is not immune Immunize postpartum if not immune
Tuberculin skin test	To screen for tuberculosis	If positive, refer for additional testing or therapy
Genetic testing (for sickle cell anemia, cystic fibrosis, Tay-Sachs disease, and other genetic conditions)	Offered if there is an increased risk for certain genetic conditions	If mother is positive, check partner Counseling appropriate to the results of testing
Hepatitis B	To detect presence of antigens in maternal blood	If present, infants should be given hepatitis immune globulin and vaccine soon after birth
Human immunodeficiency virus (HIV) screen	Voluntary test encouraged at first visit to detect HIV antibodies	Positive results require retesting, counseling, and treatment to lower infant infection
Urinalysis	To detect renal disease or infection	Requires further assessment if positive for more than trace protein (renal damage, preeclampsia), ketones (fasting or dehydration), or bacteria (infection)
Papanicolaou (Pap) test	To screen for cervical neoplasia	Treat and refer if abnormal cells are present
Cervical culture	To detect group B streptococci and sexually transmitted diseases	Treat and retest as necessary, treat group B streptococci during labor
Multiple marker screen: Maternal serum alpha-fetoprotein, human chorionic gonadotropin, and estriol. Inhibin A may also be measured. May be combined with ultrasound	To screen for fetal anomalies	Abnormal results may indicate chromosomal abnormality (such as trisomy 18 or 21) or structural defects (such as neural tube defects)
Glucose challenge test	To screen for gestational diabetes	If elevated, a glucose tolerance test is recommended

From McKinney, E., James, S., Murray, S., Nelson, K., & Ashwill, J. (2022). *Maternal-child nursing* (6th ed.). St Louis: Elsevier.

Common Laboratory Tests

INDEX

Note: Page numbers followed by "f " indicate figures, "t" indicate tables, and "b" indicate boxes.

D

L

M

R